MOSBY'S
PEDIATRIC
NURSING
REFERENCE

Sixth Edition

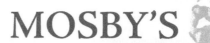

MOSBY'S

PEDIATRIC NURSING REFERENCE

Cecily Lynn Betz, PhD, RN, FAAN
Director, Nursing Training and Research
University of Southern California
University Center of Excellence in Developmental Disabilities
Childrens Hospital Los Angeles;
Editor-in-Chief
Journal of Pediatric Nursing: Nursing Care of Children and Families
Official Journal of the Society of Pediatric Nurses and the
Pediatric Endocrinology Nursing Society
Los Angeles, California

Linda A. Sowden, MN, RN
Regional Director-Florida
Prescribed Pediatric Extended Care Centers, PSA Healthcare
West Palm Beach, Florida

MOSBY

ELSEVIER

MOSBY
ELSEVIER

11830 Westline Industrial Drive
St. Louis, Missouri 63146

MOSBY'S PEDIATRIC NURSING REFERENCE   ISBN: 978-0-323-04496-7
SIXTH EDITION

Notice

Knowledge and best practice in this field are constantly changing. As new research and experience broaden our knowledge, changes in practice, treatment and drug therapy may become necessary or appropriate. Readers are advised to check the most current information provided (i) on procedures featured or (ii) by the manufacturer of each product to be administered, to verify the recommended dose or formula, the method and duration of administration, and contraindications. It is the responsibility of the practitioner, relying on their own experience and knowledge of the patient, to make diagnoses, to determine dosages and the best treatment for each individual patient, and to take all appropriate safety precautions. To the fullest extent of the law, neither the Publisher nor the Editors assumes any liability for any injury and/or damage to persons or property arising out or related to any use of the material contained in this book.

The Publisher

Previous editions copyrighted **1989, 1992, 1996, 2000, 2004**

Library of Congress Control Number 2007926826

Acquisitions Editor: Catherine Jackson
Managing Editor: Michele D. Hayden
Publishing Services Manager: Deborah Vogel
Project Manager: Brandilyn Tidwell
Designer: Margaret Reid

Printed in the United States of America
Last digit is the print number: 9   8   7   6   5   4

Contributors

Christina R. Baer-Arter, RN, BS
Pediatric Case Manager
Outpatient Pediatrics
Kaiser Permanente
Fontana, California

Roberta A. Bavin, RN, MN, CPNP
Pediatric Nurse Practitioner
Clovis Unified School District
Children's Health Centers
Clovis, California

Susan Givens Bell, RNC, MS, MABMH
Staff Nurse
Neonatal Intensive Care Unit
All Children's Hospital
St. Petersburg, Florida

Joan Calandra, RN, PhD
Clinical Nurse Specialist, Psychiatry
Behavioral Healthcare Helpline
Southern California Permanente Medical Group;
Licensed Clinical Psychologist
Los Angeles, California

April Carpenter, RN, MNSc, APN, CPNP
Pediatric Nurse Practitioner, Pulmonary
Little Rock, Arkansas

Noreene C. Clark, RN, MSN
Nurse Researcher
University of Southern California
University Center of Excellence in Developemental Disabilities
Childrens Hospital Los Angeles
Los Angeles, California

Joseph P. De Santis, ARNP, PhD, ACRN
Assistant Professor
University of Miami
School of Nursing and Health Studies
Coral Gables, Florida

Sharon DiSano, MS, ARNP, CCTC
Director, Transplant Administration
All Children's Hospital
St. Petersburg, Florida

Diane F. Dufour, RN, MS, CPNP
Pediatric Nurse Practitioner
Department of Pediatric Hematology/Oncology;
Clinical Instructor and Preceptor
College of Nursing
The Medical University of South Carolina
Charleston, South Carolina

Bonnie F. Gahn, RNC, MA, MSN
Director
Nursing Education
Ross Products Division, Abbott Laboratories
Columbus, Ohio

Patricia J. Gambol, RN, MSN, APNG
Genetic Nurse Specialist
Saddleback Memorial Medical Center
Laguna Hills, California

Anthony D. Gaston, RN, MSN, CS
Nurse Care Manager
Center for Community Mental Health
University of Southern California
University Center of Excellence in Developmental Disabilities
Childrens Hospital Los Angeles
Los Angeles, California

Angela Green, RN, PhD
Clinical Assistant Professor
University of Arkansas for Medical Sciences
College of Nursing;
Director of Nursing Research
Arkansas Children's Hospital
Little Rock, Arkansas

Valerie Hammel, RN, MSN, CNS
Department Administrator
Acute Care Pediatrics
Kaiser Permanente
Fontana, California

Deborah Hill-Rodriguez, ARNP, MSN, CS, BC
Clinical Nurse Specialist
Miami Children's Hospital
Miami, Florida

Mary C. Hooke, RN, MS, CPON
Clinical Nurse Specialist
Hematology/Oncology
Children's Hospitals and Clinics - Minnesota
Minneapolis, Minnesota

Leslie J. Humiston, RN, MNSc, PNP
Pediatric Nurse Practitioner
Department of Hematology/Oncology
University of Arkansas for Medical Sciences
Arkansas Children's Hospital
Little Rock, Arkansas

Mary M. Kaminski, RNC, MS, CNP
Clinical Instructor
The Ohio State University;
Advanced Practice Nurse
Columbus Children's Hospital
Columbus, Ohio

Sally Valentine Kimpel, RN, MN, CPN, CNS
Clinical Nurse Specialist – Pediatrics
Neonatal Intensive Care Unit
Kaiser Foundation Hospital;
Clinical Instructor
University of San Diego
San Diego, California

Bonnie Kitchen, RN, MNSc, APN
Pediatric Nurse Practitioner
Arkansas Children's Hospital
Little Rock, Arkansas

Suzanne L. Kussro, RN, MSN, A/GNP
Pediatric Clinical Coordinator
Pediatric Operating Pavilion
Mission Hospital
Mission Viejo, California

Ruth Landers, RN, MSN, CPNP, CPON
Pediatric Nurse Practitioner
Department of Hematology/Oncology
Arkansas Children's Hospital
Little Rock, Arkansas

Norma L. Liburd, RNC, MN
Pediatric Clinical Nurse Specialist
Allergy/Immunology/Rheumatology
University of South Florida
All Children's Hospital
St. Petersburg, Florida

Linda B. Madsen, RN, MS, CPON, CNP
Certified Nurse Practitioner
Hematology/Oncology
Children's Hospitals and Clinics – Minnesota
Minneapolis, Minnesota

Adele P. Moore, RN, PGD, CNRN
Clinical Manager
Neurosciences Department
Roper Hospital
Charleston, South Carolina

Wendy M. Nehring, RN, PhD, FAAN, FAAMR
Associate Dean for Academic Affairs;
Director, Graduate Program;
Associate Professor
College of Nursing
Rutgers State University of New Jersey
Newark, New Jersey

Sarah E. Plunkett, RNC, MSN, CNS
Assistant Professor of Nursing
Tulsa Community College
Nursing Division
Tulsa, Oklahoma

Trenda Ray, RN, MNSc, APN
Advanced Practice Nurse
Pediatric and Congenital Cardiac Surgery
University of Arkansas for Medical Sciences
Arkansas Children's Hospital
Little Rock, Arkansas

Gay Redcay, RN, MN, FNP
Coordinator, Transition Services
Private Practice
Los Angeles, California

Joanne Rothblum, RN, MN
Associate Professor
William Rainey Harper College
Palatine, Illinois

Sheila Savell, RN, PhD(c)
Clinical Nurse Researcher
Patient Care Services
University of Arkansas for Medical Sciences
Little Rock, Arkansas

Racquel V. Siegel, RN, MSN, ARNP
Pediatric Nurse Practitioner;
Faculty
South University
West Palm Beach, Florida;
Author
Boca Raton, Florida

Gigi Smith, APRN, MSN, CPNP
Pediatric Nurse Practitioner
Pediatric Neurology;
Instructor
College of Nursing
Medical University of South Carolina
Charleston, South Carolina

Ellen Tappero, RNC, MN, NNP
Director
Neonatal Nurse Practitioner Programs
Neonatology Associates, Ltd.
Phoenix, Arizona

Beverly Noble Vandercook, RN, MSN, CPNP, CLC
Nurse Practitioner Administrator
University of Phoenix
Southern California Campus
Costa Mesa, California

Wendy Williams, RN, MNSc, APN, CPNP
Pediatric Nurse Practitioner
University of Arkansas for Medical Sciences
Pediatric Pulmonary Department
Arkansas Children's Hospital
Little Rock, Arkansas

Michele Wolff, RN, MSN
Professor of Nursing
Saddleback College
Mission Viejo, California

Ronda M. Wood, RNC, MN, EdD
Professor of Nursing
Long Beach City College
School of Health and Science
Long Beach, California

Reviewers

Karen A. Ahearn, RN, MPA, CNAA
Director of Maternal Child Nursing
Saint Barnabas Medical Center
Livingston, New Jersey

Rachel Black, BSc
Lecturer and Practitioner
Demelza Hospice Care for Children
Sittingbourne, Kent
United Kingdom

Peggy Bozarth, RN, MSN
Professor
Hopkinsville Community College
Hopkinsville, Kentucky

Patricia Boyle Egland, RN, MSN, CPNP
Assistant Professor of Pediatric Nursing
The City University of New York
Borough of Manhattan Community College
New York, New York

Penny C. Fauber, RN, PhD
Director
School of Practical Nursing
Carilion Stonewall Jackson Hospital
Rockbridge County Schools
Lexington, Virginia

Erica Fooshee, RN, MSN
Instructor
Pensacola Junior College
Department of Nursing
Pensacola, Florida

Cenè L. Gibson, RN, MSN, ARNP
Family Nurse Practitioner
Family Healthcare and Minor Emergency Clinic
Oklahoma City, Oklahoma

H. Joyce Hendricks, RN, MS, CPNP
Adjunct Assistant Professor
Montana State University
College of Nursing
Billings, Montana

Elizabeth Kupczyk, RN, MSN
Legal Nurse Consultant
Chicago, Illinois

Adjunct Pediatric Instructor
Purdue University
Hammond, Indiana

Kristin M. Parks, RNC, MSN, CNE
Program Chair
Associate Degree Program in Nursing
Quincy College
Quincy, Massachusetts

Susan Schultz, RN, MSN, CNS
Professional Specialist
Angelo State University
Department of Nursing
San Angelo, Texas

Theresa Skybo, RN, PhD, CPNP
Assistant Professor
The Ohio State University
College of Nursing
Columbus, Ohio

Tina V. White, DSNc, FNP
Illinois Neurological Institute
Sleep Disorders Center
OSF Saint Francis Medical Center
Peoria, Illinois

Preface

Mosby's Pediatric Nursing Reference, Sixth Edition, is designed to serve as a comprehensive yet compact resource that nurses and nursing students who care for children and their families can easily use. Its small size and concise format were purposefully created for the nurse who wants an easily accessible reference.

This book is divided into two parts. Part One contains information about frequently encountered medical and surgical conditions in the pediatric population. Seven new chapters have been added that include Autism, Spectrum Disorders, Overweight and Obesity in Childhood, Down Syndrome, Fragile X Syndrome, Myringotomy with/without PE tubes, Turner Syndrome, and Diabetes Type 2. Part Two presents diagnostic procedures and tests. For the user's convenience, the chapters in each part are listed in alphabetical order. In the appendixes, the nurse will find valuable information about growth and development, immunizations, laboratory values, and guidelines for conducting complete nursing assessments for each body system. A new appendix on palliative care has also been added.

The organization of the care-planning guidelines reflects our philosophical orientation—a family-centered approach using the nursing process. The needs of the child and family are addressed from a biopsychosocial perspective. The care-planning guidelines reflect a holistic approach to the child's and the family's short-term and long-term needs using the nursing framework of care.

It is our hope that this compact yet powerful tool will prove a useful resource in the delivery of high-quality nursing care for children and the associated care required by their families.

Cecily Lynn Betz
Linda A. Sowden

Preface

Carie Lynn Herz
Linda A. Sheeba

Contents

Part II

PEDIATRIC DIAGNOSTIC PROCEDURES AND OUTPATIENT SURGERIES, 753

APPENDIXES, 803

I

❖

Pediatric Medical and
Surgical Conditions

❖

1

❖

Anorexia Nervosa

PATHOPHYSIOLOGY

Anorexia nervosa is an eating disorder that typically begins in adolescence and is characterized by the refusal to maintain a body weight within the minimal range of normal for height, weight, and body frame. The patient denies the seriousness of weight loss and has a distorted body image. Despite being dangerously thin, the individual feels fat. In addition, there may be a focus on the shape and size of particular body parts (Box 1-1).

There are two general subtypes of anorexia nervosa. The restricting type involves severe restriction of food intake and compulsive exercising. The binge eating and purging type involves restricted dietary intake coupled with intermittent episodes of binge eating, followed by purging. Self-induced vomiting and use of ipecac, laxatives, diuretics, or enemas are common means of purging. Excessive use of appetite suppressants or diet pills is seen in both types.

Purging and semistarvation may induce electrolyte imbalance and cardiac problems, which may ultimately lead to death. Starvation creates a range of medical symptoms. Changes in growth hormone levels, diminished secretion of sex hormones, defective development of bone marrow tissue, structural abnormalities of the brain, cardiac dysfunction, and gastrointestinal difficulties are common. A notable problem associated with anorexia in adolescents is the potential for growth retardation, delay of menarche, and peak bone mass reduction. When normal eating is reestablished and laxative use is stopped, the youth may be at risk for developing medical complications.

3

BOX 1-1
Diagnostic Criteria for Anorexia Nervosa

- Refusal to maintain body weight at or above a minimally normal weight for age and height (e.g., weight loss leading to maintenance of body weight less than 85% of that expected; or failure to make expected weight gain during period of growth, leading to body weight less than 85% of that expected).
- Intense fear of gaining weight or becoming fat, even though underweight.
- Disturbance in the way in which one's body weight or shape is experienced, undue influence of body weight or shape on self-evaluation, or denial of the seriousness of the current low body weight.
- Amenorrhea in postmenarchal females, i.e., the absence of at least three consecutive menstrual cycles. (A woman is considered to have amenorrhea if her periods occur only following hormone, e.g., estrogen, administration.)

Restricting Type

During the current episode of anorexia nervosa, the person has not regularly engaged in binge eating or purging behavior (i.e., self-induced vomiting or the misuse of laxatives, diuretics, or enemas).

Binge Eating and Purging Type

During the current episode of anorexia nervosa, the person has regularly engaged in binge eating or purging behavior (i.e., self-induced vomiting or the misuse of laxatives, diuretics, or enemas).

From American Psychiatric Association: *Diagnostic and statistical manual of mental disorders*, ed 4, text revision (DSM-IV-TR), Washington, DC, 2000, The Association.

A variety of psychologic factors are associated with anorexia nervosa. Personality traits of perfectionism and compulsiveness are common. Low self-esteem also plays a role. In many cases, weight loss is experienced as an achievement, and self-esteem becomes dependent on body size and weight. At the same time the adolescent may experience peer, familial, and cultural pressures to be thin. There is a high incidence of co-occurring mood disorders in anorexic patients. In some cases, major depression may result from nutritional deprivation. Individuals with anorexia nervosa may lack spontaneity in social situations and may be emotionally restrained. Family dynamics may play a role in development of symptoms. Eating behaviors ostensibly emerge in an unconscious attempt to gain control in cases where parents are perceived to be controlling and overprotective. For some adolescents, diminished weight and loss of secondary sexual characteristics are related to difficulty accepting maturation into adulthood. A reflection of the sociocultural ideal of thinness, disordered eating that is not severe enough to meet criteria for anorexia nervosa is common among adolescent girls in the United States and is on the rise in males.

INCIDENCE

1. More than 90% of individuals with anorexia are females.
2. Rate of incidence among those aged 15 through 24 years is 14.6% for females and 1.8% for males.
3. Mortality rates range between 6% and 15%; half the deaths result from suicide.
4. Prevalence continues to be higher in Western industrialized nations with predominantly white populations and among middle- and upper-class females. Increasing diversity in the ethnic and socioeconomic groups of those affected is being reported. For immigrants, degree of acculturation may play a role.
5. Cardiac complications occur in 87% of affected youth.
6. Renal complications occur in approximately 70% of affected youth.

CLINICAL MANIFESTATIONS

1. Sudden, unexplained weight loss
2. Emaciated appearance, loss of subcutaneous fat
3. Changes in eating habits, unusual eating times
4. Excessive exercise and physical activity
5. Amenorrhea
6. Dry, scaly skin

7. Lanugo on extremities, back, and face
8. Yellowish discoloration of skin
9. Sleep disturbances
10. Chronic constipation or diarrhea, abdominal pain, bloating
11. Esophageal erosion (from frequent vomiting)
12. Depressed mood
13. Excessive focus on high achievement (individual becomes distressed when performance is not above average)
14. Excessive focus on food, eating, and body appearance
15. Erosion of tooth enamel and dentin on lingual surfaces (late effects from frequent vomiting)

COMPLICATIONS

1. Cardiac: bradycardia, tachycardia, arrhythmias, hypotension, cardiac failure
2. Gastrointestinal: esophagitis, peptic ulcer disease, hepatomegaly
3. Renal: serum urea and electrolyte abnormalities (hypokalemia, hyponatremia, hypochloremia, hypochloremic metabolic alkalosis), pitting edema
4. Hematologic: mild anemia and leukopenia (common) and thrombocytopenia (rare)
5. Skeletal: osteoporosis, pathologic fractures
6. Endocrine: reduced fertility, elevated cortisol and growth hormone levels, elevated gluconeogenesis
7. Metabolic: decreased basal metabolic rate, impaired temperature regulation, sleep disturbances
8. Death caused by complications, including cardiac arrest and electrolyte imbalance, and suicide

LABORATORY AND DIAGNOSTIC TESTS

1. Electrocardiogram—bradycardia is common
2. Erect and supine blood pressure—to assess for hypotension
3. Serum urea, electrolyte, creatinine levels (in severe cases, monitor every 3 months)—may show low blood urea nitrogen level due to dehydration and inadequate protein intake; metabolic alkalosis and hypokalemia due to vomiting

4. Urinalysis, urine creatinine clearance (in severe cases, monitor annually)—pH may be elevated; ketones may be present

5. Complete blood count, platelet count (in severe cases, monitor every 3 months)—usually normal; normochromic, normocytic anemia may be present

6. Fasting blood glucose level (in severe cases, monitor every 3 months) decreased levels may be due to malnutrition

7. Liver function tests (in severe cases, perform every 3 months)—abnormal results indicate possible starvation

8. Thyroid-stimulating hormone, cortisol levels (in severe cases, monitor semiannually)

9. Bone density (in severe cases, monitor annually)—demonstrates osteopenia

10. Body composition (in severe cases, monitor annually using calipers or water immersion)—to determine loss of significant body mass

11. Presence of hypercarotenemia (causes yellowing of skin, also known as pseudojaundice)—due to vegetarian diet or decreased metabolism

MEDICAL MANAGEMENT

Treatment is provided on an outpatient basis unless severe medical problems develop. An interdisciplinary approach is needed to ensure optimal outcome. Outpatient treatment includes medical monitoring, dietary planning to restore nutritional state, and psychotherapy. Therapeutic approaches include individual, family, and group psychotherapy. Family involvement is crucial. Use of psychotropic medication should be considered only after weight gain has been established. Medication may be used to treat depression, anxiety, and obsessive-compulsive behaviors. Hospitalization is indicated if the adolescent weighs less than 20% of ideal body weight or is unable to adhere to the treatment program on an outpatient basis, or if neurologic deficits, hypokalemia, or cardiac arrhythmias are present. Hospitalization is limited to brief stays focusing on acute weight restoration and refeeding.

Psychiatric hospitalization is indicated rather than admission to a general pediatric unit, since these clients require care from nurses with experience in refeeding protocols and psychiatric illnesses. Refeeding begins with 1200 to 1500 kcal per day and is increased by 500 kcal every 4 days, until about 3500 kcal for females and 4000 kcal for males per day is reached. To some degree, refeeding reduces apathy, lethargy, and food-related obsessions. Close monitoring is required during refeeding. Vital signs should be taken regularly and attention paid to electrolyte concentrations, peripheral edema, and cardiopulmonary functioning. *Refeeding syndrome* occurs in about 6% of hospitalized adolescents. Symptoms range from the more minor transient pedal edema to, more seriously, prolonged QT intervals and weakness, confusion, and neuromuscular dysfunction resulting from hypophosphatemia. Refeeding syndrome is most likely to occur in clients whose weight is less than 70% of their ideal body weight or in those who are receiving parenteral or enteral nutrition, or when oral refeeding is too vigorous.

The following medications may be given:

1. Antidepressants—selective serotonin reuptake inhibitors (e.g., fluoxetine, sertraline, paroxetine) may be used if compulsive exercising is a component of the illness
2. Estrogen replacement—may be used for amenorrhea

NURSING ASSESSMENT

1. Assess psychologic status with psychologic inventories. The Eating Disorder Examination is designed for structured interviews. Clinical self-reports include the Eating Disorder Inventory (for ages 14 years and older). The Eating Attitudes Test and the Kids Eating Disorder Survey may be used for school-aged children. The Children's Depression Inventory may be used to assess level of depression in 7- to 17-year-olds.
2. Assess height and weight using growth charts and body mass index (weight measurements are taken after the individual has undressed and voided).
3. Assess pattern of elimination.
4. Assess exercise pattern for type, amount, and frequency.
5. Assess for signs of depression.

NURSING DIAGNOSES

- Nutrition: less than body requirements, Imbalanced
- Family process, interrupted related to situational crisis
- Fluid volume, Risk for deficient
- Activity intolerance
- Coping, Ineffective
- Self-esteem, Chronic low
- Body image, Disturbed
- Social isolation related to altered state of wellness

NURSING INTERVENTIONS

1. Participate in interdisciplinary team that uses multiple modalities such as individual and group psychotherapy, assertiveness training, music and/or art therapy, and nutritional education.
2. Support involvement of family members who are vital to recovery.
   a. Include family in developing dietary supplementation plan.
3. Provide information about adequate nutritional intake and effect of inadequate intake on energy level and psychologic well-being.
4. Organize eating of meals with others, record amount of food eaten, and monitor activity for 2 hours after eating.
5. Initiate specific plan of exercise to reinforce positive behavioral outcomes.
6. Establish trusting relationship that promotes disclosure of feelings and emotions.
7. Promote adolescent's sense of responsibility and involvement in recovery and treatment.

🏠 Discharge Planning and Home Care

1. Recommend psychotherapy for treatment of distorted body image and self-concept.
2. Refer adolescent and family to community resources, e.g., support groups and mental health professionals (see Appendix G for community services).

CLIENT OUTCOMES

1. Individual's physical health status will improve with steady, reasonable weight gain (about 1 pound every 4 days).
2. Individual will establish healthy pattern of nutritional intake.
3. Individual will establish increased self-esteem and improvement in psychologic functioning.

REFERENCES

American Psychiatric Association: *Diagnostic and statistical manual of mental disorders*, ed 4, text revision (DSM-IV-TR), Washington, DC, 2000, The Association.

American Psychiatric Association Work Group on Eating Disorders: Practice guideline for the treatment of patients with eating disorders (revision), *Am J Psychiatry;* 157(Suppl 1):1, 2000.

Carpenito L: *Handbook of nursing diagnosis*, ed 8, Philadelphia, 2005, JB Lippincott.

Ebeling H et al: A practice guideline for treatment of eating disorders in children and adolescents, *Ann Med;* 35(7):488, 2003.

Sparks S, Taylor C: *Nursing diagnostic reference manual*, ed 6, Philadelphia, 2005, Lippincott, Williams & Wilkins.

Yager J, Andersen AE: Anorexia nervosa, *N Engl J Med;* 353(14):1481, 2005.

2

❖

Aplastic Anemia

PATHOPHYSIOLOGY

Aplastic anemia occurs when bone marrow failure leads to the depletion of all marrow elements. The production of blood cells is decreased or lacking. Pancytopenia and hypocellularity of the marrow occur. The manifestation of symptoms is dependent on the extent of the thrombocytopenia (hemorrhagic symptoms), neutropenia (bacterial infections, fever), and anemia (pallor, fatigue, congestive heart failure, tachycardia). Severe aplastic anemia is characterized by a granulocyte count of less than $500/mm^3$, a platelet count of less than $20,000/mm^3$, and a reticulocyte count of less than 1%. Aplastic anemia can be acquired or inherited. Acquired forms can be caused by drugs (chloramphenicol and chemotherapeutic agents), chemicals (benzene), radiation, or viral infection (hepatitis virus, human parvovirus, Epstein-Barr virus), and in rare instances are associated with paroxysmal nocturnal hemoglobinuria. Fanconi's anemia is the most common inherited type and is associated with various physical findings and renal and cardiac abnormalities. Diamond-Blackfan anemia is a hypoplastic anemia that only affects the erythrocyte cell line; it is diagnosed in early infancy.

INCIDENCE

1. About 100 new cases of acquired aplastic anemia are diagnosed each year in children in the United States.
2. Aplastic anemia may occur at any age.
3. The majority of cases are idiopathic.
4. Long-term survival rate with bone marrow transplant from histocompatible donors is as high as 75% to 95% in

children. Without bone marrow transplant, survival is about 50%.
5. Males and females are affected equally with Fanconi's anemia. Most cases are diagnosed at about 7 years of age, although the disorder may be diagnosed in infancy or as late as 30 to 40 years of age.

CLINICAL MANIFESTATIONS

1. Petechiae, ecchymoses, epistaxis (occur first as a result of low platelet counts)
2. Oral ulcerations, bacterial infections, fever (occur later in course)
3. Anemia, pallor, fatigue, tachycardia (late signs)
4. Café-au-lait spots, melanin-like hyperpigmentation, absent thumbs, renal abnormalities, short stature (Fanconi's anemia)
5. Pallor and anemia at birth or in early infancy (Diamond-Blackfan anemia)

COMPLICATIONS

1. Sepsis
2. Sensitization to cross-reacting donor antigens resulting in uncontrollable bleeding
3. Graft versus host disease (can occur after bone marrow transplantation)
4. Failure of marrow graft (can occur after bone marrow transplantation)
5. Acute myelogenous leukemia (associated with Fanconi's anemia)

LABORATORY AND DIAGNOSTIC TESTS

1. Bone marrow aspiration and biopsy—used to assess the cells in the bone marrow; findings are marrow hypoplasia with less than 25% normal cellularity.
2. Complete blood count with differential—used to evaluate circulating numbers and sizes of red and white blood cells. Findings with aplastic anemia include macrocytic anemia and decreased absolute neutrophil count to less than 500/μL. White blood cell counts are normal in Diamond-Blackfan anemia.

3. Platelet count—used to assess the number of platelets in the blood, which are needed for blood clotting. Findings include a platelet count of less than 20,000/µL. Platelet counts are normal in Diamond-Blackfan anemia.
4. Reticulocyte count—used to indirectly analyze hematopoiesis or the forming and development of blood cell lines. Decreased reticulocyte count in the presence of anemia indicates underlying pathology.
5. Hemoglobin electrophoresis—used to detect presence of fetal hemoglobin, which is increased in Diamond-Blackfan anemia.
6. Chromosome breakage test—used to detect chromatid breaks and other abnormalities. A positive result indicates Fanconi's anemia.

MEDICAL MANAGEMENT

The first-choice treatment for severe aplastic anemia is bone marrow transplant from a sibling donor who is human lymphocyte antigen (HLA)–matched. In more than 70% of cases, there will be no sibling match. However, there is an increased chance of a match between one parent and the child with aplastic anemia. To avoid sensitization, if bone marrow transplantation is to be done, HLA typing of the family is performed immediately and blood products are used as little as possible. Further, blood should not be donated by the child's family. Blood products should always be irradiated and filtered to remove white blood cells before being given to a child who is a candidate for bone marrow transplantation. Children with severe aplastic anemia treated with bone marrow transplant recover more rapidly and with fewer complications than adults. More recent advances include using umbilical cord blood that was banked at birth or saved from a newborn sibling at birth and then typed and used. Umbilical cord blood is rich in stem cells, which then grow well in children with aplastic anemia.

Immunotherapy with either antithymocyte globulin or antilymphocyte globulin is the primary treatment for children who are not candidates for bone marrow transplantation. The child will respond within 3 months or not at all to this therapy. Cyclosporine is also an effective immunosuppressant that can be used in the treatment of aplastic anemia. Androgens, used in the past, are rarely used today unless no other treatment is available. Corticosteroids are the initial therapy in Diamond-Blackfan anemia; with a positive response, indicated by an increasing hematocrit, the dose is tapered.

Clinical trials exploring the use of granulocyte-macrophage colony-stimulating factor (GM-CSF) or granulocyte colony-stimulating factor (G-CSF) in pediatric clients continue to show some hematologic improvement with these treatments. Further research continues to determine the role of GM-CSF and G-CSF in treating aplastic anemia and Fanconi's anemia.

Supportive therapy includes use of antibiotics and administration of blood products. Antibiotics are used to treat fever and neutropenia; prophylactic antibiotics are not indicated for the asymptomatic child. Blood product administration is based on clinical findings. All products should be leukocyte-reduced and irradiated. Blood products used may include the following:

1. Platelets—to maintain platelet count appropriate for the individual child to prevent bleeding—in chronic cases the count may drop to as low as 15,000/mm^3 before transfusion is given. Use single-donor platelet pheresis to decrease the number of HLA antigens to which the child is exposed.

2. Packed red blood cells—to maintain hemoglobin level (chronic anemia is often well tolerated). For long-term therapy, deferoxamine is used as a chelating agent to prevent complications of iron overload.

NURSING ASSESSMENT

1. See the Hematologic Assessment section in Appendix A.
2. Assess for sites of bleeding and hemorrhagic symptoms.
3. Assess for signs of infection.
4. Assess activity level.
5. Assess developmental level.

NURSING DIAGNOSES

- Injury, Risk for
- Infection, Risk for
- Activity intolerance
- Fatigue

NURSING INTERVENTIONS

1. Identify and report signs and symptoms of hemorrhage.
   a. Vital signs (increased apical pulse, thready pulse, decreased blood pressure)
   b. Bleeding sites
   c. Skin color (pallor) and signs of diaphoresis
   d. Weakness
   e. Decreased level of consciousness
   f. Decreased platelet count
2. Protect from trauma and prevent/decrease bleeding.
   a. Do not administer aspirin or nonsteroidal antiinflammatory drugs.
   b. Provide good oral hygiene with soft toothbrush.
   c. Avoid use of intramuscular injections and suppositories.
   d. Administer contraceptive to decrease excessive menstruation.
3. Protect from infection.
   a. Limit contact with potential sources of infection.
   b. Use strict isolation precautions (refer to institution's policies and procedures).
4. Administer blood products and monitor child's response to their infusion (after bone marrow transplantation, to avoid sensitization to donor transplantation antigen).
   a. Observe for side effects or untoward response (transfusion reaction).
   b. Observe for signs of fluid overload.
   c. Monitor vital signs before transfusion, 15 minutes after infusion has started, as needed during infusion (or based on institution's policies), and upon completion of transfusion.
5. Provide frequent rest periods. Organize nursing care to increase activity tolerance and prevent fatigue.
6. Monitor child's therapeutic and untoward response to medications; monitor action and side effects of administered medications.
7. Prepare child and family for bone marrow transplantation.
8. Monitor for signs of bone marrow transplant complications (see the Complications section in this chapter).

9. Provide age-appropriate diversional and recreational activities.
10. Provide age-appropriate explanation before procedures.

🏠 Discharge Planning and Home Care

1. Instruct parents about measures to protect child from infection.
   a. Limit contact with infectious agents.
   b. Identify signs and symptoms of infection.
2. Instruct parents to monitor for signs of complications (see the Complications section in this chapter).
3. Instruct parents about administration of medication.
   a. Monitor child's therapeutic response.
   b. Monitor for untoward response.
4. Provide child and family with information about community support systems for long-term adaptation.
   a. School reintegration
   b. Parent groups
   c. Child and sibling groups
   d. Sources of financial advice

CLIENT OUTCOMES

1. Child will have gradual increase in red blood cells, white blood cells, and platelets.
2. Child will have minimal bleeding episodes.
3. Child will have fewer infections.
4. Child and family will understand home care and follow-up needs.

REFERENCES

Brill JR, Baumgardner DJ: Normocytic anemia, *Am Fam Physician* 62(10):2255, 2000.

D'Andrea AD et al: Marrow failure, *Hematology* (American Society of Hematology education program):58, 2002.

Lemons RS: Bone marrow dysfunction, In: Osborn LM et al, editors: *Pediatrics*, St. Louis, 2005, Mosby.

Trigg MN: Hematopoietic stem cells, *Pediatrics* 113(4):1051, 2004.

3

Apnea

PATHOPHYSIOLOGY

Apnea is the cessation of respiration for more than 20 seconds with or without cyanosis, hypotonia, or bradycardia. Apnea may be a symptom of another disorder that resolves when the latter is treated. Such disorders may include infection, gastroesophageal reflux, hypoglycemia, metabolic disorders, drug toxicity, or hydrocephalus, or thermal instability in newborns. Central apnea is a respiratory pause, the cause of which is related to the failure of the excitatory mechanisms to function properly in the respiratory center in the brain. Immaturity of the central nervous system frequently accounts for apnea of the newborn, which occurs most frequently during active sleep. Obstructive apnea occurs when an obstruction of the airway exists, usually at the level of the pharynx, and occurs most frequently during sleep. Here, there is continuation of respiratory effort without air flow in the airway because of the obstruction. This condition may be due to enlarged tonsils and adenoids, congenital disorders such as Pierre Robin syndrome, or muscular hypotonia. Apnea consisting of both central and obstructive components is mixed apnea. Apnea can also occur in premature infants during certain normal activities, such as feeding.

INCIDENCE

1. More than 50% of infants weighing less than 1.5 kg require treatment for recurrent prolonged apneic episodes.
2. About one third of infants born at less than 32 weeks' gestation have apneic episodes.
3. Idiopathic apnea rarely occurs in term infants.

4. The prevalence of obstructive sleep apnea is estimated at 1% to 3% of preschool- and school-aged children. Obstructive apnea is most often caused by hypertrophy of the adenoids and tonsils.

CLINICAL MANIFESTATIONS

1. Cessation of respiration for more than 20 seconds with or without cyanosis, bradycardia, or hypotonicity
2. Snoring

COMPLICATIONS

1. Cardiovascular: bradycardia, diminished perfusion, decreased blood pressure
2. Pulmonary: oxygen desaturation, hypoxia, hypercarbia
3. Neurologic: hypoxic-ischemic brain injury associated with prolonged apnea and bradycardia in preterm infants
4. Growth and development: failure to thrive

LABORATORY AND DIAGNOSTIC TESTS

1. Polysomnography—a sleep study that includes direct observation of the patient along with electroencephalogram (EEG), blood pressure, breathing rate, heart rhythm, oxygen saturation, eye movement, and electrical activity of muscles. Used to determine if apnea is central, obstructive, or mixed.
2. Apnea monitoring—used to monitor the frequency and duration of apneic episodes.
3. Pulse oximetry—used to assess for associated oxygen desaturation.

MEDICAL MANAGEMENT

Infants with suspected or documented apnea are monitored using either a cardiorespiratory or an apnea monitor. The immediate management of an apneic episode is to provide gentle stimulation by rubbing the child's back or feet. Do not shake infant or child vigorously to stimulate the infant. If the infant or child does not respond, the airway should be opened, and cardiopulmonary resuscitation (CPR) should be initiated. If apnea is a symptom of another disorder, the treatment of that disorder should result in the elimination of apnea.

The management of central apnea, most frequently seen in premature infants, includes minimizing potential causes such as temperature variances and feeding intolerance. Xanthine medications such as caffeine and theophylline provide central nervous system stimulation. Pulmonary function support may include the use of supplemental oxygen and continuous positive airway pressure (CPAP) at low pressures. Indications for home apnea monitoring in newborns with apnea include a history of severe apneic episodes, documentation of apnea during polysomnography, severe feeding difficulties with apnea and bradycardia, and sibling relationship with a victim of SIDS.

The management of obstructive apnea may include the use of specific positioning techniques, the use of CPAP or inspiratory and expiratory positive airway pressure (BiPAP), tracheostomy to bypass the area of obstruction, or adenotonsillectomy. Aggressive surgical management to widen the caliber of the trachea has eliminated the need for tracheostomy in some cases.

NURSING ASSESSMENT

1. See the Respiratory Assessment section in Appendix A.
2. Provide early identification of apneic event.

NURSING DIAGNOSES

- Ventilation, Spontaneous, Impaired
- Tissue perfusion, Ineffective
- Sleep pattern, Disturbed
- Family processes, Interrupted
- Caregiver role strain, Risk for

NURSING INTERVENTIONS

1. Perform routine monitoring of heart rate and respiratory rate in preterm infants.
2. Gently rub infant's back or feet, which will stop some apneic episodes if they are caught early.
3. Allow parents to verbalize feelings.
4. Provide instruction on all equipment to be used by parents, such as apnea monitor or BiPAP unit.

🏠 Discharge Planning and Home Care

1. Educate parents in use of monitor and proper application of electrodes or belt, as well as in infant safety and infant CPR.
2. Educate parents in how to position child to prevent airway obstruction.

CLIENT OUTCOMES

1. Child will maintain adequate oxygenation.
2. Child's apneic events will be identified early to minimize complications.

REFERENCES

American Academy of Pediatrics Committee on Fetus and Newborn: Apnea, sudden infant death syndrome, and home monitoring, *Pediatrics* 111 (3):914, 2003.

Goldstein NA et al: Clinical assessment of pediatric obstructive sleep apnea, *Pediatrics* 114(1):33, 2004.

Hockenberry MJ et al: *Wong's nursing care of infants and children*, ed 7, St. Louis, 2004, Mosby.

Kenner C et al: *Comprehensive neonatal nursing*, ed 3, St. Louis, 2002, Mosby.

Stokowski LA: A primer on apnea of prematurity, *Adv Neonatal Care* 5(3):155, 2005.

4

❖

Appendicitis and Appendectomy

PATHOPHYSIOLOGY

Appendicitis is the most common condition requiring emergency abdominal surgery during childhood. Acute appendicitis is caused by the obstruction of the appendiceal lumen, resulting in compression of the blood vessels. Obstruction of the lumen can be caused by hyperplasia of the submucosal lymphoid tissue, appendiceal fecaliths, foreign bodies, and/or parasites. Bacteria then invade the layers of the appendiceal wall, causing local inflammation (acute appendicitis). Perforated appendicitis occurs when the inflamed wall becomes necrotic and "bursts" (perforates), resulting in peritonitis. In most cases, no definitive cause can be identified at the time of surgery. The prognosis is excellent, especially when surgery is performed before perforation occurs.

INCIDENCE

1. Approximately 80,000 children experience appendicitis per year.
2. Occurs in 1 per 1000 children younger than 14 years old
3. Incidence highest in later childhood, age 10 to 12 years.
4. Occurrence is unusual in children younger than 4 years of age and is rare in children younger than 1 year old.
5. Likelihood of perforation is related to age—it occurs more frequently in younger children, most probably because of difficulty in diagnosis.
6. Slightly higher incidence in males.

CLINICAL MANIFESTATIONS

1. Classic triad
   a. Pain—cramping located in periumbilical area migrating to right lower quadrant, with most intense pain at McBurney's point (located midway between right anterior superior iliac crest and umbilicus)
   b. Vomiting (common early sign; less common in older children)
   c. Fever—low-grade early in disease; can rise sharply with peritonitis
2. Anorexia
3. Nausea
4. Rebound tenderness
5. Decreased or absent bowel sounds
6. Constipation
7. Diarrhea (small, watery evacuations)
8. Difficulty walking or moving
9. Irritability

COMPLICATIONS

(In the absence of proper diagnosis or delay in treatment)
1. Perforation
2. Peritonitis
3. Abscess formation
4. Adhesions
5. Bowel obstruction
6. Death

LABORATORY AND DIAGNOSTIC TESTS

1. Complete blood count—leukocytosis, neutrophilia, absence of eosinophils
2. Urinalysis—to exclude urinary tract infection
3. Abdominal radiographic study—concave curvature of spine to right, calcified fecaliths
4. Ultrasonography (test of choice)—noncalcified fecaliths, nonperforated appendix, appendiceal abscess
5. Computed tomographic (CT) scan of abdomen—provides differential diagnosis for abdominal pain

SURGICAL MANAGEMENT

Children with suspected appendicitis are admitted to hospital for observation and are given antibiotics and intravenous (IV) fluids to correct electrolyte imbalances, especially if dehydrated; the rapid progression of symptoms will make the diagnosis obvious. A nasogastric tube is inserted if the child is vomiting. The child is taken to surgery, where the appendix is removed by one of two ways: (1) by open appendectomy, through an incision in the right lower quadrant; or (2) laparoscopically, which has been shown to reduce length of hospital stay. Perforated appendicitis is generally treated surgically: the appendix is removed, and the abdominal cavity is irrigated. A drain may be inserted and the wound left open to prevent wound infection and abscess formation. In some cases, a small catheter may be left in place to instill antibiotics. Postoperatively the child is put in semi-Fowler position for the first 24 hours. Gastric drainage and administration of IV fluids and antibiotics are continued. Narcotic and/or analgesic medications are used for pain. Oral feedings are started within 1 or 2 days and increased as tolerated when bowel function has returned. Interval appendectomy (medical therapy) is another treatment for perforated appendicitis: the child receives IV antibiotics for a determined length of time and is then scheduled to return for an elective appendectomy 4 weeks to 3 months after completion of antibiotic therapy.

NURSING ASSESSMENT

1. See the Gastrointestinal Assessment section in Appendix A.
2. Assess for rapid progression in severity of symptoms.
3. Assess for preoperative and postoperative pain.
4. Assess for symptoms of perforation, including sudden relief from pain.
5. Assess postoperatively for bowel sounds and abdominal distention.
6. Assess wound for drainage and signs of infection.

NURSING DIAGNOSES

- Pain, Acute
- Fluid volume, Risk for deficient

- Infection, Risk for
- Injury, Risk for
- Nutrition: less than body requirements
- Anxiety
- Knowledge, Deficient
- Family processes, Interrupted

NURSING INTERVENTIONS
Preoperative Care

1. Provide pain relief and comfort measures.
   a. Positioning for comfort.
   b. Avoidance of unnecessary movements and unnecessary palpation of abdomen.
   c. Administration of pain medications as ordered.
2. Maintain fluid and electrolyte balance.
   a. Maintain nothing by mouth (NPO) status.
   b. Monitor infusion of IV solution at maintenance rate.
   c. Monitor and record output of vomitus, urine, stool, and nasogastric drainage.
3. Monitor child's status for progression of symptoms and complications.
   a. Signs of shock—decreased blood pressure, decreased respiratory rate, pallor, diaphoresis, rapid and thready pulse.
   b. Perforation or peritonitis—sudden relief from pain with subsequent increase of diffuse pain with rigid guarding of abdomen, absent bowel sounds, increased apical pulse, increased temperature, rapid and shallow breathing, abdominal splinting, pallor, chills, irritability, restlessness.
   c. Intestinal obstruction—decreased or absent bowel sounds, abdominal distention, pain, vomiting, no stools.
4. Prepare child for surgery.
   a. Maintain NPO status.
   b. Administer antibiotics if ordered.
   c. Collect specimens preoperatively for analysis.
   d. Prepare child for and support child during laboratory and diagnostic testing.
   e. Explain anticipated preoperative and postoperative events (e.g., dressing, nasogastric tube).

Postoperative Care

1. Assess pain and institute pain relief measures as needed.
   a. Administer analgesics as needed.
   b. Use distraction to alleviate pain.
   c. Use comfort measures such as cold and positioning (e.g., right side–lying or low Fowler's to semi-Fowler position).
2. Prevent and monitor for abdominal distention.
   a. Maintain NPO status.
   b. Maintain patency of nasogastric tube.
   c. Monitor output of nasogastric tube (amount, color).
   d. Assess abdominal tenseness (firm, soft).
3. Monitor hydration and nutritional status.
   a. Monitor intake and output.
   b. Maintain NPO status; then advance as tolerated.
   c. Maintain total parenteral nutrition if child is unable to eat for several days.
   d. Maintain IV infusions and IV site as ordered.
4. Promote and maintain respiratory function.
   a. Have child turn, cough, and deep breathe.
   b. Perform postural drainage and percussion.
   c. Change child's position every 2 hours.
   d. Keep head of bed in semi-Fowler position.
5. Monitor for signs of infection, and prevent spread of infection.
   a. Monitor vital signs as ordered.
   b. Observe wound for signs of infection—warmth, drainage, pain, swelling, and redness.
   c. Administer antibiotics; monitor child's response.
   d. Perform wound care as indicated and dispose of dressings appropriately.
   e. Encourage ambulation and have child ambulate when able.
6. Promote wound healing.
   a. Perform wound care—maintain site, keeping it clean and dry.
   b. Position child in semi-Fowler position to promote drainage if drain is present.

7. Support child and parents to help them deal with emotional stresses of hospitalization and surgery.
   a. Provide age-appropriate information before and after procedures.
   b. Encourage quiet diversional activities.
   c. Promote family contacts and visits with peers.
   d. Incorporate child's home routine into daily activities.

🏠 Discharge Planning and Home Care

1. Instruct parents to observe for and report signs of complications.
   a. Infection
   b. Obstruction
2. Instruct parents regarding wound care.
3. Involve discharge planning team (such as social worker) if patient is to be discharged with orders for home IV antibiotic therapy.
4. Instruct parents to have child avoid strenuous activities for a few weeks.
5. Instruct parents about follow-up appointment.
   a. Name and phone number of physician.
   b. Date and time of follow-up appointment.

CLIENT OUTCOMES

1. Child will have return to normal gastrointestinal function, including presurgery dietary intake and normal bowel function.
2. Child will have minimal pain.
3. Child will be free from infection.
4. Child and family will understand home care and follow-up needs.

REFERENCES

Behrman RE, Kiegman R, Jenson HB: *Nelson textbook of pediatrics*, ed 17, Philadelphia, 2004, WB Saunders.

Chen C et al: Current practice patterns in the treatment of perforated appendicitis in children, *J Am Coll Surg* 196(2):212, 2003.

Hockenberry MJ et al: *Wong's nursing care of infants and children,* ed 7, St. Louis, 2004, Mosby.

McCollough M, Sharieff GQ: Abdominal pain in children, *Pediatr Clin North Am* 53(1):107, 2006.

McCollough M, Sharieff GQ: Abdominal surgical emergencies in infants and young children, *Emerg Med Clin North Am* 21(4):909, 2003.

Meguerditchian AN et al: Laparoscopic appendectomy in children: A favorable alternative in simple and complicated appendicitis, *J Pediatr Surg* 37 (5):695, 2002.

Vasavada P: Ultrasound evaluation of acute abdominal emergencies in infants and children, *Radiol Clin North Am* 42(2):445, 2004.

5

Asthma

PATHOPHYSIOLOGY

Asthma, also known as reactive airway disease (RAD), is a disease of the lower airway in which there is airway obstruction, airway inflammation, and airway hyperresponsiveness or spasm of the bronchial smooth muscle, increasing mucus formation. Symptoms usually include wheezing, coughing, shortness of breath, a feeling of tightness in the chest, and fatigue, as well as feeding difficulties in very young children. Clients may have retractions, a prolonged expiratory phase, and decreased breath sounds or poor air movement. An exacerbation of asthma may be precipitated by specific allergens (e.g., pollen, mold, animal dander, dust, or cigarette smoke) or by other factors such as weather changes, respiratory infections, exercise, gastroesophageal reflux, or emotional factors. Although the specific cause of asthma is not known, it is well known that the disease may "run in families," and genetic investigations are underway.

INCIDENCE

1. Asthma affects over 9 million children under the age of 18 in the United States.
2. Asthma is the number one cause of hospitalization for children under the age of 15, with children under the age of 4 having greater admission rates.
3. Asthma accounts for 25% of school absences caused by chronic illness.
4. Asthma death rates are increasing by 6% per year.

CLINICAL MANIFESTATIONS

1. Clinical evidence of airway obstruction—obstruction may be gradual or acute; severity of acute exacerbations is classified as mild intermittent, mild persistent, moderate persistent, or severe persistent
2. Dyspnea with prolonged expiration
3. Expiratory wheezing, progressing to inspiratory and expiratory wheezing, progressing to inaudibility of breath sounds
4. Grunting respirations in infancy
5. Nasal flaring
6. Cough
7. Accessory muscle use
8. Anxiety, irritability, decreasing level of consciousness
9. Cyanosis
10. Drop in arterial partial pressure of carbon dioxide ($Paco_2$) initially from hyperventilation; then rise in $Paco_2$ as obstructive process worsens

COMPLICATIONS

1. Status asthmaticus
2. Pneumonia
3. Gastroesophageal reflux
4. Atelectasis
5. Pneumothorax
6. Cor pulmonale with right-sided heart failure
7. Death

LABORATORY AND DIAGNOSTIC TESTS

1. White blood cell count—increased with infection
2. Arterial blood gas values (for severe cases)—initially increased pH, decreased Pao_2, and decreased $Paco_2$ (mild respiratory alkalosis from hyperventilation); subsequently decreased pH, decreased arterial partial pressure of oxygen (Pao_2), and increased $Paco_2$ (respiratory acidosis)
3. Eosinophil count—increased in blood, sputum
4. Chest radiographic study—to rule out infection or other cause of worsening respiratory status

5. Pulmonary function tests—decreased tidal volume, decreased vital capacity, decreased maximal breathing capacity
6. Peak flow meter monitoring—decreased peak expiratory flow volumes (less than 50% of personal best during acute episode)

MEDICAL MANAGEMENT

Medical management is targeted at preventing asthma exacerbations by avoiding asthma triggers and by decreasing airway obstruction, inflammation, and reactivity with medications. Medication choices and combinations depend on the severity classifications indicated in the Clinical Manifestations section in this chapter. Medications include corticosteroids (by oral, inhaled, intramuscular [IM], or intravenous [IV] routes) to decrease inflammation, bronchodilators (nebulized form or by metered dose inhaler). Oxygen may be required during an acute episode to maintain adequate levels of oxygenation. The National Asthma Education Prevention Program (NAEPP) recommended in 2002 that young children be placed on a daily preventive medication if they have had more than three episodes of wheezing within the past year and have risk factors of developing asthma. Risk factors include eczema, parent history of asthma, and the presence of two of the following: allergic rhinitis, wheezing with no upper respiratory symptoms, and/or increased eosinophils shown on the complete blood count (CBC). Prevention of exacerbations is the mainstay of treatment of this chronic illness, and two medication classifications have emerged: long-term control and acute control.

Long-Term Control

1. Inhaled corticosteroids—antiinflammatory; either inhaled form or metered dose inhaler (MDI) such as Pulmicort or Flovent
2. Cromolyn sodium and nedocromil—antiinflammatory; inhaled form; used to reduce exercise-induced asthma
3. Long-acting β-agonists—bronchodilator; inhaled form such as Serevent, Foradil, or Advair is used to reduce exercise-induced asthma and nocturnal symptoms

4. Leukotriene receptor antagonist—improve lung function and reduce need for short-acting β_2-agonists; oral form such as Singulair

Acute Control

1. Inhaled corticosteroids—short-acting bronchodilator; nebulized form such as Xopenex or Albuterol
2. Oral corticosteroids—antiinflammatory; oral form such as prednisolone

NURSING ASSESSMENT

1. See the Respiratory Assessment section in Appendix A.
2. Assess for anxiety and/or agitation.
3. Assess fluid volume status.
4. Assess child and family coping strategies.

NURSING DIAGNOSES

- Airway clearance, Ineffective
- Gas exchange, Impaired
- Fluid volume, Risk for deficient
- Anxiety
- Family processes, Interrupted

NURSING INTERVENTIONS

1. Promote pulmonary function.
   a. Administer and assess response to oxygen for respiratory distress.
   b. Administer and assess response to aerosolized bronchodilators and antiinflammatory agents.
   c. Elevate head of bed.
   d. Avoid use of sedatives in child with asthma experiencing respiratory distress.
2. Assess and monitor child's hydration status.
   a. Monitor intake and output.
   b. Assess for signs of dehydration.
   c. Monitor infusion of intravenous solution.
   d. Monitor urine specific gravity.
3. Alleviate or minimize child's and parents' anxiety, in manner appropriate for developmental level.

4. Assess child's and parents' feelings about child's having asthma and taking medications.
5. Provide and reinforce asthma education

🏠 Discharge Planning and Home Care

1. Begin client education at time of diagnosis and integrate it with continuing care.
2. Reinforce understanding of asthma.
3. Provide specific instructions about medications, equipment, and adverse effects.
4. Instruct on monitoring signs and symptoms and peak expiratory flow rate, and recognizing indications for treatment modifications.
5. List steps in managing an acute episode of asthma, and instruct on when to seek emergency medical care.
6. Instruct in how to identify asthma triggers and how to avoid, eliminate, or control them.
7. Discuss fears and misconceptions concerning treatments.

CLIENT OUTCOMES

1. Child will have optimal pulmonary function.
2. Child will be able to perform daily activities.
3. Child will be able to participate in endurance activities (e.g., swimming, tennis).

REFERENCES

Behrman R, Kiegman R, Jenson HB: *Nelson textbook of pediatrics*, ed 17, Philadelphia, 2004, WB Saunders.

Corjulo M: Telephone triage for asthma medication refills, *Pediatr Nurs* 32 (2):116, 2005.

Guidelines for the diagnosis and management of asthma: National asthma education program—expert panel report 2, Bethesda, Md, February 1997, National Institutes of Health.

Hockenberry MJ et al: *Wong's nursing care of infants and children*, ed 7, St. Louis, 2004, Mosby.

National Asthma Education Prevention Program (NAEPP): Panel Report 2: Guidelines for the diagnosis and management of asthma, *J Allergy Clin Immunol* 110(5):S142, 2002.

Vazquez D, Philotas R: Peds respiratory emergencies, *Adv for Nurses* 5(20):17, 2004. Florida Edition.

6

❖

Attention-Deficit/ Hyperactivity Disorder

PATHOPHYSIOLOGY

Attention-deficit/hyperactivity disorder (ADHD) is a chronic neurobiologic disorder characterized by problems in regulating activity (hyperactivity), inhibiting behavior (impulsivity), and attending to tasks (inattention). The Diagnostic and Statistical Manual of Mental Disorders, fourth edition, text revision (DSM-IV-TR), outlines specific observable behavioral symptoms in these three areas (Box 6-1). To meet the criteria for ADHD, symptoms must be present across settings. In other words, if the child is hyperactive at home but not at school, ADHD is not diagnosed.

Although ADHD symptoms are present before age 7 years, a diagnosis is not usually made until the child begins school, when behavior interferes with academic and social functioning. Children with ADHD are prone to physical injury. Sensorimotor coordination may be impaired, and clumsiness and problems with spatial orientation are common. Disruptiveness, temper outbursts, and aimless motor activity often irritate peers and family members. Secondary problems such as oppositional behavior, mood and anxiety disorders, and communication problems are common. Learning may be delayed as a result of chronic inability to attend to educational tasks.

As children enter adolescence, observable symptoms are less obvious. Restlessness and jitteriness replace the excessive activity seen during childhood. Adolescents with ADHD have difficulty complying with behavioral expectations or rules normally

BOX 6-1

Diagnostic Criteria for Attention-Deficit/ Hyperactivity Disorder

A. Either (1) or (2):
  (1) Six (or more) of the following symptoms of **inattention** have persisted for at least 6 months to a degree that is maladaptive and inconsistent with developmental level:
  Inattention
    (a) Often fails to give close attention to details or makes careless mistakes in schoolwork, work, or other activities
    (b) Often has difficulty sustaining attention in tasks or play activities
    (c) Often does not seem to listen when spoken to directly
    (d) Often does not follow through on instructions, and fails to finish schoolwork, chores, or duties in the workplace (not as a result of oppositional behavior or failure to understand instructions)
    (e) Often has difficulty organizing tasks and activities
    (f) Often avoids, dislikes, or is reluctant to engage in tasks that require sustained mental effort (such as schoolwork or homework)
    (g) Often loses things necessary for tasks or activities (e.g., toys, school assignments, pencils, books, or tools)
    (h) Is often easily distracted by extraneous stimuli
    (i) Is often forgetful in daily activities
  (2) Six (or more) of the following symptoms of **hyperactivity-impulsivity** have persisted for at least 6 months to a degree that is maladaptive and inconsistent with developmental level:
  Hyperactivity
    (a) Often fidgets with hands or feet or squirms in seat
    (b) Often leaves seat in classroom, or in other situations in which remaining seated is expected
    (c) Often runs about or climbs excessively in situations in which it is inappropriate (in adolescents or adults, may be limited to subjective feelings of restlessness)
    (d) Often has difficulty playing or engaging in leisure activities quietly
    (e) Is often "on the go" or often acts as if "driven by a motor"
    (f) Often talks excessively

BOX 6-1

Diagnostic Criteria for Attention-Deficit/
Hyperactivity Disorder—cont'd

Impulsivity

    (g) Often blurts out answers before questions have been completed

    (h) Often has difficulty awaiting turn

    (i) Often interrupts or intrudes on others (e.g., butts into conversations or games)

B. Some hyperactive-impulsive or inattentive symptoms that caused impairment were present before age 7 years.

C. Some impairment from the symptoms is present in two or more settings (e.g., at school [or work] and at home).

D. There must be clear evidence of clinically significant impairment in social, academic, or occupational functioning.

E. The symptoms do not occur exclusively during the course of a pervasive developmental disorder, schizophrenia, or other psychotic disorder and are not better accounted for by another mental disorder (e.g., mood disorder, anxiety disorder, dissociative disorder, or personality disorder).

Code based on type:

314.01: Attention-deficit/hyperactivity disorder, combined type: if both criteria A1 and A2 are met for the past 6 months

314.00: Attention-deficit/hyperactivity disorder, predominantly inattentive type: if criterion A1 is met but criterion A2 is not met for the past 6 months

314.01: Attention-deficit/hyperactivity disorder, predominantly hyperactive-impulsive type: if criterion A2 is met but criterion A1 is not met for the past 6 months

Coding Note: For individuals (especially adolescents and adults) who currently have symptoms that no longer meet full criteria, "in partial remission" should be specified

From American Psychiatric Association: *Diagnostic and statistical manual of mental disorders,* ed 4, text revision (DSM-IV-TR), Washington, DC, 2000, The Association.

observed in educational and work settings. Conflicts with authority figures are also noted. Symptoms may persist into adulthood. These individuals may be described as "on the go," always busy, and unable to sit still.

No signal cause of ADHD exists. Genetic influences are likely, but to date, no specific genetic link has been found.

Neurodevelopmental and genetic risk factors do exist. Most notable are fetal risk factors, which include exposure to alcohol, nicotine, and lead, and nutrient deficiencies (e.g., iron, calcium).

INCIDENCE

1. Studies suggest a higher incidence of ADHD in children with first-degree biologic relatives with diagnosed ADHD.
2. The incidence rate among school-aged children is 3% to 5%.
3. Incidence is higher in males than in females (roughly 3 times higher in boys than in girls).

CLINICAL MANIFESTATIONS

Clinical manifestations are listed in Box 6-1.

COMPLICATIONS

1. Secondary diagnoses—conduct disorder, depression, and anxiety disorder
2. Scholastic: academic underachievement, school failure, reading and/or arithmetic difficulties (frequently resulting from attentional problems)
3. Social: poor peer relationships (frequently due to impulsive behaviors such as aggressive behavior and verbal outbursts)

LABORATORY AND DIAGNOSTIC TESTS

1. For accurate diagnosis of ADHD, symptoms must meet specific criteria outlined in DSM-IV-TR (see Box 6-1).
2. Take behavioral history—obtain historical data from parents and teachers.
3. Use ADHD teacher and parent assessment tools (e.g., Conners Rating Scales—Revised; Swanson, Nolan, and Pelham-IV Questionnaire; SKAMP Rating Scale; ADHD Rating Scale IV; Vanderbilt ADHD Teacher Rating Scale and Vanderbilt ADHD Parent Rating Scale).
4. The following neuropsychologic tests may be used as a baseline and to assess and monitor treatment (no neuropsychologic instrument can be relied upon exclusively to diagnose):
   - Continuous Performance Test
   - Matching Familiar Figures Test
   - Paired Associates Learning Task

5. Intelligence and achievement testing provides information about overall intellectual functioning and academic achievement (ADHD is likely to affect achievement and cognitive performance). The assessment report should include the child's strengths and weaknesses.

MEDICAL MANAGEMENT

The treatment plan for ADHD should be carefully tailored to each child and includes no single intervention. Treatment options generally include medications (most commonly stimulants) and specific behavioral treatments. The various behavioral treatments include psychotherapy, behavioral therapy, social skills training, support groups, and parent skills training. Behavioral rating scales and neuropsychologic tests may be used for baseline measurement and monitoring of treatment effectiveness.

Medication

Stimulants are the most widely used medications for treating ADHD. Examples of stimulants approved by the United States Food and Drug Administration (FDA) for use in children include amphetamine (Adderall), methylphenidate (Concerta, Ritalin), and dextroamphetamine (Dexedrine). Stimulants reduce hyperactivity and impulsivity and improve ability to focus. They have been used for decades and are considered relatively safe. Newer sustained-release stimulants can be taken before school, and administration by the school nurse is therefore no longer required. Side effects from stimulants are usually related to dosage (higher doses produce more side effects). The most common side effects include decreased appetite, insomnia, and increased anxiety and/or irritablity. Mild stomach aches or headaches are also common. When taken as prescribed for ADHD, stimulants are neither addictive, nor do they lead to substance abuse.

For children who do not respond to or are unable to tolerate stimulants, atomoxetine (Strattera) a nonstimulant medication recently approved by the FDA for treatment of ADHD may be prescribed. So called "off label" such as antidepressant medications may also be used in such incidences. However, their safety and efficacy have not been established in children. Antidepressants may also be used to treat comorbid symptoms.

Parents may express concern about using medication. Risks and benefits of medication must be explained to parents, including prevention of potentially ongoing scholastic and social problems through the use of medications. For most children, medication alone may not be the best strategy.

NURSING ASSESSMENT

1. Assess family history via interview and/or genogram.
2. Assess child's behavioral history.

NURSING DIAGNOSES

- Therapeutic regimen management, Ineffective
- Self-concept, Disturbed
- Parenting, Risk for impaired
- Social interaction, Impaired
- Violence, Risk for other-directed
- Injury, Risk for

NURSING INTERVENTIONS

Nursing interventions are generally implemented in outpatient and community settings.

1. Assist parents in implementing a behavior program, including positive reinforcement.
2. Provide daily structure.
3. Administer stimulant medication as ordered.
   a. Stimulants may be temporarily discontinued on weekends and holidays.
   b. Stimulants are not given after 3 or 4 pm.

🏠 Discharge Planning and Home Care

1. Educate and support parents and family members.
2. Collaborate with teachers and involve parents. Encourage parents to ensure that teacher and school nurse are aware of medication name, dosage, and times of administration.
3. Ensure that child receives necessary academic evaluation and tutoring. Placement in special education class is often required.
4. Monitor child's progress and response to medication.

5. Refer to behavioral and parenting specialists to develop and implement a behavior plan.
6. Refer child or youth to child psychologist, counselor, or child mental health nursing specialist as indicated for ongoing counseling.
7. Refer child or youth as appropriate for social skills training and/or peer support groups.

CLIENT OUTCOMES

1. School performance will improve, as evidenced by classroom grades and work completed.
2. Improvement of child's behavior according to teacher and parent rating will be noted.
3. Child will display positive peer relationships.
4. Child will acquire developmental appropriate competencies.

REFERENCES

American Psychiatric Association: *Diagnostic and statistical manual of mental disorders*, ed 4, text revision (DSM-IV-TR), Washington, DC, 2000, The Association.

Daley D: Attention deficit hyperactivity disorder: A review of the essential facts, *Child Care Health Dev* 32(2):193, 2006.

Collett BR, O'Phan JL, Myers KM: Ten-year review of rating scales. V: Scales assessing attention-deficit/hyperactivity disorder, *J Am Acad Child Adolesc Psychiatry* 42(9):1015, 2003.

Magyary D, Brandt P: A decision tree and clinical paths for the assessment and management of children with ADHD, *Issues Ment Health Nurs* 23(6):553, 2002.

Prince, JB (2006). Pharmacotherapy of attention-deficit hyperactivity disorder in children and adolescents: Update on new stimulant preparations, atomoxetine, and novel treatments, *Child Adolesc Psychiatr Clin N Am* 15 (1):13, 2006.

Strock M: Attention deficit hyperactivity disorder, *National Institute of Mental Health*, NIH Publication No. 3572, 2003.

7

❖

Autism Spectrum Disorders (Pervasive Developmental Disorders)

PATHOPHYSIOLOGY

Autism spectrum disorders (ASDs), also known as pervasive developmental disorders, comprise a group of neuropsychiatric disabilities involving varying degrees of restricted, repetitive, and stereotyped patterns of behavior as well as impairment in communication skills and social interaction. ASD diagnoses range from the milder Asperger's disorder to the more severe autistic disorder. The *Diagnostic and Statistical Manual of Mental Disorders,* fourth edition, text revision (DSM-IV-TR) outlines specific observable behavioral components related to social interactions, communication, and repetitive and stereotypical behaviors and other indicators, presented for Asperger's disorder in Box 7-1 and autistic disorder in Box 7-2. Intact language skills distinguish Asperger's disorder from autism. Rare forms of ASD include Rett syndrome (Box 7-3) and childhood disintegrative disorder (CDD) (Box 7-4). In both disorders there is normal development followed by a profound regression of cognitive abilities. Rett syndrome occurs only in girls and is likely genetically based. The DSM criteria for pervasive developmental disorder, not otherwise specified, are presented in Box 7-5.

The exact cause of autism is unknown. Some studies show abnormal brain development beginning in the first months of life. In spite of popular belief, there is no scientific evidence

BOX 7-1
Diagnostic Criteria for Asperger's Disorder

A. Qualitative impairment in social interaction, as manifested by at least two of the following:
   (1) Marked impairments in the use of multiple nonverbal behaviors such as eye-to-eye gaze, facial expression, body postures, and gestures to regulate social interaction
   (2) Failure to develop peer relationships appropriate to developmental level
   (3) A lack of spontaneous seeking to share enjoyment, interests, or achievements with other people (e.g., by a lack of showing, bringing, or pointing out objects of interest to other people)
   (4) Lack of social or emotional reciprocity
B. Restricted repetitive and stereotyped patterns of behavior, interests, and activities, as manifested by at least one of the following:
   (1) Encompassing preoccupation with one or more stereotyped and restricted patterns of interest that is abnormal either in intensity or focus
   (2) Apparently inflexible adherence to specific, nonfunctional routines or rituals
   (3) Stereotyped and repetitive motor mannerisms (e.g., hand or finger flapping or twisting, or complex whole-body movements)
   (4) Persistent preoccupation with parts of objects
C. The disturbance causes clinically significant impairments in social, occupational, or other important areas of functioning
D. There is no clinically significant general delay in language (e.g., single words used by age 2 years, communicative phrases used by age 3 years)
E. There is no clinically significant delay in cognitive development or in the development of age-appropriate self-help skills, adaptive behavior (other than social interaction), and curiosity about the environment in childhood
F. Criteria are not met for another specific pervasive developmental disorder of schizophrenia

From American Psychiatric Association: *Diagnostic and statistical manual of mental disorders*, ed 4, text revision (DSM-IV-TR), Washington, DC, 2000, The Association.

BOX 7-2
Diagnostic Criteria for Autistic Disorder

A. A total of six (or more) items from (1), (2), and (3), with at least two from (1), and one each from (2) and (3)

   (1) Qualitative impairment in social interaction, as manifested by at least two of the following:

      (a) Marked impairments in the use of multiple nonverbal behaviors such as eye-to-eye gaze, facial expression, body posture, and gestures to regulate social interaction

      (b) Failure to develop peer relationships appropriate to developmental level

      (c) A lack of spontaneous seeking to share enjoyment, interests, or achievements with other people, (e.g., by a lack of showing, bringing, or pointing out objects of interest to other people)

      (d) Lack of social or emotional reciprocity (Note: The DSM description gives the following as examples: not actively participating in simple social play or games, preferring solitary activities, or involving others in activities only as tools or "mechanical" aids)

   (2) Qualitative impairments in communication as manifested by at least one of the following:

      (a) Delay in, or total lack of, the development of spoken language (not accompanied by an attempt to compensate through alternative modes of communication such as gesture or mime)

      (b) In individuals with adequate speech, marked impairment in the ability to initiate or sustain a conversation with others

      (c) Stereotyped and repetitive use of language or idiosyncratic language

      (d) Lack of varied, spontaneous make-believe play or social imitative play appropriate to developmental level

   (3) Restricted repetitive and stereotyped patterns of behavior, interests, and activities, as manifested by at least two of the following:

      (a) Encompassing preoccupation with one or more stereotyped and restricted patterns of interest that is abnormal either in intensity or focus

      (b) Apparently inflexible adherence to specific, nonfunctional routines or rituals

BOX 7-2
Diagnostic Criteria for Autistic Disorder—cont'd

    (c) Stereotyped and repetitive motor mannerisms (e.g.,
        hand or finger flapping or twisting, or complex whole-
        body movements)
    (d) Persistent preoccupation with parts of objects
B. Delays or abnormal functioning in at least one of the following
   areas, with onset before age 3 years:
    (1) Social interaction
    (2) Language as used in social communication
    (3) Symbolic or imaginative play
C. The disturbance is not better accounted for by Rett syndrome
   or Childhood Disintegrative Disorder.

From American Psychiatric Association: *Diagnostic and statistical manual of mental disorders*, ed 4, text revision (DSM-IV-TR), Washington, DC, 2000, The Association.

BOX 7-3
Diagnostic Criteria for Rett Syndrome (Females Only)

A. All of the following:
    (1) Apparently normal prenatal and postnatal development
    (2) Apparently normal psychomotor development
    (3) Normal head circumference at birth
B. Onset of all of the following after a period of normal
   development:
    (1) Deceleration of head growth between ages 5 and 48
        months
    (2) Loss of previously acquired purposeful hand skills between
        ages 5 and 30 months with subsequent development of
        stereotyped hand movements (e.g., hand wringing or
        hand washing)
    (3) Loss of social engagement early in the course (although
        social interaction often develops later)
    (4) Appearance of poorly coordinated gait or trunk
        movements
    (5) Severely impaired expressive and receptive language
        development with severe pyschomotor retardation

From American Psychiatric Association: *Diagnostic and statistical manual of mental disorders*, ed 4, text revision (DSM-IV-TR), Washington, DC, 2000, The Association.

BOX 7-4

Diagnostic Criteria for Childhood Disintegrative Disorder*

A. Apparently normal development for at least the first 2 years after birth as manifested by the presence of age-appropriate verbal and nonverbal communication, social relationships, play, and adaptive behavior

B. Clinically significant loss of previously acquired skills (before age 10 years in at least two of the following areas):
   (1) Expressive or receptive language
   (2) Social skills or adaptive behavior
   (3) Bowel or bladder control
   (4) Play
   (5) Motor skills

C. Abnormalities of functioning in at least two of the following areas:
   (1) Qualitative impairment in social interaction (e.g., impairment in nonverbal behaviors, failure to develop peer relationships, lack of social or emotional reciprocity)
   (2) Qualitative impairments in communication (e.g., delay or lack of the development of spoken language, inability to initiate or sustain a conversation, stereotyped and repetitive use of language, lack of verbal make-believe play)
   (3) Restricted repetitive and stereotyped patterns of behavior, interests, and activities, including motor stereotypes and mannerisms

D. The disturbance is not better accounted for by another specific pervasive developmental disorder or by schizophrenia.

*Childhood disintegrative disorder is much rarer than autism.
From American Psychiatric Association: *Diagnostic and statistical manual of mental disorders*, ed 4, text revision (DSM-IV-TR), Washington, DC, 2000, The Association.

to date that immunizations (e.g., measles, mumps, and rubella vaccine) cause autism. The co-occurrence of seizure disorders and some degree of mental retardation is common.

INCIDENCE

1. One in every 500 children has some form of pervasive developmental disorder (PDD).

BOX 7-5

Diagnostic Criteria for Pervasive Developmental Disorder, Not Otherwise Specified (including Atypical Autism)

This category should be used when there is a severe and pervasive impairment in the development of reciprocal social interaction or in verbal and nonverbal communication skills, or when the stereotyped behavior, interests, and activities are present, but the criteria are not met for a specific pervasive developmental disorder, schizophrenia, schizotypal personality disorder, or avoidant personality disorder. For example, this category includes "atypical autism"—presentations that do not meet the criteria for autistic disorder because of late age at onset, atypical symptomatology, or subthreshold symptomology (i.e., fewer than six items), or because of all three reasons.

From American Psychiatric Association: *Diagnostic and statistical manual of mental disorders*, ed 4, text revision (DSM-IV-TR), Washington, DC, 2000, The Association.

2. Prevalence rate of autistic disorder is approximately 2 to 5 in 10,000 births.
3. Asperger's disorder is more common in males.
4. Prevalence rate of Asperger's disorder is not established.
4. Prevalence rate of Rett syndrome is 1 in 10,000 to 15, 000 births.
5. Prevalence rate of CDD is low, 2 in 100,000 births.

CLINICAL MANIFESTATIONS

A diagnosis of an ASD is made based on behavioral symptoms. Possible indicators of ASDs are as follows:

Communication

1. Does not babble, point, or make meaningful gestures by 1 year of age
2. Does not speak one word by 16 months
3. Does not combine 2 words by 2 years
4. Does not respond to name

5. Loses language or social skills
6. May remain mute throughout life
7. May use language in unusual ways
8. Repeats certain phrases over and over
9. Speaks in single words
10. May have large vocabulary but difficulty sustaining conversation
11. Has difficulty understanding body language and tone of voice
12. Tone of voice and body language may not reflect what person is saying
13. High pitched or sing-song voice

Social Symptoms

1. Appears indifferent to others and prefers being alone
2. May resist or passively accept hugs and cuddling
3. Seldom seeks comfort (at older age)
4. Slow to learn to interpret what others are thinking and feeling
5. Misses subtle social cues (e.g., grimace or wink)
6. Difficulty regulating emotions (i.e., may be disruptive and aggressive, cries easily or inappropriately, has verbal outbursts)

Repetitive, Stereotypical Behaviors

1. Exhibits odd repetitive motions (e.g., flapping arms, walking on toes)
2. Suddenly freezes in position
3. Spends hours lining up toys
4. Needs absolute consistency
5. Becomes distressed with change in routine (e.g., times for dressing, taking a bath, going to school)
6. May focus intently on one thing (e.g., learning about vacuum cleaners, train schedules, numbers, symbols, or science topics)

Other Indicators

1. Poor eye contact
2. Does not seem to know how to play with toys
3. Is attached to one particular toy or object
4. Does not smile

5. Seems to be hearing-impaired at times
6. Lacks imaginative play
7. Hyper-sensitive senses (e.g., sounds, textures, tastes, smells; covers ears and screams at certain sounds such as ringing telephone)

COMPLICATIONS

Autism is not associated with complications; however, the child with autism may have secondary diagnoses such as depression, obsessive-compulsive disorders, and anxiety.

LABORATORY AND DIAGNOSTIC TESTS

1. Developmental assessments—Ages and Stages Questionnaire (ASQ), Greenspan Social-Emotional Growth Chart, Temperament and Atypical Behavior Scale (TABS).
2. Screening tools specific to autism.
   a. Autism Diagnostic Interview-Revised (ADI-R) is a semi-structured interview conducted with parents or caregivers to obtain information about the child's behavior related to social interactions, communication, and repetitive, stereotypical behaviors.
   b. Pervasive Developmental Disorder Screening Test-II (PDDST-II) is used to screen for ASD (autism, pervasive developmental delay, Asperger's disorder) in children aged 18 months and older.
   c. Modified Checklist for Autism in Toddlers (M-CHAT) is used to screen children for autism.
   d. Childhood Autism Rating Scale (CARS) is an observational tool used to assess the child (aged 2 years and older) on social interactions, intellectual functioning, visual and auditory responsiveness, environmental adaptation, anxiety, and activity level.
   e. Autism Diagnostic Observation Schedule (ADOS) is an observational tool used to assess social interactions, communication, and play behaviors of children aged 3 years and older for autism or PDD.
   f. Social Communication Questionnaire (SCQ) is a short screening tool used with the parent or caregiver to assess

social functioning and communication in children ages 4 and older (mental age of 2 years).

3. Parent or caregiver interviews may include semistructured format or structured formats such as ADI-R.

4. Child observations in various settings and times are conducted in the home, the school, and other community settings familiar to the child (ADOS).

5. Medical assessment.
   a. Medical history.
   b. Physical examination.
   c. Developmental and neurologic assessment (see developmental assessment material under Laboratory and Diagnostic Tests, earlier).

6. Assessment of adaptive functioning.
   a. Vineland Adaptive Behavior Scales are used to measure adaptive individual and social skills (i.e., communication, daily living skills, socialization, motor skills) from birth to adulthood using interview (with parent or caregiver) and/or classroom observational (teacher) formats.

7. Assessment of cognitive functioning.

8. Assessment of verbal and nonverbal language—SCQ, Peabody Picture Vocabulary Test-Revised (PPVT-R).

MEDICAL MANAGEMENT

Many behavioral programs exist to treat ASDs, applied behavioral analysis (ABA) being the most widely accepted. The objective of any good program is to reduce inappropriate behavior and increase communication and appropriate social behaviors. Behavioral plans should be structured and individualized. Parental involvement is essential. In some cases, medication is used. Antipsychotic medications are prescribed for severe behavioral problems. Medications are also used to treat co-occurring symptoms of anxiety, depression, and obsessive-compulsive disorders. Many medications are currently used "off label" (not approved by the United States Food and Drug Administration [FDA] for use in children), but psychopharmacologic studies are underway.

NURSING ASSESSMENT

1. Assess child social behaviors including interactions with others, communication skills, repetitive and stereotypical behaviors, play, and affect.
2. Assess family adaptation and coping.

NURSING DIAGNOSES

- Caregiver role strain
- Development, Risk for delayed
- Family processes, Interrupted
- Growth and development, Delayed
- Parenting, Impaired
- Self-care deficit, Bathing/Hygiene
- Self-care deficit, Dressing/Grooming
- Self-care deficit, Feeding
- Self-care deficit, Toileting
- Social interaction, Impaired
- Therapeutic regimen management, Ineffective family

NURSING INTERVENTIONS

Interventions for Inpatient Treatments, Hospitalizations, or Outpatient Visits

1. Provide quiet, structured environment.
2. Take vital signs with sense of calmness, with as little distraction as possible.
3. Give one instruction at a time.
4. Tell child or youth what to expect, and use simple explanations.
5. Talk in a soft, low voice.
6. Have child or youth visit same clinician on each outpatient medical appointment.
7. Use same routine each visit.
8. Remain composed even when child or youth is screaming.
9. Encourage parents to be present.
10. Avoid touching clients who are hypersensitive to touch.
11. Don't try to engage in eye contact.

Infants, Toddlers, and Preschoolers

1. Refer to early intervention program for development of individualized family service plan (IFSP) and interdisciplinary treatment plan; or, if child, refer to preschool program for individualized education plan (IEP) (see Appendix G) that provides opportunities for developmental learning (Appendix B):
   a. Social development.
   b. Fine motor development.
   c. Gross motor development.
   d. Sensory integration development.
   e. Communication and language development.
2. Refer parents and caregivers to family resource centers and/ or parent information centers that provide early intervention services to parents of infants and toddlers with disabilities for parental support and assistance with informational needs and respite services.
3. Collaborate with other interdisciplinary professionals to formulate IFSP and/or IEP that is based upon individual needs, is family-centered, has measurable objectives, and includes periodic evaluations.
4. Serve as health resource consultant to community service coordinator.
5. Assist family in navigating service systems to obtain needed services for child and family.
6. Refer to the Discharge Planning and Home Care section in this chapter.

School-Age Children

1. Collaborate with other interdisciplinary professionals to formulate IEP that is based upon individual needs, is individual- and family-centered, has measurable objectives, and includes periodic evaluations.
2. Collaborate with IEP team on identification of health-related needs and development of IEP objectives.
3. Assist family in navigating service systems to obtain needed services for child and family.
4. Refer to the Discharge Planning and Home Care section in this chapter.

Adolescents

1. Collaborate with other interdisciplinary professionals to formulate transition IEP that is based upon individual needs, is youth-centered, has measurable objectives, and includes periodic evaluations.
2. Collaborate with IEP team on identification of health-related transition needs and development of IEP objectives.
3. Provide input on transition plan related to health-related needs.
   a. Facilitate access to adult primary and specialty health care providers.
   b. Promote the development of self-reliance in managing healthcare self-care.
   c. Assist with obtaining health insurance in anticipation of termination of pediatric eligibility.
4. Assist family in navigating service systems to obtain needed services for child and family.
5. Refer to the Discharge Planning and Home Care section in this chapter.

🏠 Discharge Planning and Home Care

1. Instruct parents, family members, and child or youth and reinforce information about the behavioral and speech and language manifestations (social difficulties, speech and language limitations, characteristic repetitive and stereotypic behaviors), and long-term outcomes and prognosis of the autism diagnosis.
2. Educate parents, family members, and child or youth about long-term management strategies and community resources needed to access services (refer to Appendix G).
   a. Early intervention.
   b. Special education program (IEP).
   c. Specialized medical and therapy services.
   d. Community support services (e.g., rehabilitation, recreational, daily living skills, social skills).
   e. Vocational rehabilitation (joint programs with schools when in high school).
   f. Transportation.
   g. Housing.

3. Refer families to early intervention programs to address child's needs for treatment services.
4. Participate as a member of an interdisciplinary team to develop plan of services to address family-centered goals and objectives based on child's individual needs.

CLIENT OUTCOMES

1. Child will be diagnosed early, enabling participation in early treatment and intervention.
2. Child or youth will achieve highest potential of biopsycho-social functioning.
3. Child or youth will achieve highest possible level of self-sufficiency.
4. Child or youth will demonstrate highest achievable level of autonomy, self-determination, and self-advocacy.
5. Family will demonstrate ability to cope with child's or youth's behaviors and needs and to access needed services.
6. Parents will demonstrate attachment and responsive parenting behaviors.
7. Parents will demonstrate ability to accept child's limitations and recognize child's strengths.

REFERENCES

American Psychiatric Association: *Diagnostic and statistical manual of mental disorders,* ed 4, text revision (DSM-IV-TR), Washington, DC, 2000, The Association.

Chez MG, Chin K, Hung PC: Immunizations, immunology and autism, *Semin Pediatr Neurol* 11(3):214, 2004.

Masi G: Pharmacotherapy of pervasive developmental disorders in children and adolescents, *CNS Drugs* 18(14):1031, 2004.

National Institute of Mental Health: *Autism spectrum disorders (pervasive developmental disorders)* (website): www.nimh.nih.gov/publicat/autism.cfm. Accessed December 15, 2006.

Souders MC et al: Caring for children and adolescents with autism who require challenging procedures, *Pediatr Nurs* 28(6):555, 2002.

Sparks SM, Taylor CM: *Nursing diagnosis reference manual,* ed 6, Philadelphia, 2005, Lippincott, Williams & Wilkins.

Spence SJ, Sharifi P, Wiznitzer M: Autism spectrum disorder: Screening, diagnosis, and medical evaluation, *Semin Pediatr Neurol* 11(3):186, 2004.

Vastag B: Autism interventions come of age, *JAMA* 291(23):2807, 2004.

8

❖

Bulimia Nervosa

PATHOPHYSIOLOGY

Bulimia nervosa is a nutritional and psychologic disorder characterized by rapid consumption of large quantities of food (bingeing), followed by any of a number of behaviors used to prevent weight gain. Eating occurs during discrete periods of time. Self-induced vomiting is the most commonly used method to avoid weight gain. Other purging methods include use of laxatives, enemas, and diuretics, as well as of cathartics, thyroid medications, diet pills and appetite suppressants, stimulants, and nutritional supplements; diabetics may neglect to take their insulin.

Complications are related to the method of purging. Purging is ineffective when large quantities are consumed, because digestion begins rapidly and much of the food is digested and absorbed. Fluids and electrolytes are lost in the large intestine with laxative use, but digestion takes place in the small intestine. Fasting and excessive exercise may also be used as an attempt to compensate for intake and prevent weight gain. Most individuals develop a chronic pattern of binge/purge behavior. Bingeing may be triggered by dysphoria, stress, or negative feelings related to body image. Because of associated feelings of shame, bingeing is often done in secrecy. Individuals typically feel out of control during bingeing episodes. For some, vomiting becomes the goal in and of itself.

Impulse control problems such as alcohol abuse and shoplifting often coexist with bulimia. As in individuals with anorexia nervosa, there is an excessive focus on one's body. Self-worth is connected to physical appearance. Unlike the individual with anorexia, the bulimic individual is likely to be within the normal weight range for age and height, but weight may also vary by 10 pounds or more. The diagnostic criteria of the *Diagnostic and Statistical Manual of Mental Disorders*, fourth edition, text revision (DSM-IV-TR), are presented in Box 8-1.

BOX 8-1
Diagnostic Criteria for Bulimia Nervosa

1. Recurrent episodes of binge eating occur. An episode of binge eating is characterized by both of the following:
   a. Eating, in a discrete period of time (e.g., within any 2-hour period), an amount of food that is definitely larger than most people would eat during a similar period of time and under similar circumstances
   b. A sense of lack of control over eating during the episode (e.g., a feeling that one cannot stop eating or control what or how much one is eating)
2. Recurrent inappropriate compensatory behavior occurs to prevent weight gain, such as self-induced vomiting; misuse of laxatives, diuretics, enemas, or other medications; fasting; or excessive exercise.
3. The binge eating and inappropriate compensatory behaviors both occur, on average, at least twice a week for 3 months.
4. Self-evaluation is unduly influenced by body shape and weight.
5. The disturbance does not occur exclusively during episodes of anorexia nervosa.

Purging Type
During the current episode of bulimia nervosa, the person has regularly engaged in self-induced vomiting or the misuse of laxatives, diuretics, or enemas.

Nonpurging Type
During the current episode of bulimia nervosa, the person has used other inappropriate compensatory behaviors, such as fasting or excessive exercise, but has not regularly engaged in self-induced vomiting or the misuse of laxatives, diuretics, or enemas.

From American Psychiatric Association: *Diagnostic and statistical manual of mental disorders*, ed 4, text revision (DSM-IV-TR), Washington, DC, 2000, The Association.

Bulimia nervosa is difficult to diagnose because bulimics are normal or above average in weight, may not show any physical signs, and are not forthcoming about their condition; symptoms are typically concealed, and the family may be in denial. Minorities and men are largely overlooked, because clinicians see eating disorders as upper socioeconomic female disorders. Males are even more reluctant to disclose eating disorders behavior because of guilt and shame; the course is the same as for females in terms of secrecy and physical health problems.

The risk factors for men include athletic sports that require low body fat or are weight sensitive (swimming, gymnastics, and wrestling), negative life experiences, teasing, physical abuse, homosexuality, and the presence of a comorbid psychiatric condition. During the wrestling season, 17% of high school wrestlers meet short-term criteria for an eating disorder; a small minority do not recover after the season. Males generally use excessive exercise after bingeing rather than purging. In female clients, distorted body image leads to an overestimation of weight. Being a gay male is a documented risk, not because of sexual orientation but because of the value placed on lean muscularity. Because the ideal male form is lean and muscular, males are more likely to underestimate their weight. The reverse of anorexia, with body dismorphia at its core, is bigarexia. Often steroids are abused in an attempt to gain defined muscle mass and impossibly low body fat.

INCIDENCE

1. Bulimia nervosa affects about 2% to 4% of adolescent girls and fewer than 1% to 5% of adolescent boys.
2. Most individuals with bulimia manifest symptoms in the latter half of adolescence.
3. Female/male ratio is 10:1; there are community-based epidemiologic studies citing a 3:1 ratio.
4. Bulimia is independent of social class, unlike anorexia, which occurs predominantly in higher socioeconomic classes.
5. There is high comorbidity with anxiety and affective disorders and obsessive-compulsive disorder.

6. Fifty percent of bulimic individuals have an alcoholic relative and relatives with a high incidence of eating disorders, obesity, and affective disorders.
7. Large numbers of adolescents do not meet full DSM-IV-TR criteria for bulimia or anorexia but experience psychologic and physiologic consequences of eating disorders.

CLINICAL MANIFESTATIONS

1. Some bulimic individuals are in the normal range for their height and weight, some a few pounds overweight, and some a few pounds underweight
2. Secret and solitary binge eating as means of dealing with anxiety and stress
3. In one episode, an individual may consume thousands of calories
4. A feeling of inability to stop eating or loss of control after the binge has begun
5. Though eating may be viewed as pleasurable, afterward there is depressed mood, guilt, and self-criticism.
6. Hiding or stealing of food
7. Excusing of self to use bathroom during or after meals
8. Compulsive dieting and exercise
9. Preoccupation with weight and physical appearance. Clients may display concern for how they appear to others and undue concern for sexual attractiveness
10. Impaired body image and self-concept
11. Depression and dysthymia
12. Food cravings may be for any food, but typically for junk food or carbohydrates
13. Bingeing alternates with periods of fasting and normal eating

COMPLICATIONS

1. Integumentary: dry skin, dry mucous membranes, poor skin turgor, Russell's sign—scarring of and callous formation on knuckles
2. Facial/ophthalmic: facial fullness, parotid and submaxillary gland swelling (sialadenosis, "chipmunk" facial appearance), conjunctival hemorrhages

3. Mouth and throat: acute or chronic esophagitis, esophageal rupture, discoloration of teeth, erosion of tooth enamel, multiple caries
4. Cardiopulmonary: arrhythmias, bradycardia, tachycardia, hypertension, palpitations, postural hypotension, myocardial toxicity from ipecac, aspiration pneumonia
5. Gastrointestinal: abdominal tenderness or pain, gastritis, gastric distention, irritable bowel syndrome, melanosis coli, delayed gastric emptying
6. Genitourinary: constipation, diarrhea, hemorrhoids, rectal bleeding, rectal prolapse, acute and chronic renal failure, hematuria, proteinuria
7. Musculoskeletal: tetany, cramps, poor abdominal muscle tone, weakness
8. Endocrine: hypercortisolism
9. Neuropsychiatric: seizures, peripheral neuropathy, insomnia, impairment of school and social functioning resulting from preoccupation with food, depression, dysthymia, anxiety, impulsivity, obsessive-compulsive disorder, substance abuse, suicidal ideation
10. Hematologic: anemia, leukopenia
11. Peripheral vascular: edema

LABORATORY AND DIAGNOSTIC TESTS

Refer to Appendix D for normal values and ranges of laboratory and diagnostic tests.

Most test results will be within normal limits, but that does not mean that these individuals do not have a high morbidity or mortality risk.

1. Serum electrolyte levels—to detect electrolyte imbalances due to purging such as hypokalemia, hyponatremia, hypochloremia, hypocalcemia, hypoglycemia, hypomagnesemia, metabolic alkalosis
2. Serum amylase level—possible elevation indicates client is practicing vomiting (increases 2 hours after vomiting and remains elevated for 2 weeks)
3. Lipid panel—assess for elevated levels; during fasting, stored triglycerides may be hydrolyzed into glycerol and fatty acids and released into blood

4. Electrocardiogram—perform to assess for the complications of cardiac arrhythmias
5. Complete blood count—to assess for anemia due to nutritional deficiencies
6. Renal function test—to assess for diuretic abuse
7. Stool test—to detect phenolphthalein in laxative abuse
8. Drug screen—to assess for methamphetamine that is taken for weight loss, appetite control, and thrill seeking
9. Blood gases—to assess for metabolic alkalosis (with vomiting) or metabolic acidosis (when laxatives are taken)
10. Other tests may be ordered to rule out or confirm comorbid conditions (e.g., hyperthyroidism, Crohn's disease, neurologic disease, diabetes mellitus)

MEDICAL MANAGEMENT

Treatment is provided on an outpatient basis unless severe medical problems emerge. The factors that influence treatment modality are length and severity of illness, previous treatment approaches and outcomes, specific manifestations of disease, program availability, insurance, and financial resources. An interdisciplinary approach is needed to ensure optimal outcomes. The team is optimally composed of a pediatrician, nutritionist, nurse, psychiatrist, and therapist who specialize in eating disorders. Outpatient treatment includes medical monitoring, initiation of a dietary plan to restore nutritional state, and individual and family psychotherapy.

Family therapy is very helpful for younger adolescents; older adolescents may benefit more from both individual and family therapy. Treatment involves helping the individual learn to self-monitor and to identify distorted thinking patterns about weight, food, body image, and relationships. The goal of treatment is to restore normal eating. Fluoxetine (Prozac) has been shown to be effective in reducing binge behavior. It is likely, if fluoxetine is not tolerated, that another selective serotonin reuptake inhibitor (SSRI) would be as effective. Prognosis is better if the condition is treated early, before purging is reinforced by weight loss. Day treatment and residential treatment are used only when outpatient and short hospitalization fail, because these treatments are costly, and some insurance benefits do not adequately cover treatment, leaving parents and practitioners with difficult and limited options.

NURSING ASSESSMENT

1. Perform thorough nursing history taking and assessment, including history of bulimic episodes, information related to family dynamics, and psychosocial functioning.
2. Screen all teenagers for body image perception and dieting history. Ask direct questions about purging, prefacing with the fact that it is not an unusual way for teenagers to lose weight. Other questions include gathering information on perception of body image, disclosure of frequent dieting, weight dissatisfaction, and preoccupation with food.
3. Conduct thorough physical examination that includes height, postvoiding weight in simple hospital gown (to prevent the carrying of hidden weights), and vital signs (to assess for orthostatic hypotension, hypertension, and bradycardia).
4. Gather data on family history and family's communication styles and attitudes, degree of family support, and family's fostering of adolescent's independence and separation. Bulimic patients may report family history of affective disorders, especially depression.
5. Assess the adolescent's peer and intimate relationships.
6. Evaluate the adolescent's ability to express emotions, especially anger and fear, since the youth likely has difficulty identifying and expressing feelings.
7. Determine the adolescent's method of coping with stress and anxiety, since the youth may have problems with impulsivity, stealing, drug and alcohol abuse, self-mutilation, and suicide attempts.
8. Assess psychologic status to determine the level of awareness that behavior is abnormal, which may be expressed as depression, isolation, guilt, self-criticism, difficulty concentrating, and/or insomnia.
9. Administer psychologic inventories as appropriate:
   a. Beck Depression Inventory (adolescent version) can be used to assess level of depression.

b. Eating Disorder Examination can be used for structured interviews.

c. Eating Disorder Inventory is a self-report measure that can be used for youths 14 years and older.

d. Eating Attitudes Test and the Kids Eating Disorder Survey are applicable for school-aged and middle school–aged children, respectively.

NURSING DIAGNOSES

- Nutrition: less than body requirements, Imbalanced
- Fluid volume, Risk for deficient
- Body image, Disturbed
- Self-esteem, Chronic low
- Coping, Ineffective
- Family processes, Interrupted
- Social interaction, Impaired

NURSING INTERVENTIONS

1. Provide information about adequate nutritional intake and effect of inadequate intake on energy level and psychologic well-being.

2. Teach the importance of daily fluid intake of 2000–3000 ml. Monitor laboratory serum levels and report significantly abnormal values to physician.

3. Help adolescent reexamine negative perceptions of self and recognize positive attributes.

4. Assist adolescent to develop a realistic perception of body image.

5. Establish trusting relationship that promotes disclosure of feelings and emotions about body image, self-concept, frustrations, and fears.

6. Assist in the development and use of effective problem-solving and coping strategies.

7. Teach, practice, and role-play appropriate social skills. Set up group activity opportunities to use social skills.

8. Incorporate family-centered approach in providing services; include family in treatment decisions.

🏠 Discharge Planning and Home Care

1. Recommend psychotherapy for treatment of distorted body image and self-concept.
2. Stress the importance of adherence with counseling and follow-up visits for patient and family.
3. Refer to local eating disorder support group.
4. Review medication regimen, side effects, discontinuation, and emergency protocol.

CLIENT OUTCOMES

1. Adolescent will maintain weight within normal range for age.
2. Adolescent will use more effective mechanisms to cope with negative emotions.
3. Adolescent will practice normal patterns of eating.
4. Adolescent will be able to demonstrate increase in self-esteem as manifested by verbalizing positive aspects of self and misperceptions of body image.
5. Adolescent will engage in developmentally appropriate activities.

REFERENCES

American Academy of Pediatrics (Committee on Adolescence): Identifying and treating eating disorders, *Pediatrics* 2003;111;204–211 2003 (serial online): http://pediatrics.aappublications.org/cgi/reprint/111/1/204. Accessed March 7, 2007.

American Psychiatric Association: *Diagnostic and statistical manual of mental disorders*, ed 4, text revision (DSM-IV-TR), Washington, DC, 2000, The Association.

Bean P et al: Eating disorders in men: Update, *J Men's Health Gender* 2(2):186, 2005.

Bryant-Waugh R, Gowers S: Management of child and adolescent eating disorders: Current evidence base and future directions, *J Child Psychol Psychiatry* 45(1):63, 2004.

Kondo D, Sokol M: Eating disorders in primary care: A guide to identification and treatment, *Postgrad Med Online* (serial online): www.postgradmed.com/issues/2003/11_03/kondo.htm. Accessed December 16, 2006.

Shannon R: Eating disorders in adolescent males, *Prof School Counsel* (serial online): www.findarticles.com/p/articles/mi_m0KOC/is_1_8/ai_n6335450. Accessed December 16, 2006.

Townsend MC: Eating disorders. In: Townsend MC, editor: *Nursing diagnosis in psychiatric nursing: Care plans and psychotropic medications,* ed 6, Philadelphia, 2004, FA Davis.

Willcutts S: Nutritional problems. In: Nettina S: *Lippincott manual of nursing practice,* ed 8, Ambler, PA, Lippincott, Williams & Wilkins, 2006.

9

Burns

PATHOPHYSIOLOGY

Burns are the tissue damage that results from contact with thermal, chemical, electrical, or radiation agents. Thermal burns are the most common type of injury. A thermal burn occurs when the skin is damaged by heat. Tissue under the skin may also be damaged. Chemical burns occur upon contact with acid, alkali, or organic compounds. Electrical burns occur upon contact with high- or low-voltage electricity. In children, this contact is most often with electrical cords. Radiation burns are least common and are infrequent in children. Burn severity is determined by (1) the depth of burn injury, (2) percentage of body surface area affected, and (3) involvement of specific body parts. See Box 9-1 and Figure 9-1 for descriptions of burn severity and depth.

The severity of the burn determines the degree of change seen in the body's organs and systems. A thermal injury creates an open wound as a result of destruction of the skin. Following the burn, skin perfusion is decreased as blood vessels are occluded and vasoconstriction occurs. Intravascular volume decreases as fluids are leaked from the intravascular to the interstitial space as a result of increased capillary permeability. Pulmonary injury may occur as a result of inhalation of smoke, steam, or irritants. With a major burn, cardiac output decreases and blood flow to the liver, kidney, and gastrointestinal tract is compromised. The child with a major burn is in a hypermetabolic state, consuming oxygen and calories at a rapid rate. Prognosis is dependent on the severity of the burn.

BOX 9-1

Burn Classification According to Depth

First Degree (Superficial)
- Superficial; involves only superficial epidermis (e.g., sunburn)
- Symptoms: pain, redness, no tissue or nerve damage

Second Degree (Partial Thickness)
- Superficial to deep dermal; involves entire epidermis and varying amounts of dermis (e.g., scald)
- Symptoms: pain; red, edematous skin; vesicles

Third Degree (Full Thickness)
- Epidermis and dermis destroyed; involves subcutaneous adipose tissue, fascia, muscle, and bone (e.g., fire)
- Symptoms: no pain; white, red, or black skin; edematous skin

INCIDENCE
1. Burns are the second leading cause of accidental injury and death in children younger than 14 years of age.
2. Children account for 35% of all burn injuries.
3. Mortality from burns is 2500 children annually; 10,000 experience severe permanent disability.
4. Toddlers account for 85% of children with burn injuries.
5. Burns caused by scalds are the most common and usually occur in the kitchen or the bathroom.
6. Electrical and chemical burns are common in the toddler age group.

CLINICAL MANIFESTATIONS
The following are initial manifestations of second to third degree burns over more than 20% of the body surface area:
1. Tachycardia
2. Decreased blood pressure
3. Cold extremities and poor perfusion
4. Change in level of consciousness
5. Dehydration (decreased skin turgor, decreased urinary output, dry tongue and skin)

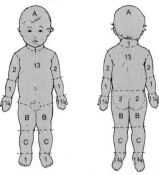

RELATIVE PERCENTAGES OF AREAS AFFECTED BY GROWTH

AREA	BIRTH	AGE 1 YR	AGE 5 YR
A = ½ of head	9½	8½	6½
B = ½ of one thigh	2¾	3¼	4
C = ½ of one leg	2½	2½	2¾

A

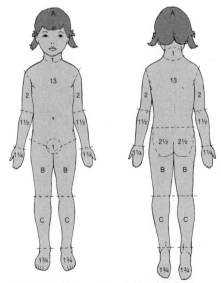

RELATIVE PERCENTAGES OF AREAS AFFECTED BY GROWTH

AREA	AGE 10 YR	AGE 15 YR	ADULT
A = ½ of head	5½	4½	3½
B = ½ of one thigh	4½	4½	4¾
C = ½ of one leg	3	3¼	3½

B

Figure 9-1 Estimated distribution of burns in children. **A,** Children from birth to age 5 years. **B,** Older children. (From Hockenberry M: *Wong's nursing care of infants and children,* ed 8, St. Louis, 2007, Mosby.)

6. Increased rate of respirations
7. Pallor (not present with second- and third-degree burn)

COMPLICATIONS

1. Renal failure
2. Metabolic acidosis
3. Hyperkalemia
4. Hyponatremia
5. Hypocalcemia
6. Pulmonary problems
   a. Pulmonary edema
   b. Pulmonary insufficiency
   c. Pulmonary embolus
   d. Bacterial pneumonia
7. Infection
8. Scarring and joint contractures

LABORATORY AND DIAGNOSTIC TESTS

1. Complete blood count—decreased
2. Arterial blood gas values—metabolic acidosis (decreased pH, increased partial pressure of carbon dioxide [Pco_2], and decreased partial pressure of oxygen [Po_2])
3. Serum electrolyte levels—decreased because of loss to traumatized areas and interstitial spaces
4. Serum glucose level—increased because of stress-invoked glycogen breakdown or glyconeogenesis
5. Blood urea nitrogen level—increased because of tissue breakdown and oliguria
6. Creatinine clearance—increased because of tissue breakdown and oliguria
7. Serum protein levels—decreased because of protein breakdown for massive energy needs
8. Chest radiographic study

MEDICAL MANAGEMENT

Burn treatment is based on the size and severity of the burn along with consideration as to its cause. Burn care can be divided into three phases: emergent, acute, and rehabilitative. Emergent care occurs for the first 72 hours of injury. Fluid resuscitation is critical in remedying intravascular fluid losses. Inadequate correction during this time may result in inadequate regional blood flow to the skin, the kidney, the gastrointestinal tract, the heart, and the brain, in that order. Oxygen is delivered by mask or artificial ventilation. The acute phase accounts for the majority of time the patient spends in the hospital. Care is focused on wound care, pain management, infection prevention, nutritional support, and psychosocial support. The burn itself may be covered with either moist or dry sterile dressings. Addition of topical antimicrobial medications such as silver sulfadiazine, mafenide acetate, bacitracin, gentamicin, or mupirocin may also be indicated. The child will receive analgesics or narcotics for pain. The rehabilitative phase lasts from complete wound healing to scar maturation. Depending on the severity of the burn, this may include reconstructive procedures, contracture releases, and reintegration into family, school, and social life.

NURSING ASSESSMENT

1. See Appendix A.
2. Assess fluid volume status.
3. Assess for adequate oxygenation and tissue perfusion.
4. Assess for pain; see Appendix I.
5. Assess cause, extent, and depth of burns.

NURSING DIAGNOSES

- Gas exchange, Impaired
- Fluid volume, Deficient
- Pain, Acute
- Infection, Risk for
- Skin integrity, Impaired
- Nutrition: less than body requirements, Imbalanced
- Disuse syndrome, Risk for
- Anxiety
- Family processes, Interrupted

NURSING INTERVENTIONS
First Aid and Emergency Care
Prevent further injury.
1. Scald burn—stop burning process; remove individual's clothing and jewelry; apply moist or dry sterile dressing.
2. Flame burn—have individual drop and roll to extinguish; remove nonadherent clothing; apply moist or dry sterile dressing.
3. Chemical burn—flush eyes and skin for 20 minutes with water.
4. Electrical burn—turn off power sources; initiate cardiopulmonary resuscitation.

Hospital Care
1. Maintain patent airway.
   a. Monitor and report signs of respiratory distress (dyspnea, increased respiratory rate, air hunger, nasal flaring).
   b. Provide thorough pulmonary care.
   c. Elevate head of bed—administer oxygen as necessary; keep intubation kit at bedside.
   d. Administer corticosteroids as prescribed to reduce swelling.
2. Monitor child for signs and symptoms of hypovolemic shock.
   a. Monitor vital signs and capillary refill time every hour, or more frequently, until stable.
   b. Monitor input and output hourly (output—20 to 30 ml/hr, >2 years; 10 to 20 ml/hr, <2 years).
   c. Administer fluids as ordered.
3. Monitor child for signs and symptoms of electrolyte imbalances (Box 9-2).
4. Monitor child for signs and symptoms of hemorrhage.
5. Provide pain relief measures to alleviate or control child's pain (see Appendix I).
   a. Use comfort measures (pillow, bed, cradle).
   b. Position for comfort.
   c. Medicate before wound care or dressing changes.

BOX 9-2
Electrolyte Imbalances

Hyperkalemia
- Oliguria or anuria
- Diarrhea
- Muscle weakness
- Arrhythmias
- Intestinal colic

Hyponatremia
- Abdominal cramps
- Diarrhea
- Apprehension

Hypocalcemia
- Tingling in fingers
- Muscle cramps
- Tetany
- Convulsions

    d. Use distraction, guided imagery, hypnosis.
    e. Monitor child's therapeutic response to medications.
  6. Protect child from potential infections.
    a. Administer tetanus booster as ordered.
    b. Monitor child's therapeutic and untoward response to antibiotics.
    c. Maintain and monitor use of protective isolation.
    d. Use sterile technique during wound care.
    e. Monitor for wound infections (offensive odor, redness at site, increased temperature, warmth, purulent drainage).
  7. Promote adequate nutritional intake to counteract nitrogen loss and potential gastrointestinal complications.
    a. Provide diet high in calories and protein (total caloric requirement = 60 calories × weight in kg + 60 calories × percentage of burn).
    b. Monitor for signs of Curling's ulcer (decreased hemoglobin level, decreased red blood cell count [anemia], coffee-ground emesis, abdominal distention).

   c. Administer antacids as needed.

   d. Monitor bowel sounds for ileus.

8. Promote optimal healing of wounds (see Medical Management section in this chapter).

   a. Use sterile technique when dressing wound.

   b. Observe for cellulitis or area that is trapping pus.

9. Promote maximal function of joints.

   a. Use splints appropriately to prevent contractures.

   b. Check splints every 4 hours for pressure sores.

   c. Direct performance of range of motion exercises and passive range of motion exercises for extremities.

   d. Encourage ambulation when child is able.

   e. Encourage participation in self-care activities.

10. Encourage verbalization of feelings regarding altered body image.

   a. Depression (associated with injury and pain).

   b. Anxiety (associated with treatments).

   c. Shame (associated with appearance).

11. Provide for child's developmental needs during hospitalization.

   a. Encourage use of age-appropriate toys; modify according to child's condition (e.g., use passive coloring—child directs nurse in coloring pictures).

   b. Encourage contact with peers (as appropriate).

   c. Provide age-appropriate roommate as dictated by condition.

   d. Encourage academic pursuits.

12. Provide emotional and other support to family.

   a. Encourage airing of concerns.

   b. Refer to social services as necessary.

   c. Refer to other parents in comparable situation as appropriate.

   d. Provide for physical comforts (e.g., place to sleep and bathe).

   e. Refer to support group (e.g., parent, religious) as needed.

🏠 Discharge Planning and Home Care

1. Instruct child and/or parents in wound care.
2. Provide burn prevention education.
3. Make referrals for outpatient physical and occupational therapies as indicated.

CLIENT OUTCOMES

1. Child will be free from infection.
2. Child will have adequate intravascular fluid volume.
3. Child will demonstrate adequate respiratory function.
4. Child will experience little to no pain.

REFERENCES

Behrman R, Kleigman R, Jenson HB, editors. *Nelson textbook of pediatrics*, ed 17, Philadelphia, 2004, WB Saunders.

Hockenberry M et al: *Wong's nursing care of infants and children*, ed 7, St. Louis, 2004, Mosby.

Supple K: Burn injury care, *Advance for Nurses* 6(26):15, 2005. Florida Edition.

10

❖

Cellulitis

PATHOPHYSIOLOGY

Cellulitis is an infection that affects the skin and subcutaneous tissue. The site of involvement is most commonly an extremity, but cellulitis may also occur on the scalp, the head, and the neck. Organisms causing cellulitis include *Staphylococcus aureus,* group A streptococci, and *Streptococcus pneumoniae.* Once common, invasive infection caused by *Haemophilus influenzae* type B is now rare as a result of childhood immunization. A history of trauma or, in young children, an upper respiratory tract infection or sinusitis, is often reported. The site of infection is characterized by a swelling with indistinct margins that is tender and warm. Infection may extend to deeper tissues or spread systemically. See Box 10-1 for orbital and periorbital cellulitis symptoms. Outcome is excellent with treatment.

INCIDENCE

1. Most children with periorbital or facial cellulitis are under the age of 2 years.
2. Cellulitis of the extremities occurs at a median age of 5 years.

CLINICAL MANIFESTATIONS
Local Reaction

1. Edematous area with indistinct margins
2. Usually red, warm, and painful site of involvement
3. Indurated tissue; skin surface may have appearance of an orange peel
   Note: For orbital and periorbital reactions, see Box 10-1.

BOX 10-1
Orbital and Periorbital Cellulitis Symptoms

Orbital Cellulitis
- Infection easily spreads from sinuses because orbit shares common wall with ethmoid, maxillary, and frontal sinuses (caused by group A streptococci, *Staphylococcus aureus*, and *Streptococcus pneumoniae*)
- Symptoms: exophthalmos, ophthalmoplegia, and loss of visual acuity

Periorbital Cellulitis
- Generally caused by trauma, infected wound, or insect bite
- Symptoms: rapid onset of fever and swelling; area is warm, indurated, and tender

Systemic Reaction
1. Fever
2. Malaise
3. Chills
4. Red streak along lymphatic drainage path
5. Enlarged and painful lymph glands

COMPLICATIONS
1. Systemic involvement: septicemia
2. Musculoskeletal: osteomyelitis, septic arthritis
3. Neurologic: meningitis, loss of visual acuity (orbital cellulitis), potential for brain abscess (orbital, periorbital cellulitis)

LABORATORY AND DIAGNOSTIC TESTS
1. Complete blood count—used to assess elevation of white blood cell count, which indicates underlying pathology. Refer to Appendix D for normal values and ranges of this test.
2. Blood cultures—used to identify organism and to determine appropriate antibiotic therapy. Blood cultures are positive in fewer than 5% of patients with cellulitis and are obtained in more severe cases.

3. Culture of needle aspirate from tissue—used to identify organism and to determine appropriate antibiotic therapy. Needle aspirate culture is positive in 5% to 40% of patients with cellulitis.
4. Radiographic study of paranasal sinuses—used in periorbital cellulitis to assess severity of condition by identifying opacification of sinuses.
5. Computed tomographic scan of orbit and paranasal sinuses—used to rule out orbital involvement.

MEDICAL MANAGEMENT

Children with cellulitis may be treated with oral antibiotics as outpatients if they have localized symptoms without fever. When systemic symptoms are present, the child is admitted to the hospital for a course of intravenous (IV) antibiotics. Warm compresses are applied to the site. The site is elevated and immobilized whenever possible. Acetaminophen is given as needed to manage fever and pain. For the first 24 to 36 hours after effective antibiotic therapy is begun, it is not unusual for the cellulitis to appear to progress. Antibiotic administration may be changed from IV to oral administration when symptoms of redness, warmth, and swelling have significantly improved. A total 10- to 14-day course of antibiotics is given. Incision and drainage may be performed if the area becomes suppurative.

NURSING ASSESSMENT

1. Assess for local and systemic reactions.
2. Assess for pain.

NURSING DIAGNOSES

- Tissue integrity, Impaired
- Pain, Acute
- Anxiety

NURSING INTERVENTIONS

1. Monitor child's status for progression of symptoms and complications.
   a. Assess skin locally for changes; minimize palpation, since it will increase pain.

    b. Assess for signs of systemic infection.

    c. Monitor therapeutic and untoward responses to antibiotics.

2. Provide pain relief and comfort measures.

    a. Elevate affected extremity, immobilize as appropriate.

    b. Apply warm compresses to site for 10 to 20 minutes daily or more frequently.

    c. Administer pain medications as needed.

3. Provide emotional support to child and family to decrease anxiety.

    a. Provide age-appropriate explanations before procedures.

    b. Incorporate home routine into care.

    c. Encourage parental verbalization of concerns.

    d. Refer to social services as needed.

🏠 Discharge Planning and Home Care

1. Instruct parents about importance of continuing full course of antibiotics even though symptoms have resolved.

2. Instruct parents to elevate involved extremity until swelling is reduced.

3. Instruct parents to observe for and report signs of infection spread.

4. Instruct parents about follow-up appointment.

CLIENT OUTCOMES

1. Child will have decreased redness, swelling, and warmth at cellulitis site.

2. Child will be free of pain.

3. Child and family will understand home care and follow-up needs.

REFERENCES

Stevens DL et al: Practice guidelines for the diagnosis and management of skin and soft-tissue infections, *Clin Infect Dis* 41(15 November):1373, 2005.

Vu BLL et al: Development of a clinical severity score for preseptal cellulitis in children, *Pediatr Emerg Care* 19(5):302, 2003.

Wald ER: Periorbital and orbital infections, *Pediatr Rev* 25(9):312, 2004.

11

Cerebral Palsy

PATHOPHYSIOLOGY

Cerebral palsy (CP) is a nonspecific term used to characterize abnormal muscle tone, posture, and coordination caused by a nonprogressive lesion or injury that affects the immature brain. CP may result from a variety of prenatal, perinatal, and postnatal factors, although CP results most commonly from either existing perinatal brain abnormalities or postnatal injury. The actual brain abnormality may arise from a variety of causes: anatomical malformations of the brain, atrophy, vascular occlusion, loss of neurons, or low brain weight. Anoxia, which is often secondary to other causative mechanisms, is the most significant factor in the pathologic state of brain damage. Predisposing risk factors include multiple-gestation births, maternal infections, and maternal and fetal thrombophilic conditions. CP is frequently classified according to the functional categories used to describe the neuromuscular abnormalities or dysfunction. Clinical classification of CP is presented in Box 11-1.

INCIDENCE

1. CP is the most common permanent physical disability of childhood.
2. Incidence is 1.5 to 3 infants in every 1000 live births.
3. The prevalence of CP has risen with the improved survival of extremely low birth weight and very low birth weight infants.
4. Spastic CP is the most common type.

BOX 11-1
Clinical Classification of Cerebral Palsy

1. Spastic cerebral palsy (CP) is the most common form (80% of cases). It is characterized by hypertonicity and poor postural control, balance, and coordination. Gross and fine motor skills are impaired. Spastic CP is further classified according to the part of the body affected:
   a. Hemiparesis—most common form of spastic CP. One side of the body is affected. Motor deficit is usually greater in upper extremity; most children are able to walk; affected limbs are underdeveloped.
   b. Diplegia—involves the legs and occurs most often in those who were premature infants and who had an intraventricular hemorrhage or ischemic leukomalacia. Mild lack of upper extremity uncoordination may also be seen.
   c. Monoplegia—involves only one extremity.
   d. Quadriparesis—involves all extremities, with the legs having more impairment. Carries highest incidence of severe disability.
2. Dyskinetic/Athetoid CP is characterized by a movement disorder and results from Rh incompatibility and hypoxic ischemic encephalopathy. Characteristics include the following:
   a. Athetosis—slow writhing, wormlike movements involving the extremities, the trunk, the neck, the facial muscles, and the tongue.
   b. Drooling and dysarthria due to involvement of the pharyngeal, laryngeal, and oral muscles.
   c. Chorea-like movements (irregular, jerky movements) that increase in intensity with emotional stress and at adolescence.
3. Ataxic CP is characterized by a wide-based gait, and rapid, repetitive movements that are poorly performed.
4. Mixed type/dystonic—combination of spasticity and athetosis.

CLINICAL MANIFESTATIONS

1. Delay in reaching motor developmental milestones as evidenced by poor head control after 3 months of age; cannot sit up without support by 8 months of age
2. Abnormal motor performance and loss of selective motor control

3. Alterations of muscle tone
4. Abnormal posture
5. Reflex abnormalities
6. Extreme irritability or crying
7. Persistent gagging or choking when fed

COMPLICATIONS

1. Impaired intellectual function
2. Seizures
3. Communication disorders
4. Drooling and feeding and swallowing difficulties
5. Joint contractures
6. Perceptual dysfunction
7. Learning disabilities
8. Attention deficit/hyperactivity disorder

LABORATORY AND DIAGNOSTIC TESTS

Refer to Appendix D for normal values and ranges of laboratory and diagnostic tests.

1. Clinical examination to identify tone abnormalities; frequently hypotonicity followed by hypertonicity, postural abnormalities, and delayed motor development
2. Cranial ultrasonography to detect hemorrhagic and hypoxic ischemic insults
3. Computed tomography to detect central nervous system lesions
4. Magnetic resonance imaging to detect small lesions
5. Positron emission tomography and single photon emission computed tomography—to visualize brain metabolism and perfusion

MEDICAL MANAGEMENT

The overall goal of medical management is to develop a rehabilitation plan to promote optimal functioning. This includes assisting the child to gain new skills and anticipating potential complications. A multidisciplinary team approach is required. Most children identified with a delay or risk for delay are enrolled in an early intervention program (EIP) and receive physical, occupational, and speech therapy as indicated (Appendix G).

As children grow from the infancy and toddler stages, treatments support the functional goals set. These treatments include therapeutic exercises, splinting, serial casting, bracing, and use of mobility aids and adaptive devices to provide functional independence. Surgical procedures such as osteotomies or tendon lengthening or tendon transfer may be performed. Antispasmodic drugs may be given orally or injected into the nerves to decrease spasticity. Neurologic procedures are used only in selected cases. Dorsal rhizotomy and botulinum toxin type A have been used successfully in the treatment of spasticity. Intrathecal baclofen administration via an implanted infusion pump has also been effective in the treatment of spasticity.

NURSING ASSESSMENT

1. See the Musculoskeletal Assessment section in Appendix A.
2. Assess for delay in motor skills.

NURSING DIAGNOSES

- Growth and development, Delayed
- Injury, Risk for
- Mobility, Impaired physical
- Social interaction, Impaired

NURSING INTERVENTIONS

1. Promote maximal functioning of joints.
2. Provide and instruct parents and child on the use of adaptive equipment for activities of daily living.
3. Ensure adherence with use of ambulatory aids (i.e., walker, crutches, orthoses).
4. Anticipate and assess for pain and fatigue from increased muscle tone and spasticity.
5. Position to prevent contractures.
6. Direct performance of active and passive range of motion exercises.
7. Make appropriate referrals to speech, physical, occupational, and nutritional therapy, social services and child life specialist, and hospital teacher as needed.

8. Encourage verbalization of feelings about altered body image.
9. Encourage social interaction with peers.
10. Collaborate with educational specialist in individualized education plan (IEP) and/or 504 planning to promote achievement of educational goals (see Appendix G).

🏠 Discharge Planning and Home Care

1. Refer to IEP educator or outpatient physical, occupational, and/or speech therapy.
2. Obtain adaptive equipment.
3. Teach individual and family how to maintain individual's optimum functional independence.
4. Identify appropriate support groups for individual and family.

CLIENT OUTCOMES

1. Child will achieve flexibility, alignment, and locomotion within defined capabilities.
2. Child will be safe from injury.
3. Child's and family's needs for psychosocial support will be met.
4. Child will acquire developmental competencies appropriate for age and capabilities.

REFERENCES

Gormley ME Jr: Treatment of neuromuscular and musculoskeletal problems in cerebral palsy, *Pediatr Rehabil* 4(1):5, 2001.

Jacobs JM: Management options for the child with spastic cerebral palsy, *Orthop Nurs* 20(3):53, 2001.

Volpe JJ: *Neurology of the newborn,* ed 4, Philadelphia, 2001, WB Saunders.

12

❖

Child Abuse and Neglect

PATHOPHYSIOLOGY

The Federal Child Abuse Prevention and Treatment Act, as amended by the Keeping Children and Families Safe Act of 2003, defines child abuse and neglect as, at a minimum, "any recent act or failure to act on the part of a parent or caretaker, which results in death, serious physical or emotional harm, sexual abuse or exploitation, or an act or failure to act which presents an imminent risk of serious harm." There are four major types of abuse: physical abuse, sexual abuse, emotional abuse (psychologic, verbal, or mental injury), and child neglect. It is of interest to note that emotional abuse is almost always present when other forms are identified. The most recent research suggests several other types or subcategories of maltreatment, including congenital child abuse, sibling abuse, and child abandonment.

Child maltreatment crosses all areas of society and all cultural, racial or ethnic, religious, socioeconomic, and professional groups. It is most common, however, among adolescent parents and in low-income families. Risk factors and statistics associated with child maltreatment are categorized as they relate to parents, children, families, and the environment.

Perpetrators of child maltreatment are the persons responsible for a child's well-being, such as parents or caretakers, who have abused or neglected the child. Maltreating parents consistently report having been physically, sexually, or emotionally abused or neglected as children. However, not all maltreated children grow up to be abusive parents. Approximately 80% of perpetrators are parents. Other relatives account for 6%,

81

and unmarried partners of parents account for 4% of perpetrators. The remaining perpetrators include persons with other relationships (e.g., camp counselor, school employee) or unknown relationships to the child victims. Common characteristics identified in abusive parents include low self-esteem, low intelligence, social isolation, depression, low frustration tolerance, immaturity, lack of parenting and/or coping skills, lack of knowledge of child development, marital problems, single or adolescent parenthood, closely spaced pregnancies, substance abuse, physical illness, and criminal behavior.

A number of characteristics have been associated with children who are victims of abuse. Children at greater risk for abuse are those who are born prematurely and/or with congenital anomalies or who have difficult-to-soothe temperaments, frequent illness, or special needs. Children from birth to 3 years of age are at highest risk for physical abuse. Girls are slightly more likely to be victims than boys (52% to 48% of victims). Children are consistently vulnerable to sexual abuse from age 3 years and up. More recently, public attention has been directed to recognizing the vulnerabilities that youth may encounter with adult sexual predators through the Internet and from adult authority figures in schools, social organizations, and even religious institutions. Pacific Islander, American Indian, Alaska Native, and African-American children have the highest rate of victimization according to the national population.

Some known characteristics are associated with families at high risk for abusing children. Children in single-parent families had a 77% higher risk of physical abuse, an 87% higher risk of physical neglect, and an 80% higher risk of serious injury or harm from abuse or neglect than children living with both parents. Children in the largest families were physically neglected nearly 3 times more often than those from single-child families. Children from families with annual incomes below $15,000 were more than 22 times more likely to suffer some form of maltreatment as defined by the Harm Standard and more than 25 times more likely to experience some form of maltreatment as defined by the Endangerment Standard than were children from families with annual incomes above $30,000. Harm Standard refers to child maltreatment as identification of children who have experienced observable harm; endangerment standard refers to child maltreatment as identification of children based on risk for being harmed.

Children from the lowest-income families were 18 times more likely to be sexually abused, almost 56 times more likely to be educationally neglected, and over 22 times more likely to suffer serious injury as defined by the Harm Standard than were children from higher-income families. Children living in the same home for less than 2 years and living in the same community less than 5 years have a 60% higher risk of being abused.

Environmental factors related to child abuse include ethnic and/or racial prejudices, poor living conditions, lack of community and family resources, poor access to health care and follow-up services, economic pressure, varied cultural beliefs concerning the role of the child in the family, and varied cultural attitudes toward use of physical punishment. Ineffective child protection laws are another culprit in the environment. Studies have shown that nearly half of the children killed by caretakers are killed after they come to the attention of the child welfare service. Keeping the family intact may no longer be the goal if maltreatment is significant.

INCIDENCE

1. In 2003, child protective services investigated more than 2.9 million reports alleging maltreatment of more than 5.5 million children.
2. Two thirds (68%) of these reports prompted investigations, which resulted in the identification of 906,000 victims.
3. An estimated 1500 child maltreatment fatalities occurred in the 50 states and the District of Columbia in 2003. Children younger than 1 year of age accounted for 44% of all deaths, and 79% of child fatalities were in children younger than 4 years of age.
4. More than half of all victims (60%) suffered neglect (including medical neglect), 20% suffered physical abuse, and about 10% of victims were sexually abused. Victims of emotional maltreatment accounted for 5% of all victims. Other types of maltreatment including abandonment,

congenital drug addiction, and threats to harm the child accounted for 16% of victims. (Percentage totals are higher than 100% because some children suffered multiple types of abuse.)

5. Sexual abuse is most common among girls, stepfamilies, and children living with one parent or a primary caregiver who is an unrelated male.

6. Abuse occurs in 11 per 1000 white, 21 per 1000 Pacific Islander, 21 per 1000 American Indian and Native Alaskan, and 20 per 1000 African-American children.

CLINICAL MANIFESTATIONS

See Box 12-1 for a list of the clinical manifestations of child abuse.

COMPLICATIONS

1. Developmental and neurologic: attention-deficit/hyperactivity disorder (ADHD), developmental delays

2. Academic: learning difficulties and low academic achievement

3. Mental health: aggressive behaviors (fighting or cruelty to animals), substance abuse, other mental health problems (e.g., depression, post-traumatic stress disorder, eating disorders), suicide attempts

4. Psychosocial: difficulties with social relationships, developmental delays, inappropriate sexual behaviors and teen pregnancy, increased risk for sexually transmitted diseases (e.g., acquired immunodeficiency syndrome [AIDS])

LABORATORY AND DIAGNOSTIC TESTS

1. Skeletal (bone) survey radiographic studies, in two planes, for all children with suspected abuse injuries. Repeat in 2 weeks for children for whom there is a strong suspicion of abuse—RATIONALE: metaphyseal ("corner-chip") fractures have high specificity for abuse but may be difficult to see initially. Healing fractures form a callus (bump of bone) that is apparent within 2 weeks of an acute injury. Skeletal surveys also provide information about the age of the

BOX 12-1
Clinical Manifestations of Child Abuse and Neglect

Skin Injuries

Skin injuries are the most common and easily recognized signs of maltreatment in children. Human bite marks appear as ovoid areas with tooth imprints, suck marks, or tongue-thrust marks. Multiple bruises or bruises in inaccessible places are indications that the child has been abused. Bruises in different stages of healing may indicate repeated trauma. Bruises that take the shape of a recognizable object are generally not accidental.

Traumatic Hair Loss

Traumatic hair loss occurs when the child's hair is pulled or used to drag or jerk the child. The result of the pulling on the scalp can cause the blood vessels under the skin to break. An accumulation of blood can help differentiate between abusive and nonabusive loss of hair.

Falls

If a child is reported to have had a routine fall but has what appear to be severe injuries, the inconsistency of the history with the trauma sustained raises the suspicion of child abuse.

External Head, Facial, and Oral Injuries

Cuts, bleeding, redness, or swelling of the external ear canal; facial fractures; tears or scarring of the lip; oral, perioral and/or pharyngeal lesions; loosened, discolored, or fractured teeth; dental caries; tongue lacerations; unexplained erythema or petechiae of the palate; and bilateral black eyes without trauma to the nose all may indicate abuse.

Deliberate or Unexplained Thermal Injuries

The following suggest intentional harm: immersion burns, with clear line of demarcation; multiple small, circular burns, in varying stages of healing; iron burns (show iron pattern); diaper area burns; and rope burns.

Shaken Baby Syndrome

A shaken baby may suffer only mild ocular or cerebral trauma. The infant may have a history of poor feeding, vomiting,

Continued

BOX 12-1

Clinical Manifestations of Child Abuse and Neglect—cont'd

lethargy, and/or irritability that occurs periodically for days or weeks before the initial health care consultation. In 75% to 90% of cases, unilateral or bilateral retinal hemorrhages are present, but they may be missed unless the child is examined by a pediatric ophthalmologist. Shaking produces an acceleration-deceleration (shearing) injury to the brain, causing stretching and breaking of blood vessels that results in subdural hemorrhage. Subdural hemorrhage may be most prominent in the interhemispheric fissure. However, cerebral edema may be the only finding. Serious insult to the central nervous system may result, without external evidence of injury.

Unexplained Fractures and Dislocations

Posterior rib fractures in different stages of healing, spiral fractures, or dislocation from twisting of an extremity may provide evidence of nonaccidental injury in children.

Sexual Abuse

Abrasions or bruising of the inner thighs and genitalia; scarring, tearing, or distortion of the labia and/or hymen; anal lacerations or dilation; lacerations or irritation of external genitalia; repeated urinary tract infections; sexually transmitted disease; nonspecific vaginitis; pregnancy in the young adolescent; penile discharge; and sexual promiscuity may provide evidence of sexual abuse.

Neglect

The symptoms of neglect reflect a lack of both physical and medical care. Manifestations include failure to thrive without a medical explanation, multiple cat or dog bites and scratches, feces and dirt in the skin folds, severe diaper rash with the presence of ammonia burns, feeding disorders, and developmental delays.

injuries. Multiple fractures at various stages of healing are common in child abuse

2. Computed tomography and/or magnetic resonance imaging of affected areas—to verify presence of injuries

3. Ophthalmologic examination—to detect retinal hemor-rhages (result from severe shaking or slamming of head)
4. Color photographs of injuries—for legal and clinical documentation
5. Head circumference, abdominal circumference—to determine skeletal and/or abdominal injuries due to physical abuse
6. Examination of cerebrospinal fluid—to detect presence of blood in children who sustained head trauma from physical abuse
7. Pregnancy test—to determine pregnancy status in children who have been sexually abused
8. Screens for sexually transmitted infections (STIs), human immunodeficiency virus (HIV)—to detect STIs in children who have been sexually abused
9. Evidentiary examination—to collect specimens and reveal signs and symptoms of abuse (should comply with the recommendations of child protective services or local coroner or medical examiner)

MEDICAL MANAGEMENT

The first priority in the care of the abused child is resuscitation and stabilization as deemed necessary according to the injuries sustained. Confirmation of the abuse is achieved through thorough history taking, complete physical examination with detailed inspection of the child's entire body, and collection of laboratory specimens. All injuries should be documented with color photographs and recorded carefully in the written medical record.

Every state has a child abuse law that specifies legal responsibilities for reporting suspected abuse. Suspected abuse must be reported to the local child protective service agency. Mandated reporters include nurses, physicians, dentists, podiatrists, psychologists, speech pathologists, coroners, medical examiners, child day care center employees, children's services workers, social workers, clergy, film and photographic print processors, law enforcement officers, and schoolteachers. Failure to report suspected child abuse can result in a fine or other punishment, depending on individual statutes.

NURSING ASSESSMENT

1. Conduct comprehensive history taking and parent (or caregiver) interview. Verification and documentation of circumstances associated with the injury event are critical. Therefore nurse should make a written checklist of who, what, when, where, why, and how questions and answers.
2. Perform comprehensive physical examination as well as social, emotional, and cognitive assessment.
3. Observe parent-child interactions, including frequency of contact and length of time parent visits child.
4. Assess emotional status of parents.
5. If a child is initially seen in the emergency room and a sexual assault is suspected, a sexual assault nurse examiner may be contacted to conduct the examination (Box 12-2).

NURSING DIAGNOSES

- Injury, Risk for
- Pain
- Fear
- Growth and development, Delayed
- Coping, Compromised family

NURSING INTERVENTIONS

1. Resuscitate and stabilize as necessary.
2. Protect child from further injury.
3. Assist with diagnosis of abuse.

BOX 12-2
Training for Sexual Assault Nurse Examiner

Training (40 hours) for a sexual assault nurse examiner (S.A.N.E) certificate is available through the International Association of Forensic Nurses:

The International Association of Forensic Nurses
East Holly Avenue, Box 56
Pitman, NJ 08071–0056
Phone: 856–256–2425
Fax: 856–589–7463
Website: www.forensicnurse.com

4. Report suspected abuse.
5. Provide supportive care to child (refer to supportive care section in Appendix F).
6. Document assessment of physical findings, parent interactions, and child's verbal disclosures.
7. Provide explanations of normal child growth and development, and compliment parent for behaviors that indicate appropriate responses to child's needs (refer to Appendix B).
8. Discuss, encourage, and role-model behaviors that foster maternal-child attachment and positive parenting skills.
9. Discuss alternative methods of discipline, and encourage positive reinforcement for good behavior in child.
10. Discuss family stress and review coping strategies (positive versus negative).
11. Discuss need for community resources and make appropriate referrals (e.g., child life specialist; child protective services; social worker; home visiting nurse; parenting classes; women, infants, and children [WIC] services; fuel assistance; Section 8 housing assistance; Parents Anonymous; Parents United International) (refer to Appendix G).

🏠 Discharge Planning and Home Care

1. Refer parents to multidisciplinary community resources that will assist with improving impulse control, increase knowledge of child's growth and development, aid in setting realistic expectations, and provide alternatives to physical abuse (Box 12-3).
2. Refer family to support groups, family therapy, or parenting effectiveness classes.

CLIENT OUTCOMES

1. Child will be protected from further injury, neglect, or harm.
2. Child will demonstrate minimal long-term sequelae as a result of abuse.
3. Parents will develop effective parenting skills.
4. Parents will receive assistance for problems.

BOX 12-3
Resources

- American Academy of Pediatrics website: www.AAP.org
- Child Help USA
  Phone: 800–4-A-Child
  Website: www.childhelpusa.org
- National Child Abuse Reporting Hotline: 800–522-3511
- National Clearinghouse on Child Abuse and Neglect Information
  330 C St., SW
  Washington, DC 20447
  Phone: 800–394-3366 or 703–385-7565
  Fax: 703–385-3206
  E-mail: nccanch@caliber.com
  Website: www.nccanch.acf.hhs.gov
- National Data Archive on Child Abuse and Neglect website: www.ndacan.cornell.edu

REFERENCES

Child Welfare Information Gateway (2006): *Child abuse and neglect information packet* (website): www.childwelfare.gov/pubs/can_info_packet.pdf. Accessed March 22, 2007.

Flaherty EG et al: Assessment of suspicion of abuse in the primary care setting, *Ambul Pediatr* 2:120, 2002.

International Child Abuse Network: *Child abuse statistics* (website): www.yesican.org/stats.html. Accessed December 28, 2006.

Oliver WJ, Kuhns LR, Pomeranz ES: Family structure and child abuse, *Clin Pediatr* 45(2):111, 2006.

U.S. Department of Health and Human Services, Children's Bureau, Administration for Children and Families: *Child maltreatment 2003* (website): http://acf.hhs.gov/programs/cb/pubs/cm03/index.htm. Accessed April 25, 2006.

13

Chronic Lung Disease of Infancy

PATHOPHYSIOLOGY

Chronic lung disease (CLD) of infancy, formerly known as bronchopulmonary dysplasia (BPD), is a disorder seen in infants born with severe respiratory distress syndrome. The disease occurs in both full-term and preterm infants who have been treated with prolonged positive pressure ventilation and/or oxygen therapy. Susceptibility to CLD is influenced by the degree of prematurity, the severity of respiratory distress syndrome, the need for mechanical ventilation and supplemental oxygen, and concurrent diseases. It is the most common complication in the care of very low birth weight infants (less than 1000 g) at birth. CLD is a pathologic process related to alveolar damage from lung disease, prolonged exposure to high peak inspiratory pressures and oxygen, and immature alveoli and respiratory tract. The clinical presentation is characterized by ongoing respiratory distress, persistent oxygen requirement (with or without ventilatory support) at 28 days postpartum and/or 36 weeks' postconceptual age, and a classically abnormal chest radiographic study. The major risk factors that contribute to the development of CLD are prematurity, presence of respiratory distress or failure, severe initial respiratory illness, congenital heart disease, oxygen supplementation, prolonged use of positive pressure ventilation, and lack of antenatal treatment with steroids. Other important risk factors include history of air leaks, fluid overload, poor vitamin A status, sepsis, meconium aspiration, and a patent ductus arteriosus. Pulmonary changes typical of infants with CLD include alterations in lung structure, increased airway and/or vascular resistance, increased airway reactivity, decreased lung compliance, increased mucus production, and increased work of breathing. Although pulmonary function often improves significantly in early childhood, recent research demonstrates that some pulmonary problems may persist for many years. The survival rate is dependent on the infant's birth weight and gestational age and the severity of the infant's CLD.

INCIDENCE

1. Incidence varies because of differences in diagnostic criteria, client populations, and client management.
2. There is questionable research indicating that white, male infants are at greater risk for developing CLD.
3. It is estimated that 80% of infants of less than 30 weeks' gestation develop CLD, and 10,000 infants are treated annually with home oxygen in the United States.
4. The suggestion has been made that the incidence has increased as a result of improved infant survival rates.
5. Mortality has been reported as greater than 40% in hospitalized infants with CLD and is usually due to infection or respiratory failure.

CLINICAL MANIFESTATIONS

1. Hypoxia
2. Hypercapnia
3. Tachypnea
4. Retractions (progression of retractions from sternal to substernal, supraclavicular, intercostal, and subcostal)
5. Paradoxic or "seesaw" breathing (due to decreased lung compliance)
6. Wheezing
7. Crackles
8. Cough
9. Bronchospasm
10. Mucus plugging
11. Increased work of breathing (nasal flaring, grunting, irritability)

COMPLICATIONS

1. Pulmonary: persistent changes in pulmonary function, respiratory infections, and long-term need for supplemental oxygen, tracheostomy, and prolonged mechanical ventilation
2. Cardiovascular: pulmonary hypertension, electrocardiogram (ECG) changes, right ventricular hypertrophy, cor pulmonale, and systemic hypertension
3. Neurologic: cognitive delay
4. Gastrointestinal and fluid, electrolytes, and nutrition: oral feeding aversions, gastroesophageal reflux, and constipation; altered growth and nutrient needs
5. Head, eyes, ears, nose, and throat: hearing loss requiring amplification, bilateral blindness, delayed tooth eruption, altered oral and dental structures from prolonged intubation, and enamel effects

LABORATORY AND DIAGNOSTIC TESTS

Refer to Appendix D for normal values and ranges of laboratory and diagnostic tests.
1. Chest radiographic studies—may include spectrum of findings including bilateral diffuse hazy lung fields, interstitial thickening (mild to very severe), inflammation, normal to increased lung expansion, and chronic findings that change little over time
2. Arterial and venous blood gas values—hypercapnia and compensated respiratory acidosis are common findings
3. Pulmonary function testing—used to assess respiratory status and severity of condition, and to determine therapy
4. Serum electrolyte levels—useful when monitoring effects of long-term diuretic therapy
5. Serial ECGs/echocardiograms—useful to monitor for cor pulmonale and pulmonary hypertension

MEDICAL MANAGEMENT

The goals of medical management for infants with CLD are (1) treatment of the complications and symptoms with oxygen therapy and medication, and (2) enhancement of lung healing through adequate nutrition and promotion of respiratory stability (stable oxygenation and prevention of infection). Therapies commonly used include oxygen, bronchodilators (which decrease pulmonary resistance and increase lung compliance), diuretics to prevent fluid overload and pulmonary edema, and corticosteroids, which decrease inflammatory responses and promote lung healing. Adequate nutrition promotes lung and total body healing, growth, and development. Early supplementation of vitamin A, which plays a role in lung development, has been shown to be an effective preventive treatment. Gastric tubes may be inserted to assist in the infant's nutrition. Palivizumab, used prophylactically, protects against respiratory syncytial virus (RSV). Currently there are several controversial therapies including continuous positive airway pressure (CPAP), high-frequency oscillatory ventilation (HFOV), and permissive hypercapnia, intended to minimize barotrauma or volutrauma. Research has shown that early surfactant therapy and daily doses of caffeine allow more rapid weaning from the ventilator and earlier extubation. Early studies of inhaled nitric oxide (INO) showed no benefit for prevention of CLD but found improved outcomes associated with greater lung volumes, dynamic lung compliance, and decreased expiratory resistance.

NURSING ASSESSMENT

1. See the Respiratory Assessment section in Appendix A.
2. Assess infant's cardiorespiratory status.
3. Assess for signs and symptoms of fluid overload.
4. Assess infant's oral intake and growth.
5. Assess developmental level.
6. Assess infant-parent interactions.
7. Assess parents' discharge readiness and ability to manage home care and access community resources.

NURSING DIAGNOSES

- Gas exchange, Impaired
- Fluid volume, Excess
- Nutrition: less than body requirements, Imbalanced
- Growth and development, Delayed

- Activity intolerance
- Family processes, Interrupted
- Parent-infant attachment, Risk for impaired
- Knowledge, Deficient
- Therapeutic regimen management, Ineffective

NURSING INTERVENTIONS

1. Maintain cardiorespiratory stability.
   a. Establish infant's baseline respiratory assessment, and monitor for changes.
   b. Monitor responsiveness to medical interventions.
   c. Monitor trends in oxygenation through oximetry.
   d. Monitor action and side effects of medications.
      i. Bronchodilators
      ii. Corticosteroids
      iii. Diuretics
2. Evaluate for signs and symptoms of fluid overload.
   a. Monitor intake (ml/kg/day) and output (ml/kg/hr).
   b. Administer diuretic and/or fluid-restrictive therapy as ordered.
3. Monitor for adequate caloric intake and growth over time.
   a. Weight gain should be approximately 20 to 30 g/day.
   b. Monitor infant's ability to maintain adequate oral intake. (Infants who are tachypneic and have increased work of breathing may not be able to take in food orally because of risk of aspiration.)
   c. Monitor for increased oxygen requirements during and immediately after oral feedings; provide increased oxygen as needed.
   d. Provide supplementation to oral feedings through enteral tube feedings.
4. Promote growth and development through integration of play and positive stimulation into care routine (see relevant section of Appendix B).
   a. Provide opportunities for developmentally appropriate visual, auditory, tactile, and kinesthetic stimulation—when infant is alert and stable.

b. Integrate pattern and routine into care, including undisturbed night sleep and predictable daytime activities.

5. Monitor infant's response to caregiving and developmental activities.
   a. Assess for increased oxygen requirements during and immediately following activity.
   b. Assess for patterns of response to activities and care-givers.
   c. Develop list of likes, dislikes, and comfort measures from assessed patterns of response.
   d. Decrease environmental and caregiver stimulation during periods of agitation and/or stress.

6. Facilitate integration of infant into his or her family.
   a. Assist parents in recognizing infant's responses to activity.
   b. Teach parents how they can best interact with and provide care for their child.
   c. Develop parents' confidence in caring for their child.
   d. Promote visitation and caregiving by other key family members, including siblings, as soon as appropriate.

7. Prevent infection
   a. Provide RSV prophylaxis as recommended.
   b. Ensure that immunizations are given on schedule.
   c. Ensure proper handwashing.

🏠 Discharge Planning and Home Care

1. Evaluate readiness for discharge. Factors to assess include presence of the following:
   a. Stable respiratory status
   b. Adequate nutritional intake and growth
   c. Stable medication needs
   d. Medical treatment plan that is realistic for the home
      i. Parents or other caregivers can provide needed care
      ii. Needed home equipment and monitoring are provided
      iii. Parents have necessary social and/or financial supports
      iv. Provision is made for respite or home nursing needs

2. Provide discharge instruction for parents covering the following:
   a. Explanation of CLD (BPD)
   b. Monitoring for signs of respiratory distress and other medical problems
   c. Individualized feeding needs
   d. Well-baby needs
   e. Guidelines on when to call doctor
   f. Method of performing infant/child cardiopulmonary resuscitation
   g. Use of home equipment and monitoring
   h. Administration of medications and monitoring of their effects
   i. Infection prevention—hand hygiene
   j. Importance of smoke-free environment
   k. Appropriate developmental activities
   l. Recognition of infant's stress and interaction cues
   m. Available community resources and supportive services (see Appendix G)
3. Provide follow-up to monitor ongoing respiratory, nutritional, and developmental needs; administer RSV prophylaxis; and address other specialized needs.
   a. Help parents make first follow-up appointments; provide written documentation of when appointments are scheduled.
   b. Make referral for in-home nursing visits or care based on needs of infant and family.
   c. Ensure that infant is referred to an early intervention program.

CLIENT OUTCOMES

1. Infant will have optimal lung functioning, with gas exchange and oxygenation sufficient for tissue perfusion, growth, and healing.
2. Infant will reach maximum potential for growth and development.
3. Parents will be competent in the care of their child.

REFERENCES

American Lung Association BPD: *Bronchopulmonary dysplasia* (website): www.lungusa.org. Accessed May 24, 2006.

Ball JW, Bindler RC: *Clinical handbook for pediatric nursing,* Upper Saddle River, NJ, 2006, Pearson Education.

Ballard PL et al: Surfactant composition and function in a primate model of infant chronic lung disease: Effects of inhaled nitric oxide, *Pediatr Res* 59 (1):157, 2006.

Ellsbury D et al: Variability in the use of supplemental oxygen for bronchopulmonary dysplasia, *J Pediatr* 140(2):247, 2002.

Huether SE, McCance KL: *Understanding pathophysiology,* ed 3, St. Louis, 2006, Mosby.

Nievas F, Chernick V: Bronchopulmonary dysplasia (chronic lung disease of infancy): An update for the pediatrician, *Clin Pediatr* 41(2):77, 2002.

Romanko EA: Caring for children with bronchopulmonary dysplasia in the home setting, *Home Healthcare Nurse* 23(2):95, 2005.

Stenmark KR, Balasubramaniam V: Angiogenic therapy for bronchopulmonary dysplasia: Rationale and promise, *Circulation* 112(16):2383, 2005.

Van Marter LJ: Strategies for preventing bronchopulmonary dysplasia, *Curr Opin Pediatr* 17(2):174, 2005.

14

❖

Cleft Lip and Cleft Palate

PATHOPHYSIOLOGY

Cleft lip and cleft palate are the outcomes of the failure of the soft tissue and/or bony structure to fuse during embryonic development. Cleft lip is a separation of the two sides of the lip. It may affect both sides of the lip as well as the bone and soft tissue of the alveolus. Cleft palate is a midline opening of the palate that results from the failure of the two sides to fuse during embryonic development. The exact cause is unknown, but in most cases it is thought to be multifactorial (a combination of environmental and genetic factors). Clefting is usually an isolated event but may occur as part of a syndrome. A good physical examination is very important to identify any other malformations.

INCIDENCE

1. Cleft lip with or without cleft palate occurs in 1 in 700 live births.
2. Clefting is more common in Hispanic and Asian groups but may be seen in all ethnic groups.

CLINICAL MANIFESTATIONS

1. Visible unilateral or bilateral cleft lip (may be a complete cleft through the nares or an incomplete cleft of part of the lip)
2. Palpable and/or visible cleft palate
3. Cleft of the alveolus (gum line, may affect bone and soft tissue)
4. Nasal distortion
5. Feeding difficulties

COMPLICATIONS

1. Speech and language: speech difficulties may include hypernasality, hyponasality, and compensatory articulation.
2. Dental: malocclusion may occur, with abnormal tooth eruption pattern and abnormal development of the way the mandible and the maxilla meet; excessive dental decay is not unusual.
3. Auditory: chronic otitis media, secondary to eustachian tube dysfunction, may result in hearing loss and speech delay.
4. Psychosocial: altered self-esteem and body image may occur.

LABORATORY AND DIAGNOSTIC TESTS

1. Multidisciplinary team evaluation to counsel parents on clefting and to prepare them for the treatment plan including the surgical plan.
2. Evaluation by a geneticist including laboratory and diagnostic tests if other anomalies exist.
3. Audiologic evaluation to determine if hearing loss is present and if the use of pressure-equalizing tubes is warranted.

SURGICAL MANAGEMENT: CLEFT LIP AND CLEFT PALATE REPAIR

Cleft lip is repaired at 8 to 12 weeks of age if the baby has demonstrated good weight gain. The usual suggestion is that the baby weigh 10 pounds at the time of cleft lip repair. Cleft lip repair is usually done by a plastic surgeon specially trained in the repair of clefts. The plastic surgeon may choose among several methods for repair of the cleft lip, depending on his or her training and experience. Some surgeons choose the Millard repair, which results in a zigzag scar on the lip. Others choose to place the suture lines where the lines of the columella would have been if the clefting had not occurred. Still others choose among other types of repairs. The goal of all cleft lip surgery is the same, however—to achieve lip competence and to create the most natural-appearing lip.

Cleft palate repair is usually performed when the child is 9 to 12 months of age, weighing 18 to 20 pounds. Palatoplasty involves reconstruction of the palatal musculature with the goal of creating an intact palate in order to develop normal speech.

NURSING ASSESSMENT

1. Assess feeding to determine if the baby is receiving adequate caloric intake for growth. Work with the family to develop the best feeding method for that baby. The following are broad guidelines for determining infant calorie requirements:
   a. Newborns require about 100 kcal/kg/day to grow. (Multiply the weight in kilograms by 100 to obtain the daily calorie requirements. For example, 2.87 kg × 100 kcal/kg/day = 287 kcal/day.) Standard infant formula and breast milk have 20 kcal/oz.
   b. Daily intake (number of ounces needed in a 24-hr period) is determined by first calculating total kilocalories needed per day (as indicated earlier), then dividing by 20. For example, 287 kcal/day ÷ 20 kcal/oz = 14.35 oz/day.
   c. Most infants feed every 3 or 4 hours, which amounts to six to eight feedings per day. To determine the volume of each feeding, calculate the number of ounces needed per day and divide by the number of feedings. For example, 14.35 oz divided by 6 (feeding every 4 hr) is 2.4 oz or about 2.5 oz every 4 hours. If the infant is fed more frequently—every 3 hours—divide the ounces per day by 8. In this example, feedings would be 1.8 oz, or about 2 oz, every 3 hours.
2. Assess parents' interactions with infant for signs of healthy attachment.
3. Screen for maternal depression.
4. Assess respiratory status (respiratory effort, rate, oxygenation, tachycardia).
5. Assess for signs of infection.

NURSING DIAGNOSES

- Parenting, Risk for impaired
- Knowledge, Deficient (regarding clefting)

- Nutrition: less than body requirements, Imbalanced
- Gas exchange, Impaired
- Airway clearance, Ineffective
- Breathing pattern, Ineffective
- Pain, Acute (related to surgical procedure)

NURSING INTERVENTIONS
Preoperative Care

1. Facilitate parents' positive adjustment to infant.
   a. Assist parents in dealing with their feelings about having a child with a visible difference. Encourage expression of feelings.
   b. Discuss treatment plan for child, answering parents' questions.
   c. Provide information that instills hope and positive feelings for infant (e.g., comment on infant's positive features, note positive aspects of parent-child interactions).
   d. Encourage parents to engage in caregiving activities.
   e. Model acceptance of and delight in the baby, congratulate family on birth of their baby.
   f. Arrange meeting with parents of other babies who have undergone surgical and medical treatment.
2. Explain concept of team care and refer to local cleft palate team. Local team listings may be found by contacting the American Cleft Palate–Craniofacial Association (ACPA/CPF), 104 South Estes Drive, Suite 204, Chapel Hill, NC 27514, 919–933–9044, www.info@cleftline.org.
3. Provide information and resources to families regarding cause and treatment of clefting.
   a. Provide information on etiology of cleft lip and palate that explains when, during embryonic development, clefting occurred.
   b. Explain timing of surgical intervention.
   c. Educate parents on feeding techniques.
4. Maintain adequate nutritional intake to promote optimal growth.
   a. Babies with isolated cleft lips can usually feed at the breast. It is important to encourage and provide support

to a new mother in breast-feeding her baby with a cleft lip.

b. Babies with cleft palates have a difficult time breast-feeding. Most babies with cleft palates cannot generate enough suction at the breast to obtain the necessary nutrition. Mothers of babies with cleft palates are encouraged to pump their breast milk and feed it to their babies via a special nipple and bottle.

c. A variety of bottle-nipple combinations may be used. No single method is best. What is best is what works for the family and allows the infant to finish feeding within 20 to 30 minutes, so that the feeding experience is satisfying for the family.

  i. Most babies with a cleft palate can be fed successfully using a soft nipple with an added crosscut (about $\frac{1}{8}$ inch each way).

  ii. Another feeding system is the Pigeon nipple-bottle system. The Pigeon system has a squeeze bottle and a soft nipple with a valve, which prevents the baby from ingesting excess air during the feeding.

  iii. The Mead Johnson cleft lip/palate nurser can also be used. It is a compressible bottle.

d. Feeding instructions are as follows:

  i. Place the infant in an upright position (almost sitting).

  ii. Place the nipple in the baby's mouth, trying to position the nipple where there is more palatal tissue.

  iii. Support chin with your pinky finger to improve the oral seal.

  iv. Assess the infant's response to feeding.

  v. If the baby arches and turns away, the flow of milk may be too rapid. The X cut may be too large. Use a nipple with a smaller X cut. If the baby does not get enough milk, you may need to enlarge the X cut or compress the bottle.

  vi. If a squeeze bottle is used, parents are taught to compress the bottle in time with the infant's chewing motions and allow for rest periods when the infant rests. The parents should be taught to read their infant's cues.

    vii. Burp the baby about halfway through the feeding. The feeding should not last more than 20 to 30 minutes; otherwise the calories taken in will be expended by the feeding effort.

    viii. Monitor weight at least twice weekly until weight gain is at least an ounce per day.

5. Monitor respiratory status (respiratory effort, breath sounds, vital signs).

Preoperative Home Care

1. There is no special instruction for preoperative care. Bathe infant as usual.
2. Refer to institutional regimen for preoperative procedure, including when to stop feeding before surgery.

Postoperative Care

Cleft Lip Repair

1. Promote adequate nutritional fluid intake.
   a. Give breast milk or formula as tolerated (or per institution policy).
2. Promote healing and maintain integrity of child's incision site.
   a. Cleanse suture line gently if required by institutional protocol.
   b. Many surgeons use Dermabond skin adhesive to close outer layer of lip (skin). Antibiotic ointment and hydrogen peroxide should not be used in such cases, since they break down the Dermabond.

Cleft Palate Repair

1. Offer clear liquid (when recovered from anesthesia) with same feeding device used before surgery (or per surgeon's orders). Advance to blenderized or soft diet as tolerated.
2. Avoid placing objects in child's mouth (suction catheters, tongue depressors, straws, ice chips).
3. Remove toys that are hard or pointed.
4. Monitor for signs of infection or bleeding.
5. Observe for respiratory difficulty.

Both Types of Repair

1. Monitor infant's level of pain and need for nonpharmacologic interventions (e.g., holding, rocking) and/or pharmacologic interventions (see Appendix I). Ensure that you have a current infant pain scale, either the FLACC (face, legs, activity, cry, consolability) or NPASS (Neonatal Pain, Agitation, and Sedation Scale).

🏠 Discharge Planning and Home Care

1. Instruct parents about care of surgical site.
2. Instruct parents about feeding techniques.
3. Instruct parents about signs of infection.
4. Instruct parents on how to position child for feeding.
5. Encourage parents to discuss feelings and concerns about caring for baby at home, as well as about long-term care.
6. Reinforce to parents importance of long-term team care for early treatment of problems, which may include abnormalities in speech, language, hearing, dentition, and occlusion.
7. Inform parents of agencies and support groups for children with cleft lip and/or palate (refer to Appendix G).

CLIENT OUTCOMES

1. Infant's or child's incision will heal properly without complications.
2. Infant or child will have appropriate weight gain.
3. Feeding will be pleasurable experience for infant and parent.
4. Parents will demonstrate correct feeding techniques.
5. Parents will demonstrate attachment to their infant or child.

REFERENCES

Andrews-Casal M et al: Cleft lip with or without cleft palate: Effect of family history on reproductive planning, surgical timing, and parental stress, *Cleft Palate Craniofac J* 35(1):52, 1998.

Behrman RE, Kiegman R, Jenson, HB, editors: *Nelson textbook of pediatrics,* ed 17, Philadelphia, 2004, WB Saunders.

Golden AS: Cleft lip and cleft palate. In: Hoekelman RA et al, editors: *Primary pediatric care,* ed 3, St. Louis, 1997, Mosby.

Grow JL, Lehman JA: A local perspective on the initial management of children with cleft lip and palate by primary care physicians, *Cleft Palate Craniofac J* 39(5):535, 2002.

Heidbuchel KL et al: Dental maturity in children with a complete bilateral cleft lip and palate, *Cleft Palate Craniofac J* 39(5):509, 2002.

Hockenberry MJ et al: *Wong's essentials of pediatric nursing,* ed 7, St. Louis, 2004, Mosby.

Resnick JI, Zarem HA: Diseases and injuries of the oral region. In: Burg FD et al, editors: *Gellis and Kagan's current pediatric therapy,* ed 16, Philadelphia, 1999, WB Saunders.

Savage HE: An early intervention guide to infants born with clefts. Infant-toddler intervention, *Transdisciplinary J* 7(4):271, 1997.

Smahel Z et al: Changes in craniofacial development due to modifications of the treatment of unilateral cleft lip and palate, *Cleft Palate Craniofac J* 35(3):240, 1998.

15

Coarctation of the Aorta

PATHOPHYSIOLOGY

Coarctation of the aorta is a localized narrowing or obstruction of the aortic lumen. The narrowing usually occurs adjacent to the site of insertion of the ductus arteriosus. Narrowing increases pressure in the ascending aorta, which results in higher pressure to the coronary arteries and vessels that arise from the aortic arch. Pressure is decreased distal to the site of obstruction. Coarctation of the aorta is often associated with bicuspid aortic valve. Other associated defects include other forms of left-sided obstruction, patent ductus arteriosus, and ventricular septal defect. Prognosis is excellent with surgical intervention.

INCIDENCE

1. Accounts for 8% to 10% of individuals with congenital cardiac defects
2. Male-female ratio is 2:1
3. More common in families of European descent
4. Known familial clustering of left ventricular outflow tract obstructions, including coarctation of the aorta
5. Occurs in 30% of patients with Turner's syndrome

CLINICAL MANIFESTATIONS

1. Absent or diminished femoral pulses
2. Cool lower extremities with prolonged capillary refill time
3. Blood pressure differential between upper and lower extremities
4. May have systolic or diastolic murmurs
5. May have an ejection click

6. Two patterns of presentation:
   a. Neonatal—asymptomatic until ductus arteriosus closes or until onset of left ventricular failure. Present with severe congestive heart failure that can progress to shock if untreated
   b. Postneonatal—typically, asymptomatic and present with hypertension. Other symptoms are sequelae of coarctation of the aorta and include calf pain, headache, epistaxis, dizziness, and fainting

COMPLICATIONS

1. Cardiovascular: hypertension, recurrent coarctation of the aorta, aortic aneurysm, cerebrovascular accident
2. Infectious disease: bacterial endocarditis

LABORATORY AND DIAGNOSTIC TESTS

1. Electrocardiogram (ECG)—normal or may reveal left ventricular hypertrophy or right bundle branch block.
2. Chest radiograph—neonates with severe coarctation of the aorta may have cardiomegaly and pulmonary edema; infants and older children may have normal or slightly enlarged heart with visible dilation of the ascending aorta. Rib notching may be present in older children.
3. Echocardiogram—reveals site and extent of coarctation, presence of other abnormalities, left ventricular dysfunction.
4. Cardiac catheterization—required to evaluate other defects or if echocardiography provides insufficient information.
5. Magnetic resonance imaging—most useful in older children and adults to assess for recurrent coarctation.
6. Preoperative laboratory data—refer to Appendix D for normal values and ranges of laboratory and diagnostic tests.
   a. Complete blood count—used to screen hematologic status preoperatively, including evaluation of baseline white blood cell count, hemoglobin, and hematocrit.
   b. Baseline electrolyte levels and renal function panels—to assess renal function and metabolic status preoperatively: sodium, potassium, chloride, carbon dioxide, blood urea nitrogen, and creatinine.

c. Blood coagulation studies—prothrombin time, partial thromboplastin time, platelet count.

d. Type and cross-match—in the event that transfusion is required.

MEDICAL AND SURGICAL MANAGEMENT

Management strategies vary by age of child and severity of the coarctation of the aorta. Neonates with critical coarctation of the aorta require intravenous infusion of prostaglandin E_1 to reopen the ductus arteriosus. They may also require stabilization with inotropic agents and respiratory support, and are scheduled for repair when medically stable. Traditionally, defects in children with hypertension who were otherwise asymptomatic were repaired between the age of 3 and 5 years. At present, many centers schedule for repair at presentation to decrease the risk of residual hypertension and postoperative complications.

Repair refers to using one of several methods including resection with end-to-end anastomosis, subclavian flap aortoplasty (ligation and use of the subclavian artery to enlarge the aorta), patch aortoplasty, or conduit insertion. The team selects the method of repair most appropriate for the child's age and anatomy. The overall mortality rate for repair of isolated coarctation of the aorta is less than 5% and in older children is less than 1%. Balloon dilation is an effective treatment for recurrent coarctation of the aorta and is being used in some institutions to treat native coarctation of the aorta. Finally, stents may be placed in the aorta for mild native or recurrent coarctation of the aorta in older children and adults.

Postoperative Complications

1. Cardiovascular
   a. Hypertension is the most common postoperative problem and is more common in older children
   b. Recurrent coarctation occurs in 6% to 33% of those whose defects are repaired in infancy, 3% in children whose defects are repaired after 3 years of age

2. Hematologic
   a. Hemorrhage as demonstrated by chest tube output, presence of blood clots, or bleeding from other sites such as nose, mouth and gastrointestinal (GI) tract
3. Pulmonary
   a. Laryngeal nerve damage leading to stridor
   b. Phrenic nerve damage leading to paralysis of the diaphragm
   c. Chylothorax—refers to lymphatic fluid in the pleural space
4. Gastrointestinal
   a. Postcoarctectomy syndrome—This is more common in older children and in those with preoperative hypertension. Symptoms include vomiting, abdominal distention, and fever
5. Neurologic
   a. Spinal cord ischemia leading to paraplegia (rare)

Antihypertensive Medications

1. Sodium nitroprusside (Nipride)—continuous infusion used to treat acute postoperative hypertension; acts on the smooth muscle to produce peripheral vasodilation, causing decreased arterial pressures
2. Propranolol (Inderal)—used to treat postoperative hypertension; acts as a beta-blocker of cardiac and bronchial adrenoreceptors, decreasing heart rate and myocardial irritability and potentiating contraction and conduction pathway
3. Captopril (Capoten)—used to treat postoperative hypertension; works on the renin-angiotensin system to reduce afterload

NURSING ASSESSMENT

1. See the Cardiovascular Assessment section in Appendix A.
2. Ascertain blood pressure in four extremities to assess pressure gradient above and below coarctation of the aorta.
3. Assess the child's growth and development.

NURSING DIAGNOSES

- Cardiac output, Decreased
- Gas exchange, Impaired
- Deficient fluid volume
- Risk for feeding intolerance
- Pain
- Anxiety
- Activity intolerance
- Coping, Ineffective
- Infection, Risk for
- Family processes, Interrupted
- Therapeutic regimen management, Ineffective
- Knowledge, Deficient

NURSING INTERVENTIONS
Preoperative Care

1. Monitor cardiac status.
   a. Color of mucous membranes and nail beds
   b. Quality and intensity of peripheral pulses in upper and lower extremities
   c. Capillary refill time
   d. Temperatures of extremities
   e. Apical pulse
   f. Blood pressure in upper and lower extremities
   g. Respiratory rate
2. Promote child's understanding by use of age-appropriate terminology (see Appendix F).
3. Provide information to assist parents in understanding child's condition.
4. Stress the importance of normal well-child care and immunizations.
5. Stress the importance of age-appropriate social and recreational activities (see Appendix D).

Postoperative Care

1. Monitor cardiac status frequently per institutional policy.
   a. Apical pulse, respiratory rate, core and skin temperature.

    b. Arterial blood pressure—hypertension often present initially (no blood pressure present in left arm if subclavian artery used for surgery).

    c. Capillary refill time.

    d. Cardiac rhythm.

2. Control hypertension if present. Since pain or anxiety can increase blood pressure, ensure adequate treatment of pain and/or anxiety before starting antihypertensive medications.

3. Use no cuff pressure or arterial punctures in left arm if left subclavian flap was performed, because only collateral vessels are providing arterial circulation.

4. Promote optimal respiratory status.

    a. Have child turn, cough, and deep breathe.

    b. Perform chest physiotherapy.

    c. Humidify air.

    d. Monitor chest tube for patency and color and consistency of drainage.

5. Monitor for signs and symptoms of hemorrhage.

    a. Measure chest tube output per institutional policy.

    b. Assess for clot formation in chest tube (increased output of blood followed by abrupt decrease).

    c. Assess bowel sounds and monitor for abdominal distention.

    d. Assess for bleeding from other sites (e.g., nose, mouth, GI tract).

    e. Strictly record input and output.

6. Monitor and correct hydration status.

    a. Dry mucous membranes.

    b. Bulging or depressed fontanelles.

    c. Decreased tearing, dry mouth.

    d. Poor skin turgor.

    e. Specific gravity.

    f. Daily weight.

    g. Intake and output.

    h. Administer intravenous fluids as ordered.

7. Monitor child's response to medications and blood products.

    a. See the Antihypertensive Medications section in this chapter.

    b. Assist with collection of laboratory data.

8. Resume oral feedings slowly; monitor tolerance and abdominal status.
9. Relieve postoperative pain and anxiety using medication, parental presence, and age-appropriate interventions (see Appendix I).
10. Provide age-appropriate diversional activities (see the relevant section in Appendix F).
11. Provide age-appropriate explanations before treatments and painful procedures (see the Preparation for Procedures and Surgery section in Appendix F).
12. Perform wound care according to instutitional policy.
13. Assess for signs and symptoms of infection.
14. Encourage parental presence and involvement in care.
15. Provide parent support and education.

🏠 Discharge Planning and Home Care

Review the following points with parents and caregivers before discharge:

1. Appropriate wound care according to institutional policy
2. Observe for signs and symptoms of infection
3. Activity limitations as instructed by the health care team
4. Appropriate lifting techniques for infants and toddlers: avoid grabbing child under the arms, support child's head and shoulders with one arm and the lower body with the other
5. Pain management (refer to Appendix I)
6. Administration of medications and monitoring child's response
7. Importance of follow-up to screen for hypertension, recurrent coarctation, and other complications
8. Good dental hygiene and antibiotic prophylaxis before and after invasive procedures to prevent bacterial endocarditis
9. Importance of routine well-child care and immunizations
10. Importance of developmentally appropriate social and recreational activities (refer to Appendix B)
11. Importance of maintaining expectations for behavior and discipline, and supporting the child's complete recovery

CLIENT OUTCOMES

1. Child will be free of postoperative complications.
2. Child will have adequate pain management.
3. Child will demonstrate sense of mastery of the surgical experience as evidenced by expression of feelings and resumption of normal activity level.
4. Child will participate in physical activities appropriate for age.
5. Parent will verbalize home care and follow-up instructions.

REFERENCES

Craig J et al: Cardiovascular critical care problems. In: Curley MAQ, Moloney-Harmon PA, editors: *Critical care nursing of infants and children,* ed 2, Philadelphia, 2001, WB Saunders.

Koenig P, Hijazi ZM, Zimmerman F: *Essential pediatric cardiology,* New York, 2004, McGraw-Hill.

Mavroudis C, Backer CL: *Pediatric cardiac surgery,* ed 3, St. Louis, 2003, Mosby.

McBride KL et al: Inheritance analysis of congenital left ventricular outflow tract obstruction malformations: Segregation, multiplex relative risk, and heritability, *Am J Med Genet* 134(2):180, 2005.

McConnaha M: Surgery for congenital heart defects: A different world, *Semin Periop Nurs* 6(3):170, 1997.

Park M: *Pediatric cardiology* for *practitioners,* ed 4, St. Louis, 2002, Mosby.

Pye S, Green A: Caring for your baby after heart surgery, *Adv Neonatal Care* 3(3):157, 2003.

Pye S, Green A: Parent education after newborn congenital heart surgery, *Adv Neonatal Care* 3(3):147, 2003.

Wood MK: Acyanotic cardiac lesions with normal pulmonary blood flow, *Neonatal Network* 17(3):5, 1998.

16

Congestive Heart Failure

PATHOPHYSIOLOGY

Congestive heart failure (CHF) occurs when the heart cannot pump the blood returning to the right side of the heart, provide adequate circulation to meet the needs of organs and tissues in the body, or a combination of the two. The component factors in CHF include preload and circulating volume, afterload, and contractility. Causes include congenital and acquired heart diseases with pressure and/or volume overload, and myocardial insufficiency.

1. Congenital heart disease with pressure or volume overload is a common cause of CHF in pediatric patients. The timing of onset varies fairly predictably with the type of defect (Table 16-1). It is important to note the following:

   a. Children with tetralogy of Fallot (TOF) do not develop CHF unless they have undergone a large aorta-to-pulmonary artery shunt procedure such as a Waterston or Potts operation. These procedures are no longer performed.

   b. Atrial septal defects (ASD) rarely cause CHF in children.

   c. Large left-to-right shunts such as ventricular septal defect and patent ductus arteriosus (PDA) do not cause CHF before 6 to 8 weeks of age in full-term infants, because pulmonary vascular resistance (PVR) does not fall low enough to allow the left-to-right shunt until this time. However, CHF may occur earlier in premature infants with these lesions as a result of an earlier fall in PVR.

TABLE 16-1

Causes of Congestive Heart Failure Due to Congenital Heart Disease According to the Time of Occurrence

Age or Time of Occurrence	Cause
At birth	a. HLHS b. Volume overload lesions (e.g., severe TR or PR, large systemic AV fistula)
First week	a. TGA b. PDA in small premature infants c. HLHS (with more favorable anatomy) d. TAPVR, particularly those with pulmonary venous obstruction
1–4 weeks	a. COA (with associated anomalies) b. Critical AS c. Large L-R shunt lesions (e.g., VSD, PDA) in premature infants d. All other lesions listed above
4–6 weeks	a. Some L-R shunt lesions, such as ECD
6 weeks to 4 months	a. Large VSD b. Large PDA c. Others: anomalous left coronary artery from PA

Reprinted with permission from Park MK: *The pediatric cardiology handbook*, St. Louis, 2003, Mosby.

AS, Aortic stenosis; *AV,* arteriovenous; *COA,* coarctation of the aorta; *ECD,* endocardial cushion defect; *HLHS,* hypoplastic left heart syndrome; *L-R,* left to right; *PA,* pulmonary artery; *PDA,* patent ductus arteriosus; *PR,* pulmonary regurgitation; *PS,* pulmonary stenosis; *TAPVR,* total anomalies pulmonary venous return; *TGA,* transposition of the great arteries; *TR,* tricuspid regurgitation; *VSD,* ventricular septal defect.

2. Acquired heart disease of various etiologies can result in CHF. The age of onset of CHF is less predictable with acquired heart disease than with congenital heart disease; however, there are some general considerations:
   a. Metabolic abnormalities in newborns including severe hypoxia and acidosis, hypoglycemia, and hypocalcemia

b. Endocardial fibroelastosis, a rare primary myocardial disease, causes CHF in infants. In 90% of the cases, signs of CHF are evident in the first 8 months of life.

c. Viral myocarditis can occur in small children, usually over 1 year of age; it may occur in newborns with sudden onset and severe illness.

d. Acute rheumatic carditis is an occasional cause of CHF primarily in school-aged children.

e. Rheumatic valvular diseases with volume overload lesion such as mitral regurgitation (MR) or aortic regurgitation (AR) cause CHF in older children. Uncommon in industrialized countries.

f. Idiopathic dilated cardiomyopathy may cause CHF at any age during childhood and adolescence.

g. Cardiomyopathies associated with muscular dystrophy and Friedreich's ataxia may cause CHF in older children and adolescents.

h. Doxorubicin-associated cardiomyopathy may occur months to years after completion of chemotherapy in children with malignancies.

3. Other causes:

a. Complete heart block associated with structural heart defects in the newborn period and early infancy.

b. Supraventricular tachycardia (SVT) in early infancy.

c. Severe anemia at any age.

d. Hydrops fetalis in the newborn.

e. Sicklemia beyond the newborn period.

f. Acute hypertension following acute infectious glomerulonephritis in school-aged children. Hypertension is related to fluid retention with poor renal function.

g. Bronchopulmonary dysplasia in premature infants causes predominantly right-sided heart failure in the first few months of life.

h. Acute cor pulmonale due to airway obstruction as seen with large tonsils can cause CHF at any age, but is most common during early childhood.

If the heart fails for any reason and cardiac output is not sufficient to meet the metabolic needs of the body, the sympathetic nervous system responds by trying to increase circulating blood volume by diverting blood from nonessential organs. This decreases renal blood flow, activates the renin-angiotensin-aldosterone mechanism, and increases sodium and water retention. Catecholamine release with decreased cardiac output causes increased heart rate, increased vascular tone, and sweating. These initial compensatory mechanisms for maintaining cardiac output (increased circulating blood volume, increased heart rate, and vascular tone) eventually lead to clinical manifestations of CHF.

INCIDENCE

1. Of infants with congenital heart defects, 90% develop CHF within the first year of life.
2. The majority of affected infants manifest symptoms within the first few months of life.
3. Incidence varies depending on cause.

CLINICAL MANIFESTATIONS

1. Tachycardia
2. Cardiomegaly
3. Increased respiratory effort
4. Tachypnea
5. Wheezing and crackles may be present
6. Hepatomegaly
7. Edema, puffy eyelids (in infants)
8. Diaphoresis
9. Feeding difficulty and poor weight gain
10. Irritability

COMPLICATIONS

Low cardiac output syndrome refractory to medications may develop.

LABORATORY AND DIAGNOSTIC TESTS

Diagnosis is made on the basis of physical examination revealing signs and symptoms previously noted. The following can assist in further evaluation:

1. Electrocardiogram (ECG)—for diagnosis of tachycardia or bradycardia arrhythmias, may be helpful in determining type of defect; is not helpful in determining presence of CHG.
2. Chest radiographic study—heart will be enlarged, and pulmonary infiltrates will be present. Children with large left-to-right shunts have cardiomegaly without CHF.
3. Echocardiogram—may confirm enlarged heart chamber(s) and/or impaired left ventricular (LV) function. Useful in determining cause of CHF and in ongoing evaluation of efficacy of therapy.

MEDICAL MANAGEMENT

The initial management of CHF is accomplished by the use of pharmacologic agents that act to improve the function of the heart muscle and/or reduce the workload on the heart. Digitalis is given to increase cardiac output by slowing conduction through the atrioventricular node and make each contraction stronger. Diuretics decrease preload volume because their actions result in decreased extracellular fluid volume. Venous, arterial, and mixed dilators may be given to decrease preload volume by reducing systemic or pulmonary vascular resistance. Fluids are usually restricted to two thirds of maintenance levels, and attention is given to nutrition and rest. Medical management continues with the plan for interventional cardiac catheterization or surgical intervention, if indicated.

NURSING ASSESSMENT

1. See the Cardiovascular Assessment and Respiratory Assessment sections in Appendix A.
2. Assess activity level.
3. Assess extremities for edema.
4. Assess feeding pattern and weight gain history.
5. Assess family coping patterns.

NURSING DIAGNOSES

- Cardiac output, Decreased
- Breathing pattern, Ineffective
- Activity intolerance
- Fluid volume, Excess

- Nutrition: less than body requirements, Imbalanced
- Knowledge, Deficient
- Family processes, Interrupted

NURSING INTERVENTIONS

1. Promote cardiac output.
   a. Continue cardiovascular assessments, including evaluation of vital signs, pulses, color, capillary refill, and lung sounds.
   b. Administer medications, and assess and record effects.
2. Promote oxygenation and ventilation.
   a. Maintain patent airway, and assess effect of oxygen if provided.
   b. Elevate head of bed, or place infant in infant seat, to promote systemic venous return.
3. Provide rest and comfort measures.
   a. Maintain quiet environment with quick response to crying of infant or child.
   b. Swaddle infants.
   c. Provide neutral thermal environment, maintaining constant temperature for least oxygen consumption.
   d. Schedule activities to provide extended rest periods.
4. Promote and maintain child's fluid and electrolyte balance.
   a. Assess intake and output.
   b. Assess edema.
   c. Measure and record child's weight daily.
   d. Restrict fluids, usually to two thirds of maintenance fluid levels.
   e. Follow potassium levels closely if child is on diuretic therapy.
5. Promote child's nutritional status.
   a. Assess and record infant's tolerance of and response to feedings.
   b. Provide small, frequent feedings for conservation of energy.
   c. Collaborate with nutrition services to provide optimal diet for maximal calories and minimal fluids.
6. Assist family in understanding, accepting, and working through emotions of having a child with a chronic condition.

🏠 Discharge Planning and Home Care

1. Educate on specific condition.
2. Provide specific instructions about medications and adverse effects.
3. Although caregivers of infants with chronic CHF are usually quite skilled in assessing for signs and symptoms of CHF, reinforce as necessary.
4. Instruct in feeding techniques and nutritional requirements.
5. Refer as indicated to infant stimulation programs or parent support groups.

CLIENT OUTCOMES

1. Child will have adequate cardiac output.
2. Child will have normal growth and development.
3. Caregivers will demonstrate ability to handle all facets of infant's home care.

REFERENCES

James SR et al: *Nursing care of children: Principles and practice,* Philadelphia, 2002, WB Saunders.

Park MK: *Pediatric cardiology for practitioner,* St. Louis, 2002, Mosby.

Park MK: *The pediatric cardiology handbook,* St. Louis, 2003, Mosby.

17

Cystic Fibrosis

PATHOPHYSIOLOGY

Cystic fibrosis (CF), inherited as an autosomal-recessive trait, is caused by a mutation of the CF gene on chromosome 7. This results in absence or decreased function of a protein called cystic fibrosis transmembrane regulator (CFTR), which leads to abnormal sodium and chloride transport across the epithelium. The disorder affects the exocrine glands and causes the production of viscous mucus, which leads to obstruction of the small passageways of the bronchi, the small intestine, and the pancreatic and bile ducts. The effects of this biochemical defect on the involved organs are as follows:

1. Lungs
   a. Bronchial and bronchiolar obstruction from excessive pooling of secretions causes generalized hyperinflation and atelectasis.
   b. Pooled mucous secretions increase the susceptibility to bacterial infections. (*Pseudomonas aeruginosa* and *Staphylococcus aureus* are the predominant organisms found in sputum and lungs. *Burkholderia cepacia* is associated with later-life infection in the CF-affected lung, causing devastating infection. *B. cepacia* is highly transmissible from the infected person with CF to others with CF, and those with known infection should not have contact with an uninfected individual with CF.)
   c. Altered oxygen and carbon dioxide exchange can cause varying degrees of hypoxia, hypercapnia, and acidosis.

   d. Fibrotic lung changes take place and, in severe cases, pulmonary hypertension and cor pulmonale can occur.
2. Pancreas
   a. Degeneration and fibrosis of acini occur.
   b. Secretion of pancreatic enzymes is inhibited, which causes impaired absorption of fats, proteins and, to a limited degree, carbohydrates.
3. Small intestine—absence of pancreatic enzymes (trypsin, amylase, lipase) causes impaired absorption of fats and proteins, which results in steatorrhea and azotorrhea.
4. Liver—biliary obstruction, fibrosis
5. Skeleton
   a. Growth and onset of puberty are retarded.
   b. Retardation of skeletal maturation results in delayed bone aging and shortness of stature (38% to 42% of children with CF).
6. Reproductive system
   a. Female—late menses; possible infertility because of thickness of cervical mucus
   b. Male—vas deferens often absent; sterility but not impotence

INCIDENCE

1. CF affects 1 in every 3700 infants born in the United States, with the birth prevalence varying based on race and ethnicity:
   a. 1 in 2500 to 3500 births of non-Hispanic white infants each year
   b. 1 in 4000 to 10,000 births of Hispanic infants
   c. 1 in 15,000 to 20,000 non-Hispanic blacks
2. CF rarely affects infants of Asian descent (1 in 31,000).
3. Odds are 1 in 4 (25%) that each subsequent pregnancy after the birth of a child with CF will result in a child with CF.
4. CF affects males and females equally.
5. Newborn screening for CF is available and, when positive, could lead to an earlier age at diagnosis compared with

when diagnosis is symptom-based. This would lead to earlier nutritional management and result in improved growth and development. At present, newborn screening for CF has improved outcomes for the child with CF but has not been universally adopted.

6. Symptoms vary greatly, resulting in variable life span—95% survival to age 16 years, with a median predicted age of survival of 35.1 years. About 42% of patients with cystic fibrosis are 18 years of age or older. Infants born in the 1990s or later have a predicted median survival age of 40 years.

7. Length and quality of life have greatly increased in recent years, but the disease is ultimately terminal.

CLINICAL MANIFESTATIONS

1. Meconium ileus (at birth in 15% to 20% of infants with CF)
2. Cough—initially dry and nonproductive, changing to loose and productive
3. Viscous sputum, increasing in amount, normally yellow-gray and greenish during infection
4. Wheezy respirations, moist crackles
5. Cyanosis, clubbed fingers and toes, increased anteroposterior diameter of chest (later signs)
6. Steatorrhea
7. Bulky, loose, foul-smelling stools
8. Distended abdomen
9. Thin extremities
10. Failure to thrive (below norms for height and weight despite large food intake)
11. Profuse sweating in warm temperatures
12. Salty-tasting skin
13. Excessive loss of sodium and chloride

COMPLICATIONS

1. Pulmonary: emphysema, pneumothorax, pneumonia, bronchiectasis, hemoptysis, cor pulmonale, respiratory failure

2. Gastrointestinal: cirrhosis, portal hypertension, esophageal varices, fecal impactions, enlarged spleen, intussusception, cholelithiasis, pancreatitis, rectal prolapse
3. Endocrine: CF-related diabetes mellitus, poor bone mineralization leading to osteopenia and osteoporosis, poor growth, heat prostration

LABORATORY AND DIAGNOSTIC TESTS

1. Genetic blood testing for CF marker
2. Sweat test—to measure concentration of sodium and chloride in sweat; most definitive diagnostic test; not reliable for newborns younger than 1 month old (two positive results on sweat tests are diagnostic; value higher than 60 mEq/L represents positive result for CF)
3. Pulmonary function testing—used to assess respiratory status and severity of condition, and to determine therapy
4. Chest radiographic study—for evaluation of pulmonary complications

MEDICAL MANAGEMENT

The child with symptoms of CF is hospitalized for the diagnostic work-up, initiation of treatment, clearing of any symptoms of respiratory tract infection, and education of the child and family. The goal of this hospitalization is to stabilize the child's condition so that care can be managed for long periods at home.

Antibiotics are given based on the suspected organisms, sensitivity to antibiotics, the severity of infection, and the child's response to therapy. The course of therapy is usually at least 14 days. After the initial admission, when respiratory tract infections are not responsive to intensive home treatment measures or oral antibiotic therapy, the child may either be readmitted for intravenous (IV) antibiotic therapy or have home IV antibiotic therapy.

Pulmonary toilet includes adequate hydration to loosen secretions and chest percussion and postural drainage to clear mucus from the small airways. Breathing exercises and devices designed to loosen and mobilize pulmonary secretions are also used. Aerosol generators may be used to administer normal saline, bronchodilators (such as albuterol or other β-agonist drugs), antibiotics (such as tobramycin), and mucolytics. Dornase alfa is used to reduce the viscosity of sputum and improve lung function in children with CF. Some bronchodilators are administered through a metered-dose inhaler, with or without a spacer. Intermittent positive pressure breathing does not improve drug delivery and may aggravate the pulmonary status.

Pancreatic enzyme supplements are given with meals and snacks; dosages are individualized for the child and generally increase as the child gets older. Supplements of fat-soluble vitamins (A, D, E, and K) are needed in greater than the normal dosage because they are not well absorbed. Diet is modified to increase the number of calories provided (up to 150% more than normal needs based on age, weight, and activity). High levels of protein and normal amounts of fat (about 40%) should be included in the child's diet.

Lung or heart-lung transplantation may be an option for end-stage CF lung disease. The waiting period for donor organs is between 6 months and 2 years; it is increasing at all transplant centers. Transplant criteria include progressive respiratory function impairment with severe hypoxemia and hypercarbia, increasing functional impairment, major life-threatening pulmonary complications, and antibiotic resistance of bacteria infecting the lungs. Individual transplant centers may have additional criteria or restrictions. On behalf of the federal government, in the spring of 2005, United Network for Organ Sharing (UNOS) put priority guidelines into place for deciding who should get available donor lungs, which eliminated the first-come-first-served system for persons older than age 12. A twice-yearly evaluation serves to determine the person's health status before transplant and what his or her projected health will be after the transplant; then a mathematical formula is used to arrive at a "lung allocation score" that allows donor lungs to be given to the person who needs them the most at the time. The current 5-year survival rate for lung transplant in individuals with CF is 50%. The child with CF who undergoes transplantation is at risk for the same complications as other child transplant recipients (effects of immunosuppression, infection, acute rejection, and bronchiolitis obliterans). In addition, because of CF, such a child may have malabsorption of the immunosuppressive agents.

NURSING ASSESSMENT

1. See the Respiratory Assessment and Gastrointestinal Assessment sections in Appendix A.
2. Assess amount of sputum and its color and characteristics.
3. Assess activity level.
4. Assess nutritional intake.
5. Assess height and weight for age of child.

NURSING DIAGNOSES

- Airway clearance, Ineffective
- Activity intolerance, Risk for
- Nutrition: less than body requirements, Imbalanced
- Infection, Risk for
- Coping, Compromised family
- Growth and development, Delayed

NURSING INTERVENTIONS

1. Monitor respiratory status and report any significant changes (in respiratory rate, presence of intercostal retractions, presence of cyanosis, and color and amount of sputum).
2. Monitor effects of aerosolized treatment (performed before postural drainage).
3. Administer and evaluate effects of postural drainage and percussion.
4. Administer and monitor side effects and actions of medications.
   a. Antibiotics
   b. Pancreatic enzymes
   c. Vitamin A, D, E, and K supplements
   d. Mucolytic agents (dornase alfa)
   e. Bronchodilators
5. Teach and supervise breathing exercises (exhalation, inhalation, coughing), although these are not a substitute for percussion and postural drainage.

6. Encourage physical activity and a regular exercise program as condition permits.
7. Obtain baseline information about dietary habits (food preferences and dislikes, eating attitudes, developmental abilities).
8. Monitor and record characteristics of stool (color, consistency, size, frequency).
9. Promote nutritional status.
   a. Administer high-protein, high-calorie (120% to 150% recommended daily allowance) diet, with about 40% of the calories coming from fat.
   b. Administer supplemental fat-soluble vitamins.
   c. Administer pancreatic enzymes before meals and snacks.
   d. Assess need for supplemental protein formula or tube feeding.
10. Observe for and report signs of complications (see the Complications section in this chapter).
11. Provide emotional support to child and parents during hospitalization and in the ambulatory setting.
12. Provide guidance related to independence, self-care, sexuality, and educational planning as adolescent undergoes transition to adulthood.

🏠 Discharge Planning and Home Care

1. Instruct parents and child about techniques of home management.
   a. Dietary needs
   b. Postural drainage and percussion
   c. Aerosol treatments
   d. Breathing exercises
   e. Administration of medications
   f. Avoidance of exposure to respiratory tract infections
   g. Management of constipation or diarrhea
2. Monitor family's compliance with home management.
   a. Monitor child's clinical course.
   b. Monitor frequency of hospital admissions.
   c. Assess family's level of knowledge.

3. Assist family in contacting support systems for financial, psychologic, and medical assistance (e.g., Cystic Fibrosis Foundation).
4. Provide genetic counseling.
5. Immunize the child and all household members annually against influenza.

CLIENT OUTCOMES

1. Child's ability to clear airway will improve.
2. Child will gain weight.
3. Parents will administer home care regimen and provide for medical follow-up.

REFERENCES

Centers for Disease Control and Prevention: Newborn screening for cystic fibrosis: Evaluation of benefits and risks and recommendations for state newborn screening programs, *MMWR* 53(RR-13):1, 2004.

Cystic Fibrosis Foundation: *Patient registry annual data report 2004* (website): www.cff.org/living_with_cf. Accessed April 1, 2006.

Orenstein DM, Higgins LW: Update on the role of exercise in cystic fibrosis, *Curr Opin Pulm Med* 11(6):519, 2005.

Powers SW et al: Randomized clinical trial of behavioral and nutrition treatment to improve energy intake and growth in toddlers and preschoolers with cystic fibrosis, *Pediatrics* 116(6):1442, 2005.

Stark LJ, Powers SW: Behavioral aspects of nutrition in children with cystic fibrosis, *Curr Opin Pulm Med* 11(6):539, 2005.

Starner TD, McCray PB: Pathogenesis of early lung disease in cystic fibrosis: A window of opportunity to eradicate bacteria, *Ann Intern Med* 143 (11):816, 2005.

Zindani GN et al: Adherence to treatment in children and adolescent patients with cystic fibrosis, *J Adolesc Health* 38(2006):13, 2006.

18

Cytomegaloviral Infection

PATHOPHYSIOLOGY

Cytomegalovirus (CMV) is the leading cause of congenital viral infections in North America. A number of related strains of CMV exist. The virus is a member of the herpes family. CMV is probably transmitted through direct person-to-person contact with body fluids or tissues, including urine, blood, saliva, cervical secretions, semen, and breast milk. The period of incubation is unknown. The following are estimated incubation periods: after delivery, 3 to 12 weeks; after transfusion, 3 to 12 weeks; after transplantation, 4 weeks to 4 months. The urine often contains CMV months to years after infection. The virus can remain dormant in individuals and be reactivated. Currently, no immunizations exist to prevent infection with the virus.

Three types of CMV infection exist:

1. Congenital—acquired transplacentally in utero. The likelihood of congenital infection and the extent of the disease in the newborn depend on maternal immune status. Approximately 30% to 40% of infants born to women experiencing a primary (first) CMV illness during pregnancy will have clinical disease at birth. With recurrent maternal infection, (i.e., CMV infection that occurs repeatedly, leading to preconceptual immunity), the risk of transmission to the fetus is lower, ranging from 0.5% to 1.5%. Most of these infants appear normal at birth. The most severe form of congenital infection is referred to as cytomegalic inclusion disease.

2. Acute acquired—acquired anytime during or after birth through adulthood. Symptoms resemble those of

mononucleosis (malaise, fever, pharyngitis, splenomegaly, petechial rash, respiratory symptoms). Infection is not without sequelae, especially in young children it can result from transfusions.

3. Generalized systemic disease—occurs in individuals who are immunosuppressed, especially if they have undergone organ transplantation. Symptoms include pneumonitis, hepatitis, and leukopenia, which can occasionally be fatal. Previous infection does not produce immunity and may result in reactivation of the virus.

INCIDENCE

1. Among live births, 0.4% to 2.5% of infants have congenital infection.
2. Premature infants are affected more often than full-term infants.
3. Of infected infants, 10% are symptomatic at birth; 90% suffer long-term sequelae (e.g., deafness, mental retardation, or ocular abnormalities).
4. Of severely infected infants, 4% to 30% die by 3 months of age; the remaining 60% to 75% will have some form of intellectual impairment or developmental delay.
5. Approximately one third of infected infants are normal in late childhood.
6. Prevalence of CMV infection is approximately 80% in children younger than 2 years of age who attend child care centers.
7. Seroprevalence of CMV approximates 50% in young adults of middle-upper socioeconomic status.
8. Incidence is higher in lower socioeconomic groups.
9. Of susceptible women, the seroconversion rate during pregnancy is 0.7% to 4.1%.
10. Both sexes are equally susceptible to infection and morbidity from CMV.

CLINICAL MANIFESTATIONS

In the newborn period, an infant infected with CMV is usually asymptomatic. Onset of symptoms from congenitally acquired infection can occur immediately after birth or as late as 12 weeks after birth.

There are no predictable indicators, but the following symptoms are common:

1. Petechiae and ecchymoses
2. Hepatosplenomegaly
3. Neonatal jaundice; direct hyperbilirubinemia
4. Microcephaly with periventricular calcifications
5. Intrauterine growth retardation
6. Prematurity
7. Small size for gestational age

Other symptoms can occur in the newborn or older child:

1. Purpura
2. Hearing loss
3. Chorioretinitis; blindness
4. Fever
5. Pneumonia
6. Respiratory distress
7. Brain damage

COMPLICATIONS

1. Neurologic: variable hearing loss (7% to 15% in asymptomatic infants), lower intelligence quotient, visual impairment (rare in asymptomatic infants), microcephaly, sensorineural handicaps.

LABORATORY AND DIAGNOSTIC TESTS

1. Viral cultures of urine, pharyngeal secretions, and peripheral blood leukocytes. The most sensitive detection system is growth of the virus from urine in tissue culture, usually positive in 3 to 7 days.
2. A more rapid method of viral isolation is called the shell vial assay; after enhancing viral attachment to cells and staining, results are available in 24 hours.
3. Polymerase chain reaction and DNA hybridization or DNA amplification testing—to detect CMV in urine, amniotic fluid, fetal blood, and cerebrospinal fluid.

4. Microscopic examination of urinary sediment, body fluids, and tissues—to detect virus in large quantities (examining urine for intranuclear inclusions is not helpful; verification of congenital infection must be accomplished within first 3 weeks of life).
5. Toxoplasmosis, other infections, rubella, CMV infection, and herpes (TORCH) screen—used to assess presence of other viruses.
6. Serologic tests: Detection of immunoglobulin M (IgM) antibody should not be used to diagnose congenital CMV because it is less sensitive and more subject to false-positive results than culture or PCR. Only about 50% of congenitally infected infants produce IgM antibody.
7. Radiologic studies—skull radiographic studies or computed tomographic scans of head used to reveal intracranial calcifications, ventriculomegaly, cerebella hypoplasia, and, less commonly, myelination delay.

MEDICAL MANAGEMENT

The CMV virus differs from herpes and varicella viruses in that it lacks a specific enzyme. This feature renders it resistant to antiviral agents that depend on the enzyme for their action, such as acyclovir. Currently there are three antivirals licensed for treatment of CMV: ganciclovir, foscarnet, and cidofovir. There is limited experience using these agents in the setting of congenital and perinatal CMV infection; however, encouraging data from a controlled clinical trial indicate that ganciclovir therapy may be of value in limiting the neurodevelopmental injury caused by congenital infection, particularly sensorineural hearing loss. Clinical evaluation of vaccines against CMV is now underway. A vaccine using a construct of the glycoprotein B of the virus has been shown to be immunogenic and well tolerated by healthy adults and by children. CMV vaccines, once available, may ultimately be the best control strategy for this public health problem. The most important means of prevention are basic hygiene and handwashing for pregnant women, especially after contact with urine, diapers, oral secretions, and other body fluids. Caregivers should wear gloves, employ good handwashing techniques, and use universal precautions.

NURSING ASSESSMENT

1. See the Respiratory Assessment and Neurologic Assessment sections in Appendix A.
2. Assess nutritional status.
3. Assess developmental level.
4. Assess for history of impaired vision and hearing.

NURSING DIAGNOSES

- Infection, Risk for
- Nutrition: less than body requirements, Imbalanced
- Growth and development, Delayed
- Sensory perception, Disturbed
- Home maintenance, Impaired

NURSING INTERVENTIONS

1. Monitor action and side effects of medications.
2. Monitor response to and side effects of blood transfusions.
3. Review and reinforce with parents importance of maintaining adequate caloric intake.
4. Weigh child upon admission and daily.
5. Monitor urine and serum electrolyte and glucose levels as needed.
6. Assess age and developmental level.
7. Provide age-appropriate stimulation.
8. Promote process of attachment between parents and infant.
9. Identify community resources that may be helpful in dealing with long-term sequelae.

🏠 Discharge Planning and Home Care

1. Instruct parents about methods to prevent spread of infection.
   a. Advise parents of possibility that virus is secreted for more than 1 year.
   b. Pregnant friends should not perform child care (e.g., changing child's diapers).
   c. Care should be taken to perform thorough handwashing after each diaper change and to dispose of diapers properly.
2. Instruct parents about long-term management of condition.
   a. Reinforce information about virus.

b. If neurologic, cognitive, or developmental sequelae are evident, refer for community-based services.
c. Emphasize importance of medical monitoring after an acute episode.

Presence of sequelae will necessitate further interventions beyond the scope of this section.

CLIENT OUTCOMES

1. Child will have consistent weight gain.
2. Child will have maximal level of developmental functioning.
3. Parents will verbalize understanding of child's condition, home care, and follow-up needs.

REFERENCES

American Academy of Pediatrics: Cytomegalovirus infection. In: Pickering LK, editor: *2003 Red book: report of the Committee on Infectious Diseases,* ed 26, Elk Grove Village, Ill, 2003, The Academy.

Griffiths PD, Walter S: Cytomegalovirus, *Curr Opin Infect Dis* 18(3):241, 2005.

Pan ES: Viral infections of the fetus and newborn. In: Taeusch HW, Ballard RA, Gleso CA, editors: *Avery's diseases of the newborn,* ed 8, 2005, Philadelphia, WB Saunders.

Pass RF: Congenital cytomegalovirus infection following first trimester maternal infection: Symptoms at birth and outcome, *J Clin Virol* 35(2):216, 2006.

Schleiss MR: Antiviral therapy of congenital cytomegalovirus infection, *Semin Pediatric Infect Dis* 16(1):50, 2005.

Yudin MH, Gonik B: Perinatal infections. In: Martin RJ, Fanaroff AA, Walsh MC, editors: *Fanaroff and Martin's Neonatal-perinatal medicine: Diseases of the fetus and infant,* ed 8, St. Louis, 2006, Mosby.

19

Diabetes Type 1: Insulin-Dependent

PATHOPHYSIOLOGY

Type 1 diabetes, previously called insulin-dependent diabetes mellitus (IDDM), or juvenile-onset diabetes, is an autoimmune disease that destroys the beta cells of the pancreas, which results in insulin deficiency. Complete insulin deficiency necessitates the use of exogenous insulin to promote appropriate glucose use and to prevent complications related to elevated glucose levels, such as diabetic ketoacidosis and death.

Insulin is necessary for the following physiologic functions: (1) to promote the use and storage of glucose for energy in the liver, muscles, and adipose tissue; (2) to inhibit and stimulate glycogenolysis or gluconeogenesis, depending on the body's requirements; and (3) to promote the use of fatty acids and ketones in cardiac and skeletal muscles. Insulin deficiency results in unrestricted glucose production without appropriate use, which leads to hyperglycemia and increased lipolysis and production of ketones and, in turn, to hyperlipidemia, ketonemia, and ketonuria. The insulin deficiency also heightens the effects of the counterregulatory hormones—epinephrine, glucagon, cortisol, and growth hormone (see Box 19-1 for these hormones' functions).

INCIDENCE

1. Type 1 diabetes accounts for the majority of new diabetes cases in youth.

BOX 19-1
Functions of Counterregulatory Hormones

Epinephrine
- Inhibits uptake of glucose by muscle
- Activates glycogenolysis and gluconeogenesis
- Activates lipolysis, causing release of fatty acids and glycerol

Glucagon
- Promotes production of glucose through glycogenolysis and gluconeogenesis

Cortisol
- Limits glucose use by inhibiting muscle uptake
- Increases glucose production by stimulating gluconeogenesis

Growth Hormones
- Impede glucose uptake

2. The onset most commonly occurs around puberty (ages 10–14 years).
3. Among preschool-aged children, the disease is more commonly diagnosed in boys.
4. Among children 5 to 10 years of age, the disease is more commonly diagnosed in girls.
5. The disease is diagnosed more often in winter than in summer.
6. Diabetic ketoacidosis is a frequent cause of morbidity and sometimes of death.

CLINICAL MANIFESTATIONS
Initial Effects
1. Polyuria
2. Polydipsia
3. Polyphagia
4. Recent weight loss (during a period of less than 3 weeks)
5. Fatigue
6. Headaches
7. Yeast infections in girls
8. Fruity breath odor

9. Dehydration (usually 10% dehydrated)
10. Diabetic ketoacidosis (Box 19-2)—hyperglycemia, ketonemia, ketonuria, metabolic acidosis, Kussmaul respirations
11. Abdominal pain
12. Change in level of consciousness (due to progressive dehydration, acidosis, and hyperosmolality, which results in decreased cerebral oxygenation)

Diagnosis is confirmed by the presence of symptoms combined with an elevated blood glucose level (higher than 200 mg/dl) and glycosuria.

Long-Term Effects

1. Failure to grow at normal rate and delayed maturation
2. Neuropathy
3. Recurrent infection

BOX 19-2
Signs of Diabetic Ketoacidosis

- Kussmaul respirations (deep, sighing respirations)
- Hyperglycemia (serum glucose level higher than 300 mg/dl)
- Ketonuria (moderate to large amounts; positive Ketostix result)
- Metabolic acidosis (pH <7.3; increased partial pressure of carbon dioxide [Pco_2]; decreased partial pressure of oxygen [Po_2]; sodium bicarbonate [$NaHCO_3$] <15 mEq/L)
- Dehydration (as a result of polyuria and polydipsia)
- Fruity breath odor
- Electrolyte imbalance (falsely elevated potassium and sodium levels)
- Potential for life-threatening cardiac arrhythmias (as a result of electrolyte imbalance)
- Cerebral edema (caused by overzealous infusion of fluids)
- Coma (caused by electrolyte imbalance and acidosis)
- Death (infrequent)

Time Periods of Insulin Activity

- AM: Regular insulin works from breakfast to lunch
- AM: Neutral protamine Hagedorn (NPH) works from breakfast to dinner
- PM: Regular insulin works from dinner to bedtime
- PM: NPH works from bedtime to the next morning

4. Retinal and/or renal microvascular disease
5. Ischemic heart disease or arterial obstruction

COMPLICATIONS

1. Diabetic ketoacidosis
2. Coma
3. Hypokalemia and hyperkalemia
4. Hypocalcemia
5. Hypoglycemia
6. Osteopenia
7. Limited joint mobility
8. Microvascular changes resulting in retinopathy (maintaining a high degree of metabolic control is associated with delay in and possible prevention of microvascular changes)
9. Cardiovascular disease
10. Thromboemboli
11. Overwhelming infections

LABORATORY AND DIAGNOSTIC TESTS
For the Individual Newly Diagnosed with Diabetes:

1. Randomly determined plasma glucose level—200 mg/dl or higher
2. Fasting plasma glucose level—higher than or equal to 126 mg/dl
3. Glycosylated hemoglobin (hemoglobin A_{1c}) level—reflects percentage of hemoglobin to which glucose is attached
4. Blood urea nitrogen, creatinine levels—increased because of interference of ketones in measurement
5. Serum calcium, magnesium, phosphate levels—decreased as a result of diuresis
6. Serum electrolyte (potassium [K^+] and sodium [Na^+]) levels—may be falsely elevated as a result of hyperosmolarity
7. Complete blood count—white blood cells may be increased, with predominance of polymorphonuclear lymphocytes
8. Immunoassay—to measure level of C-peptides after glucose challenge (to verify endogenous insulin secretion)

9. Twenty-four-hour urine analysis for glucose—considered a more reliable measure of urine glucose level
10. Urinalysis—glucose in urine

For Diabetic Ketoacidosis:

1. Plasma glucose level—higher than 300 mg/dl
2. Serum bicarbonate ($NaHCO_3$) level—less than 15 mEq/L
3. Arterial pH—less than 7.3
4. Electrocardiogram—increased T wave with hyperkalemia
5. Serum ketone level—higher than 3 mm/L

MEDICAL MANAGEMENT

Children with the initial diagnosis of Type 1 diabetes are usually admitted to the hospital for stabilization and education but may be treated on an outpatient basis. Medical management includes the regulation of serum glucose, fluid, and electrolyte levels. This is accomplished through monitoring of laboratory results, administration of insulin, and intravenous (IV) administration of fluids containing the indicated additives. Secondary problems (i.e., infections) are also treated accordingly. Once glucose levels are stabilized, insulin doses are given to maintain serum glucose level. The management of these children requires a multidisciplinary approach. The child and family need ongoing education and support regarding nutrition, exercise, and daily diabetes self-management.

NURSING ASSESSMENT

1. See the Measurements section in Appendix A.
2. Assess hydration status.
3. Assess for hyperglycemia.
4. Assess for hypoglycemia.
5. Assess dietary patterns.
6. Assess activities and exercise patterns.
7. Assess self-administration of insulin and ability to monitor blood glucose levels.

NURSING DIAGNOSES

- Fluid volume, Deficient
- Infection, Risk for

- Nutrition: less than body requirements, Imbalanced
- Knowledge, Deficient (related to lack of information about the disease)
- Home maintenance, Impaired

NURSING INTERVENTIONS
Diabetic Ketoacidosis

1. Monitor and observe child for change in status of diabetic ketoacidosis (see Box 19-2).
2. Promote child's hydration status.
   a. Accurately record intake, output, and specific gravity.
   b. Monitor for dehydration.
      i. Dry or doughy skin
      ii. Increased specific gravity
      iii. Dry mucous membranes
      iv. Depressed fontanelles (infants)
   c. Monitor for fluid overload.
      i. Decreased specific gravity
      ii. Peripheral edema
   d. Administer and monitor IV solutions as ordered based on laboratory results and clinical appearance. (Saline bolus 10 to 20 ml/kg is usually given before maintenance IV.)
3. Monitor child's glucose level hourly.
   a. Blood glucose level should not fall below 250 mg/dl during the first 12 hours of treatment; glucose level should not fall more than 100 mg/dl/hr, because too rapid a decline in osmolarity predisposes child to cerebral edema.
   b. Regular insulin is preferably administered by IV route for treatment of diabetic ketoacidosis; typically, bolus dose (0.1 units/kg) is given, followed by continuous infusion (0.1 units/kg/hr).
      i. Prime tubing with insulin solution before starting infusion.
      ii. Insulin administration is switched to subcutaneous route once serum glucose level reaches 250 mg/dl, serum pH is 7.35, dehydration is corrected, and child is no longer on nothing-by-mouth status.

    c. Monitor urine for glucose and ketones with each voiding (dipstick).
4. Monitor child's neurologic status hourly until stable.
5. Monitor for signs of complications.
    a. Acidosis
    b. Coma
    c. Hyperkalemia and hypokalemia
    d. Hypocalcemia
    e. Cerebral edema
    f. Hyponatremia

Recovery and Maintenance

1. Monitor and observe for signs of hypoglycemia and hyperglycemia.
2. Promote glucose control.
    a. Monitor urine and blood glucose levels as needed to assess effectiveness of insulin.
    b. Insulin dose is given to maintain serum glucose level; typically, total insulin dose consists of two-thirds neutral protamine Hagedorn (NPH) insulin and one-third regular insulin; two thirds of total dose is administered before breakfast and one third before dinner (Box 19-3).
3. Promote adequate nutritional intake (see Box 19-3 for nutritional recommendations).
4. Monitor and establish appropriate relationship between insulin dose, dietary requirements, and exercise.
5. Provide emotional support to individual and family to promote psychosocial adaptation to diabetes.

🏠 Discharge Planning and Home Care

1. Instruct child and parents about management of diabetes.
    a. Insulin administration
    b. Dietary pattern
    c. Blood glucose monitoring at least 4 times per day
    d. Urine glucose monitoring
    e. Prevention of complications
    f. Care of hypoglycemic and hyperglycemic states

BOX 19-3
Nutritional Requirements in Diabetes

Purpose of Dietary Plan
- The dietary plan provides the necessary intake of calories for energy requirements and appropriate distribution of nutrients (carbohydrates, fats, and proteins).

Energy Requirements
- Carbohydrates: 40% to 60% of total calories
- Fats: 25% to 40% of total calories
- Proteins: 15% to 30% of total calories
- Ratio of polyunsaturated to saturated fat should be at least 2:1. Total daily fat intake should be 42 g.

Dietary Plans
Two exchange systems are used by diabetic individuals: the American Diabetic Association (ADA) exchange group and the British Diabetic Association exchange system.
- The ADA exchange group has six exchange lists, which are for milk, fruit, vegetables, bread, meat, and fat. The exchange lists give the equivalent amounts of calories and nutrients.
- The British Diabetic Association exchange focuses on carbohydrate intake only. A liberal intake of protein is allowed and fats are less restricted. Many children and adolescents prefer carbohydrate counting because it allows for more flexibility in dietary management than the exchange system.

General Information
- Foods high in fiber retard carbohydrate absorption.
- Foods have different glycemic responses (glycemic index).
- Long periods between eating must be avoided.
- Extra food must be consumed for increased activity (10 to 15 g of carbohydrate for every 30 to 45 minutes of activity).
- Quantity of food needed between meals will vary according to increase or decrease in physical activity.

    g. Skin care
    h. Activity regimen
    i. Illness management

2. The onset most commonly occurs around puberty (ages 10–14 years).
3. Type 2 diabetes occurs disproportionately in American Indian, African American, Mexican American, and Pacific Islander youth.
4. Type 2 diabetes accounts for up to half of all diagnosed cases of diabetes in children and adolescents.

CLINICAL MANIFESTATIONS

1. Fatigue
2. Blurry vision
3. Frequent urination
4. Yeast infections in girls
5. Hypertension
6. Elevated low-density lipoproteins (LDLs) and triglycerides
7. Polycystic ovary syndrome
8. Acanthosis nigricans—velvety patches of skin that most often occur where skin bends or rubs together

COMPLICATIONS

1. Hypertension
2. Dyslipidemia
3. Obstructive sleep apnea as a result of increased weight

LABORATORY AND DIAGNOSTIC TESTS

For the individual newly diagnosed with diabetes, the following tests are indicated:

1. Randomly determined plasma glucose level—200 mg/dl or higher
2. Fasting plasma glucose level—higher than or equal to 126 mg/dl

Prediabetes is diagnosed for children with fasting glucose levels of 100 mg/dl to 125 mg/dl

MEDICAL MANAGEMENT

Children with the initial diagnosis of Type 2 diabetes do not require insulin injections, because the pancreas is still producing insulin. The focus of therapy is to decrease insulin resistance. This is done through increased exercise and healthier eating. Should this therapy regimen prove to be ineffective, then medications and/or insulin therapy may be needed. At this time, the only approved oral medication for children aged 10 years and older is metformin (Glucophage). If ineffective to reduce glucose levels, insulin may be used. The management of these children requires a multidisciplinary approach for lifestyle changes. Hypertension is managed with weight management, reduced sodium intake, and increased intake of fruits and vegetables. If unsuccessful, blood pressure medications are used. Hyperlipidemia should improve with increased exercise, weight loss, and glucose control. Additional serum lipid screening is done at diagnosis and every 2 years afterward. The goal is keep atherogenic LDL cholesterol below 100 mg/dl, protective high-density lipoproteins (HDLs) above 35 mg/dl, and triglycerides below 150 mg/dl. The child and family need ongoing education and support regarding nutrition, exercise, and daily diabetes self-management. To evaluate the effectiveness of the necessary lifestyle changes, blood glucose levels are monitored regularly.

NURSING ASSESSMENT

1. See the Measurements section in Appendix A.
2. Assess for hyperglycemia.
3. Assess for hypoglycemia.
4. Assess dietary patterns.
5. Assess activities and exercise patterns.

NURSING DIAGNOSES

- Nutrition: more than body requirements, Imbalanced
- Knowledge, Deficient (related to lack of information about the disease)
- Home maintenance, Impaired

NURSING INTERVENTIONS

1. Institute a healthy diet to manage weight.
    a. Focus on healthy eating as opposed to placing child on a diet.
    b. Avoid high calorie foods and snacks.
    c. Use appropriately sized portions.
    d. Substitute water for juice and soda.

2. Blood glucose monitoring
3. Encourage exercise
   a. Thirty minutes of aerobic exercise daily
   b. Make exercise a family activity
   c. Limit television and videogame time
4. Use age-appropriate written materials to facilitate learning.
   a. Disease overview
   b. Lifestyle changes: eating and exercise needs
5. Involve entire family in lifestyle changes

🏠 Discharge Planning and Home Care

1. Institute lifestyle changes throughout the entire family.
   a. Eating habits
   b. Exercise
2. Routine health assessments to include height and weight assessments
3. Routine blood glucose monitoring

CLIENT OUTCOMES

1. Child will achieve normal growth and development.
2. Child will maintain normal serum glucose levels.
3. Child and family will demonstrate care required at home and have support system in place.
4. Child will have minimal complications: hypertension, hyperlipidemia, neuropathy, nephropathy, and retinopathy.

REFERENCES

Berman RE, Kliegman RM, Jenson HH, editors: *Nelson textbook of pediatrics,* ed 17, Philadelphia, 2004, WB Saunders.

Law T: Type 2 diabetes mellitus in youth, *Adv for Nurses* (Florida edition) 7(8):13, 2006.

Scott LK: Insulin resistance syndrome in children, *Pediatr Nurs* 32(2):119, 2006.

Thomassian BD: Type 2 diabetes among youth reaches epidemic proportions, *Nurs Spectrum* (Florida edition) 14(24):22, 2004.

Children's Health-Related Websites

www.KeepKidsHealthy.com
www.NutritionForKids.com
www.Kidnetic.com
www.YourChildsHealth.com/Nutrition.html

21

Down Syndrome

PATHOPHYSIOLOGY

Down syndrome, the most common chromosomal condition that results in intellectual disabilities, is associated with an extra chromosome on chromosome 21. Current genetic studies have found that this chromosome consists of 329 genes. Understanding how these genes work will provide a real opportunity to understand how this condition occurs and how the characteristics of this condition result.

Down syndrome may occur by one of three mechanisms: a free trisomy or nondisjunction (about 95% of cases), translocation (about 3% to 5%), or mosaicism (about 1% to 2%). Free trisomy or nondisjunction occurs when three copies of chromosome 21 result in 100% of the cells. This situation arises from an unequal distribution of chromosomes in anaphase 1 or 2 during meiosis or in the anaphase of mitosis. The phenotype for nondisjunction and translocation is the same.

Nondisjunction occurs by maternal meiotic origin in approximately 90% of cases; it results in three copies of chromosome 21. Nondisjunction usually occurs spontaneously and is not familial. Approximately 8% of cases are caused by paternal factors, most often advanced paternal age, of 55 years or older. Factors that can influence the occurrence of nondisjunction Down syndrome are maternal age, earlier menopause, and gene polymorphisms that influence folate metabolism.

Translocation happens when all or part of a chromosome is exchanged with another chromosome. This can result in a balanced or unbalanced translocation, depending upon the amount of chromosomal material involved. In Down syndrome, translocations are unbalanced; the most common combination of chromosomes involved is 14 and 21 (14;21), followed by both copies of the chromosome 21 (21;21). In 75% of all cases of unbalanced translocations, the cause is not familial, but it is in 25% of the cases. The cause is considered to be multifactorial and independent of parental age.

Mosaicism is characterized by the absence of trisomy (three copies) of chromosome 21 in 100% of the cell lines. This form of Down syndrome is most frequently caused by maternal meiotic nondisjunction. Individuals with mosaic Down syndrome have fewer phenotypic features. Diagnosis of the genotype of Down syndrome is made through a chromosome analysis (American Academy of Pediatrics Committee on Genetics, 2001; Lashley, 2005).

There are many physical features of Down syndrome, also called the phenotype, that do not exist in every child who has the condition. Presence or absence of a physical feature usually does not indicate severity of the condition. The exception is the degree of mental retardation, which would affect developmental outcomes. For information on the complications and secondary problems associated with Down syndrome, refer to Complications in this chapter.

INCIDENCE

1. The incidence of Down syndrome is approximately 1 in 800 live births, and the prevalence is generally accepted to be 1 in 650 to 1000 live births.
2. The availability of prenatal diagnosis, especially in women of advanced maternal age, has influenced these figures.
3. The incidence of having a child with Down syndrome for a woman in her twenties is approximately 1 in 2000 live births. This figure increases to approximately 34 in every 1000 live births for the woman who is age 45.
4. Down syndrome may occur three ways: nondisjunction, translocation, or mosaicism.
5. Down syndrome is found in all ethnic groups and races. Incidences are higher in Hispanic and African American mothers who are age 35 years and older.

6. The risk of recurrence varies by the type of transmission.
   a. In general, the recurrence risk for nondisjunction Down syndrome is approximately 1%.
   b. In translocation Down syndrome, the recurrence risk is approximately 10% if the translocation was 14;21, and if the translocation carrier was the father, the recurrence risk is approximately 5%. If the translocation was 21;21, the recurrence risk is 100%.
   c. The risk of recurrence of mosaic Down syndrome is extremely rare.

CLINICAL MANIFESTATIONS

1. Down syndrome is diagnosed at birth because of distinctive phenotype, but confirmed by karyotype (see more under Laboratory and Diagnostic Tests in this chapter).
2. Visual diagnosis may be more difficult in newborns of color since the phenotypic characteristics may not be obvious and other signs such as Mongolian spots, common in African Americans, may not be identified as part of a syndrome.
3. There are more than 50 characteristic features of Down syndrome occurring on the skull, the eyes, the ears, the nose, the mouth, the neck, the chest, the abdomen, and the extremities, and affecting physical growth and development in all domains. No one feature is diagnostic, and not every characteristic feature is present in any one person with Down syndrome.
4. The most common features are generalized hypotonia, mental retardation, incurved fifth finger, simian crease, flattened occipital, small nose with flat nasal bridge, epicanthic folds, Brushfield's spots, absent Moro reflex, wide spaces between the first and second toes, hearing impairment, ocular problems, thyroid problems, dental problems, and/or orthodontic problems.

COMPLICATIONS

1. Premature aging is present and affects development throughout life; early-onset Alzheimer's disease may be a factor.

2. Congenital anomalies that occur with greater frequency in Down syndrome include congenital cardiac disease (endocardial cushion defects and septal defects most common), gastrointestinal malformations (duodenal or esophageal atresia and congenital megacolon most common), celiac disease, and leukemia (transient myeloproliferative disorder, in particular).

3. Mental health problems: behavioral problems, depression, and/or attention deficit hyperactivity disorder (ADHD) can also occur in children with Down syndrome (Crocker, 2006; Lashley, 2005; Nehring, 2004).

LABORATORY AND DIAGNOSTIC TESTS

1. The best practice to obtain an accurate diagnosis is to offer pregnancy screening by blood test for chromosomal anomalies and neural tube defects, followed by cytogenic diagnosis. This combination serum test, often called a quadruple screen, includes alpha fetoprotein, human chorionic gonadotropin, unconjugated estriol, and dimeric inhibin-A in maternal serum. This blood test is done during weeks 16 to 18 of pregnancy. Researchers are currently examining the use of the quadruple screen with a fetal ultrasound for nuchal translucency during gestational week 11 and adding the quadruple screen during the second trimester for confirmation, as a more efficacious screening protocol.

2. Invasive screening tests include chorionic villi sampling during gestational week 12 and amniocentesis during week 16.

3. Diagnosis of Down syndrome is made through chromosome analysis.

4. Ocular defects are common; the child with Down syndrome should see an ophthalmologist by 6 months of age and then, beginning around age 3 years, every 2 years. Vision should be checked yearly.

5. Auditory defects are also common. Auditory brainstem response testing should be completed by 3 months of age, followed by evaluation by a specialist every 6 months up through age 3 years and annually thereafter.

6. Otoscopy and tympanometry should be done at each visit by the specialist.
7. Periodontal disease is common, so the child with Down syndrome should see a dentist every 6 months beginning at age 18 months.
8. A full cardiac evaluation should be completed in infancy, with follow-up as needed according to occurrence of cardiac conditions.
9. Thyroid-stimulating hormone levels should be measured at 6 and 12 months and annually thereafter, since thyroid dysfunction is a common condition.
10. Children with Down syndrome should first be checked for atlantoaxial instability between 3 and 5 years and then as needed before athletic involvement.
11. The risk for hip dislocation is present, so the child should be checked for this condition during well-child visits through 10 years of age and if a gait abnormality is present.
12. Because of the risk of mitral value prolapse, this condition should be checked for, beginning in adolescence.
13. IgA-antiendomysium antibodies of immunoglobulin A class should be assessed when the child is between 2 and 3 years old because of the higher prevalence of celiac disease.

MEDICAL MANAGEMENT

At present, it is not possible to reverse Down syndrome and cure this condition through treatment(s) of the genetic cause. Medical advancements, genetic discoveries, and interdisciplinary best practices in recent years have directed current standards of practice, which include genetic counseling, treatment and/or surgical correction of congenital anomalies and sensory defects, prevention and/or maintenance of secondary conditions, participation in early intervention programs, and inclusion in school settings from ages 3 through 21 years. An interdisciplinary approach, based on best practices, is recommended to (a) treat or correct congenital anomalies and sensory defects; (b) prevent periodontal disease and obesity; (c) prevent or maintain secondary conditions such as arthritis, atlantoaxial instability, behavior problems, celiac disease, constipation, dermatologic problems, diabetes, feeding problems, leukemia, obstructive sleep apnea, seizures, sensory defects, thyroid dysfunction, and/or upper respiratory infections; and (d) provide sex education and assess for contraception needs in adolescence. Alternative therapies such as use of piracetam, nutritional supplements, human growth hormone therapy, and antioxidants should not be prescribed, since current research evidence has not found these therapies to be beneficial or efficacious (American Academy of Pediatrics Committee on Genetics, 2001; Cohen, 1999).

NURSING ASSESSMENT

1. Assess for feeding problems.
2. Assess for sleep disorders.
3. Assess growth and development, and refer as needed to other disciplines.
4. Assess child's ability to perform age-appropriate self-care skills.
5. Assess child's ability to get along with others, make friends, and participate in social activities.
6. Assess child's and adolescent's school experiences.
7. Assess child's and adolescent's exercise habits.
8. Assess presence of "self-talk" in older child and adolescent.
9. Assess knowledge of condition and its effect on child's and adolescent's life.
10. Assess sexual knowledge and need for contraception during adolescence.
11. Assess for behavioral problems, ADHD, and/or depression (especially in adolescence).
12. Assess for health-related self-care skills, vocational skills, and ability to live independently during adolescence in preparation for transition to adulthood.
13. Assess for need for guardianship once the age of majority is reached during adolescence.
14. Assess parental response to birth of infant with Down syndrome. Throughout childhood and adolescence, assess meaning of child to parents and impact on their life.
15. Assess whether parents' expectations for their child are developmentally age-appropriate.

16. Assess parents' understanding of the condition throughout their child's life.
17. Assess the impact of the child with Down syndrome on siblings and other family members.
18. Assess cultural and religious influences on family responses and impact of having a family member with Down syndrome.
19. The nurse should assess his or her own feelings and attitudes toward caring for a child with an intellectual disability and providing education, support, and advocacy to family members.

NURSING DIAGNOSES

- Breastfeeding, Ineffective
- Caregiver role strain, Risk for
- Communication, Impaired verbal
- Growth and development, Delayed
- Infection, Risk for
- Nutrition, more than body requirements, Risk for imbalanced
- Self-care deficit, Bathing/Hygiene
- Self-care deficit, Dressing/Grooming
- Self-care deficit, Feeding
- Self-care deficit, Toileting
- Self-esteem, Risk for situational low
- Skin integrity, Risk for impaired
- Social interaction, Impaired
- Sorrow, Chronic

NURSING INTERVENTIONS
Infancy, Toddler, Preschool

1. Assist mothers if breastfeeding, or parents if bottle feeding, if hypotonia affects sucking ability. Different strategies may be suggested, such as more frequent and shorter feedings. Blended or chopped foods may be needed when solid foods are introduced. If aspiration or serious problems occur, an occupational therapist should be consulted or a referral made.
2. Assist the parents and siblings in making a realistic appraisal of what the infant with Down syndrome should

be expected to do and when. Together, across time, identify the child's strengths and limitations.

3. Identify formal and informal supports available to the parents, and suggest that they visit with a member of a local Down syndrome support group.

4. Monitor growth and development using Down syndrome growth charts.

5. Refer parents to area early intervention programs.

6. Serve as child and parent advocate in individualized family service plan (IFSP) meetings (refer to Appendix G).

7. Inform parents about federal and state laws affecting children with intellectual disabilities.

8. Provide anticipatory guidance to the parents for typical infant milestones, and provide information on average ages for infants with Down syndrome based on research literature.

9. Use a life-span approach to providing anticipatory guidance on child's developmental milestones.

10. Advise parents that toilet training will be delayed; the median age is 3 years. Normal methods of training may be used.

11. Encourage parents to use discipline methods that are developmentally appropriate. Parents should not be overly protective or allow their child to be manipulative because of having Down syndrome.

12. Assist parents in finding a medical "home" if their current pediatrician has not had experience in caring for a child with Down syndrome.

13. Monitor for constipation. Use age-appropriate treatment methods.

14. Teach parents about common secondary conditions for infants. In infancy, this includes eye, ear, heart, intestinal, and upper respiratory conditions. Discuss additional screening and testing that will be done for the infant and child with Down syndrome to check for these conditions.

15. Refer for sleep study, if symptoms of sleep apnea appear.

16. Discuss alternative and complementary treatments with parents, and provide up-to-date information on the value

of each type of method. There is no cure for Down syndrome, and parents must sometimes be assisted to understand why something may or may not work. This discussion could also include the use of plastic surgery to make the child "appear more normal."

17. Provide up-to-date information and relevant references including Internet sites as needed.

Childhood

1. Monitor impact of parenting and living with a child with Down syndrome on each parent and sibling.

2. Assist family as needed in finding insurance, dental care, and other, related services.

3. Ask parents if they have any questions about appropriate developmental milestones, behavior, or health concerns. Follow through as needed with further assessment or referral.

4. Monitor growth and development. In particular, screen the child's expressive and receptive language skills. Refer to speech therapist if necessary.

5. Encourage parents to enroll child in inclusive child care setting, preferably one that has had previous experience with a child with Down syndrome.

6. Refer to inclusive preschool for 3- to 5-year-olds, and assist parents, if necessary, to interview school officials and teachers to make sure child's academic needs are met. Serve as an advocate for the child and parents in individualized education plan (IEP) and individualized health plan (IHP) meetings.

7. Assist parents with choosing an appropriate school system that provides for inclusive education. Nurses can assist in educating parents on federal laws concerning the education of children with intellectual disabilities.

8. Monitor child's diet, and provide nutritional education as needed. Referral to a nutritionist may be needed, especially if celiac disease is diagnosed, necessitating a gluten-free diet.

9. Monitor presence of secondary conditions, including behavioral and mental health issues, and intervene as needed.
10. Allow child to be a partner in making decisions about needed health care. Such planning should be centered on the persons involved, not on the requirements of the health care system.
11. Assist the child and parents to identify community programs, such as Boy and Girl Scouts, 4-H, YMCA, Special Olympics, music-related programs, based upon their individual needs, interests, and preferences.

Adolescence

1. Ascertain parents' goals and plans for adolescent and his or her transition to adulthood.
2. Identify differences between adolescent's and parents' goals and plans, and discuss with all. Make appropriate plans for transition, including participating in the development and implementation of the adolescent's individualized transition plan (ITP), and collaborate as needed with other professionals.
3. Discuss school experiences, especially during junior high or middle school, since this time period appears to be the most difficult for this age group. Teasing is a frequent complaint among persons in this age group who have disabilities.
4. Monitor presence of any secondary conditions and adherence with treatment. Adolescents should be as responsible as possible with their own health. Reinforcement of proper techniques or education should be provided as needed.
5. Be aware of diagnostic overshadowing, which occurs when a health professional attributes health-related signs and symptoms to Down syndrome and not to the underlying cause. An example is a complaint of "feeling down and sad," or depressed, being attributed to having Down syndrome, as opposed to the professional probing and finding out that the adolescent just broke up with a boyfriend.

6. Provide any needed sexual education and information about contraception. Discuss risks of having a child with Down syndrome, should the female adolescent with Down syndrome become pregnant. May refer adolescent to program that discusses these topics.

7. Discuss with adolescent and parents that "self-talk" (talking to self out loud) is often present in adolescents with Down syndrome, and teach when this behavior is appropriate.

8. Assist adolescent to become own health self-advocate.

9. Plan for transition to adult medical care that includes selection of adult medical providers.

10. Monitor adolescent's diet. Discuss proper nutrition. Watch for signs and symptoms of overweight and obesity.

11. Identify regular inclusive social interactions such as sports and social clubs.

12. Identify area self-advocacy groups, and assist adolescent to determine whether to participate in such groups.

13. Identify adolescent's goals and plans for the future, including school, work, residential settings, and lifelong care.

🏠 Discharge Planning and Home Care

1. Make appropriate referrals to professionals and agencies for specific health-related and service-related needs.

2. Family members should be referred to appropriate community agencies for insurance, recreation, respite, counseling, and/or supportive services.

3. Facilitate transition into different settings throughout childhood, such as early intervention, preschool, school, recreational, and health care agencies.

4. Facilitate parents' understanding of developmental milestones and realistic expectations for a child with Down syndrome. In turn, assist child and adolescent with Down syndrome to set their own realistic goals and meet them.

5. Facilitate parents' ability to become advocates for their child and the adolescent's ability to become a self-advocate in relation to health and all other facets of life.

6. Provide coordination of services and communication between services, as needed, to serve as a resource to parents for "the total picture."

CLIENT OUTCOMES

1. Child or adolescent will grow up in a supportive and educated environment.
2. Child or adolescent with Down syndrome will have a positive impact on and meaning for all who interact with him or her, as well as a positive self-meaning.
3. Child or adolescent will experience inclusive settings throughout childhood in the least restrictive environment possible.
4. Child and adolescent will meet IEP objectives and annual goals.
5. Parents and adolescent will be adept at identifying needs and accessing needed resources.
6. Adolescent will become an educated health advocate.
7. Adolescent will graduate from high school and enter further education or obtain employment in an area of his or her interest.
8. Adolescent will have a satisfactory social life, which includes mobility and independence.
9. Plans will be identified for care of adolescent across the life span, including residential choices, insurance, primary health care providers, and finances.
10. Make sure that outcomes correspond to the nursing diagnoses and interventions listed in this chapter.

REFERENCES

American Academy of Pediatrics Committee on Genetics: Health supervision for children with Down syndrome, *Pediatrics* 107(2):442, 2001.

Bosch JJ: Health maintenance throughout the life span for individuals with Down syndrome, *J Am Acad Nurse Pract* 15(1):5, 2003.

Capone GT: Down syndrome: Advances in molecular biology and the neurosciences, *J Devel Behavior Pediatr* 22(1):4059, 2001.

Cohen WI, editor: Health care guidelines for individuals with Down syndrome: 1999 revision, *Down Syndrome Quarterly* (serial online): www.denison.edn/collaborations/dsq/health99.html. Accessed May 10, 2004.

Crocker AC: Down syndrome. In: Rubin IL, Crocker AC, editors: *Medical care for children & adults with developmental disabilities,* ed 2, Baltimore, 2006, Paul H Brookes.

Day SM et al: Mortality and causes of death in persons with Down syndrome in California, *Devel Med Child Neurol* 47(3):171, 2005.

Hecht CA, Hook EB: Rates of Down syndrome at live birth at one-year maternal age intervals in studies with apparent close to complete ascertainment in populations of European origin: A proposed revised rate schedule for use in genetic and prenatal screening, *Am J Med Genet* 62(4):376, 1996.

Lashley FR: *Clinical genetics in nursing practice,* ed 3, New York, 2005, Springer.

Nehring WM: Down syndrome. In: Aller PJ, Vessey JA, editors: *Primary care of the child with a chronic condition,* ed 4, St. Louis, 2004, Mosby.

Palomaki GE, Bradley LA, McDowell GA: Down Syndrome working Group, ACMG Laboratory Quality Assurance Committee: Technical standards and guidelines: Prenatal screening for Down syndrome, *Genet Med* 7(5):344, 2005.

Roizen NJ: Complementary and alternative therapies for Down syndrome, *Mental Retardation Devel Disabil Res Rev* 11(2):149, 2005.

Roizen NJ, Patterson D: Down's syndrome, *Lancet* 361(9365):1281, 2003.

Tolmie JL: Down syndrome and other autosomal trisomies. In: Rimoin DL, et al, editors: *Emery and Rimoin's principles and practices of medical genetics,* ed 4, New York, 2002, Churchill Livingstone.

Wenstrom KD: Evaluation of Down syndrome screening strategies, *Semin Perinatol* 29(4):219, 2005.

Yang Q, Rasmussen SA, Friedman JM: Mortality associated with Down's syndrome in the USA from 1983–1997: A population-based study, *Lancet* 359 (9311):1019, 2002.

FURTHER READING

Aitken DA, Crossley JA, Spencer K: Prenatal screening for neural tube defects and aneuploidy. In: Rimoin DL et al, editors: *Emery and Rimoin's principles and practices of medical genetics,* ed 4, New York, 2002, Churchill Livingstone.

Malone FD et al: First-trimester or second-trimester screening, or both, for Down's syndrome, *N Engl J Med* 353(19):2001, 2005.

Morris JK et al: Risk of a Down syndrome live birth in women 45 years of age and older, *Prenatal Diagnosis* 25(4):275, 2005.

22

Drowning and Near-Drowning

PATHOPHYSIOLOGY

Each year, between 4000 and 5000 people drown in the United States, and the number of near-drownings is estimated to be 3 to 4 times that figure. Drowning is defined as death from asphyxia while submerged, or within 24 hours of submersion. Near-drowning occurs when the child survives longer than 24 hours after submersion, regardless of the final outcome.

The physiologic events that occur after submersion are sequential. After the initial panic and struggle, victims will hold their breath, and some will swallow a small amount of water, vomit, then aspirate the vomitus. Laryngospasm follows, which leads to hypoxia and death (dry drowning). In most children laryngospasm occurs initially; this leads to hypoxia, which causes cardiac arrest and relaxation of the airway, so that the lungs are permitted to fill with large amounts of water (wet drowning). Regardless of whether the child aspirates water, hypoxia is the most important physiologic consequence of submersion injuries and affects all organ systems. Submersion also results in hypothermia. The child's relatively large body surface area leads to a rapid decrease in body temperature when the child is in cold water. Severe hypothermia in young children may protect the brain when the diving reflex occurs, causing bradycardia and shunting of blood away from the periphery and thereby increasing the cerebral and coronary circulation.

Prognosis is affected by a variety of factors, such as duration of submersion, extent of hypothermia, physiologic response of the victim, and length of time until effective cardiopulmonary resuscitation is provided. Irreversible brain damage usually occurs after 4 to 6 minutes of submersion, but some children have experienced complete recovery after a much longer period (10 to 30 minutes) in very cold water. Morbidity and death are directly related to the degree of neuronal damage.

INCIDENCE

1. Drowning is the second leading cause of accidental death in children.
2. Preschool children and teenagers have the highest risk for drowning and near-drowning.
3. Boys are 5 times more likely to drown than girls.
4. Peak incidence is during summer months, on weekends, and between 4 pm and 6 pm.
5. Most drownings occur in residential swimming pools.
6. Younger children most often drown in pools, bathtubs, hot tubs, toilets, and buckets.
7. Older children most often drown in lakes, rivers, and oceans while boating or diving, or in association with alcohol ingestion.

CLINICAL MANIFESTATIONS

Clinical manifestations are directly related to the extent of injury and level of consciousness following rescue and resuscitation.

1. Respiratory distress—ranging from rapid, shallow breathing to apnea
2. Cyanosis
3. Pink, frothy sputum
4. Pulmonary edema
5. Flaccidity
6. Decorticate or decerebrate posturing
7. Coma
8. Seizures
9. Shock
10. Arterial blood gas abnormalities
11. Abnormal chest radiographic studies
12. Arrhythmias

13. Metabolic acidosis
14. Hyperkalemia
15. Hyperglycemia
16. Hypothermia

COMPLICATIONS

1. Hypoxic encephalopathy
2. Aspiration pneumonia
3. Pulmonary interstitial fibrosis
4. Ventricular arrhythmias
5. Renal failure
6. Disseminated intravascular coagulation
7. Pancreatic necrosis
8. Infection

LABORATORY AND DIAGNOSTIC TESTS

1. Chest radiographic study—variable findings (from scattered parenchymal infiltrates to extensive pulmonary edema)
2. Arterial blood gas values—to detect respiratory and metabolic acidosis
3. Electroencephalogram—to assess seizure activity and document brain death
4. Complete blood count, hematocrit, hemoglobin—to determine extent of hemodilution or hemoconcentration and need for fluid resuscitation
5. Serum electrolyte levels—to determine need to correct any imbalances caused by submersion
6. Blood urea nitrogen level—to determine renal function
7. Creatinine clearance—to determine renal function
8. Blood culture and sensitivity—to detect superimposed respiratory infection

MEDICAL MANAGEMENT

Aggressive basic and advanced life support at the scene is essential, because the full extent of the central nervous system injury cannot be accurately assessed at the time of rescue. Ensuring an adequate airway, breathing, and circulation is the top priority. Other injuries must be considered, and the need for hospitalization is determined by the severity of the event and clinical evaluation. Individuals with respiratory symptoms, decreased oxygen saturation, and altered level of consciousness must be admitted to the hospital. Ongoing attention to oxygenation, ventilation, and cardiac function is the priority. Protecting the central nervous system and reducing cerebral edema are of paramount importance and directly relate to outcome.

Treatments used include high-flow oxygen therapy and positive end-expiratory pressure for adequate oxygenation; administration of crystalloid solution for fluid resuscitation; dopamine and dobutamine for cardiac therapy; furosemide (Lasix) for diuresis; and mannitol (Mannitor) for control of intracranial hypertension and for sedation.

NURSING ASSESSMENT

1. See the Respiratory Assessment section in Appendix A.
2. Assess for spontaneous respirations.
3. Assess cardiovascular status.
4. Assess core temperature.
5. Assess for level of consciousness.
6. See the Neurologic Assessment section in Appendix A.

NURSING DIAGNOSES

- Gas exchange, Impaired
- Cardiac output, Decreased
- Tissue perfusion, Ineffective (related to cerebral insult)
- Fluid volume, Excess
- Hypothermia
- Nutrition: less than body requirements, Imbalanced
- Family processes, Interrupted

NURSING INTERVENTIONS

1. Monitor respiratory system.
   a. Assess respiratory status, including breath sounds and work of breathing.
   b. Maintain patent airway.
   c. Suction airway as needed.
   d. Insert nasogastric tube to prevent aspiration.
   e. Monitor oxygen therapy.
   f. Monitor oxygen level.

2. Monitor cardiovascular system.
   a. Assess cardiovascular status, including vital signs, perfusion, skin temperature and color, and urine output.
   b. Monitor fluid lines and fluid resuscitation efforts.
3. Monitor and record child's level of neurologic functioning.
   a. Perform neurologic assessment (frequency depends on status).
   b. Observe and report signs of increased intracranial pressure (IICP) (lethargy, increased blood pressure, decreased respiratory rate, increased apical pulse, dilated pupils).
   c. Prevent IICP by positioning head at midline, elevating head of bed 30 degrees, and preventing or managing elevated body temperature.
4. Monitor and maintain fluid balance.
   a. Record intake and output.
   b. Maintain patency of and care for Foley catheter.
   c. Maintain fluids as ordered.
      Observe for signs and symptoms of alteration in fluid balance, including performing laboratory testing.
5. Monitor and maintain homeostatic temperature regulation.
   a. Monitor temperature.
   b. Initiate and continue rewarming techniques, including use of warming lights, warm mattress, and warm intravenous fluids.
   c. Check skin perfusion.
6. Provide and maintain adequate nutritional intake.
   a. Assess nutritional status.
   b. Assess child's capacity to tolerate nasogastric or oral feedings (monitor weight, and check for residuals and vomiting).
   c. If total parenteral nutrition is ordered, monitor infusion, side effects, and blood chemistry results.
7. Provide emotional and other support to family.
   a. Provide calm reassurance and realistic progress reports of child's status, including hope.
   b. Provide for physical needs of family such as privacy and access to bathroom and telephone, and identify a staff member to contact with questions.
   c. Explain all treatments.

d. Allow parents and family members to be with child
   as appropriate.

🏠 Discharge Planning and Home Care

1. Instruct parents about instituting preventive measures:
   learning cardiopulmonary resuscitation; providing water
   safety and swimming lessons for child; accident-proofing
   backyard (e.g., pool cover, fence enclosures); and
   appropriately supervising children during pool use.
2. Instruct parents regarding developmental level of child and
   safety issues.
3. Instruct parents on follow-up care.

CLIENT OUTCOMES

1. Child will return to optimal level of neurologic function.
2. Respiratory distress will be reduced or eliminated.
3. Child will maintain adequate perfusion, and vital signs will
   be within normal ranges.

REFERENCES

Behrman RE, Kiegman R, Jenson HB, editors: *Nelson textbook of pediatrics,*
ed 17, Philadelphia, 2004, WB Saunders.
Burford A et al: Drowning and near-drowning in children and adolescents:
A succinct review for emergency physicians and nurses, *Pediatr Emerg Care*
21(9):610, 2005.
Hockenberry M et al: *Wong's nursing care of infants and children,* ed 7, St. Louis,
2004, Mosby.
Lassman J: Injury prevention. *Water safety, J Emerg Nurs* 28(3):241, 2002.

23

Epiglottitis

PATHOPHYSIOLOGY

Epiglottitis is an acute bacterial infection of the epiglottis and the surrounding areas (the aryepiglottic folds and the supraglottic area) that causes airway obstruction. The infection is caused by *Haemophilus influenzae* type B or, on rare occasions, by staphylococci, streptococci, pneumococci, or *Candida albicans*. The use of *H. influenzae* type B vaccine in infants has resulted in a dramatic reduction in the incidence of epiglottitis. Onset is sudden, and infection progresses rapidly, causing acute respiratory difficulty. This condition requires emergency airway stabilization and medical measures, since a complete airway obstruction may occur due to swelling of the epiglottis. If left untreated, the outcome can be fatal.

INCIDENCE

1. Children under the age of 2 are most often affected.
2. Incidence is highest in winter, but infection can occur anytime.

CLINICAL MANIFESTATIONS

1. Respiratory difficulty, which can progress to severe respiratory distress in a matter of minutes or hours (dyspnea)
2. Dysphagia, constant drooling
3. Inspiratory stridor
4. Edematous, cherry-red epiglottis
5. Sore throat
6. Breathing in upright position with head extended forward (classic "tripod" position)

7. High fever
8. Muffled voice
9. Pale color
10. Substernal or suprasternal and intercostal retractions
11. Bilateral cervical adenitis

COMPLICATIONS

1. Airway obstruction
2. Laryngospasm
3. Death

LABORATORY AND DIAGNOSTIC TESTS

1. Oxygen saturation—decrease in the amount of oxygen
2. Arterial blood gas values—decreased pH, decreased partial pressure of oxygen (Po_2), increased partial pressure of carbon dioxide (Pco_2)
3. Lateral neck radiographic study—to confirm diagnosis. The epiglottis will be swollen, and the hypopharynx will be dilated. This is known as the "thumb" sign.
4. Throat and blood cultures—to rule out other bacterial infections
5. Direct laryngoscopy—to confirm diagnosis; performed in operating room to prevent complications

MEDICAL MANAGEMENT

Children suspected of having epiglottitis should be examined where personnel and equipment are available for an emergency tracheal intubation or tracheostomy. Visual examination of the throat is contraindicated until this requirement is met. Keep child as calm and comfortable as possible. Lateral neck radiographic studies may help confirm the diagnosis but should be performed in the least distressing manner possible, usually with the child being held in the parent's lap. Endotracheal intubation or tracheostomy is performed in the operating room along with blood draws for laboratory testing, collection of throat culture specimen, and placement of intravenous lines. The child is observed in the intensive care area until swelling of the epiglottis decreases, usually by the third day. Antibiotics are given for a total of 7 to 10 days following extubation.

The child is extubated when the epiglottis appears normal and the child is able to breathe around the tube (usually 48 to 72 hours after antibiotic treatment is started).

NURSING ASSESSMENT

Caution: Do not examine the throat if epiglottitis is suspected because of the risk of reflex laryngospasm, which will result in complete airway obstruction.

1. See the Respiratory Assessment section in Appendix A.
2. Assess hydration status.
3. Assess anxiety level.

NURSING DIAGNOSES

- Suffocation, Risk for
- Airway clearance, Ineffective
- Breathing pattern, Ineffective
- Tissue perfusion, Ineffective
- Anxiety
- Family processes, Interrupted

NURSING INTERVENTIONS

1. Monitor respiratory status (including vital signs).
   a. Temperature, apical pulse, respiratory rate, blood pressure
   b. Presence of inspiratory stridor
   c. Presence of intercostal retractions
   d. Presence of circumoral cyanosis
   e. Use of accessory muscles
   f. Ability to handle oral secretions
   g. Oxygen saturation—noninvasive monitoring
   h. Arterial blood gas values—defer until child is in operating room
2. Observe and report signs of increased respiratory distress or changes in respiratory status.
3. Maintain position of comfort and security for child, to facilitate breathing (usually upright in parent's lap). Never leave child unattended.
4. Prepare child preoperatively for airway insertion (endotracheal tube or tracheostomy) if condition allows.

5. Assist and support physician during emergency procedure.
   a. Ventilate through bag-valve-mask if child experiences obstruction of breathing before reaching operating room.
   b. Observe and monitor respiratory status during intubation.
6. Maintain patency of airway and ventilator function.
7. Provide tracheostomy care (if tracheostomy is performed).
   a. Maintain patent airway.
   b. Monitor cardiopulmonary status.
   c. Use aseptic technique when suctioning.
   d. Clean tracheostomy site.
   e. Observe tracheostomy tube for incrustation.
8. Monitor action and side effects of prescribed medications.
   a. Sedate as needed.
   b. Restrain as needed.
9. Assess hydration status: monitor input and output and specific gravity.
10. Provide for child's developmental needs during hospitalization.
    a. Provide age-appropriate toys.
    b. Incorporate home routines into hospital care (e.g., feeding practices and bedtime rituals).
    c. Encourage expression of feelings through age-appropriate means.
11. Provide consistent nursing care to promote trust and alleviate anxiety.

🏠 Discharge Planning and Home Care
1. If child is discharged on regimen of oral antibiotics, provide teaching regarding administration and side effects.
2. Educate family on value of *H. influenzae* type B vaccine.

CLIENT OUTCOMES
1. Child's respiratory status will return to normal.
2. Child and family will demonstrate understanding of home care and follow-up needs.

REFERENCES

Behrman RE, Kiegman R, Jenson HB: *Nelson textbook of pediatrics*, ed 17, Philadelphia, 2004, WB Saunders.

Chiocca E: Epiglottitis, *Nursing* 36(4):88, 2006.

Rotta A, Wiryawan B: Respiratory emergencies in children, *Respir Care* 48 (3):248, 2003.

Vazquez D, Philotas R: Peds respiratory emergencies, *Adv for Nurses* (Florida edition). 5(20):17, 2004.

24

❖

Fetal Alcohol Syndrome

PATHOPHYSIOLOGY

The term fetal alcohol spectrum disorder (FASD) has been used to describe the diagnostic variations of alcohol-related birth defects that occur as a result of in utero alcohol exposure. FASD refers to "the range of effects that can occur in a person whose mother drank alcohol during pregnancy, including physical, mental, behavioral, and learning disabilities, with possible lifelong implications" (Centers for Disease Control and Prevention, 2005). Besides the diagnosis of fetal alcohol syndrome (FAS), there are other nondiagnostic variations that include fetal alcohol effects (FAE), alcohol-related birth defect (ARBD), and alcohol-related neurodevelopmental disorders (ARND).

FAS, first described as a syndrome in 1973, refers to the multiple birth defects evident in children as a result of in utero exposure to alcohol during pregnancy. FAS is responsible for the highest number of preventable birth defects and developmental disabilities. FAS is characterized by a triad of symptoms as presented in Box 24-1: (a) three dysmorphic facial features (Figure 24-1), (b) growth retardation, and (c) central nervous system (CNS) problems. Children with FAS may manifest other symptoms in addition to the symptom triad. FAS may be difficult to accurately diagnose since symptoms can be affected by the child's age and developmental level. Children born with FAE do not have the physical characteristics seen in FAS. The manifestations of FAE are fewer than seen in FAS. Children with FAE demonstrate similar problems observed in children with FAS, such as cognitive, social, and behavioral limitations.

BOX 24-1

Characteristics for Diagnosing Fetal Alcohol Syndrome

Facial Dysmorphia

In keeping with racial norms (i.e., those appropriate for a person's race), the person exhibits all three of the following characteristic facial features:

- Smooth philtrum (University of Washington Lip-Philtrum Guide* rank 4 or 5)
- Thin vermillion border (University of Washington Lip-Philtrum Guide* rank 4 or 5)
- Small palpebral fissures (at or below the 10th percentile)

Growth Problems

Confirmed, documented prenatal or postnatal height, weight, or both, at or below the 10th percentile, adjusted for age, sex, gestational age, and race or ethnicity

Central Nervous System Abnormalities

Structural

- Head circumference at or below the 10th percentile, adjusted for age and sex
- Clinically meaningful brain abnormalities observable through imaging (e.g., reduction in size or change in shape of the corpus callosum, cerebellum, or basal ganglia)

Neurologic

- Neurologic problems (e.g., motor problems or seizures) not resulting from a postnatal insult or fever, or other soft neurologic signs outside normal limits

Functional

Test performance substantially below that expected for a person's age, schooling, or circumstances, as evidenced by either of the following:

1. Global cognitive or intellectual deficits representing multiple domains of deficit (or substantial developmental delay in younger children), with performance below the 3rd percentile (i.e., two standard deviations below the mean for standardized testing)
2. Functional deficits below the 16th percentile (i.e., one standard deviation below the mean for standardized testing) in at least three of the following domains:

BOX 24-1
Characteristics for Diagnosing Fetal Alcohol Syndrome—cont'd

- Cognitive or developmental deficits or discrepancies
- Executive functioning deficits
- Motor functioning delays
- Problems with attention or hyperactivity
- Social skills
- Other (e.g., sensory problems, pragmatic language problems, or memory deficits)

Source: Bertrand J et al: Fetal alcohol syndrome: Guidelines for referral and diagnosis, *U.S. Department of Health and Human Services, CDC* (serial online): www.cdc.gov/ ncbddd/fas/documents/FAS_guidelines_accessible.pdf. Accessed January 10, 2007.
*Astley SJ: *Diagnostic guide for fetal alcohol spectrum disorders: The 4-digit diagnostic code,* ed 3, Seattle, WA, 2004, University of Washington Publication Services.

In 1981, the Surgeon General of the United States issued a national report, warning of the dangerous consequences for the fetus of ingesting alcohol during pregnancy. In 1989, federal legislation was passed requiring that all alcohol containers contain warning labels about the deleterious effects of alcohol on the fetus.

The extent to which a child is affected by FAS is dependent on the duration, amount, and pattern of prenatal alcohol exposure and the family situation. The threshold level of alcohol

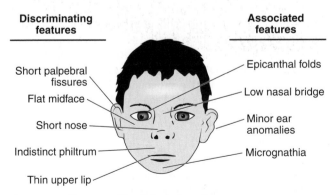

Discriminating features	Associated features
Short palpebral fissures	Epicanthal folds
Flat midface	Low nasal bridge
Short nose	Minor ear anomalies
Indistinct philtrum	Micrognathia
Thin upper lip	

Figure 24-1   Features of fetal alcohol syndrome.

needed to cause FAS is not known; any amount of alcohol consumption is considered unsafe. Damage can occur at any time during pregnancy, even when the woman is not aware that she is pregnant; this is an important factor, since 50% of pregnancies are not planned. Large amounts of alcohol are known to result in harmful fetal effects. The ingestion of seven or more drinks per week and/or of three or more drinks on multiple occasions is considered to have destructive fetal effects.

Alcohol-related risk factors associated with FAS are family member or partner who consumes alcohol, alcohol intake during pregnancy, alcohol dependence, and previous pregnancies with alcohol exposure. Psychosocial factors associated with FAS are low socioeconomic status, parental unemployment, child abuse and neglect, placement of children in foster care, and limited or no prenatal care.

Several challenges are associated with the identification and diagnosis of children with FAS. These challenges include (a) lack of clinical guidelines, (b) the provider's lack of knowledge, (c) limitations in differentiating FAS from other variations of prenatal alcohol exposure, and (d) the lack of candor with the health care provider on the part of women who consume alcohol during pregnancy. A number of factors have been shown to reduce the long-term consequences of FAS: early diagnosis and intervention, stable home environment, and supportive family environment.

The child with FAS may be first identified in community settings (early intervention program, preschool program) or clinical settings (pediatrician's office or with a pediatric nurse practitioner in the primary care setting) and then referred to an interdisciplinary team for diagnostic evaluation and treatment. Early diagnosis is essential to implementing programs and services needed to improve long-term outcomes. Diagnosis can be difficult, since the characteristic features of FAS may not be evident.

INCIDENCE

1. Prevalence rates of FAS are 0.2 to 1.5 cases per 1000 births.
2. Prevalence rates of FAE are 3 cases per 1000 births.
3. It is estimated that between 1000 to 6000 children are born with FAS annually.

4. Prevalence rates are higher in disadvantaged, Native American, and culturally diverse populations, amounting to 3 to 6 cases per 1000 births.
5. Most children with FASD do not have cognitive disabilities.
6. Approximately 25% of children diagnosed with FAS score two deviations below the mean on measures of cognitive functioning.
7. Approximately 4 million infants are born with fetal alcohol effects.
8. Of women who become pregnant, 13% to 15% continue to ingest alcohol during pregnancy.
9. Of pregnant women, 3% report engaging in binge or heavy drinking of alcohol.
10. Women who have given birth to a child with FAS are at high risk for giving birth to second child with FAS.

CLINICAL MANIFESTATIONS

1. Triad of symptoms associated with FAS (see Figure 24-1 and Box 24-1):
   a. Three characteristic dysmorphic facial features
   b. CNS problems
   c. Prenatal and postnatal growth retardation at or below the 10th percentile
2. Cognitive limitations according to one of the two following parameters:
   a. IQ is less than normal range (below the 3rd percentile)
   b. Deficits in three or more of the following areas (below the 16th percentile):
      i. Cognitive limitations and/or developmental delays
      ii. Limitations in executive functioning
      iii. Delays in fine and/or gross motor functioning
      iv. Problems with attention and hyperactivity
      v. Deficits with social skills
      vi. Other problems such as memory deficits, language delays, sensory problems
3. Level of daily functioning below what is expected for age
4. Inability to follow social rules and authority figures

COMPLICATIONS

FASD is not associated with complications; however, the infant born with FAS may have other secondary diagnoses and long-term problems such as the mental health diagnoses of depression, oppositional defiant disorders, and conduct disorders (Box 24-2). Adaptation problems may occur such as unemployment, dropping out of school, and criminality.

The following problems have been noted in association with FASD:

1. Mental health problems
   a. Conduct disorders
   b. Anxiety disorders
   c. Adjustment disorders
   d. Oppositional defiant disorders
   e. Depression
   f. Substance abuse disorders
2. Adaptation problems
   a. Criminality
   b. School dropout

BOX 24-2

Fetal Alcohol Spectrum Disorder (FASD) Throughout the Life Span

Infants: Low birth weight; irritability; sensitivity to light, noises and touch; poor sucking; slow development; poor sleep-wake cycles; increased ear infections

Toddlers: Poor memory capability, hyperactivity, lack of fear, no sense of boundaries, need for excessive physical contact

Grade-school years: Short attention span, poor coordination, difficulty with both fine and gross motor skills

Older children: Trouble keeping up with school, low self-esteem from recognition that they are different from their peers

Teenagers: Poor impulse control, cannot distinguish between public and private behaviors; must be reminded of concepts on a daily basis

National Organization on Fetal Alcohol Syndrome: *FASD Intervention* (website): www.nofas.org/MediaFiles/PDFs/factsheets/intervention.pdf. Accessed January 10, 2007.

c. Unemployment
d. Inability to live independently
e. Sexual promiscuity
f. High-risk behaviors
3. Sleep disorders
4. Autism
5. At risk status for sexual abuse
6. Low self-esteem

LABORATORY AND DIAGNOSTIC TESTS

1. Confirmation of alcohol use during pregnancy
   a. Self-report
   b. Clinical observation
   c. Blood alcohol levels (may be documented in medical records)
2. Diagnosis is made based on following symptoms (see Figure 24-1 and Box 24-1):
   a. Documentation of three dysmorphic facial features
   b. Growth deficits—height and weight less than or equal to the 10th percentile, adjusted for age, gestational age, sex, ethnicity and/or race
   c. CNS problems—diagnosis depends on type: structural, neurologic, or functional (see Box 24-1)
3. Comprehensive neuropsychologic testing
4. Additional diagnostic testing depends on the individualized needs of the child.
   a. Speech and language assessment
   b. Occupational and physical therapy assessment
   c. Complete medical and health history and physical examination
   d. Family assessment
5. Comprehensive family and social history of child
   a. Current or prior foster care placement
      i. Lack of documentation of alcohol use during pregnancy
   b. Living with alcoholic mother
   c. Current or prior abuse, neglect
   d. Previous referrals to child protection services
   e. Maternal death due to alcoholism

   f. Birth history
      i. May be unknown or suspected, in terms of alcohol use during pregnancy
      ii. Exposure to alcohol in utero is highly suspected in children who are in foster care.

MEDICAL MANAGEMENT

A preventive approach is key to reducing the prevalence of FASD. Preventive strategies include (a) encourage contraception for women who consume alcohol, (b) provide counseling to discourage alcohol consumption, (c) identify at-risk women (those with depression, with history of childhood abuse) of childbearing age who may be inclined to ingest alcohol, and (d) educate providers to assess women of childbearing age who are pregnant who are at risk of having or who have problems with alcohol abuse.

Members of the interdisciplinary team to treat children with FAS include geneticist, developmental pediatrician, nurse, social worker, child psychiatrist, child psychologist, special education specialist, speech and language specialist, and social worker. The extent of interventions will be dependent on the area of the brain affected, the family situation, and the child's age and developmental level.

Medications may be prescribed, depending on behaviors demonstrated, such as behaviors of impulsivity and hyperactivity, sleep disorders, and oppositional behaviors.

NURSING ASSESSMENT

The assessment process is comprehensive in scope and based on the dimensions of biophysical, psychosocial, behavioral, and educational needs.

1. Assess for the triad cluster of symptoms associated with FAS (see Box 24-1 and Figure 24-1).
   a. Dysmorphic facial characteristics
   b. Measurement of growth (height and weight identified on growth charts)
   c. CNS involvement
      i. Observation of CNS manifestations

    ii. Review of diagnostic testing; medical interpretation of testing and physical examination

2. Assessment consists of comprehensive evaluation of deficits and strengths related to the following adaptive skills:
   a. Communication
   b. Self-care
   c. Social interactions
   d. Use of community resources
   e. Self-direction
   f. Maintenance of health and safety
   g. Functional academics
   h. Development of leisure and recreational skills, and work skills
   i. Influence of the child's cultural and linguistic background, interests, and preferences
3. Assess for the manifestations of secondary problems.
   a. Mental health problems
4. Assess for long-term adaptation problems.
   a. Unemployment
   b. Criminality
   c. School dropout
5. Assess child social behaviors including interactions with others, communication skills, repetitive and stereotypical behaviors, play, and affect.
6. Assess family adaptation and coping.

NURSING DIAGNOSES

- Development, Risk for delayed
- Growth and development, Delayed (related to genetic condition)
- Caregiver role strain (related to unrelenting care requirements secondary to FAS)
- Family processes, Interrupted (related to the impact of raising a child with FAS)
- Parenting, Impaired (related to lack of knowledge)
- Social interactions, Impaired (related to communication barriers and lack of social skills secondary to FAS)
- Therapeutic regimen management, Ineffective family (related to complexity of therapeutic regimen, financial cost of regimen, insufficient social support)

NURSING INTERVENTIONS
Infants, Toddlers, and Preschoolers

1. Refer to early intervention program for development of individualized family service plan (IFSP) and interdisciplinary treatment plan; or, if child, refer to preschool program for individualized education plan (IEP) (see Appendix G) that provides opportunities for developmental learning (Appendix G):
   a. Social development
   b. Fine motor development
   c. Gross motor development
   d. Sensory integration development
   e. Communication and language development
2. Refer parents and caregivers to family resource centers and/or parent information centers that provide early intervention services to parents of infants and toddlers with disabilities for parental support and assistance with informational needs and respite services.
3. Collaborate with other interdisciplinary professionals to formulate IFSP and/or IEP that is based upon individual needs, is family-centered, has measurable objectives, and includes periodic evaluations (refer to the Medical Management section in this chapter).
4. Serve as health resource consultant to community service coordinator.
5. Assist family and child in navigating service systems to obtain needed services for child and family.
6. Refer to the Discharge Planning and Home Care section in this chapter.

School-Aged Children

1. Collaborate with other interdisciplinary professionals to formulate IEP that is based upon individual needs, is individual- and family-centered, has measurable objectives, and includes periodic evaluations.
2. Collaborate with IEP team on identification of health-related needs and development of IEP objectives.

3. Assist family in navigating service systems to obtain needed services for child and family.
4. Provide information and answer family's questions about strategies to promote the child's acquisition of developmental milestones (refer to Appendix B).
5. Make suggestions to the family for promotion of the child's development of self-reliance and sense of mastery.
6. Refer to the Discharge Planning and Home Care section in this chapter.

Adolescents

1. Collaborate with other interdisciplinary professionals to formulate transition IEP that is based upon individual needs, is youth-centered, has measurable objectives, and includes periodic evaluations.
2. Collaborate with IEP team on identification of health-related transition needs and development of IEP objectives.
3. Provide input on transition plan related to health-related needs.
   a. Facilitate access to adult primary and specialty health care providers.
   b. Promote the development of self-reliance in managing health self-care.
   c. Assist with obtaining health insurance in anticipation of termination of pediatric eligibility.
4. Assist family in navigating service systems to obtain needed services for child and family.
5. Serve as health consultant to community service co-ordinator.
6. Provide information and answer family's questions about strategies to promote the youth's acquisition of developmental milestones (refer to Appendix B).
7. Provide the family with suggestions to promote the youth's development of self-reliance and sense of mastery.
8. Emphasize the importance of creating and taking advantage of socialization opportunities to engage in peer and community activities.
9. Refer to the Discharge Planning and Home Care section in this chapter.

🏠 Discharge Planning and Home Care

1. Instruct parents, family members, caregivers, foster parents, and child or youth, and reinforce information, about the short-term and long-term outcomes and prognosis of the FAS diagnosis.

2. Educate parents, family members, and child or youth about long-term management strategies, and community resources needed to access services needed (refer to Appendix G).
   a. Early intervention
   b. Special education program (IEP)
   c. Specialized medical and therapy services
   d. Community support services (rehabilitation, recreational, daily living skills, social skills)
   e. Vocational rehabilitation (joint programs with schools when in high school)
   f. Housing, transportation
   g. Peer and family support programs

3. Refer families to early intervention and/or special education and/or transition programs to address child's or youth's needs for treatment services.

4. Participate as a member of an interdisciplinary team in school and/or community settings to develop plan of services to address family- and/or youth-centered goals and objectives based on the child's or youth's individualized needs.

5. As appropriate, refer parent to social worker and/or alcohol treatment programs.
   a. Training curriculum available for foster care, parents, and education professionals available at www.cdc.gov/ncbddd/fas/awareness.htm

CLIENT OUTCOMES

1. Child will be diagnosed early, enabling participation in early treatment and intervention.

2. Child or youth will achieve highest potential of biopsychosocial functioning.

3. Child or youth will achieve highest level of self-sufficiency possible.
4. Child or youth will demonstrate highest achievable level of autonomy, self-determination, and self-advocacy.
5. Family and caregivers will demonstrate ability to cope with child's or youth's behaviors and needs and to access needed services.
6. Parents and caregivers will demonstrate attachment and responsive parenting behaviors.
7. Parents and caregivers will demonstrate ability to accept child's limitations and recognize child's or youth's strengths.

REFERENCES

Centers for Disease Control and Prevention: Guidelines for identifying and referring persons with fetal alcohol syndrome, *MMWR* 54(No. RR-11):1, 2005.

Gerberding JL, Cordeo J, Floyd RL: *Fetal alcohol syndrome: Guidelines for referral and diagnosis*, Washington, DC, 2004, National Center on Birth Defects and Developmental Disabilities, Centers for Disease Control, Department of Health and Human Services.

National Organization on Fetal Alcohol Syndrome: *FASD Identification* (website): www.nofas.org/MediaFiles/PDFs/factsheets/identification.pdf. Accessed January 10, 2007.

National Organization on Fetal Alcohol Syndrome: *FASD Intervention* (website): www.nofas.org/MediaFiles/PDFs/factsheets/intervention.pdf. Accessed January 10, 2007.

National Organization on Fetal Alcohol Syndrome: *FASD What school systems should know about affected students* (website): www.nofas.org/MediaFiles/PDFs/factsheets/students%20school.pdf. Accessed January 10, 2007.

National Organization on Fetal Alcohol Syndrome: *FASD What the health care system should know* (website): www.nofas.org/MediaFiles/PDFs/factsheets/healthcare.pdf. Accessed January 10, 2007.

U.S. Surgeon General: *United States Surgeon General releases advisory on alcohol use in pregnancy* (website): www.surgeongeneral.gov/pressreleases/sg02222005.html. Accessed January 10, 2007.

25

Foreign Body Aspiration

PATHOPHYSIOLOGY

Foreign body aspiration refers to the lodgment of an object or substance in the airway. The foreign body tends to lodge most often in the cricopharyngeal area because of the strong propulsive pharyngeal muscles that move it to this location. Obstruction may be partial or complete. Complete airway obstruction usually occurs in the upper airway and is life threatening. Most objects aspirated by children are small enough to pass through the larynx and trachea and lodge in either of the main bronchi. Examples of items may be poorly chewed hot dog pieces, peanuts, small toys, coins, or disk (button cell) batteries. The right main bronchus is a more common site because it is larger, receives greater airflow, and has a straighter line of entry than the left bronchus. The mechanisms of airway obstruction depend on the site of obstruction and whether the foreign body is partially or completely obstructing an airway. Atelectasis occurs distal to the area where air can no longer enter. Air trapping or hyperinflation occurs when air is inhaled but can be only partially exhaled.

In many cases, foreign bodies are spontaneously expelled from the tracheobronchial tree, and symptoms that persist are from residual irritation and bronchial edema. When foreign body aspiration is diagnosed quickly and the object or substance is removed in a prompt manner, the condition follows a benign course. Aspiration of foreign bodies containing saturated fats, such as peanuts, is more problematic because of the resulting irritation and inflammation of mucosal tissue. The longer a foreign body remains lodged in place, the more complications can develop, related to increasing edema, inflammation, and threat of infection.

INCIDENCE

1. Foreign body aspiration most commonly occurs in children 9 months to 5 years of age.
2. Foreign body aspiration is the leading cause of accidental death in children younger than 1 year of age.
3. Peanuts and other nuts account for about half of all aspirated foreign bodies; vegetable pieces, seeds, and raisins are also common culprits.
4. Large objects such as hot dog pieces, grapes, balloon fragments, and popcorn may obstruct the glottic inlet and lead to respiratory arrest.

CLINICAL MANIFESTATIONS

Clinical manifestations vary according to the site at which the foreign body lodges and the degree of obstruction that occurs.

1. Initial coughing, gagging, or choking episode, which may or may not be observed
2. Acute coughing or wheezing or respiratory arrest
3. Subtle, chronic cough or wheeze
4. Dyspnea
5. Retractions
6. Cyanosis
7. Decreased breath sounds over affected side
8. Fever
9. Hoarseness, stridor, or aphonia (larynx)

COMPLICATIONS

Complications most often result from delayed diagnosis and removal.

1. Bronchospasm
2. Atelectasis
3. Bronchitis
4. Bronchiectasis
5. Pneumonia
6. Pneumothorax
7. Lung abscess

8. Bronchopulmonary fistula
9. Death

LABORATORY AND DIAGNOSTIC TESTS

1. Chest radiographic study—anterior, posterior, lateral, and oblique views, to evaluate for opaque foreign body location; for nonopaque foreign body, assess x-ray films for area of atelectasis or, with inspiratory and expiratory x-ray films, assess for air trapping

2. Laryngoscopy and bronchoscopy—performed with general anesthesia in the operating room; provide direct visualization of the upper trachea (a telescope can be used to locate the foreign body, and removal is accomplished by inserting optical forceps)

3. Fluoroscopy—provides a dynamic image of the structures under radiographic study; gives an advantage over radiographic study alone in showing trapped air distal to the foreign body site

4. Xeroradiography (a radiographic technique that uses specially coated x-ray film)—provides higher resolution of images such as of nonmetallic foreign bodies

MEDICAL MANAGEMENT

Emergency management of foreign body aspiration may begin before hospitalization for a life-threatening obstruction when attempts at relief via the Heimlich maneuver or blows to the back cannot be delayed. Initiation of CPR may be required. Provide oxygen via mask or bag-valve mask. Once foreign body aspiration is suspected, immediate attention is warranted, with aggressive diagnostic work-up including bronchoscopy for identification and removal to prevent complications.

Medications that may be used are as follows:

1. Inhaled bronchodilators for laryngospasm or broncho-spasm
2. Corticosteroids to decrease airway edema
3. Systemically acting antibiotics in cases in which fragment retention is suspected, purulent secretions are noted in the airway, or signs and symptoms of pneumonia are present

NURSING ASSESSMENT
1. See the Respiratory Assessment section in Appendix A.
2. Assess level of anxiety.

NURSING DIAGNOSES
- Airway clearance, Ineffective
- Anxiety
- Gas exchange, Impaired
- Knowledge, Deficient (related to child safety)

NURSING INTERVENTIONS
Emergency Measures
In cases of total airway obstruction or ineffective airway clearance, an airway must be established.
1. Deliver back blows followed by chest thrusts for infants 1 year and younger.
2. Perform Heimlich maneuver (abdominal thrusts) in children older than 1 year.
3. Administer oxygen.
4. Perform CPR.

Preoperative Care
1. Provide continuous respiratory monitoring; be prepared to assist with emergency airway management if partial obstruction becomes complete.
2. Monitor vital signs and oxygen saturation.
3. Provide position (of comfort) to ensure adequate airway.
4. Provide nothing by mouth before surgery.
5. Prepare child for bronchoscopy and/or thoracotomy.
6. Provide consistent nursing care to promote trust and to alleviate anxiety.

Postoperative Care
1. Perform frequent respiratory assessments to detect signs and symptoms of respiratory distress from secondary airway edema.
2. Assess effects of administered medications.

🏠 Discharge Planning and Home Care

1. Instruct parents to observe for, and report immediately, signs of respiratory distress.
2. Provide list of resources for parents in case of emergency.
3. Instruct parents in foreign body airway obstruction removal and cardiopulmonary resuscitation.
4. Instruct in prevention of foreign body aspiration.
   a. Offer types and sizes or portions of food appropriate for age of child.
   b. Discourage child from eating during performance of other activities.
   c. Restrict access to toys or other objects small enough to fit through standard toilet paper roll, as they could cause choking in young children.
   d. Provide anticipatory guidance to parents regarding direct inspection of toys and reading of warning labels to assure that toys are age-appropriate.
5. Make referral for home safety assessment if indicated.

CLIENT OUTCOMES

1. Child will achieve and maintain patent airway.
2. Child will return to safe home environment.

REFERENCES

Behrman R, Kiegman R, & Jenson HB, editors: *Nelson textbook of pediatrics*, ed 17, Philadelphia, 2004, WB Saunders.

Hockenberry M et al: *Wong's nursing care of infants and children*, ed 7, St. Louis, 2004, Mosby.

Rotta A, Wiryawan B: Respiratory emergencies in children, *Respir Care* 48(3):248, 2003.

Vazquez D, Philotas R: Peds respiratory emergencies, *Adv for Nurses* (Florida Edition) 5(20):17, 2004.

26

Fractures

PATHOPHYSIOLOGY

Fractures can have a variety of causes, including (1) a direct force applied to the bone; (2) an underlying pathologic condition, such as rickets, that leads to spontaneous fracturing; (3) abrupt, intense muscle contractions; and (4) an indirect force applied from a distance (e.g., being hit by a flying object). Other causes of fractures include child abuse, metastatic neuroblastoma, Ewing's sarcoma, osteogenic sarcoma, osteogenesis imperfecta, copper deficiency, osteomyelitis, overuse injuries, and immobilization resulting in osteoporosis.

There are a variety of fractures, which can be categorized using the Salter-Harris classification system (Box 26-1). The most common type seen in children younger than 3 years of age is the greenstick fracture. This type is characterized by an incomplete break of the cortex, which occurs because the bone is softer and more pliable than the bones of older children. Other fractures (and their related sites) include upper epiphyseal and supracondylar fractures, lateral condylar humeral fractures, and medial epicondylar fractures (humerus); proximal radial physis and radial neck fractures, and nursemaid's elbow (elbow); fractures of the shaft of the radius and ulna (forearm); and fractures of the femoral shaft and tibia (lower limb). Abuse should be considered in all children younger than 15 months of age with humeral fractures, including supracondylar and spiral fractures. In one study of 215 children, 60% of femur fractures in children younger than 1 year of age were due to abuse. Child abuse can also be suspected with rib and skull fractures.

BOX 26-1

Salter-Harris Classification

Type I
- Fracture passes through growth plate without involvement of metaphysis or epiphysis
- Occurs with mild traumatic injuries
- Seen most often in distal fibula

Type II
- Fracture extends through growth plate, involving metaphysis
- Occurs as a result of severe trauma such as car accident, fall from skateboard
- Seen most often in distal radius and proximal humerus

Type III
- Fracture extends through growth plate, involving epiphysis and joint
- Occurs during moderately severe trauma
- Seen most often in distal tibia

Type IV
- Fracture involves metaphysis, extending through growth plate into epiphysis
- Occurs as a result of falls, skateboard, and bicycle accidents
- Seen most often in humerus
- Can result in serious damage

Type V (Rare)
- Growth plate is crushed
- Compression fracture, resulting from falling or projectile impact

INCIDENCE

1. Most fractures occur to pedestrians.
2. Upper-extremity fractures account for 75% of all fractures sustained by children and frequently occur during a fall onto an outstretched hand.
3. Skull fracture ranks first in terms of morbidity and mortality.

4. Pelvic fractures constitute a small portion of skeletal fractures in children; they rank second in terms of morbidity and mortality.
5. Injuries to the growth plate occur in one third of skeletal traumas.

CLINICAL MANIFESTATIONS

1. Pain, relieved with rest
2. Tenderness
3. Swelling
4. Impaired function, limping
5. Limited motion
6. Ecchymosis surrounding site
7. Crepitus at site of fracture
8. Decreased neurovascular function distal to site of fracture
9. Distal atrophy

COMPLICATIONS

1. Orthopedic: deformity of limb, limb length discrepancy, potential for growth arrest, joint incongruity, limitation of movement, and refracture
2. Neurologic: nerve injury resulting in numbness and/or nerve palsy
3. Cardiovascular: circulatory compromise, Volkmann's contracture, gangrene, and compartment syndrome

LABORATORY AND DIAGNOSTIC TESTS

Refer to Appendix D for normal values and ranges of laboratory and diagnostic tests.
1. Radiographic study—to examine extent of the injury site
2. Bone scan—performed if radiographic studies are normal
3. Magnetic resonance imaging—to assess for pathologic interosseous features and growth plate injuries
4. Complete blood count—to determine presence of blood dyscrasias and/or anemia
5. Erythrocyte sedimentation rate—to determine level of inflammation
6. Ultrasonography—to assess intraarticular, extraarticular, and soft tissue abnormalities

MEDICAL MANAGEMENT

Management varies according to the type of fracture. Management modalities include open reduction, traction, casting, percutaneous pinning, and remodeling. Analgesics are used for pain relief. The dosage and type depend on the intensity of the child's pain.

NURSING ASSESSMENT

1. Assess site of injury for pain, swelling, change in skin color, and neurovascular impairment.
2. Assess for cause of injury.
3. Assess child's need for pain relief.
4. Assess for signs and symptoms of infection.
5. Assess for wound healing (if open reduction was performed).
6. Assess for skin irritation (if casted).
7. Assess for cast or traction integrity.
8. Assess for hydration status.
9. Assess for signs and symptoms of complications such as fat emboli and compartment syndrome.
10. Assess child's and family's ability to adhere to treatment regimen.
11. Assess child's ability to participate in self-care activities.
12. Assess child's need for diversional activities.

NURSING DIAGNOSES

- Injury, Risk for
- Mobility, Impaired physical
- Tissue integrity, Impaired
- Peripheral neurovascular dysfunction, Risk for
- Pain
- Self-care deficit, bathing/hygiene
- Self-care deficit, dressing/grooming
- Self-care deficit, feeding
- Self-care deficit, toileting
- Diversional activity, Deficient
- Knowledge, Deficient
- Therapeutic regimen management, Ineffective

NURSING INTERVENTIONS
Admission
1. Monitor and document condition and cause of injury.
   a. Amount of swelling.
   b. Amount of pain.
   c. Change in skin color.
   d. Circulatory status of limb distal to injury (color, warmth, pulses).
   e. Neurologic status of limb distal to injury (tingling, numbness).
   f. Factors associated with injury.
2. Apply splint or Jones dressing to affected limb to alleviate pain and prevent further injury (traction may be used).
   a. Apply to one side of affected limb.
   b. Immobilize fracture site and joints above and below it.
   c. Stabilize splints with bandages.
   d. Apply Jones dressing—wrap extremity with two or three layers of cotton and cover with Ace bandage; repeat process 3 or 4 times.
   e. Refer to Appendix I for additional pain relief measures.
3. Maintain nothing-by-mouth status until after treatment; child may have to be anesthetized.
4. Prepare child and family for selected treatment modality.

Later Treatment
1. Observe and report status of limb distal to fracture site.
   a. Neurovascular status
      i. Upper limbs—radial and ulnar pulses
      ii. Lower limbs—dorsalis pedis and posterior tibial pulses
      iii. Motor function and sensation
   b. Edema and swelling
   c. Skin color and warmth
2. Alleviate edema and swelling of trauma site and area distal to it.
   a. Elevate limb for 24 to 48 hours.
   b. Apply ice if necessary.

     c. Monitor every hour immediately after treatment, then every 4 hours for 48 hours.

3. Promote skin integrity.
   a. Apply alcohol to reddened areas.
   b. Petal cast edges to prevent skin irritation.
   c. Reposition every 2 hours to alleviate increased pressure on bony prominences.
   d. Observe for reddened areas every 4 hours.
4. Observe and report signs of infection.
   a. Elevated temperature
   b. Offensive odors
   c. Drainage
5. Observe for and record bleeding; note and outline amount.
6. Provide cast care (as indicated).
7. Maintain traction (as indicated).
8. Provide age-appropriate diversional activities to alleviate or minimize effects of sensory deprivation and immobilization (see Appendix F).
9. Promote adequate fluid and nutritional intake.
   a. Encourage fluid intake; maintenance fluids—0 to 10 kg: 100 ml/kg; 11 to 20 kg: 50 ml/kg (plus 100 ml/kg for the first 10 kg); above 20 kg: 20 ml/kg.
   b. Provide high-fiber and high-roughage diet to promote peristalsis.
   c. Provide well-balanced diet to promote healing.
10. Prevent complications of unaffected limb; provide daily exercises.
11. Refer case to child protective services if child abuse is suspected (see Chapter 12).

🏠 Discharge Planning and Home Care

1. Monitor child's and family's ability to keep follow-up appointments.
2. Instruct parents and child about care of cast, use of crutches, movement, weight bearing, and return to school or home teaching.

3. Instruct parents and child to monitor and report signs of complications (as described in Nursing Interventions section in this chapter).
   a. Skin breakdown
   b. Signs of infection
   c. Signs of bleeding
   d. Signs of neurovascular compromise: decreased perfusion, decreased sensation, contractural deformity of distal limb
4. Review home safety precautions to help prevent further injuries.
5. Review vehicular safety precautions such as proper use of seat belts and car seats.
6. Review recreational safety precautions such as using knee pads and helmets while skateboarding or bicycling.

CLIENT OUTCOMES

1. Child's fracture will heal without complications.
2. Child's pain will be minimized or alleviated.
3. Child will participate in self-care activities as fully as possible.

REFERENCES

Battaglia TC et al: Factors affecting forearm compartment pressures in children with supracondylar humeral fractures, *J Pediatr Orthop* 22(4):431, 2002.

Horner, Gail: Physical abuse; recognition and reporting, *J Pediatr Health Care* 19 (1):4, 2005.

Kocher MS, Mininder S, Sarwark JF: What's new in pediatric orthopaedics, *J Bone Joint Surg Am* 86-A(6):1337, 2004.

Sofka CM, Potter HG: Imaging of elbow injuries in the child and adult athlete, *Radiol Clin North Am* 40(2):251, 2002.

Starling SP et al: Pelvic fractures in infants as a sign of physical abuse, *Child Abuse Negl* 26(5):475, 2002.

Townsend DJ, Bassett GS: Common elbow fractures in children, *Am Fam Physician* 53(6):2031, 1996.

Wiss D: What's new in orthopaedic trauma, *J Bone Joint Surg Am* 83(11):1762, 2001.

Zalavras C et al: Pediatric fractures during skateboarding, roller skating and scooter riding, *Am J Sports Med* 33(4):568, 2005.

27

Fragile X Syndrome

PATHOPHYSIOLOGY

Mutations in the fragile X mental retardation *(FMR1)* gene are associated with fragile X syndrome, fragile X–associated tremor/ataxia syndrome (FXTAS), and *FMR1*-related premature ovarian failure. Individuals with fragile X syndrome have an intellectual disability; individuals with FXTAS and *FMR1*-related premature ovarian failure usually do not have an intellectual disability, but they are at high risk for having children or grandchildren with fragile X syndrome.

The *FMR1* gene is located on the X chromosome; thus women inherit two copies (alleles) of the *FMR1* gene and men inherit one allele. A particular region on the *FMR1* gene (often referred to as the fragile site) has three DNA bases (cytocine [C], guanine [G], guanine) that are repeated (trinucleotide repeat) many times. There are essentially four allelic categories that define repeat length.

A normal allele is characterized by 5 to 40 CGG repeats. An intermediate (gray zone) allele has 41 to 58 repeats. A premutation allele has 59 to 200 CGG repeats. A premutation allele is not associated with intellectual disability, but does convey an increased risk for FXTAS and *FMR1*-related premature ovarian failure. Women who have 59 to 200 CGG repeats are considered to be at risk for having children affected with fragile X syndrome. Individuals who have more than 200 hypermethylated CGG repeats (usually several hundred to several thousand) have full mutations; they have fragile X syndrome. The number of repeats is unstable from generation to generation, making the pattern of inheritance difficult to predict.

The *FMR1* gene codes for a protein called the FMR protein, made in many tissues and having a high concentration in the brain and testes. The FMR protein plays a role in the development of synapses between nerve cells in the brain where cell to cell communication occurs. The connection between nerve cells can change and adapt over time in response to experience (synaptic plasticity). The FMR protein is thought to help regulate synaptic plasticity, which is important for learning and memory. Consequently, an individual born with a full mutation in his or her *FMR1* gene suffers from cognitive and neuropsychologic problems.

The more profound intellectual disability (formerly known as mental retardation) seen in males can be explained by X inactivation that occurs during embryogenesis. A female embryo inherits two X chromosomes; two active X chromosomes are not compatible with life, and thus one X chromosome in every cell has to be inactivated. The inactivation process is random; in a female embryo, it does not automatically inactivate the X chromosome that has a defective *FMR1* gene.

For example, if a female inherits a defective *FMR1* gene from her father, it could work out that 80% of his X chromosomes will be inactivated. That, in turn, means that 80% of her cells will be making adequate FMR1 protein; she will probably not have a severe intellectual disability, and perhaps not any. On the other hand, if 80% of her mother's X chromosomes were inactivated, the child would most likely have an intellectual disability.

INCIDENCE

1. Fragile X syndrome is the number one cause of inherited intellectual disability.
2. Fragile X affects 1 in 4000 males and 1 in 8000 females.
3. The prevalence is similar in most ethnic and racial groups.
4. High repeat numbers (41 to 199 CGG repeats) occur in 4% of all males and 8% of all females; they are considered carriers.
5. Approximately 15% of women with premature ovarian failure have 35 to 54 CGG repeats.

6. Approximately 3% of men over age 50 years with unexplained ataxia have 83 to 109 CGG repeats.

CLINICAL MANIFESTATIONS

1. Family history
   a. Multiple male relatives with intellectual disability
   b. Mother with learning disabilities and family members with ataxia and/or tremors
   c. Female infertility secondary to premature ovarian failure
   d. Dizygotic twinning is more common in fragile X carriers.
2. Developmental characteristics
   a. Developmental milestones are normal or slightly delayed.
      i. Sits alone (10 months)
      ii. Walks (about 21 months)
      iii. First word (20 months)
   b. Speech delays noted during the second year of life.
   c. As the patient ages, perseveration and echolalia may dominate.
   d. Delayed continence is common.
   e. Average age at diagnosis is 8 years.
3. Cognitive limitations
   a. Has intelligence quotient (IQ) ranging from mild to severe intellectual disability (20 to 70). Females can have IQ reaching 80.
   b. IQ may be higher in childhood than in adulthood.
4. Neuropsychologic problems are common.
   a. Autistic-like behavior in approximately 20% of affected individuals
   b. Attention deficit hyperactivity disorder (ADHD)
   c. Seizure disorder in approximately 20% of affected individuals
5. Physical
   a. Early growth spurt, but adult height is slightly below normal.
   b. Feeding problems are evident.
      i. Infants may have failure to thrive.
      ii. Obsessive eating may result in obesity in older children.

c. Head and facial characteristics: adolescents and adults have long, thin face, with prominent ears.
d. Mouth: characterized by dental overcrowding and high-arched palate.
e. Eyes: strabismus is frequently noted.
f. Extremities: hyperextensibility, double-jointed thumbs, a single palmar crease, and pes planus.
g. Musculoskeletal: pectus excavatum and scoliosis are common.
h. Genitals: macroorchidism is universal in adult males.
i. Cardiac: heart murmur or click consistent with mitral valve prolapse.
6. Affected individuals have a normal life span.

COMPLICATIONS

1. Intellectual: intellectual disability
2. Orthopedic: scoliosis
3. Cardiovascular: mitral valve prolapse
4. Sensory: recurrent sinusitis, otitis media, and decreased visual acuity

LABORATORY AND DIAGNOSTIC TESTS

Refer to Appendix D, Laboratory Values, for normal values and ranges of laboratory and diagnostic tests.
1. Laboratory tests
   a. Polymerase chain reaction (PCR)—a technique that replicates the first and last nucleotides of the *FMR1* gene to a person's DNA. The DNA is heated and cooled until the gene fills in. The gene has been sequenced, and the CGG repeats can now be counted.
   b. Southern blot—a functioning *FMR1* gene has a certain weight; it will fall through a gel and leave a mark. Think of putting a fleck of sand (dyed black) into honey and then measuring where it ends. Scientists know how heavy the *FMR1* gene is and where it should end in a gel.
   c. Methylation status—replacement of a hydrogen atom with CH_3. In order to accurately diagnose fragile X–related disorders, the gene has to have over 200 repeats, and it must have considerable CH_3 attached to it

(think of 100 hands in an assembly line, 50 of which have handcuffs on).

2. Prenatal genetic testing is conducted when a mother is a known carrier.
   a. Cultured amniocytes via amniocentesis at 15 weeks' gestation
   b. Chorionic villus sampling (CVS) at 10 to 12 weeks' gestation
   c. CVS may not be accurate; methylation of the *FMR1* gene not established this early in gestation
3. Preimplantation genetic testing (see Box 27-1 for CLIA-approved clinics in the United States)
4. Standardized intelligence tests (see Chapter 44)
5. Measurements of adaptive behaviors (see Chapter 44)

MEDICAL MANAGEMENT

Medical management is directed to providing care that addresses primary care needs and provides supports for long-term management. For additional information on the long-term management of the child with fragile X syndrome, refer to Chapter 44. The child with fragile X syndrome will require long-term monitoring to detect secondary conditions that may

BOX 27-1

CLIA-Approved Clinics for Preimplantation Diagnosis

1. Reproductive Genetics Institute
   Chicago, IL
   Phone: 773-472-4900
   Website: www.reproductivegenetics.com/index.html
2. Wake Forest University School of Medicine
   Winston-Salem, NC
   Phone: 336-713-7572 or 336-713-7573
   Website: www1.wfubmc.edu/medicalgenetics/
3. Go to www.genetests.org to find CLIA-approved laboratory in your area.

develop. Medical treatment includes pharmacologic management for hyperactivity, depression, sleep disorders, and seizures.
Methylphenidate and dextroamphetamine are prescribed to treat
hyperactivity, and antidepressants (selective serotonin reuptake
inhibitors [SSRIs]) for depression; traxodone and melatonin
are used to treat sleep disorders. Carbamazepine is commonly
prescribed, and it may help with behavior problems. Carbamazepine is altered by macrolide antibiotics, cimetidine, pro-
poxyphene, and isoniazid. Estimated average lifetime cost of
care for a patient with fragile X syndrome is $957,000.

NURSING ASSESSMENT

1. Accurate assessment of the family's cognitive development
   and disease conditions is imperative.
2. Construct a four-generation pedigree to elucidate suspicious
   diseases (Figure 27-1).
3. Ask focused questions about parents, children, siblings,
   aunts, uncles, and grandparents (Box 27-2).
4. If answers to questions raise suspicion for fragile X–related
   disorders, refer to genetic specialist for risk assessment (Box
   27-3) (cost of antenatal screening per carrier detected is
   estimated to be $46,400).
5. Assess for ethical, legal, and social implications (ELSI).
   a. Potential for genetic discrimination, since adverse treat-
      ment may be based on genotype (Box 27-4).
   b. Assess harm to self.
      i. Fragile X carrier may not feel desirable for dating or
         marriage.
      ii. Child may suffer if, after testing, his family's percep-
          tion of him changes.
   c. Assess ethical issue—family's values regarding termina-
      tion of a pregnancy.
6. Assess for legal ramifications.
   a. Mutation-positive family member may not want to share
      information with other family members.
   b. If primary prevention is to occur, this information must
      be shared.
   c. Federal requirements on the issue of "duty to warn" of
      inherited health risk are still being formulated.

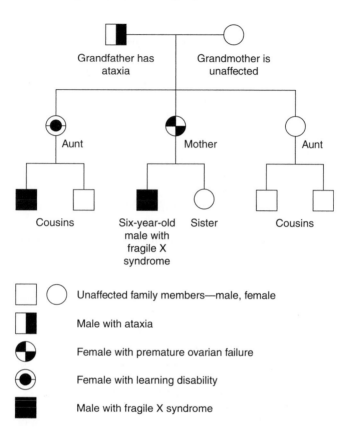

Figure 27-1 Fragile X–related disorders.

NURSING DIAGNOSES

- Knowledge of fragile X–related disorders, Readiness for enhanced
- Conflict, decisional, secondary to proceeding with DNA testing for fragile X mutation
- Conflict, decisional, secondary to sharing testing results with other family members
- Conflict, decisional, secondary to terminating pregnancy
- Family processes, Interrupted
- Health-seeking behaviors

BOX 27-2

Focused Family Nursing Assessment
Questions for Pregnant Couples, Parents, and Adults Who Are Concerned about Fragile X–Related Disorders

1. Did you ever receive special education services?
2. Did any of your family members receive special education services?
3. Is this family member still menstruating?
4. Does this family member suffer from tremors, rigidity, slow movements, or balance problems?
5. Is this infant or child developmentally delayed?
6. Is this child hyperactive?

BOX 27-3

Risk Assessment: Patients Who May Benefit from Genetic Counseling and/or Testing

A. Family/Medical History Risk Assessment

a. Patients of either sex with intellectual disability, developmental delay, or autism
b. Family history of fragile X syndrome
c. Patient or family member has undiagnosed intellectual disability or tremor/ataxia syndrome
d. Individuals seeking reproductive counseling who have a family history of intellectual disability
e. Fetuses of known carrier mothers
f. Women under forty who have elevated follicle-stimulating hormone (FSH) levels

B. Genetic Patterns of Inheritance Risk Assessment

a. FMR1-related disorders are inherited in an X-linked dominant manner
b. Parents of a child with fragile X syndrome
   i. Mother is a carrier of a premutation or a full mutation.
   ii. Premutation mother may have a father or mother who is a premutation carrier.

Continued

BOX 27-3

Risk Assessment: Patients Who May Benefit from Genetic Counseling and/or Testing—cont'd

   iii. Mother of a male with a premutation also has a premutation.
   iv. Mother with premutation is at risk for *FMR1*-related premature ovarian failure and FXTAS.
   v. Father with premutation is at risk for developing FXTAS.

C. Risk Assessment for Siblings of Child with Fragile X Syndrome

a. Risk depends on
   i. Gender
   ii. Gender of carrier parent
   iii. Size of the trinucleotide repeat in the carrier parent

D. Risk Assessment for Offspring of an Individual with a Full Mutation

a. Male with a full mutation has an intellectual disability; generally does not reproduce.
b. Female with a full mutation; ~50% risk she will have an intellectual disability; X-inactivation may provide her protection.

E. Risk Assessment for Family Premutation

   a. Male who is a premutation carrier—all his daughters will be premutation carriers.
   b. Male who is a premutation carrier—None of his sons inherit the premutation because they inherit his Y chromosome.
      i. Offspring of a female with a premutation—50% risk of inheriting a premutation or a full mutation.
      ii. Maternal aunts (of an affected child) and their offspring may be at risk of being carriers or being affected.
      iii. Grandchildren (through daughters) of premutation carriers are at risk for fragile X syndrome.

- Self-care deficit, bathing/hygiene
- Self-care deficit, dressing/grooming
- Self-care deficit, feeding
- Self-care deficit, toileting
- Social interaction, impaired

BOX 27-4
Nondiscrimination Genetics Laws

1. Americans with Disabilities Act of 1990—protects individuals with genetic disabilities.
2. Health Insurance Portability and Accountability Act of 1996 (HIPPA)—applies to employer-based group health insurance. It prohibits employers from using genetics information to exclude anyone or charge more for the same services; a genetic abnormality without illness is not a preexisting condition.
3. HIPPA National Standards to Protect Patients' Personal Medical Records (December 2002)—Improper use or disclosure of health information has criminal and civil penalties.

Visit www.hhs.gov/ocr/hipaa/ for more information.

NURSING INTERVENTIONS

1. Instruct family and reinforce information on knowledge of fragile X–related disorders.
   a. Explain to family that many health care providers have a poor understanding of these disorders.
   b. Assist the family in self-education.
   c. Inform family of available fragile X resources (Box 27-5).
2. Answer family concerns regarding the decision to have DNA testing for fragile X mutation.
   a. Refer for genetic counseling.
   b. Consult with advanced practice nurse in genetics, genetic counselor, or medical geneticist.
3. Address family concerns regarding the decision to share testing results with other family members.
   a. Nurses should encourage but not coerce the sharing of genetic information in families.
4. Address parental concerns about the decision to terminate a fragile X–affected fetus.
   a. Inform family that most states prohibit termination of pregnancy after the twentieth or the twenty-first week.
   b. Validate the family's religious convictions surrounding abortions.

5. Provide reproductive and contraceptive counseling.
   a. Coordinate age-appropriate sex education and birth control, especially for females.
   b. Fertility is normal in men, but reproduction is rare as a result of cognitive delay.

🏠 Discharge Planning and Home Care

1. Refer family to community resources for support and assistance.
   a. Assist family with access to care services such as genetic counseling and family counseling therapy.
   b. Assist family with finding local advocacy groups.
   c. Refer to Appendix G for community services.
2. Promote the infant's, child's, or youth's development (see Chapter 44).
3. Serve as health care resource and/or consultant to child's disability service coordinator and/or care manager.
   a. Assist family in obtaining access to health care services.
   b. Assist family in obtaining accommodations in educational, work, and community settings.
   c. Educate care providers and family about sexual self-stimulation, which is common.
   d. Address issues of sexuality and reproductive concerns as developmentally appropriate (see section on psychosexual development in Appendix B).

CLIENT OUTCOMES

1. Family will be educated about fragile X–related disorders.
2. Family will seek genetic counseling and, if appropriate, genetic testing.
3. Family will attend family counseling therapy.
4. Family will understand inheritance patterns of fragile X–related disorders.
5. Family will be adept in accessing community resources.
6. Family will be adept and adjust to the long-term management needs of child.

7. Child or youth will acquire developmental competencies appropriate for age and level of cognitive and adaptive functioning.
8. Child or youth will demonstrate autonomy, self-determination, and self-advocacy behaviors.
9. Youth will graduate from high school or obtain high school certificate.
10. Youth will have acquired school-based work experience as precursor for adult employment.
11. Child or youth will have participated in inclusive school and community-based activities.
12. Child or youth will have age-appropriate social relationships.

BOX 27-5
Resources

Fragile X Foundations
- National Fragile X Foundation
  PO Box 190488
  San Francisco, CA 94119
  Phone: 925-938-9300
  Website: www.nfxf.org
- FRAXA Research Foundation
  PO Box 935
  West Newbury, MA 01985-0935
  Phone: 978-462-1866, 978-463-9985 (fax)
  Website: www.fraxa.org

Fragile X Newsletters
- National Fragile X Foundation newsletter—Call 800-688-8765 or email www.nfxf.org.
- FRAXA Research Foundation newsletter—Call 978-4462-1866 or email www.fraxa.org.

Fragile X Reading for Children
- O'Connor R: *Boys with Fragile X Syndrome*, San Francisco, 1995, National Fragile X Foundation. Can be obtained from the National Fragile X Foundation by calling 800-688-8765.
- Steiger C: *My Brother Has Fragile X Syndrome*, Chapel Hill, NC, 1998, Avanta. Call 800-434-0322.

REFERENCES

Biancalana V et al: *FMR1* premutations associated with fragile X-associated atrophy, *Arch Neurol* 62(6):962, 2005.

Ensenauer RE, Michels VV, Reinke SS: Genetic testing: Practical, ethical, and counseling consideration, *Mayo Clin Proc* 80(1):63-73, 2005.

Hagerman RJ: Fragile X syndrome. In: Jackson P, Vessey J, editors: Primary care of the child with a chronic health condition, ed 4, St. Louis, 2004, Mosby.

Human Genome Project Information: *Ethical, legal and social issues* (website): www.ornl.gov/sci/techresources/Human_Genome/elsi/legistat.shtml. Accessed January 16, 2006.

National Human Genome Research Institute, National Institutes of Health: *Genetic discrimination in health insurance* (website): www.genome.gov/10002328. Accessed January 16, 2006.

Sherman R, Pletcher BA, Driscoll DA: Fragile X syndrome: Diagnostic and carrier testing, *Genet Med* 7(8):584, 2005.

28

Gastroenteritis

PATHOPHYSIOLOGY

Gastroenteritis or acute infectious diarrhea is defined as inflammation of the mucous membranes of the stomach and intestines. Acute gastroenteritis is characterized by diarrhea and, in some cases, vomiting; the resulting fluid and electrolyte losses lead to dehydration and electrolyte imbalances. The major causes of acute gastroenteritis include viruses (rotavirus, enteric adenovirus, Norwalk virus, and others), bacteria or their toxins (*Campylobacter, Salmonella, Shigella, Escherichia coli, Staphylococcus, Yersinia,* and others), and parasites *(Giardia lamblia, Cryptosporidium)* (Table 28-1). These pathogens cause illness by infecting the cells, producing enterotoxins or cytotoxins that damage the cells, or adhering to the walls of the intestines. In acute gastroenteritis, the small intestine is the most often affected.

Rotavirus, which is the most common causative agent for gastroenteritis, has an incubation period of 24 to 48 hours. Vomiting is the first symptom in 80% to 90% of patients, followed by low-grade fever and voluminous watery diarrhea. Diarrhea usually lasts 4 to 8 days but may last longer. In young infants or immunocompromised patients, rotavirus acute gastroenteritis may be preceded by mild upper respiratory infection (URI) symptoms.

Acute gastroenteritis is transmitted by the fecal-oral route, from person to person or through contaminated water and food supplies. Spending time in day-care facilities increases the risk for gastroenteritis, as does travel to developing countries. Replacement of fluid and electrolyte insufficiency

TABLE 28-1
Characteristics of Acute Gastroenteritis

Pathogen	Vomiting	Diarrhea	Fever	Stool Characteristics	Abdominal Pain	Epidemiologic Features
Rotavirus	Very common	5-7 days; organism shed in stool even with mild or no symptoms	Common	Profuse, watery; green, yellow, or clear; no blood or pus	Some, with tenesmus	1- to 3-day incubation period
Enteric adenovirus	Occasionally	About 14 days	Occasionally, low-grade	Watery	Some, with/ without tenesmus	3- to 10-day incubation period
Norwalk virus	Very common	Less common, lasts 1-3 days	Common	Watery	Moderate to severe cramping	12- to 48-hour incubation period; outbreaks in school-aged children common

Salmonella	Sometimes, nausea common	2–7 days; 40% of cases excrete organisms in stool for 4 weeks; 45% of children under 5 yrs of age continue to excrete organisms for 12 weeks or more	Very common	Green, watery, and foul smelling; blood may or may not be present	Very common, with tenesmus	6- to 72-hour incubation period; 1% to 2% become chronic carriers
Shigella	Uncommon	≥1 week; organisms shed for 7–30 days, rarely longer; if	Common	Mucoid, bloody, green with pus (dysentery form characterized by watery	Tenderness very common; cramps sometimes occur	1- to 7-day incubation period; easily transmitted; increased incidence in

Continued

TABLE 28-1
Characteristics of Acute Gastroenteritis—cont'd

Pathogen	Vomiting	Diarrhea	Fever	Stool Characteristics	Abdominal Pain	Epidemiologic Features
		antibiotics are given shedding is reduced		diarrhea, high fever, malaise followed in 24 hours by tenesmus and colitis)		day care facilities—child should have negative stool culture results and no diarrhea before return to school or day care
Campylobacter jejuni	Nausea but seldom vomiting	3 days to1 week	Common	Starts as watery, frequently with blood or mucus; onset may be gradual or explosive	Cramping very common; tenderness common	2- to 4-day incubation period, sometimes as long as 7 days; breast-

Organism						
Escherichia coli—enterotoxigenic	None	5 days, sometimes as long as 10 days	Uncommon	Profuse watery stool, sometimes with mucus but no pus or blood	Cramping very common	feeding may be protective 10-hour to 6-day incubation period; seen in developing countries
Escherichia coli—enteroinvasive	Common	7–10 days	Common	Watery stool, may or may not be bloody (less volume than with enterotoxigenic strain)	Abdominal pain common	10-hour to 6-day incubation period
Escherichia coli—enteropathogenic	Common	1 week in older child or adult; may	Sometimes	Profuse watery stool, no	Cramping common	10-hour to 6-day incubation period

Continued

TABLE 28-1
Characteristics of Acute Gastroenteritis—cont'd

Pathogen	Vomiting	Diarrhea	Fever	Stool Characteristics	Abdominal Pain	Epidemiologic Features
Yersinia entero colitica	Not in children < 4 years; common in older child	Few days to 6 weeks	Very common (up to 40° C)	Mucoid or watery, often with leukocytes or blood	Abdominal tenderness common	Typically has a 4-to 6-day incubation period; sometimes confused with appendicitis

(continued from previous row) last 2 weeks or longer in infants — blood or mucus

and ongoing losses is critical, especially for small infants. Metabolic acidosis results from bicarbonate loss in the stool, ketosis from poor intake, and lactic acidemia from hypotension and hypoperfusion. Most infections are self-limited, and prognosis is favorable with treatment. Malnourished children may have more severe infections and take longer to recover.

INCIDENCE

1. Acute viral gastroenteritis is the second most common condition affecting children (the common cold is the first).
2. About half of all cases of gastroenteritis occur during a 3- to 4-month winter peak.
3. The highest rate of illness occurs in children between 3 months and 2 years of age.
4. Viral agents are thought to account for 80% of reported community diarrhea and repeated exposures to agents like rotavirus. Rotavirus is the causative agent in approximately 50% of hospital admissions for acute gastroenteritis. The seasonal peak occurs approximately between November and May each year, with prevalence in the United States beginning in the Southwest and spreading to the Northeast. Between 5% and 10% of admissions result from infection with enteric adenoviruses, and another 15% are due to bacterial causes.
5. Breast-fed infants contract gastroenteritis less often than formula-fed infants; maternal antibodies to some enteric pathogens are transferred in breast milk.

CLINICAL MANIFESTATIONS

1. Loose consistency of stools (diarrhea) with increased frequency, with and/or without blood or mucus
2. Anorexia, nausea, and/or vomiting (usually of short duration)
3. Fever (may or may not be present)
4. Abdominal cramping, tenesmus
5. Evidence of dehydration such as dry mucous membranes, sunken fontanelle in infants
6. Tachycardia
7. Weight loss
8. Malaise, general "sick" feeling

COMPLICATIONS

1. Severe dehydration, electrolyte imbalance
2. Decompensated hypovolemic shock (hypotension, metabolic acidosis, poor systemic perfusion)
3. Febrile seizures
4. Bacteremia

LABORATORY AND DIAGNOSTIC TESTS

1. Fecal occult blood test—to check for presence of blood (more common with bacterial origin)
2. Stool evaluation for volume, color, consistency, presence of mucus or pus
3. Complete blood count with differential
4. Enzyme immunoassay antigen tests—to confirm presence of rotavirus
5. Stool culture (if hospitalized, pus is present in stool, or course of diarrhea is prolonged)—to determine pathogen
6. Stool evaluation for ova and parasites; performed 3 times, 24 hours apart
7. Duodenal aspiration (if *G. lamblia* is suspected)
8. Urinalysis and culture (specific gravity increases with dehydration; *Shigella* organisms are shed in urine)

MEDICAL MANAGEMENT

When the child is mildly dehydrated, rehydration may be accomplished orally on an outpatient basis with commercially available oral rehydration solutions (ORSs such as Pedialyte, Ricelyte). ORSs boost and advance the reabsorption of sodium and water. Oral rehydration fluids are given frequently, in small volumes (5 to 30 ml), even in the event of vomiting. Breast-fed infants can continue to be nursed during periods of diarrhea. In the case of severe dehydration, the child is admitted for intravenous (IV) therapy to correct dehydration. The amount of dehydration is calculated, and fluid is replaced over 24 hours, at the same time that maintenance fluids are given.

When shock is present, fluid resuscitation commences immediately (20 ml/kg of normal saline solution or lactated Ringer's solution; repeat if needed). In these cases, when rapid peripheral IV access is unsuccessful, the intraosseous route may be used for emergency fluid administration in a child younger than 6 years of age. When systemic perfusion has been improved, correction of existing dehydration is begun.

Once rehydration is completed, the diet may be advanced to a regular diet of easily digested foods. Foods best tolerated are complex carbohydrates (rice, wheat, cereals, potatoes, and bread), yogurt, lean meats, fruits, and vegetables. The classic BRAT diet (bananas, rice, applesauce, and toast or tea), although well tolerated, is low in protein, fat, and calories for energy. Ideal foods to encourage are ones that contain complex carbohydrates (rice, baked potatoes, noodles, crackers, toast, cereals). Juices, sports beverages, and soft drinks should be avoided. Water should not be the only vehicle of oral fluids.

Feeding and oral administration of rehydration fluids have reportedly decreased the duration of diarrhea. The American Academy of Pediatrics, the World Health Organization, and the Centers for Disease Control and Prevention all recommend oral rehydration therapy (ORT) as the treatment of choice for most cases of dehydration caused by diarrhea. Early return to normal oral feedings is important, especially in cases of preexisting malnutrition.

Administration of antiemetics and antispasmodics is generally not recommended. Neither is the use of antibiotics indicated in most cases, because bacterial and viral gastroenteritis is self-limited. Antibiotics are used, however, in the treatment of diseases caused by *Shigella* organisms, *E. coli*, *Salmonella* organisms (when sepsis or localized infection is present), and *G. lamblia*. Use of antibiotics may increase the duration of the carrier state in *Salmonella* infections.

NURSING ASSESSMENT

See the Gastrointestinal Assessment section in Appendix A.

NURSING DIAGNOSES

- Fluid volume, Risk for deficient
- Diarrhea
- Skin integrity, Risk for impaired
- Knowledge, Deficient

NURSING INTERVENTIONS

1. Promote and monitor child's fluid and electrolyte balance.
   a. Monitor IV fluids.
   b. Assess intake and output (weigh diapers).
   c. Assess hydration status.
   d. Monitor daily weight.
   e. Assess child's ability to rehydrate by mouth.
2. Prevent further gastrointestinal tract irritability.
   a. Assess child's ability to take nourishment by mouth (i.e., first provide ORSs [Pedialyte, Ricelyte], then advance to regular diet of easily digested foods). A BRAT diet is contraindicated, especially for infants and children with acute diarrhea, because this diet has little nutritional value and is low in electrolytes. Encourage breast-feeding, whereas formula-fed infants should continue with formula.
   b. Assess for signs of lactose intolerance when milk is introduced.
   c. Consult with dietitian about selection of foods.
3. Prevent skin irritation and breakdown.
   a. Change diapers frequently, assessing skin condition each time.
   b. Wash perineum with mild soap and water, and expose perineum to air.
   c. Apply zinc oxide or lubricating ointment to perineum (acidic stools irritate skin).
4. Follow universal precautions and/or enteric precautions to prevent transmission of infection (refer to institution's policies and procedures).
5. Provide for child's developmental needs during hospitalization.
   a. Provide age-appropriate toys (see the relevant section in Appendix F).
   b. Incorporate home routine into hospital care (e.g., feeding practices, bedtime ritual).
   c. Encourage expression of feelings through age-appropriate means.

6. Provide emotional and other support to family.
   a. Encourage verbalization of concerns.
   b. Refer to social services as needed.
   c. Provide for physical comforts (e.g., places to sleep and bathe).

🏠 Discharge Planning and Home Care

1. Instruct parents and child about personal and environmental hygiene.
   a. Good handwashing
   b. Sanitary disposal of excreta
   c. Sanitary food preparation
   d. Good toileting practices
   e. Safe drinking water
2. Reinforce dietary information provided to parents about menu planning.
3. Instruct parents to observe for and report signs of dehydration or problems with oral rehydration and advancement of feedings.
4. Instruct parents about follow-up appointment.

CLIENT OUTCOMES

1. Child's gastrointestinal function will return to normal.
2. Child will be well hydrated.
3. Parents and child will understand home care and medical follow-up needed.

REFERENCES

American Academy of Pediatrics, Pickering LK, editor: *2003 Red book: Report of the Committee on Infectious Diseases*, ed 26, Elk Grove Village, Ill, 2000, The Academy.

Dennehy PH: Transmission of rotavirus and other enteric pathogens in the home, *Pediatr Infect Dis J* 19(10):S103, 2000.

Hay WW et al: *Current pediatric diagnosis and treatment*, ed 17, New York, 2005, McGraw-Hill.

Larson CE: Safety and efficacy of oral rehydration therapy for the treatment of diarrhea and gastroenteritis in pediatrics, *Pediatr Nurs* 26(2):177, 2000.

Perlstein PH et al: Implementing an evidence-based acute gastroenteritis guideline at a children's hospital, *Jt Comm J Qual Improv* 28(1):20, 2002.

Wong DL et al: *Maternal child nursing care*, ed 3, St. Louis, 2006, Mosby.

29

Gastroesophageal Reflux

PATHOPHYSIOLOGY

Considered as one of the vomiting disorders, gastroesophageal reflux (GER) is the retrograde passage of gastric contents into the esophagus, the upper airways, and the tracheobronchial area. Predisposing factors associated with GER are (1) muscle tonicity of the lower esophageal sphincter (LES); (2) age; (3) hiatal hernia, (4) intraabdominal pressure; (5) length of the esophagus below the diaphragm; (6) rate of gastric emptying; (7) drugs; (8) hormones; and (9) spontaneous relaxation of the LES secondary to neurologic involvement. Associated symptoms are pain and/or irritability, spitting up, regurgitation of food (especially of liquid to semiliquid consistency), vomiting, poor weight gain, and respiratory disorders. The reflux of gastric contents can lead to apneic spells in young infants and inflammation, damage (Barrett's esophagus) and stricture of the esophageal mucosa, failure to thrive, occult blood loss, anemia, aspiration pneumonia with or without wheezing, ear and sinus infection, and sleep disorder. In 85% of infants with GER, the condition is self-limiting, disappearing between ages 6 and 12 months; thus resolution of GER is often a maturational process. However, a child may require surgery (gastric fundoplication; see Medical Management in this chapter) if he or she does not respond to medical management.

INCIDENCE

1. Vomiting occurs in 18% to 40% of children with GER.
2. Failure to thrive occurs in 34% of these children.

3. Bleeding occurs in 28% of these children.
4. Pulmonary complications occur in 12% of these children.

CLINICAL MANIFESTATIONS

1. Chronic vomiting (most common)
2. Weight loss, failure to thrive
3. Apnea (in infants) due to aspiration or obstruction
4. Hematemesis or melena due to esophageal bleeding
5. Recurrent bronchitis and/or pneumonia
6. Irritability, loss of appetite

COMPLICATIONS

1. Aspiration pneumonia
2. Respiratory disease (asthma, cough, stridor)
3. Apnea and cyanosis
4. Esophagitis and/or Barrett's esophagus (precursor to esophageal cancer)
5. Chest pain and/or heartburn
6. Gastric fistula

LABORATORY AND DIAGNOSTIC TESTS

1. Esophageal pH measurement (less than 4.0 is diagnostic) for 23 hours
2. Electric impedance measurement
3. Endoscopy—to detect presence of gross and microscopic esophagitis and cellular dysplasia
4. Barium esophagram—to detect anatomic abnormalities; often fails to detect intermittent reflux
5. Nuclear medicine scintiscan—to assess gastric emptying
6. Manometry—to assess esophageal motility and LES function

MEDICAL MANAGEMENT

The treatment of GER reflects the severity of symptoms. Nonpharmacologic treatment and management consists of feeding thickened formula; feeding small, frequent meals; and positioning to avoid increased intraabdominal pressure—either upright without slouching in an infant seat or car seat or in prone position. Placement in an infant seat postprandially is contraindicated because such seats increase intraabdominal pressure. Pharmacologic treatment is primarily acid suppression and neutralization. Acid neutralization drugs such as aluminum or magnesium hydroxide are beneficial. H_2 blockers such as ranitidine, famotidine, cimetidine, and proton pump inhibitors (PPIs) such as omeprazole, lansoprazole, are used for acid suppression. Prokinetic agents (metoclopromide and erythromycin) and cholinergic agents (bethanecol) may be added to further prevent reflux activities. In some infants, continuous tube feedings may be used when conventional medical treatment has failed.

When medical management fails to control the symptoms and risk of complications of GER disease increases, the infant or child must be referred to a pediatric gastroenterologist and/or pediatric surgeon for advanced medical management, treatment, and possible surgical intervention. Nissen fundoplication is a major surgical procedure wherein the upper end of the stomach is wrapped around the lower portion of the esophagus, and the fundus is sutured in front of the esophagus to create a circular acute-angle valve mechanism. Family must be aware, depending on the age of the child, that there is a high possibility that repeat fundoplication may be necessary in 3 to 5 years as the child grows older. There is usually a reverse correlation between the age of the child and the number of antireflux surgeries performed. Placement of a gastrostomy tube ensures adequate nutrition and simplifies care.

NURSING ASSESSMENT

1. See the Gastrointestinal Assessment section in Appendix A.
2. Assess feeding history.
3. Assess hydration status.
4. Assess frequency and volume of emesis and length of time between feedings and emesis.
5. Assess weight gain.

NURSING DIAGNOSES

- Fluid volume, Deficient
- Pain

- Nutrition: less than body requirements, Imbalanced
- Gas exchange, Impaired
- Injury, Risk for
- Knowledge, Deficient
- Home maintenance, Impaired

NURSING INTERVENTIONS

1. Promote adequate nutritional and fluid intake.
   a. Maintain head of bed in 30- to 60-degree position for 30 to 40 minutes after feeding.
   b. Raise head of bed with 6-inch blocks.
   c. Provide small, frequent feedings every 2 to 3 hours.
   d. Thicken formula with cereal.
   e. Provide last meal of day several hours before bedtime.
   f. Weigh child daily.
   g. Monitor intake and output.
2. Observe, monitor, and report signs of respiratory distress; assess for changes in respiratory status.
3. Preoperatively, prepare child and family for surgery.
4. Monitor surgical site for intactness.
5. Prevent abdominal distention.
   a. Maintain patency of nasogastric (NG) or gastrostomy tube if placed.
   b. Check position of NG tube.
   c. Auscultate for bowel sounds.
6. Monitor for signs and symptoms of postoperative hemorrhage.
   a. Decreased blood pressure and increased apical pulse
   b. Gross blood in NG drainage
   c. Coffee-ground NG drainage expected for first 24 hours
7. Assist parents in verbalization of feelings—may express anger, guilt, or frustration because they feel inadequate or responsible.
8. Provide developmentally appropriate stimulation activities (see Appendix B).
9. Administer PPIs 15 to 30 minutes before the first meal of the day.

🏠 Discharge Planning and Home Care

1. Instruct parents about medication administration.
2. Instruct parents about feeding techniques.
3. Instruct parents to report any vomiting or presence of frank blood.

CLIENT OUTCOMES

1. Child will have consistent weight gain.
2. Child will have decreased frequency and volume of emesis.
3. Child will have decreased pain (heartburn).
4. Child will not aspirate gastric contents.

REFERENCES

Hay WW et al: *Current pediatric diagnosis and treatment*, ed 17, New York, 2005, McGraw-Hill.

O'Brien ZS, Schudder LE: *Pediatric nurse practitioner review and resource manual*, ed 2, Maryland, 2005, ANCC.

Sampayo EM, Adam HM: Rotavirus Infections, *Pediatr Rev* 24(1):175, 2003.

Wong DL et al: *Maternal child nursing care*, ed 3, St. Louis, 2006, Mosby.

30

Glomerulonephritis

PATHOPHYSIOLOGY

Glomerulonephritis is a term used for a collection of disorders that involve the renal glomeruli, which are responsible for filtering body fluids and wastes. Two types of this disease are seen, acute and chronic, with chronic being the progressive form. Acute glomerulonephritis is the most common form of nephritis in children. It is an inflammation of the glomeruli that usually follows a streptococcal upper respiratory tract infection. It is considered an immune-complex disease. The glomerular injury is induced by antigen-antibody complexes trapped in the glomerular filter. The glomeruli become edematous and are infiltrated with polymorphonuclear leukocytes, which occlude the capillary lumen. This condition results in decreased plasma filtration, causing excessive accumulation of water and retention of sodium. The resultant plasma and interstitial fluid volumes lead to circulatory congestion and edema. Hypertension is associated with glomerulonephritis.

INCIDENCE

1. Glomerulonephritis is most common in school-aged children.
2. Ages of peak incidence are from 2 to 6 years.
3. The disorder occurs predominantly in boys in childhood; in adolescence, no male or female predilection is seen.
4. Of children with acute glomerulonephritis, 60% to 80% have a history of a preceding upper respiratory tract infection or otitis media (typically, the child was in good health before the infection).

CLINICAL MANIFESTATIONS

1. Nephritis tends to have an average latency period of approximately 10 days, with onset of symptoms 10 days after the initial infection.
2. Initial signs are puffiness of the face, periorbital edema, anorexia, and dark urine.
3. Edema tends to be more prominent in the face in the morning; then it spreads to the abdomen and the extremities during the day (moderate edema may not be recognized by someone who is unfamiliar with the child).
4. Urinary output is decreased.
5. Urine is cloudy or smoky, or described as having the color of tea or cola.
6. The child is pale, irritable, and lethargic.
7. Younger children may appear ill but seldom express specific complaints.
8. Older children may complain of headaches, abdominal discomfort, vomiting, and dysuria.
9. Mild to moderate hypertension may be present.

COMPLICATIONS

Once acute glomerulonephritis progresses to the chronic stage, the following complications may be seen:

1. Deteriorating renal function (generally reflected by clinical manifestations and laboratory findings)
2. Proteinuria
3. Edema
4. Hypertension
5. Hematuria
6. Anemia (manifestation of progressive disease)
7. Hypertensive encephalopathy (characterized by headache, vomiting, irritability, convulsions, and coma)—can result from the chronic hypertension
8. Cardiac failure, possibly a result of an increase in blood volume secondary to retention of sodium and water—associated with pulmonary congestion
9. End-stage renal disease

LABORATORY AND DIAGNOSTIC TESTS

No diagnostic tests are specifically indicated for the diagnosis of glomerulonephritis. However, the following are commonly performed:

1. Examination of urine—proteinuria (1 to 4), hematuria; presence of casts, red blood cells, and white blood cells; decreased creatinine clearance rates
2. Blood tests—elevated blood urea nitrogen, serum creatinine, and uric acid levels; electrolyte alterations (metabolic acidosis; decreased sodium and calcium; increased potassium, phosphorus, serum albumin, and cholesterol); mild anemia and leukocytosis; elevated antibody titers (antistreptolysin, antihyaluronidase, or antideoxyribonuclease B) and erythrocyte sedimentation rate
3. Renal biopsy—may be indicated; if performed, possible findings are increased number of cells in each glomerulus and subepithelial "humps" containing immunoglobulin and complement

MEDICAL MANAGEMENT

Acute glomerulonephritis has no specific treatment; thus therapy is targeted at the symptoms. Marked hypertension may be treated with diuretics and/or antihypertensives. Appropriate antibiotics are used for acute infections. Some medicinal approaches for treatment of chronic glomerulonephritis have included administration of glucocorticoids and immunosuppressive agents.

NURSING ASSESSMENT

1. See the Renal Assessment section in Appendix A.
2. Assess nutritional intake.
3. Assess fluid status.

NURSING DIAGNOSES

- Fluid volume, Excess
- Nutrition: less than body requirements, Imbalanced
- Knowledge, Deficient

NURSING INTERVENTIONS

1. Maintain bed rest and keep child comfortable until diuresis occurs; after diuresis, encourage quiet activity.
2. Closely monitor vital signs (especially blood pressure).
3. When hypertension is present, limit sodium intake and administer ordered medications.
4. Monitor urine for protein and occult blood.
5. Promote adequate nutritional intake: encourage high-carbohydrate meals, serve preferred foods, and try small, frequent feedings.
6. Limit potassium intake if hyperkalemia occurs.
7. Record weight daily and accurately record intake and output.
8. Monitor for complications—significant changes in vital signs, change in appearance or volume of urine, excessive weight gain, visual disturbances, motor disturbances, seizure activity, severe pain, or any behavioral changes.

🏠 Discharge Planning and Home Care

1. Provide family with education about child's illness and treatment plan.
2. Instruct about any medications child will take at home.
3. Instruct parents and child to monitor blood pressure and weight, and to obtain urinalyses for several months; follow-up appointments should be arranged.
4. Instruct parents to contact physician if any change is seen in child's condition, such as signs of infection, edema, alteration in eating habits, abdominal pain, headaches, change in appearance or amount of urine, or lethargy.
5. Explain any dietary restrictions to parents.

CLIENT OUTCOMES

1. Child will have a return to normal renal function.
2. Child and family will understand home care and follow-up needs.

REFERENCES

Behrman R, Kiegman R, Jenson HB: *Nelson Textbook of Pediatrics*, ed 17, Philadelphia, 2004, WB Saunders.

Kasahara T et al: Prognosis of acute poststreptococcal glomerulonephritis is excellent in children when adequately diagnosed, *Pediatr Int* 43(4):364, 2001.

Lang MM, Towers C: Identifying post streptococcal glomerulonephritis, *Nurse Pract* 26(8):34, 2001.

Miller D, MacDonald D: Management of pediatric patients with chronic kidney disease, *Pediatr Nurs* 32(2):128, 2006.

Pan GG: Glomerulonephritis in childhood, *Curr Opin Pediatr* 9(2):154, 2001.

West CD, McAdams AJ, Witte DP: Acute non-proliferative glomerulitis: A cause of renal failure unique to children, *Pediatr Nephrol* 14: 786, 2000.

31

Hemolytic-Uremic Syndrome

PATHOPHYSIOLOGY

Hemolytic-uremic syndrome (HUS) is the leading cause of acute renal failure in infants and young children. HUS is a systemic disease that consists of the following symptomatology: (1) renal failure, (2) hemolytic anemia with fragmented red blood cells and platelets, and (3) thrombocytopenia. Although the exact cause is not known, HUS generally follows an episode of gastroenteritis caused by a strain of *Escherichia coli* O157:H7, or other enteric pathogens such as *Shigella, Salmonella,* and *Campylobacter.* Less commonly, the disease follows an upper respiratory tract infection. The clinical manifestations result from changes in the capillary endothelium caused by the etiologic agent. The endothelial changes result in the following pathologic responses: (1) mechanical trauma to erythrocytes and platelets, which shortens their life span and results in anemia and thrombocytopenia; and (2) decreased renal blood flow and glomerular filtration rate, which results in cortical necrosis and consequent renal failure and acquired hemolytic anemia in infants and children. The severity of the condition varies. The prognosis is related to the efficacy, aggressiveness, and promptness of treatment.

INCIDENCE

1. Most commonly seen in children under the age of 4 years
2. Can occur in geographic outbreaks
3. A seasonal variation exists, with an increased incidence during spring and fall

4. The incidence of hypertension as a long-term complication varies from 10% to 50%.
5. Hemolytic-uremic syndrome affects males and females equally.
6. It is uncommon for a sibling to be affected.
7. Mortality rate is 10% to 25%.

CLINICAL MANIFESTATIONS
Prodromal Phase

1. Episodes of diarrhea (may be bloody), vomiting, fever, and abdominal pain
2. In older children, may resemble an upper respiratory tract illness
3. Prodromal symptoms may last 1 to 2 weeks, whereas other symptoms may recur in children who appear to have recovered; severity varies. (See Box 31-1 for three types of clinical manifestation.)

BOX 31-1
Clinical Manifestations

Mild
- No anemia
- Oliguria*
- Hypertension*
- Seizures*

Severe
- Anuria for longer than 24 hours
- Deteriorating renal function
- Progressive oliguria
- Azotemia
- Complete renal failure—may not occur
- Severe hypertension
- Cardiac failure

Recurrent Hemolytic-Uremic Syndrome
- First occurrence—mild
- Recurrent occurrence—mild to severe

*Child may manifest one or more symptoms but not all three.

Acute Phase

1. Oliguria, amber urine
2. Oliguria or anuria for longer than 1 week, then diuresis
3. Renal failure (metabolic disturbance or acidosis; hypocalcemia or hyperkalemia)
4. Abdominal pain (caused by splenic enlargement or gastrointestinal [GI] involvement)
5. Edema
6. Hypertension
7. Mild icterus
8. Pallor
9. Irritability
10. Lethargy, weakness
11. Dehydration
12. Systemic bleeding manifestations—purpura, petechiae
13. Alteration in neurologic status
14. Anemia associated with uremia
15. Anorexia
16. Seizures
17. Moderate to severe respiratory distress caused by congestive heart failure and circulatory overload

COMPLICATIONS

1. Neurologic—mortality rate in children with neurologic symptoms (seizures, coma) is 90%
2. Disseminated intravascular coagulation—primarily affects vasculature of kidney, nervous system, and GI tract
3. Renal involvement—anemia, acidosis, hypertension, fluid overload, uremia, death
4. Congestive heart failure
5. Colitis (melena, perforation)
6. Diabetes mellitus

LABORATORY AND DIAGNOSTIC TESTS

1. Renal scan—to assess renal perfusion
2. Renal biopsy—to assess renal involvement
3. Serum protein level—increased

4. Complete blood count—decreased hemoglobin; increased white blood cell count; significant reticulocytosis; reticulocyte count higher than 2%
5. Platelet count—less than 140,000/mm^3; remains low for 7 to 14 days
6. Serum albumin level—decreased
7. Arterial blood gas values—decreased pH; acidosis with acute renal failure
8. Electrolyte levels—consistent with renal failure (hyponatremia, hyperkalemia)
9. Tests for hyperuricemia, hypocalcemia, hyperphosphatemia
10. Urinalysis—gross hematuria, proteinuria, casts
11. Blood urea nitrogen, creatinine levels—elevated; reflect severity of renal failure
12. Bilirubin—elevated serum concentrations

MEDICAL MANAGEMENT

Early diagnosis and aggressive treatment are the goals. Early intervention with peritoneal dialysis is the most effective treatment for children who have been anuric for 24 hours or who demonstrate oliguria with hypertension and seizures. Supportive care is directed toward vascular support and stabilization, focusing on fluid, electrolyte, and metabolic balances, adequate nutrition, and controlling blood pressure.

Drugs such as corticosteroids, anticoagulants, or antiplatelet agents have not been found to be effective.

NURSING ASSESSMENT

1. See the Renal Assessment section in Appendix A.
2. Assess hydration status.
3. Assess cardiovascular status.

NURSING DIAGNOSES

- Fluid volume, Excess
- Cardiac output, Decreased
- Infection, Risk for
- Injury, Risk for
- Imbalanced nutrition: Less than body requirements
- Activity intolerance

- Tissue integrity, Impaired
- Knowledge, Deficient
- Family processes, Interrupted
- Anxiety

NURSING INTERVENTIONS

1. Monitor and maintain fluid and electrolyte balance.
   a. Monitor types of fluids and administration rate to avoid fluid overload and cerebral edema.
   b. Accurately record intake and output.
   c. Record daily weights (twice per day during acute phase).
   d. Monitor blood pressure and pulse pressure.
   e. Replace fluids from urinary loss with isotonic solution (normal saline or lactated Ringer's solution).
   f. Assess hydration status every 4 to 6 hours during acute phase.
   g. Perform arterial pressure and central venous pressure monitoring.
2. Monitor electrolytes and observe for signs of imbalance.
   a. Hyperkalemia—muscular instability, electrocardiogram changes (peaked T waves, wide QRS complex, prolonged PR interval), cardiac arrhythmias
   b. Hypocalcemia—coma, seizures
   c. Hyponatremia—seizures
   d. Hypoglycemia—seizures
3. Transfuse with blood products as indicated.
   a. Washed packed red blood cells—for low hemoglobin level; transfuse slowly; do not raise hemoglobin level higher than 7 to 8 g/dl
   b. Platelets—as needed for bleeding
4. Observe and report signs and symptoms of impending complications.
   a. Shock
   b. Infection
   c. Disseminated intravascular coagulation
   d. Heart failure
   e. Potassium intoxication
   f. Overhydration

g. Seizures

h. Neurologic disturbance—lethargy, coma, hyperactivity

i. Pulmonary edema

j. Hypertension

5. Monitor for nutritional status; nasogastric feedings or hyperalimentation may be needed.

6. Prepare child and family for peritoneal dialysis or hemodialysis if indicated; indications include the following:

a. Anuria for 24 to 48 hours

b. Central nervous system disturbance

c. Congestive heart failure

d. Bleeding (GI and cutaneous)

e. Blood urea nitrogen level higher than 150 mg/100 ml

f. Uncontrollable hyperkalemia

g. Hyponatremia of less than 130 mEq/L

h. Change in neurologic status—lethargy to coma or hyperactivity

i. Hyperphosphatemia of higher than 8 mg/100 ml

j. Uncontrollable acidosis

k. Hypocalcemia of less than 8 mg/100 ml

7. Provide information about procedures before they are performed, and reinforce data provided to parents.

🏠 Discharge Planning and Home Care

1. Instruct child and family regarding dietary restrictions.

2. Instruct child and family regarding medications.

3. Consult discharge planning team, and educate child and family for home peritoneal dialysis if needed.

4. Instruct child and family regarding signs and symptoms of complications that must be reported.

CLIENT OUTCOMES

1. Child will have normal or near-normal renal function.

2. Child will have return to normal blood pressure or control of blood pressure.

3. Child will have return to normal neurologic function or control of central nervous system symptoms.

REFERENCES

Behrman RE, Kiegman R, Jenson HB: *Nelson textbook of pediatrics,* ed 17, Philadelphia, PA, 2004, WB Saunders.

Corrigan JJ, Boineau FG: Hemolytic-uremic syndrome, *Pediatr Rev* 22(11):365, 2001.

Hockenberry MJ et al: *Wong's nursing care of infants and children,* ed 7, St. Louis, 2004, Mosby.

Peacock E, Jacob VW, Fallone SM: *Escherichia coli* 0157:H7: Etiology, clinical features, complications, treatment, *Nephrol Nurs J* 28(5):547, 2001.

32

Hemophilia

PATHOPHYSIOLOGY

Hemophilia is a congenital blood coagulation disorder in which the child is deficient in clotting factor VIII (hemophilia A) or factor IX (hemophilia B, or Christmas disease). It is an inherited disorder that is transmitted by an X-linked recessive gene from the maternal side. Factor VIII and factor IX are plasma proteins that are necessary components of blood coagulation; they are needed for the formation of fibrin clots at the site of vascular injury. Severe hemophilia results when plasma concentrations of factors VIII and IX are less than 1%. Moderate hemophilia occurs with plasma concentrations between 1% and 5%. In mild hemophilia (severe bleeding only after major trauma and surgery), plasma concentrations are between 6% and 50% of the normal level. The clinical manifestations depend on the child's age and the severity of the deficiency of factors VIII and IX. Severe hemophilia is characterized by recurrent hemorrhages, occurring either spontaneously or after relatively minor trauma (20 to 30 episodes per year). The most common sites of hemorrhage are the joints, the muscles, and soft tissue. The most common joint sites are the knees, the elbows, the ankles, the shoulders, and the hips. The muscles most often affected are the forearm flexor, the gastrocnemius, and the iliopsoas. Bleeding into the joint or muscle can lead to pain, limited mobility, need for ongoing physical therapy, and some degree of impaired functioning. Life-threatening bleeding episodes can occur in the brain, the gastrointestinal tract, and the neck and throat. Because of improvements in treatment, almost all individuals with hemophilia are expected to live a normal life span. Preliminary data from experimental gene therapy are promising.

INCIDENCE

1. Incidence is 1 in 5000 male births.
2. Incidence of hemophilia A is 20.6 in 100,000.
3. Incidence of hemophilia B is 5.3 in 100,000.
4. Mild hemophilia (5% to 49% factor activity) has bleeding episodes after trauma or surgery.
5. Moderate hemophilia (1% to 5% factor activity) has bleeding after stress or overuse injury to joints or muscles.
6. Severe hemophilia (<1% factor activity) has bleeding with the above in addition to spontaneous bleeding.
7. The family histories of two thirds of affected children reveal an X-linked recessive form of inheritance.
8. About 30% of cases are the result of new mutations.
9. Central nervous system bleeding occurs in 3% of affected children.
10. Spontaneous bleeding and posttraumatic intracranial bleeding are associated with a 34% mortality rate and a 50% rate of long-term morbidity.
11. Of individuals with hemophilia A and hemophilia B, 10% develop immunoglobulin G antibodies that inhibit the activity of factors VIII and IX.

CLINICAL MANIFESTATIONS
Infancy (for Diagnosis)

1. Prolonged bleeding after circumcision
2. Subcutaneous ecchymoses over bony prominences (at 3 to 4 months of age)
3. Large hematoma after infections
4. Bleeding from oral mucosa
5. Soft-tissue hemorrhages

Bleeding Episodes (Throughout Life Span)

1. Initial symptom—pain
2. After pain—swelling, warmth, and decreased mobility

Long-Term Sequelae

Prolonged bleeding into muscle causes nerve compression and muscle fibrosis.

COMPLICATIONS

1. Progressive arthritis and/or arthropathy
2. Compartment syndrome
3. Muscle atrophy
4. Muscle contractures
5. Paralysis
6. Intracranial bleeding
7. Neurologic impairment
8. Hypertension
9. Renal impairment
10. Splenomegaly
11. Hepatitis
12. Cirrhosis
13. Hepatitis C infection from exposure to contaminated blood products
14. Formation of antibodies as antagonists to factors VIII and IX
15. Allergic transfusion reaction to blood products
16. Hemolytic anemia
17. Thrombosis and/or thromboembolism
18. Chronic pain

LABORATORY AND DIAGNOSTIC TESTS

1. Screening tests for blood coagulation
   a. Platelet count—normal in mild to moderate hemophilia
   b. Prothrombin time—normal in mild to moderate hemophilia
   c. Partial thromboplastin time—normal in mild to moderate hemophilia; prolonged in moderately severe hemophilia; measures adequacy of intrinsic coagulation cascade
   d. Bleeding time—normal in mild to moderate hemophilia; assesses formation of platelet plugs in capillaries
   e. Functional assays of factors VIII and IX—confirm diagnosis

f. Thrombin clotting time—normal in mild to moderate hemophilia
2. Liver biopsy (sometimes)—used to obtain tissue for pathologic examination and culture
3. Liver function tests (sometimes)—used to detect presence of liver disease (e.g., serum glutamic-pyruvic transaminase, serum glutamic-oxaloacetic transaminase, alkaline phosphatase, bilirubin levels)

MEDICAL MANAGEMENT

The management of hemophilia consists of the administration of factor VIII or IX on a prophylactic basis or to treat bleeding episodes. Prophylactic administration is performed 2 to 3 times a week to maintain levels of factor VIII or IX. The amount administered depends on the plasma level of the deficient factor needed to treat the specific bleeding episode, and it must be sufficient to allow for the distribution of the factor throughout the body and its clearance from plasma. Dose varies from 15 units/kg to 100 units/kg, depending on the severity of the bleeding episode, child's weight, and type of factor deficiency. It is administered by slow intravenous push or continuous intravenous infusion. Other methods used to treat bleeding episodes are the infusion of frozen plasma and cryoprecipitate (factor VIII). Desmopressin (DDAVP) is also used to increase plasma levels of factor VIII and can be used for nontransfusional treatment of individuals with mild or moderate hemophilia. The administration of oral aminocaproic acid (Amicar) may also be used at times to help stabilize clots. Before the introduction of hepatitis vaccinations and viral inactivation procedures, hepatitis A, B, and C and HIV infection were serious complications associated with treatment. Plasma-derived factors are now safer for use, and recombinant products are used in treating approximately 60% of individuals with severe hemophilia in the United States. General treatment guidelines include these five principles: treat promptly, test for blood borne viruses, keep immunizations up-to-date, remain active, and visit a hemophilia treatment center regularly. Nationwide, federally funded hemophilia treatment centers staffed by interdisciplinary teams composed of hematologists, orthopedic

specialists, dentists, nurses, social workers, and physical therapists provide comprehensive and interdisciplinary care to
individuals and their families.

NURSING ASSESSMENT

1. Refer to Appendix A.
2. Assess child for verbal and nonverbal behaviors indicating
   pain.
3. Assess site of involvement for extent of bleeding and sensory, nerve, and motor impairment.
4. Assess child's or adolescent's ability to engage in self-care
   activities (i.e., brushing teeth).
5. Assess child's or adolescent's and family's readiness for
   discharge and ability to manage home treatment
   regimen.

NURSING DIAGNOSES

- Fluid volume, Risk for deficient
- Pain, Acute
- Injury, Risk for
- Knowledge, Deficient
- Growth and development, Delayed
- Family processes, Interrupted
- Therapeutic regimen management, Ineffective
- Mobility, Impaired physical
- Caregiver role strain

NURSING INTERVENTIONS

Acute Episode

1. Monitor response to administration of plasma products and
   DDAVP. Record amount of factor received, time, and child's
   response to treatment.
2. Monitor child's pain behaviors and response to administration of pain medication and to nonpharmacologic
   measures to relieve pain (refer to Appendix I).
   a. Acetaminophen (avoid aspirin)
   b. Narcotic analgesics
   c. Application of ice to affected joint
   d. Immobilization of affected limb

3. Monitor for further bleeding episodes; observe for signs and symptoms of bleeding.
   a. Symptoms manifested depend on site of bleeding, such as muscles, joints, or brain.
4. Protect from further injury.
   a. Pad child's crib or bed.
   b. Apply pressure after venipunctures.
   c. Apply fibrin or gelatin foam to bleeding sites.
5. Encourage quiet age-appropriate play or diversional activities (see Appendix F).
6. Provide age-appropriate explanations before treatments and procedures (see the Preparation for Procedures or Surgery section in Appendix F).

Long-Term Management

1. Instruct and monitor dental care.
   a. Use of soft-bristle toothbrush
   b. Good nutritional intake
   c. Avoidance of excessive amounts of sweets
   d. Chewing of sugarless gum
   e. Need for regular dental visits
   f. Use of factor replacement before dental work
2. Provide education on hemophilia.
   a. Understanding of genetics and heredity
   b. Understanding of pathophysiology
   c. Recognition of signs and symptoms
   d. Instruction in monitoring for bleeding episodes and complications
   e. Knowledge about when to call for medical assistance
   f. Instruction in how to administer factor products and medication and monitor for side effects
   g. Avoidance of nonsteroidal antiinflammatory drugs
   h. Use of universal precautions
3. Provide emotional support to family (see the Supportive Care section in Appendix F).

🏠 Discharge Planning and Home Care

1. Instruct child or adolescent and parents on assuming self-care responsibilities for long-term management of hemophilia.

    a. Administration of replacement for deficient factor

    b. Signs and symptoms of bleeding episodes

    c. Use of universal precautions

    d. Possible side effects and complications of treatment

    e. Knowledge of how to institute emergency measures

    f. Ordering, storage, and handling of factor products and medications

    g. Care of central venous device and/or infusion site

    h. Prevention of and monitoring for complications

2. Discuss options and plan lifestyle activities to support achievement of developmentally appropriate milestones related to schooling, social relationships, and leisure and recreational pursuits, and achievement of self-care skills in activities of daily living (Appendix B).

3. Learn safety measures to prevent further injuries (avoidance of contact sports and physical play).

4. Discuss with parents and child methods to encourage autonomy and self-determination.

5. Refer family to appropriate community-based resources.

    a. Health insurance coverage

    b. Community services

    c. Counseling on psychosocial concerns related to raising child with disability

    d. Genetic screening and counseling for family members

6. Encourage parents and child to express feelings about hemophilia and limitations it imposes on activities.

    a. Feelings of inferiority associated with having disease

    b. Feelings of inadequacy associated with disease

    c. Feelings of parental guilt, overprotection

    d. Feelings of stress associated with uncertain disease course and daily management

CLIENT OUTCOMES

1. Child's or adolescent's bleeding episodes will be controlled.

2. Child or adolescent and family will adhere to long-term treatment regimen.

3. Child or adolescent will attain developmental milestones.

4. Child or adolescent will learn to become independent and self-sufficient.

REFERENCES

Behrman RE, Kiegman R, Jenson HB: *Nelson textbook of pediatrics,* ed 17, Philadelphia, 2004, WB Saunders.

Christie B, editor: *Nurses' guide to bleeding disorders,* New York, 2002, National Hemophilia Foundation.

Curry H: *Bleeding disorder basics,* Pediatr Nurs 30(5):402, 2005.

Mannucci P, Tuddenham E: Medical progress: the hemophilias—from royal genes to gene therapy, *N Engl J Med* 344(23):1773, 2001.

Nursing Working Group, National Hemophilia Foundation: *The basics of hemophilia* (website): www.hemophilia.org/resources/nurses/hemophilia.ppt. Accessed December 8, 2002.

Petrini P: Treatment strategies in children with hemophilia, *Pediatr Drug* 4(7):427, 2002.

33

Hepatitis

PATHOPHYSIOLOGY

Hepatitis, or inflammation of the liver, can be caused by a viral agent. Hepatitis viruses can be classified into six types: hepatitis A virus (HAV), hepatitis B virus (HBV), hepatitis C virus (HCV), hepatitis D virus (HDV), hepatitis E virus (HEV), and hepatitis G virus (HGV). The hepatocytes (epithelial cells of the liver) are damaged either directly by the virus or by the body's immune response to the virus; in either case, there is altered cellular function that leads to inflammation, necrosis, and autolysis of the liver. Regeneration of cells begins when damaged cells are removed by phagocytosis. Usually recovery is achieved with minimal residual damage, although chronic hepatitis and cirrhosis may develop.

Hepatitis A

Hepatitis A is the most highly contagious form of hepatitis and characteristically is an acute, self-limited illness. It is transmitted primarily through the fecal-oral route. It can also be transmitted by unsanitary food handlers, contaminated food supplies, and shellfish from sewage-contaminated waters. It is rarely transmitted through transfusions. Epidemics of hepatitis A have been reported in institutions that house or care for large numbers of children, such as day care centers, schools, and homes for the mentally retarded. The incubation period is approximately 1 month. Jaundice appears 4 to 6 weeks after exposure in older children and adolescents. The disease is transmissible 2 weeks before the onset of jaundice owing to the high concentration of virus in the stool before definitive symptoms are exhibited. The communicable state continues up to 1 week after the onset of jaundice. Hepatitis A manifests a wide spectrum of symptoms and does not lead to chronic hepatitis. Children may have minimal symptoms or be asymptomatic. The child is rarely hospitalized, and there is no known carrier state.

Hepatitis B and Hepatitis C

HBV and HCV are transmitted through blood or blood derivatives and body secretions (wound exudates, semen, saliva, breast milk, urine). HBV can be transmitted perinatally. With the improvement in blood-product screening procedures in recent years, the incidence of transfusion-related infection is decreasing. Hepatitis B occurs most commonly in the following populations of children: (1) infants whose mothers are chronic carriers of the viral antigen HBsAg, (2) children receiving frequent transfusions or hemodialysis (may also develop hepatitis C), (3) children involved in intravenous drug abuse (may also develop hepatitis C), (4) institutionalized children, and (5) children with person-to-person contact with infected individuals. The incubation period for hepatitis B averages 90 days, whereas that for hepatitis C averages 45 days. Children with hepatitis C are typically asymptomatic. In the United States, more than 60% of the cases of hepatitis C are associated with transfusions of blood or blood products. However, an improved blood screening test has greatly reduced the number of new cases. A carrier state and the development of chronic liver disease are possible with hepatitis B and C.

Hepatitis D

HDV can cause infection and clinical manifestations only in association with hepatitis B infection. The virus acts as a parasite of HBV. Coinfection with HDV increases the severity of the HBV infection, creating a more fulminating course and enhancing the potential for chronic liver disease. The incubation period for hepatitis D is 21 to 90 days. Hepatitis D is most common in hemophiliac individuals and intravenous drug abusers.

Hepatitis E

Hepatitis E transmission occurs via the fecal-oral route, primarily via contaminated water, and is often seen after natural disasters in the developing regions of the world. Incubation period averages 40 days for hepatitis E.

Hepatitis G

The primary cause of HGV infection is through transfusion and organ transplantation. Transmitted through blood, this virus has been detected in up to 2% of American blood donors. Infections may persist up to 20 years, with only rare elevation of liver enzyme levels. This type of hepatitis is usually harmless, but more research is needed to determine long-term effects.

INCIDENCE

1. Approximately 90% of young children and infants with hepatitis will not exhibit jaundice.
2. Up to 90% of children younger than 1 year of age, 30% of children 1 to 5 years of age, and 5% of children older than 5 years of age with hepatitis B develop chronic hepatitis.
3. Hepatitis A is the most common type of hepatitis in children. Incidence of hepatitis A is 2.7 cases per 100,000 in the United States (Centers for Disease Control and Prevention, 2005). Incidence has been declining since routine childhood hepatitis A immunization was recommended in 1996. Tropical and developing nations have a higher incidence of hepatitis A than do industrialized and temperate-zone nations.
4. The incidence of hepatitis B in the pediatric population younger than 12 years of age (this group was born after adoption of routine infant immunization for hepatitis B) is 0.02 cases of hepatitis B per 100,000 population in the United States (Centers for Disease Control and Prevention, 2005).
5. Hepatitis C is most common in the adult population and is commonly associated with intravenous (IV) drug use.

CLINICAL MANIFESTATIONS
Hepatitis A
1. Acute febrile illness
2. Anorexia
3. Nausea and vomiting
4. Malaise
5. Dark urine (precedes jaundice)
6. Jaundice (develops as fever drops)
7. Hepatomegaly
8. No symptoms in 70% of children under 6 years of age
9. In older children and adults, symptoms generally last about 2 months.

Hepatitis B, C, D, E, and G
1. Insidious onset
2. Jaundice
3. Anorexia
4. Malaise
5. Nausea
6. Abnormalities in liver function test results
7. Prodromal symptoms—arthralgia, arthritis, erythematous maculopapular rash
8. Polyarteritis nodosa
9. Hepatitis D—intensifies symptoms of hepatitis B and increases possibility of a chronic condition
10. Hepatitis C—characterized by mild asymptomatic infection with insidious onset of jaundice and malaise

COMPLICATIONS
Hepatitis A
Progression to fulminating disease is very rare, although some have prolonged duration of symptoms.

Hepatitis B and C
1. Carrier state (persistent viral infection without symptoms)
2. Chronic liver disease (in 50% of individuals with hepatitis C)
3. Acute liver failure can occur, but is uncommon.
4. Hepatocellular cancer; occurs in adulthood

5. Cirrhosis
6. Fulminant hepatic failure: encephalopathy, clotting disorders, massive hepatic necrosis

Hepatitis D

1. Fulminant hepatic failure
2. Liver failure
3. Carrier state

LABORATORY AND DIAGNOSTIC TESTS

1. General tests used to indicate liver function include the following:
   a. Aspartate transaminase (AST) level—used to assess liver injury; an increase indicates acute hepatitis
   b. Alanine aminotransferase (ALT) level—used to assess liver injury; would be increased in acute hepatitis
   c. Bilirubin level—elevated, peaking about 5 to 10 days after jaundice appears
2. Immunologic tests are used to determine the type of hepatitis based on identification of antigens (HBsAg, HBeAg) causing disease or antibodies (anti-HAV, anti-HBc, anti-HBs, or anti-HCV) that develop as a result—they confirm the diagnosis:
   a. Anti-HAV immunoglobulin M (IgM) antibodies are present at onset of hepatitis A and persist for 6 to 12 months—used to diagnose acute hepatitis A infection
   b. Anti-HAV immunoglobulin G (IgG) antibodies develop shortly after the anti-HAV IgM antibodies—when present without anti-HAV IgM indicate immunity or resolved past infection
   c. Hepatitis B surface antigen (HBsAg)—present in acute and chronic HBV infection; if persists longer than 6 months, indicates chronic hepatitis B infection
   d. Hepatitis B core antibody IgM (anti-HBc IgM)—presence is diagnostic of acute HBV infection. IgM antibody to the hepatitis B core antigen must be present to differentiate between acute and chronic HBV infection.
   e. Anti-HBs IgG—antibody to the surface antigen HBsAg; presence indicates hepatitis B recovery or immunization

   f. Anti-HBc IgG—presence indicates current, past, or recovery from hepatitis B infection

   g. Anti-HCV IgG—diagnostic for hepatitis C; used to evaluate chronic HCV infection, often negative for first 5 to 12 months after infection

   h. Anti-HDV IgM/IgG—used to identify antibodies to HDV that indicate past or present infection with hepatitis D virus; appears after symptoms develop and may be short-lived since it rapidly converts to IgG antibody

   i. Anti-HEV IgM/IgG—presence indicates hepatitis E infection

MEDICAL MANAGEMENT

Treatment is mainly supportive and includes rest, hydration, and adequate dietary intake. Hospitalization is indicated for severe vomiting, dehydration, abnormal clotting factor levels, or signs of fulminant hepatic failure (restlessness, personality changes, lethargy, decreased level of consciousness, and bleeding). Intravenous therapy, frequent laboratory studies, and physical examinations for progression of disease are the mainstay of hospital management.

   The following medications may be used:

1. Immunoglobulin (Ig)—used for prophylaxis before and after exposure to HAV (administered within 2 weeks of exposure)

2. Hepatitis A vaccine—used to prevent hepatitis A infection. Hepatitis A vaccine is recommended for all children at 12 months of age (Centers for Disease Control and Prevention, 2006). The vaccine is administered in a two-dose schedule, with the second dose administered 6 months after the first.

3. Hepatitis B immunoglobulin (HBIG)—given to neonates of infected mothers within 12 hours of birth; given as prophylaxis within 24 hours after exposure

4. Hepatitis B vaccine (Recombivax HB or Engerix-B)—used to prevent occurrence of hepatitis B. Both vaccines are administered in a three-dose schedule, with the first dose given at birth before hospital discharge. Unvaccinated children and adolescents receive the three-dose schedule.

NURSING ASSESSMENT

1. See the Gastrointestinal Assessment section in Appendix A.
2. Assess for areas of jaundice—skin and sclera.
3. Assess nutritional status.

NURSING DIAGNOSES

- Fluid volume, Deficient
- Nutrition: less than body requirements, Imbalanced
- Infection, Risk for (transmission to others)
- Pain, Acute
- Knowledge, Deficient

NURSING INTERVENTIONS

1. Provide and maintain adequate fluid and food intake.
   a. Monitor for signs of dehydration.
   b. Monitor and record intake and output.
   c. Provide small, frequent meals; antiemetics may be needed.
   d. Offer child's favorite foods.
2. Prevent secondary infections.
   a. Avoid contact between child and infectious sources.
   b. Use and encourage appropriate handwashing technique.
   c. Monitor for signs of infection.
   d. Provide for rest periods.
3. Prevent or control spread of hepatitis.
   a. Refer to institutional procedures for isolation techniques.
   b. Inoculate those people exposed to hepatitis during incubation period.
   c. Immunoglobulin
   d. HBIG vaccine
   e. Vaccinate all children and those individuals at high risk with hepatitis A vaccine and hepatitis B vaccine.
4. Provide pain relief and comfort measures.
   a. Place in position of comfort.
   b. Avoid unnecessary palpation of abdomen (hepatomegaly).
5. Monitor child closely for progression into fulminating hepatitis.
   a. Behavioral changes: disorientation, sleeping in excess, irritability, lethargy

   b. History of bleeding or bruising, results of coagulation
      studies
   c. Coma

🏠 Discharge Planning and Home Care

1. Ensure that all family members and others exposed to child
   receive inoculation of Ig or HBIG.
2. Identify family members needing immunizations for
   hepatitis.
3. Instruct parents and child about signs and symptoms of
   hepatitis so they can monitor for them in individuals
   exposed to child.
4. Provide instruction to parents about sanitary measures to
   institute in home including handwashing.
5. Refer to public health nurse or community nurse for
   assessment of use of preventive measures for hepatitis.

CLIENT OUTCOMES

1. Child's gastrointestinal and hepatic function will return to
   normal.
2. Child will return to normal activity levels without recurrence of illness.
3. Child and family will understand home care instructions,
   disease process, instructions for preventing transmission of
   disease to others, and importance of follow-up.

REFERENCES

Centers for Disease Control and Prevention: Recommended childhood and
   adolescent immunization schedule—United States, 2006, *MMWR* 54
   (51,52):Q1, 2006.
Centers for Disease Control and Prevention: A comprehensive immunization
   strategy to eliminate transmission of hepatitis B virus infection in the
   United States: Recommendations of the Advisory Committee on Immunization Practices (ACIP), Part 1: Immunization of infants, children and adolescents., *MMWR* 54(R16):1, 2005.
Centers for Disease Control and Prevention: Summary of notifiable diseases—
   United States, 2003, *MMWR* 52(54):1, 2005.
Kelly D, Skidmore S: Hepatitis C-Z: recent advances, *Arch Dis Children* 86: 339,
   2002.

McHutchinson JG: Understanding hepatitis C, *Am J Manage Care* 10(2 suppl): S21, 2004.

Pickering LK, editor: *Red book 2003: Report of the Committee on Infectious Diseases*, ed 26, Elk Grove Village, Ill, 2003, American Academy of Pediatrics.

Selekman J: Hepatitis update, *Pediatr Nurs* 25(5):542, 1999.

34

Hirschsprung's Disease

PATHOPHYSIOLOGY

Hirschsprung's disease, or congenital aganglionic megacolon, is a congenital anomaly characterized by the absence of ganglion cells in the rectum and extending proximally to the colon and, rarely, the small intestines. The absence of ganglion cells causes a lack of enteric nervous system stimulation, resulting in the inability of the internal sphincter to relax and thus increase intestinal tone, which in turn causes decreased peristalsis. Intestinal contents are propelled to the aganglionic segment; because of the lack of innervation, fecal material accumulates, which results in dilation of the bowel (megacolon) proximal to the aganglionic area. Along with the lack of peristalsis, there is loss of the rectosphincteric reflex; namely, the rectal sphincter fails to relax, which prevents the normal passage of stool and thereby contributes to the obstruction. Exact etiology is not known; however, genetics and environmental factors are suspected to play a role. Hirschsprung's disease generally manifests during the neonatal period; however, it may appear at any age.

INCIDENCE

1. Occurs in 1 in 5000 live births
2. Four times more common in males than in females
3. Increased familial incidence
4. May be associated with other congenital defects including Down syndrome
5. Accounts for 15% to 20% of neonatal intestinal obstructions

CLINICAL MANIFESTATIONS
Neonatal Period
1. Failure to pass meconium within 24 to 48 hours of birth
2. Bilious vomiting
3. Abdominal distention
4. Reluctance to feed, failure to thrive

Infancy and Childhood
1. Constipation
2. Recurrent diarrhea
3. Ribbonlike, foul-smelling stool
4. Abdominal distention
5. Vomiting
6. Failure to thrive
7. Chronic constipation
8. History of delayed meconium passage

COMPLICATIONS
1. Enterocolitis, life-threatening (acute)
2. Leakage at anastomosis (postsurgical)
3. Anal strictures (postsurgical)
4. Incontinence (long-term)

LABORATORY AND DIAGNOSTIC TESTS
1. Abdominal radiographic studies (supine, erect, prone, lateral decubitus)—diagnostic
2. Barium contrast studies—diagnostic
3. Anorectal manometry—determines ability of internal sphincter to relax
4. Full-thickness rectal biopsy (definitive diagnosis)—detects absence of ganglion cells

SURGICAL MANAGEMENT
Surgical treatment of Hirschsprung's disease is a two-stage process. Initially, a temporary colostomy is performed (1) to decompress the bowel and divert the fecal contents, and (2) to allow the dilated and hypertrophied portion of the bowel to regain normal tone and size. When the bowel regains normal

tone, after approximately 3 to 4 months (infants should be between 6 and 12 months of age or weigh 8 to 10 kg), a rectal pull-through procedure is performed in which all aganglionic bowel is removed and the normal bowel is reconnected to the anus. The colostomy is also closed during the second surgery.

NURSING ASSESSMENT

See the Gastrointestinal Assessment section in Appendix A.

Preoperative

1. Assess child's clinical status.
   a. Vital signs
   b. Intake and output
2. Assess for signs of bowel perforation.
3. Assess for signs of enterocolitis.
   a. Fever
   b. Tachycardia
   c. Tender abdomen
   d. Leukopenia
   e. Signs and symptoms of shock
4. Assess child's level of pain (see Appendix I).
5. Assess child's and family's ability to cope with upcoming surgery.

Postoperative

1. Assess child's postoperative status.
   a. Vital signs
   b. Bowel sounds
   c. Abdominal distention
2. Assess for signs of dehydration or fluid overload.
3. Assess fecal contents (ostomy) or return of bowel movements (after pull-through).
4. Assess for signs of infection.
5. Assess child's level of pain (see Appendix I).
6. Assess child's and family's ability to cope with hospital and surgical experience.
7. Assess parents' ability to manage treatment regimen and ongoing care.

NURSING DIAGNOSES

- Anxiety
- Infection, Risk for
- Pain
- Fluid volume, Deficient
- Altered nutrition: less than body requirements, Risk for
- Body image, Disturbed
- Skin integrity, Risk for impaired
- Knowledge, Deficient

NURSING INTERVENTIONS

Preoperative Care

1. Monitor nutritional status before surgery.
   a. Offer diet low in fiber and high in calories and protein.
   b. Administer total parenteral nutrition if needed.
   c. Use alternative route of intake if infant cannot take oral fluids.
   d. Assess intake and output accurately.
   e. Weigh infant every day.
2. Prepare infant and family emotionally for surgery (see Appendix F).
3. Monitor clinical status preoperatively.
   a. Monitor vital signs every 2 hours as needed.
   b. Monitor intake and output.
      i. Characteristics of bowel movement
      ii. Administer irrigation enemas as ordered and note stool characteristics
   c. Observe for signs and symptoms of bowel perforation.
      i. Vomiting
      ii. Increased tenderness
      iii. Abdominal distention
      iv. Irritability
      v. Respiratory distress (dyspnea)
   d. Monitor for signs of enterocolitis.
   e. Measure abdominal girth, at largest diameter, every 4 hours (to assess for abdominal distention).

4. Monitor infant's reactions to presurgical preparations.
   a. Bowel preparation
      i. Enemas until fecal content is clear (to sterilize bowel preoperatively)
      ii. GoLytely administration if ordered
   b. Intravenous (IV) tube insertion
   c. Foley catheter insertion
   d. Preoperative medication, including systemic antibiotics
   e. Diagnostic testing
   f. Decompression of stomach and bowel (nasogastric [NG] or rectal tube)
   g. Nothing by mouth for 12 hours before surgery

Postoperative Care

1. Monitor and report child's postoperative status.
   a. Auscultate for return of bowel sounds.
   b. Monitor vital signs every 2 hours until stable, then every 4 hours (depending on hospital protocol).
   c. Monitor for abdominal distention (maintain patency of NG tube).
2. Monitor child's hydration status (depending on child's status and hospital protocol).
   a. Assess for signs of dehydration or fluid overload.
   b. Measure and record NG drainage.
   c. Measure and record colostomy drainage.
   d. Measure and record Foley catheter drainage.
   e. Monitor IV infusion (amount, rate, infiltration).
   f. Observe for electrolyte imbalances (hyponatremia or hypokalemia).
3. Observe and report signs of complications.
   a. Intestinal obstruction caused by adhesions, volvulus, or intussusception
   b. Leakage from anastomosis
   c. Sepsis
   d. Fistula
   e. Enterocolitis
   f. Frequent stools
   g. Constipation

    h. Bleeding
    i. Recurrence of symptoms
 4. Promote return of peristalsis.
    a. Maintain patency of NG tube.
    b. Irrigate with normal saline solution every 4 hours and
       as needed.
    c. Encourage ambulation, in older children.
 5. Promote and maintain fluid and electrolyte balance.
    a. Record intake per route (IV, oral).
    b. Record output per route (urine, stool, emesis, stoma).
    c. Consult with physician about disparities.
 6. Alleviate or minimize pain and discomfort (see
    Appendix I).
    a. Assess pain.
    b. Provide nonpharmacologic and/or pharmacologic pain
       interventions.
    c. Monitor child's response to administration of medica-
       tions.
 7. Promote and maintain respiratory function.
    a. Have child turn, cough, and deep breathe.
    b. Perform postural drainage and percussion.
    c. Change child's position every 2 hours.
    d. Keep head of bed in semi-Fowler position.
 8. Prevent infection.
    a. Monitor incision site.
    b. Provide Foley catheter care every shift (protocols vary
       according to institution).
    c. Change dressing as needed (perianal and colostomy).
    d. Refer to institutional procedures manual for care related
       to specific procedure.
    e. Change diaper frequently to avoid fecal contamination.
 9. Promote skin integrity.
    a. Provide skin care per institutional procedures.
    b. Use appropriate ostomy supplies.
    c. Use protective skin barriers to ostomy site and perianal
       area (after return of bowel function).
10. Provide emotional support to child and family (see the
    Preparation for Procedures or Surgery section in
    Appendix F).

🏠 Discharge Planning and Home Care

1. Instruct parents to monitor for signs and symptoms of the following long-term complications:
   a. Stenosis and constrictions
   b. Incontinence
   c. Inadequate emptying
2. Provide instructions to parents and child about colostomy care:
   a. Skin preparation and care
   b. Use of colostomy equipment
   c. Stomal complications (bleeding, failure to pass stool, increased diarrhea, prolapse, ribbonlike stools)
   d. Care and cleaning of colostomy equipment
   e. Irrigation of colostomy (refer to Chapter 43 for further information)
3. Provide and reinforce instructions about dietary management:
   a. Low-fiber diet
   b. Unlimited fluid intake
   c. Signs of electrolyte imbalance or dehydration
4. Encourage parents' and child's expression of concerns related to colostomy (see Appendix F):
   a. Appearance
   b. Odor
   c. Discrepancy between parents' child and "ideal" child
5. Provide parents with information regarding enterocolitis:
   a. Signs and symptoms
   b. Immediate notification to health care provider
6. Refer to specific institutional procedures for information to be distributed to parents about home care.

CLIENT OUTCOMES

1. Child will remain without signs of infection.
2. Child will remain adequately hydrated.
3. Child's stoma site and perianal area will not show tissue breakdown.
4. Child will return to normal bowel function after full surgical process.
5. Child will not have complications such as enterocolitis.

REFERENCES

Behrman RE, Kiegman R, Jenson HB: *Nelson textbook of pediatrics,* ed 17, Philadelphia, 2004, WB Saunders.

De Lorijn F et al: Diagnosis of Hirschsprung's disease: A prospective, comparative accuracy study of common tests, *J Pediatr* 146(6):787, 2005.

Halter JM et al: Common gastrointestinal problems and emergencies in neonates and children, *Clin Fam Pract* 6(3):731, 2004.

Hockenberry MJ et al: *Wong's nursing care of infants and children,* ed 7, St. Louis, 2004, Mosby.

James SR, Ashwill JW: *Nursing care of children—principles and practice,* ed 3, Philadelphia, 2007, WB Saunders.

Swenson O: Hirschsprung's disease: A review, *Pediatrics* 109(5):914, 2002.

35

HIV Infection and AIDS

PATHOPHYSIOLOGY

Infection with the human immunodeficiency virus (HIV) occurs when the virus attaches to and enters helper T CD4 lymphocytes. The virus infects CD4 lymphocytes and other immunologic cells, and the person experiences a gradual destruction of CD4 cells. These cells, which amplify and replicate immunologic responses, are necessary to maintain immune function. When the CD^+ lymphocytes are reduced in number, immune functioning begins to fail. As $CD4^+$ lymphocytes decrease, the body is at risk for the development of opportunistic infections (OIs). When these $CD4^+$ lymphocytes have decreased to fewer than 200 cells/mm^3 (>15%), the client's HIV infection has progressed to clinical acquired immunodeficiency syndrome (AIDS).

HIV can also infect macrophages, cells that permit HIV to cross the blood-brain barrier into the brain. B lymphocyte function is also affected, with increased total immunoglobulin production associated with decreased specific antibody production. As the immune system progressively deteriorates, the body becomes increasingly vulnerable to OIs and is also less able to slow the process of HIV replication. HIV infection is manifested as a multisystem disease that may be dormant for years as it produces gradual immunodeficiency. The rate of disease progression and clinical manifestations vary from person to person.

HIV is transmitted only through direct contact with blood or blood products and body fluids, such as cerebrospinal fluid, pleural fluid, human breast milk, semen, saliva, and cervical secretions. In the United States, intravenous drug use, sexual contact, perinatal transmission from mother to infant (also referred to as vertical transmission), and breast-feeding are established modes of transmission. There is no evidence that HIV infection is acquired through casual contact. Administration of zidovudine or nevirapine to pregnant HIV-infected women significantly reduces perinatal transmission.

Currently, the majority of reported cases of HIV infection and AIDS in the United States occurs in men who have sex with men (MSM). However, the highest rates of new HIV infections are among heterosexual individuals. With advances in the screening of blood products for HIV, the incidence of new infections from blood transfusions has been greatly reduced in developed countries.

Four populations in the pediatric age group have been primarily affected:

1. Infants infected through perinatal transmission from infected mothers; this accounts for more than 90% of AIDS cases among children younger than 13 years of age
2. Children who have received blood products from HIV-infected donors (especially children with hemophilia)
3. Adolescents infected after engaging in high-risk behavior
4. Infants who have been breast-fed by infected mothers (primarily in developing countries)

INCIDENCE

1. Children account for less than 2% of all reported cases of AIDS in the United States.
2. Over 90% of infected children in the United States acquired the infection from their mothers.
3. The number of infants infected by perinatal transmission has decreased significantly as a result of diagnosis and treatment of HIV-infected pregnant women.
4. AIDS is more prevalent in ethnic minority children. Currently, African-American, non-Hispanic children account for 62% of U.S. cases of AIDS, and Hispanic children account for 22%. White children comprise 15% of the total U.S. cases of AIDS.

CLINICAL MANIFESTATIONS
Infants and Children

The majority of children who are born to HIV-infected mothers become symptomatic during the first 6 months of life, with the development of lymphadenopathy as the initial finding (Box 35-1). The most common clinical manifestations include the following:

1. Lymphadenopathy
2. Hepatomegaly
3. Splenomegaly
4. Failure to thrive
5. Recurrent upper respiratory tract infections
6. Parotitis
7. Chronic or recurrent diarrhea
8. Recurrent bacterial and viral infections
9. Persistent Epstein-Barr virus infection
10. Oropharyngeal candidiasis (thrush)
11. Thrombocytopenia
12. Neuropathy
13. Lymphoid interstitial pneumonia

A significant number of children with HIV infection have neurologic involvement that primarily manifests itself as a progressive encephalopathy, developmental delay, or loss of motor milestones.

Adolescents

Most adolescents who are infected via sexual transmission or through injection drug use may experience an extended period of asymptomatic illness that may last for years. This may be followed by signs and symptoms that begin weeks to months before the development of opportunistic infections and malignancies. The signs and symptoms include the following:

1. Fever
2. Malaise
3. Fatigue
4. Night sweats
5. Unexplained weight loss
6. Recurrent or chronic diarrhea

BOX 35-1
Clinical Categories of HIV Infection for Children Under 13 Years of Age

Category N: Not Symptomatic or One Condition Listed in Category A

Children with no signs or symptoms thought to be the result of HIV infection

Category A: Mildly Symptomatic

Children who have two or more of the following:

- Dermatitis
- Hepatomegaly
- Lymphadenopathy
- Parotitis
- Recurrent or persistent upper respiratory tract infection, sinusitis, or otitis media
- Splenomegaly

Category B: Moderately Symptomatic

Children who have symptomatic conditions that are attributed to HIV infection:

- Anemia, neutropenia, thrombocytopenia persisting >30 days
- Bacterial meningitis, pneumonia, or sepsis
- Cardiomyopathy
- Cytomegalovirus infection with onset before 1 month of age
- Diarrhea, recurrent or chronic
- Herpes stomatitis, recurrent
- Herpes simplex virus bronchitis, pneumonitis, or esophagitis with onset before 1 month of age
- Herpes zoster (shingles), two or more episodes
- Leiomyosarcoma
- Lymphoid interstitial pneumonia (LIP)
- Nephropathy
- Nocardiosis
- Persistent fever lasting for over 1 month
- Thrush lasting longer than 2 months in a child >6 months
- Toxoplasmosis with an onset before 1 month of age
- Varicella, disseminated

Category C: Severely Symptomatic (AIDS-defining conditions)

Children who have any of the following conditions:

- Bacterial infections, multiple or recurrent

Continued

BOX 35-1

Clinical Categories of HIV Infection for Children Under 13 Years of Age—cont'd

- Candidiasis of the trachea, bronchi, lungs, or esophagus
- Chronic herpes simplex ulcer (>1 month duration) or bronchitis, pneumonitis, or esophagitis with onset after 1 month of age
- Coccidioidomycosis, disseminated or extrapulmonary
- Cryptococcosis, extrapulmonary
- Cryptosporidiosis with diarrhea lasting >1 month
- Cytomegalovirus disease (other than liver, spleen, nodes), onset after age 1 month
- Cytomegalovirus retinitis (with loss of vision)
- Histoplasmosis, disseminated or extrapulmonary
- HIV encephalopathy
- Isosporiasis, chronic intestinal (>1 month duration)
- Kaposi's sarcoma
- HIV malignancies such as lymphoma (Burkitt's or immunoblastic sarcoma) or lymphoma, primary in brain
- *Mycobacterium tuberculosis* infection, disseminated or extrapulmonary
- Disseminated *Mycobacterium avium* complex (MAC)
- *Pneumocystis jiroveci* pneumonia (PCP)
- Progressive multifocal leukoencephalopathy
- Salmonella septicemia, recurrent
- Toxoplasmosis of brain, onset after age 1 month
- Wasting syndrome caused by HIV

Modified from Centers for Disease Control and Prevention: 1994 Revised classification system for human immunodeficiency virus infection in children less than 13 years of age, *MMWR* 43(RR-12):1, 1994.

7. Generalized lymphadenopathy
8. Oral candidiasis
9. Arthralgias and myalgias

COMPLICATIONS

1. High risk for development of infections, sepsis, and/or OIs
2. Severe wasting
3. Progressive encephalopathy

LABORATORY AND DIAGNOSTIC TESTS

1. Enzyme-linked immunosorbent assay (ELISA), the most commonly used initial test, detects antibody to HIV antigens (almost universally used to screen for HIV antibody in persons older than 2 years of age)
2. Western blot test, the most commonly used test to confirm the ELISA; detects antibody against several specific HIV proteins
3. HIV culture—viral culture requires up to 28 days for positive results; seldom used in the United States
4. HIV DNA polymerase chain reaction (PCR) test—detects HIV DNA; preferred test for children under 18 months of age. Infants born to HIV-infected mothers should have an HIV DNA PCR test at birth or within 48 hours of life, at 1 to 2 months of age, and again at 3 to 6 months of age
5. HIV antigen test—detects HIV antigen; seldom used in the United States

The following laboratory findings may be seen in HIV-infected infants and children:

1. Reduced absolute CD4 lymphocyte count, percentage, and CD4/CD8 ratio
2. Leukopenia
3. Anemia, thrombocytopenia
4. Hypergammaglobulinemia (immunoglobulin G, immunoglobulin A, immunoglobulin M)
5. Symptomatic children may have a poor response to vaccines

A child born to an HIV-infected mother and who is younger than 18 months of age and who has tested positive on two separate HIV laboratory tests is termed "HIV infected." A child born to an HIV-infected mother and who is younger than 18 months of age and who has not tested positive to these tests is categorized as "perinatally exposed."

MEDICAL MANAGEMENT

Currently, no cure exists for HIV/AIDS. Antiretroviral medications are used to control viral replication and to prevent disease progression by preservation of the immune system.

Management begins with a staging evaluation to determine disease progression and the appropriate course of treatment. Children are categorized according to Table 35-1 using three parameters: immune status, infection status, and clinical status. A child with mild signs and symptoms but with no evidence of immune suppression is categorized as A2. The immune status is based on the CD4 count and CD4 percentage and the child's age, according to Table 35-2.

Currently four classes of antiretroviral medications are used to control viral replication. These classes are used in a combination therapy termed highly active antiretroviral therapy (HAART) to treat HIV infection. Table 35-3 provides a summary of the drug classes and their major side effects and/or toxicities. In addition to controlling disease progression, treatment is directed at preventing and managing OIs.

Immunizations are recommended for children with HIV infection. Usually, HIV-infected children can receive all immunizations; however, children who are in the immune category III (severe suppression) should not receive the measles-mumps-rubella (MMR) vaccine. In addition, the varicella

TABLE 35-1
Categorization of Children with HIV Infection and AIDS

Immune Categories	*Clinical Categories*			
	(N) No Signs or Symptoms	(A) Mild Signs or Symptoms	(B) Moderate Signs or Symptoms	(C) Severe Signs or Symptoms
(1) No evidence of suppression	N1	A1	B1	C1
(2) Evidence of moderate suppression	N2	A2	B2	C2
(3) Severe suppression	N3	A3	B3	C3

TABLE 35-2
Determination of Immune Category Based on Age and CD4+ Count

Immune Categories	Age Groups: CD4+ Count and Percentage		
	0–11 Months	1–5 Years	6–12 Years
(1) No evidence of suppression	>1500 (>25%)	>1000 (>25%)	>500 (>25%)
(2) Evidence of moderate suppression	750–1499 (15% to 24%)	500–999 (15% to 24%)	200–499 (15% to 24%)
(3) Severe suppression	>750 (>15%)	>500 (>15%)	>200 (>15%)

Modified from Centers for Disease Control and Prevention: 1994 Revised classification system for human immunodeficiency virus infection in children less than 13 years of age, *MMWR* 43(RR-12):1, 1994.

TABLE 35-3
Antiretroviral Medication Classes and Major Side Effects and Toxicities

Medication Class	Side Effects and Toxicities
Nucleoside reverse transcriptase inhibitors (NRTIs), nucleotide reverse transcriptase inhibitor	Anemia, diarrhea, headache, allergic reactions, lactic acidosis, nausea, vomiting, pancreatitis, peripheral neuropathy
Nonnucleoside reverse transcriptase inhibitors (NNRTIs)	Dizziness, vivid dreams, liver function changes, hepatotoxicity, rash
Protease inhibitors (PIs)	Abdominal pain, diarrhea, hyperglycemia, hyperlipidemia, hepatitis, body fat redistribution, nausea, vomiting, kidney stones, rash
Fusion inhibitor	Headache, injection site reactions, pain, pneumonia

vaccine is indicated only in HIV-Infected children who are in immune category 1 (no evidence of suppression) with a $CD4^+$ lymphocyte percentage greater than 25.

NURSING ASSESSMENT

1. See Appendix A.
2. Assess nutritional status.
3. Assess for opportunistic infections and other signs and symptoms of infection.
4. Assess for knowledge of transmission—safer sex, avoidance of needle sharing, and so forth.

NURSING DIAGNOSES

- Infection, Risk for
- Growth and development, Delayed

- Nutrition: less than body requirements, Imbalanced
- Family processes, Interrupted
- Grieving, Anticipatory
- Noncompliance
- Social interaction, Impaired

NURSING INTERVENTIONS

1. Protect infant, child, or adolescent from infectious contacts (Box 35-2); although casual person-to-person contact does not permit HIV transmission, a number of recommendations have been made for children with HIV infection and AIDS.
   a. Caregivers in foster homes should be educated on precautions regarding blood exposure.
   b. Day care attendance should be evaluated on an individual basis.
   c. Child should attend school if health, neurologic development, behavior, and immune status are appropriate.
2. Prevent transmission of HIV infection.
   a. Clean spills of blood or other body fluids with bleach solution (10:1 ratio of water to bleach).
   b. Wear latex gloves when exposure to blood or body fluids is anticipated.

BOX 35-2
Preventive Measures

Preventive efforts are of vital importance in dealing with HIV/ AIDS.

Reducing the number of sexual partners each individual has would decrease the incidence of this disease in the adult and adolescent population, as would involvement in drug rehabilitation programs and avoidance of needle-sharing during drug use.

Elimination of HIV-infected blood and blood products has decreased the likelihood of transmission. Blood and blood products are screened for the HIV antibody, resulting in a blood supply that is much safer.

HIV-infected women in the United States should be instructed not to breast-feed their infants.

    c. Wear mask with protective eyewear if aerosolization or splashing with blood or body fluids is anticipated.

    d. Wash hands after exposure to blood or body fluids and after removing gloves.

    e. Place uncapped needles attached to syringes (and other sharps) in closed, puncture-proof container labeled as biohazardous and/or infectious waste.

    f. Dispose of waste contaminated with visible blood in biohazard plastic bag.

3. Protect child from infectious contacts when he or she is immunocompromised.

    a. Screen for infections.

    b. Place child in room with noninfectious children.

    c. Restrict visitors with active illnesses, especially influenza and varicella.

4. Assess child's achievement of developmental milestones and nutritional status.

    a. Provide age-appropriate, stimulating activities (see Appendix F).

    b. Monitor growth pattern (height, weight, head circumference) and refer to dietitian for assistance with nutritional interventions.

5. Involve social services, child life therapists, and other health team members to assist child and family with crisis and stresses of chronic illness.

    a. Encourage expression of feelings.

    b. Refer to clergy for spiritual support.

    c. Discuss chronic nature of HIV/AIDS. With the development of HAART, HIV infection is now considered a chronic disease.

    d. Discuss terminal stage of disease and possible death of child only when necessary. With advances in care and treatment, the death rate from AIDS in children has dramatically decreased over the past 10 years.

    e. Encourage caregivers to disclose the child's HIV status to the child when the child is developmentally ready to accept the diagnosis (usually when the child is 10 to 13 years of age); when the child begins to questions his or her diagnosis; or when the child becomes sexually active.

6. Assist family in identifying factors that impede compliance with treatment plan.
   a. Educate child and family about medical research protocols.
   b. Educate child and family about risks of nonadherence to medication therapy and treatment plan.
   c. Assist family in establishing schedule that optimizes therapeutic effect of medication and fits into family's lifestyle.
7. Encourage child to participate in activities with other children.
   a. Assist child and family in identifying personal strengths.
   b. Educate school or day care personnel and classmates about HIV infection and AIDS only with the permission of the child's caregivers.
   c. Educate adolescent about sexual transmission, abstinence, use of condoms, and dangers of unprotected sexual behaviors.
   d. Educate adolescent about relationship between substance abuse and practice of risky behaviors.
   e. Encourage use of support network of family and friends and refer to HIV/AIDS support group as needed.
   f. Collaborate with school nurse regarding child's condition only with permission of the child's caregiver.

🏠 Discharge Planning and Home Care

1. Instruct child and family to contact medical team and/or nurse case manager in case of signs or symptoms of infection.
2. Instruct child and family to observe response to medications and notify physician and/or nurse case manager of adverse reactions.
3. Instruct child and family about follow-up appointments.
   a. Name and phone number of physician and appropriate health care team members
   b. Date, time, and purpose of follow-up appointments

CLIENT OUTCOMES

1. Child will exhibit no signs or symptoms of infection.
2. Child and family will demonstrate understanding of home care and follow-up needs.
3. Child will participate in activities with family and peers.

REFERENCES

Anabwani GM, Woldetsadik EA, Kline MW: Treatment of HIV in children using antiretroviral drugs, *Semin Pediatr Infect Dis* 16(2):116, 2005.

Centers for Disease Control and Prevention: Revised classification system for human immunodeficiency virus infection in children less than 13 years of age, *MMWR* 43(RR-12):RR49, 1994.

Centers for Disease Control and Prevention: *A glance at the HIV/AIDS epidemic* (website): www.cdc.gov/hiv/pubs/Facts/At-A-Glance.htm. Accessed March 1, 2006.

Hatherill M: Sepsis predisposition in children with human immunodeficiency virus, *Pediatr Crit Care Med* 6(3):S92, 2005.

Hockenberry MJ et al: *Wong's nursing care of infants and children,* ed 7, St. Louis, 2004, Mosby.

Kirton C, editor: ANAC's core curriculum for HIV/AIDS nursing, ed 2, Thousand Oaks, CA, Sage Publications, 2003.

McKinney RE, Cunningham CK: Newer treatments for HIV in children, *Curr Opin Pediatr* 16(1):76, 2004.

Pickering LK, editor: *Red book 2003: Report of the Committee on Infectious Diseases,* ed 26, Elk Grove Village, Ill, 2003, American Academy of Pediatrics.

36

❖

Hodgkin's Disease

PATHOPHYSIOLOGY

Hodgkin's disease is a malignancy of the lymphoid system. The cause remains unknown. Hodgkin's disease is seen with a higher frequency in children with inherited immune deficiency syndromes. There has also been an association for some patients following infection with Epstein-Barr virus. Hodgkin's disease is characterized by a proliferation of Reed-Sternberg cells that are surrounded by a pleomorphic infiltrate of reactive cells. Although no tissue is exempt from involvement, Hodgkin's disease primarily affects nodal or lymphatic sites. The liver, the spleen, the bone marrow, and the lungs may also be involved. Hodgkin's disease is classified according to the predominating type of cells and is characterized by four histologic states: (1) lymphocytic predominance (rare in children, often very localized disease requiring minimal therapy), (2) nodular sclerosis (most common in children), (3) mixed cellularity, and (4) lymphocytic depletion.

High survival rates have been achieved in children with Hodgkin's disease as a result of improved staging procedures, combined therapies, and advances in supportive care. The 5-year relative survival rate for children under age 15 has gone from 78% in 1976 to 95% in 2001. However, cure often comes with significant cost secondary to the late effects of therapy. Over the past 2 decades, there has been a focus on lowering the doses and fields of radiation and limiting the exposure of certain chemotherapeutic agents. Newer treatment protocols are also evaluating therapy that is based on the individual's response to initial treatment. If there is an early complete response to treatment, then the remaining therapy is less intense. The hope is that cure rates can be maintained with fewer long-term side effects. Early results have been encouraging.

INCIDENCE

1. Hodgkin's disease accounts for 5% of malignancies in children in the United States.
2. Hodgkin's disease has been reported in infants and young children but is rare before the age of 5 years.
3. Only 10% to 15% of cases occur in children younger than 16 years of age. The majority of cases in children occur in children aged 11 years and older.
4. Before age 10 year, Hodgkin's disease is more common in males. After age 10, the ratio approaches 1:1.
5. The 5-year survival rate for stages I and II disease is 85% to 95%; for stages III and IV disease, 70% to 90%.

CLINICAL MANIFESTATIONS

1. Lymphadenopathy, usually in the cervical, supraclavicular, and mediastinal areas; mediastinal presentation common in adolescents and young adults; significant mediastinal adenopathy may cause cough, dyspnea, or superior vena cava syndrome
2. Painless, movable lymph nodes in tissues surrounding involved area
3. Unexplained fever
4. Weight loss
5. Drenching night sweats
6. Malaise

COMPLICATIONS
Common Acute Complications of Therapy

1. Bone marrow suppression—puts patient at risk for infection, bleeding, fatigue
2. Hair loss—very likely with all Hodgkin's therapy regimens for children
3. Nausea and vomiting—often can be prevented or minimized with newer and combination antiemetic regimens

4. Constipation—likely with regimens that include oncovin (vincristine); associated with decreased mobility and use of narcotic pain medications
5. Diarrhea—may occur after prolonged antibiotic use; may be secondary to infection such as *Clostridium difficile*
6. Mucositis—secondary to mucosal damage from chemotherapy or radiation—may be accompanied by fungal infection (oral candidiasis)
7. Weight loss—secondary to anorexia, altered taste
8. Pain—after procedures such as central line placement or bone marrow or node biopsy
9. Allergic or anaphylactic reactions—may occur with some chemotherapy agents such as bleomycin, or with blood products
10. Gastritis—secondary to steroids administration, stress, vomiting
11. Mood swings, fluid retention, and altered glucose metabolism—secondary to steroids administration
12. Anxiety, behavioral problems such as regression, sleep disturbances—secondary to diagnosis and necessary treatments and procedures

Potential Late Complications Related to Treatment

1. Endocrine dysfunction including hypothyroidism, premature ovarian failure, sterility in males, and osteopenia
2. Cardiac dysfunction, including pericardial effusion, valvular heart disease, coronary artery disease, and constrictive pericarditis with tamponade
3. Pulmonary dysfunction, including fibrosis or pneumonitis
4. Impaired immunity (during therapy and in the first year posttherapy)
5. Soft tissue and bone growth impairment in irradiated fields
6. Secondary malignancy, including thyroid carcinoma, basal cell carcinoma, osteosarcomas, breast and colon carcinomas, soft tissue sarcomas, non-Hodgkin's lymphoma, and leukemia

LABORATORY AND DIAGNOSTIC TESTS

1. Complete blood count—diagnostic (anemia may indicate advanced disease)
2. Erythrocyte sedimentation rate (ESR)—may be elevated at diagnosis
3. Serum copper, iron, calcium, and alkaline phosphatase levels—also may be elevated at diagnosis
4. Liver and renal function tests—to assess organ involvement
5. Urinalysis—to determine renal involvement
6. Chest radiographic study—to determine mediastinal or hilar node involvement
7. Computed tomography—to evaluate mediastinal, pulmonary, and abdominal disease
8. Gallium and/or positron emission tomography (PET) scan to determine the extent of involvement
9. Excisional lymph node biopsy—essential to diagnosis and staging
10. Bone marrow biopsy if patient has stage 3 or 4 disease according to imaging studies

MEDICAL MANAGEMENT

Staging is used to determine the anatomic extent of the disease at the time of diagnosis and to select the most appropriate therapy (Box 36-1). Staging includes biopsy, history, physical examination, and radiographic data collection. With advances in radiographic techniques, a staging laparotomy that formerly would have been done is not routinely recommended. Even with the best radiographic techniques, false positives and false negatives occur. Also, because all children and adolescents on treatment protocols receive chemotherapy now (and not just local radiation), staging laparotomy is no longer routinely performed.

At the time of diagnosis, approximately 60% of children with Hodgkin's disease have stage I or II disease. Stage III disease is diagnosed in approximately 30% of children, and 10% have stage IV disease. Approximately 30% of children have B symptoms (unexplained fever, more than 10% weight loss, night sweats). Those with B symptoms are treated more intensively. The absence of these B symptoms is known as A classification.

BOX 36-1
System for Hodgkin's Disease: Ann Arbor Staging

Stage	Description*
I	Involvement of a single lymph node region or a single extralymphatic organ or site
II	Involvement of two or more lymph node regionson the same side of the diaphragm or localized involvement of an extralymphatic organ or site and one or more lymph node regions on the same side of the diaphragm
III	Involvement of lymph node regions or extralymphatic organs or sites or spleen on both sides of the diaphragm
IV	Diffuse involvement of one or more extralymphatic organs or tissues with or without associated lymph node involvement

*Subdivision A has no defined symptoms; subdivision B symptoms include unexplained recent weight loss or fever or night sweats.

The treatment approach is guided by the stage of the disease at diagnosis. The goal of treatment is cure of the disease with minimal treatment-related toxicities and sequelae.

Over the last 30 years, the treatment for Hodgkin's disease has evolved significantly. In the 1960s, radiation was the mainstay of therapy. Though this was curative for localized disease, those with advanced disease were rarely cured. In the 1960s a drug combination known as MOPP (nitrogen mustard, oncovin, prednisone, procarbazine) was used for those with advanced disease. In combination with radiation, more patients with advanced disease were cured. However, these patients often suffered significant side effects such as infertility, secondary leukemia, and other secondary malignancies. In the 1970s, a new drug combination known as ABVD (adriamycin, bleomycin, velban, and dacarbazine) was developed. This regimen was determined to be effective, with fewer problematic side effects than MOPP. In the 1980s, these two drug combinations were alternated to minimize the dose-related side effects of each regimen. Protocols were subsequently developed using chemotherapy with reduced radiation doses and fields. Today, the treatment for Hodgkin's disease continues to evolve and is now risk-adapted. The most intensive regimens are used only for patients with advanced disease. Several new drug combinations are being used: BEACOPP (bleomycin, etoposide, adriamycin, cytoxan, oncovin, prednisone, and procarbazine), and COPP/ABV (cytoxan, oncovin, prednisone, procarbazine, adriamycin, bleomycin, and velban). More combinations are being explored in clinical trials. Reduction of radiation doses and fields is also being explored in pediatric trials. With very strict criteria, some patients are randomized to not receive radiation following chemotherapy.

NURSING ASSESSMENT

1. Assess child's physiologic status (see Appendix A).
   a. Signs and symptoms of Hodgkin's disease
   b. Involvement of other body systems (e.g., respiratory, gastrointestinal)
   c. Adverse effects of treatment
2. Assess family's psychosocial needs (see Appendix F).
   a. Knowledge and education level
   b. Body image
   c. Family structure
   d. Family stressors
   e. Coping mechanisms
   f. Support systems
3. Assess child's developmental level (see Appendix B).
4. Assess family's ability to manage home care.

NURSING DIAGNOSES

- Tissue integrity, Impaired
- Anxiety
- Fluid volume, Deficient
- Nutrition: less than body requirements, Imbalanced
- Skin integrity, Impaired
- Oral mucous membrane, Impaired
- Pain
- Fatigue

- Growth and development, Delayed
- Therapeutic regimen management, Ineffective
- Body image, Disturbed

NURSING INTERVENTIONS
Staging Procedure
1. Provide preprocedural education to child and family (see Appendix F).
2. Prepare child for clinical staging procedures with age-appropriate approach (see Appendix F).
3. Assist and support child in collection of laboratory specimens.
4. Provide instruction, support, and family crisis intervention.

Radiation and/or Chemotherapy Phase
1. Provide sedation for radiation treatments if needed.
2. Monitor cardiorespiratory status during treatments.
3. Prepare for treatment-induced emergencies.
   a. Metabolic disturbances, though Hodgkin's disease is generally low risk for tumor lysis syndrome
   b. Hematologic disturbances, such as febrile neutropenia, severe anemia
   c. Space-occupying tumors, specifically superior vena cava syndrome
4. Assess for signs of extravasation of chemotherapeutic agents.
   a. Edema, erythema, pain at infusion site
   b. Tissue sloughing
5. Monitor for signs and symptoms of infection.
6. Assess skin integrity.
7. Minimize side effects of radiotherapy and/or chemotherapy.
   a. Bone marrow suppression
   b. Nausea and vomiting
   c. Anorexia and weight loss
   d. Oral mucositis
   e. Pain

8. Provide ongoing emotional support to child and family (see Appendix F).
9. Refer to child life specialist to assist with continued coping strategies.
10. Provide ongoing education about treatment and follow-up care, medications—both chemotherapy and supportive care medications.
11. Refer family to social services for support and resource utilization.
12. If school age, refer to hospital or homebound teacher or obtain lessons for teaching.

🏠 Discharge Planning and Home Care

Instruct child and parents about home care management, including the following:
1. Signs of infection and guidelines on when to seek medical attention
2. Care of child's central venous access device, including site care, dressing change, flushing, and emergency care
3. Medication administration (provide written information); review side effects and indications for medications
4. Adherence to treatment regimen and medical appointments, as well as future late effects follow-up
5. Proper nutrition for optimal weight gain and health maintenance
6. School attendance and/or activity restrictions
7. Potential behavioral changes in child and/or siblings
8. Stress importance of oral hygiene; discuss dental care and appointments while on therapy
9. Assess transportation needs
10. Provide and review staff phone numbers; that is, who to contact with questions, and who to contact for emergencies

CLIENT OUTCOMES

1. Child and family will demonstrate ability to cope with life-threatening illness.

2. Infectious complications will be minimized.
3. Child and family will understand home care, current treatment plan, and long-term follow-up needs.

REFERENCES

Baggott CR et al, editors: *Nursing care of children and adolescents with cancer,* ed 3, Philadelphia, 2002, WB Saunders.

Devita V and Hellman S, Rosenberg S, editors: *Cancer: Principles and practice of oncology,* ed 7, Philadelphia, 2005, Lippincott, Williams & Wilkins.

Jemal A et al: Cancer Statistics 2006, *CA Cancer J Clin* 56(2):106, 2006.

Lin H, Teitell M: Second malignancy after treatment of pediatric Hodgkin disease, *J Pediatr Hematol Oncol* 27(1):28, 2005.

Max A et al: Developing nursing care guidelines for children with Hodgkin's disease, *Eur J Oncol Nurs* 7(4):253, 2003.

Yung L et al: Long-term outcome in adolescents with Hodgkin's lymphoma: Poor results using regimens designed for adults, *Leuk Lymphoma* 45 (8):1579, 2004.

37

❖

Hydrocephalus

PATHOPHYSIOLOGY

Hydrocephalus may be congenital or acquired. Congenital hydrocephalus is frequently associated with other congenital neurologic disorders or malformations. Some of the most commom associated diagnoses are myelomeningocele, Arnold-Chiari malformation, and aqueduct stenosis. The genetic factors that lead to hydrocephalus are unknown, with the exception of congenital X-linked hydrocephalus, which accounts for less than 4% of all cases. Acquired hydrocephalus may be caused by maternal malnutrition, intrauterine infections, tumors, vascular malformations, abscesses, intraventricular cysts, intraventricular hemorrhage, meningitis, and cerebral trauma. Causes of hydrocephalus are commonly labeled as idiopatic, infectious, hemorrhagic, posttraumatic, or tumor-related. Regardless of the cause, the result is a blockage of cerebral spinal fluid (CSF) flow and absorption secondary to microscopic changes in the CNS tissue or mechanical obstruction of the CSF circulation. Less than 0.5% of all cases of hydrocephalus are caused by overproduction of CSF. Excessive accumulation of CSF leads to ventricular enlargement and increased intracranial pressure (ICP) that may contribute to further CNS tissue damage. Children with hydrocephalus are at risk for both physical and cognitive delays; however, many benefit from physical and educational interventions and go on to live happy, healthy lives.

INCIDENCE

Congenital hydrocephalus occurs in 3 or 4 of 1000 live births.

CLINICAL MANIFESTATIONS
Signs and symptoms are the results of ICP and vary with the child's age and the skull's ability to expand.

Infants
1. Progressive head enlargement (above 95th percentile); enlarged, bulging, tense fontanelles, split sutures; distention of superficial scalp veins; prominence of frontal portions of skull
2. Irritability or lethargy
3. Poor feeding, vomiting
4. Seizure activity
5. Delay or regression in developmental milestones
6. Symmetrically increased transillumination over skull
7. "Sunsetting" eyes
8. Infants younger than 2 weeks of age may have no symptoms

Older Children
1. Headache
2. Nausea and vomiting
3. Drowsiness
4. Irritability
5. Ataxia
6. Urinary incontinence
7. Diplopia, blurred vision
8. Papilledema
9. "Sunsetting" eyes
10. Change in mental status or personality; behavioral changes

COMPLICATIONS
1. Infection
2. Increased ICP
3. Shunt malfunction
4. Delays in cognitive, psychosocial, and physical development
5. Decreased intelligence quotient

Surgical Complications
1. Shunt malfunction (blockage, disconnection, fracture, migration)

2. Shunt infection, meningitis
3. Overdrainage of CSF

LABORATORY AND DIAGNOSTIC TESTS

See Appendix F for normal values and ranges of laboratory and diagnostic tests.

1. Computed tomographic scan—used to determine the degree of venticular enlargement and the etiology of the hydrocephalus; also used to evaluate shunt for possible malfunction if symptoms return
2. Magnetic resonance imaging—used to determine the degree of ventricular enlargement and the etiology of the hydrocephalus; also used to evaluate shunt for possible malfunction if symptoms return
3. Ultrasound may be used in very young infants who have open fontanelles.

SURGICAL MANAGEMENT

The traditional management is surgical shunt insertion. The shunt removes the excess CSF and decreases ICP. The proximal end of the shunt is inserted in the lateral ventricle; the distal end is extended to the peritoneal cavity or the right atrium as a means of draining excessive fluid into another body cavity. The ventricular-peritoneal (VP) shunt is used most frequently, because the atrioventricular shunt is associated with higher risks. An endoscopic third ventriculostomy creates an outlet for the CSF in the floor of the third ventricle, but is indicated only in a limited number of patients. Even though first-year failure rates of VP shunts are as high as 40%, this is still the treatment of choice in most patients.

NURSING ASSESSMENT

1. See the Neurologic Assessment and Musculoskeletal Assessment sections in Appendix A.
2. Assess for increased ICP.
3. Assess for signs and symptoms of infection.

NURSING DIAGNOSES

- Injury, Risk for
- Infection, Risk for

- Skin integrity, Risk for impaired
- Growth and development, Risk for delayed
- Pain
- Knowledge, Deficient related to therapuetic regimen

NURSING INTERVENTIONS

Preoperative Care

1. Monitor for, prevent, and intervene in case of increased ICP.
   a. Place child in position of comfort; raise head of bed to 30 degrees and maintain head in neutral position (to promote venous return).
   b. Monitor for signs of increased ICP.
      i. Decreased respiratory rate, decreased heart rate, increased blood pressure, and increased temperature
      ii. Decreased level of consciousness (LOC)
      iii. Seizure activity
      iv. Vomiting
      v. Alteration in pupil size, symmetry, and reactivity
      vi. Fullness of fontanelles—tense to bulging
   c. Decrease external stimuli.
   d. Maintain oxygen and suction at bedside.
2. Prepare child and parents for surgical procedure.
   a. Provide age-appropriate explanations (see the Preparation for Procedures or Surgery section in Appendix F).
   b. Provide and reinforce information given to parents about child's condition and treatment.

Postoperative Care

1. Monitor child's vital signs and neurologic status; report signs of increased ICP (decreased LOC, anorexia, poor or ineffective sucking, vomiting, convulsions, seizures, or sluggishness).
2. Monitor and report signs of infection (fever, tachycardia, general malaise, tenderness, inflammation, nausea, and vomiting).

3. Monitor and maintain functioning of shunt.
   a. Report signs of shunt malfunction (irritability, decreased LOC, vomiting).
   b. Position according to surgeon's order, based on type of shunt.
   c. Position child on nonoperative side, turn according to surgeon's order.
   d. If VP shunt was placed, then child will be on nothing-by-mouth (NPO) status with nasogastric tube in place because of placement of abdominal catheter. Administer intravenous (IV) fluids as ordered. Assess intake and output closely. Check for return of bowel sounds.
   e. Monitor for seizure activity.
4. Monitor for pain and provide nonpharmacologic and pharmacologic measures to relieve pain (refer to Appendix I).
5. Support child and parents to help them deal with emotional stresses of hospitalization and surgery (refer to the Supportive Care section in Appendix F).
   a. Provide age-appropriate information before procedures (refer to the Preparation for Procedures or Surgery section in Appendix F).
   b. Encourage participation in age-appropriate developmental, recreational, and diversional activities.
   c. Incorporate child's home routine into daily activities.

🏠 Discharge Planning and Home Care

1. Instruct parents to monitor for and report signs of shunt complications.
   a. Shunt malfunction
   b. Shunt infection
2. Provide parents with assistance in contacting community resources.
   a. Follow-up by home health nurse
   b. Support group for parents of children with hydrocephalus (see Appendix F)
   c. Referral to early intervention programs (see Appendix G)
   d. Selection of preschool and recreational programs

3. Encourage parents to increase fluid and roughage in child's diet to prevent constipation, because straining at passing stool causes increased ICP.
4. Assess cognitive, linguistic, adaptive, and social behaviors to determine development; use developmental history to assess achievement of early milestones and refer to appropriate specialists as needed.

CLIENT OUTCOMES

1. Child will not have signs or symptoms of increased ICP.
2. Child will not have signs or symptoms of infection.
3. Child's skin will remain clean, dry, and intact, without signs of erythema or ulceration.
4. Child and parents will understand how to monitor for and report shunt complications.
5. Child will demonstrate regular, observable growth and achieve age-appropriate developmental milestones.
6. Parents will be able to describe hydrocephalus and how it affects their child; identify measures used to treat the disorder; and state realistic expectations about their child's condition following shunt insertion.

REFERENCES

Kestle JRW: Pediatric hydrocephalus: Current management, *Neurol Clin North Am* 21:883, 2003.

National Institute of Neurological Disorders and Stroke (NINDS): *Hydrocephalus fact sheet* (website): www.ninds.nih.gov. Accessed April 26, 2006.

Pattisapu JV: Etiology and clinical course of hydrocephalus, *Hydrocephalus* 36(4):351, 2001.

Simpkins CJ: Ventriculoperitoneal shunt infections in patients with hydrocephalus, *Pediatr Nurs* 31(6):457, 2005.

38

Hyperbilirubinemia

PATHOPHYSIOLOGY

Neonatal hyperbilirubinemia or physiologic jaundice, a total serum bilirubin level higher than 5 mg/dl, is due to the neonate's predisposition for bilirubin production and limited ability to excrete it. By definition, there is no other abnormality or pathologic process present to account for the jaundice. The yellow coloration of the skin and mucous membranes is due to the deposition of unconjugated bilirubin pigment. The primary source of bilirubin is the breakdown of hemoglobin in aging or hemolyzed red blood cells (RBCs). In the neonate, RBCs have a higher turnover and a shorter life span, which enhances the higher production rate of bilirubin. The immaturity of the neonatal liver is a limiting factor in bilirubin excretion.

Unconjugated or indirect bilirubin is lipid soluble and binds to plasma albumin. The bilirubin is then taken up by the liver, where it is conjugated. Conjugated or direct bilirubin is excreted in the bile into the intestines. In the intestines, bacteria convert the conjugated bilirubin into urobilinogen. The majority of the highly soluble urobilinogen is reexcreted by the liver and is eliminated in the feces; the kidneys excrete 5% of the urobilogen. Not only do increased RBC destruction and liver immaturity promote increased bilirubin levels, but other intestinal bacteria can deconjugate bilirubin, which allows it to be reabsorbed into the circulation and further raises bilirubin levels.

INCIDENCE

1. Up to 60% of term newborns have clinical evidence of jaundice.

2. Age of onset is 2 to 3 days.
3. Severity differs among different races, with Asian and Native American infants manifesting higher bilirubin levels.
4. Infants from certain geographic areas, particularly areas around Greece, have an increased incidence of hyperbilirubinemia.
5. Birth trauma (cephalohematoma, cutaneous bruising, instrumented delivery) increases risk for hyperbilirubinemia.
6. Incidence is higher in male infants.

CLINICAL MANIFESTATIONS

1. Jaundice is first noted on head and trunk and progresses downward.
2. Jaundice is noted on sclera, skin, and mucous membranes.
3. Urine becomes dark gold to brown color.
4. Bilirubin levels decline by fifth day and are usually within normal limits by tenth day of life.

COMPLICATIONS

1. Neurologic: lethargy, kernicterus or encephalopathy resulting from deposition of unconjugated bilirubin in brain cells
2. Gastrointestinal: poor feeding, dehydration

LABORATORY AND DIAGNOSTIC TESTS

1. Complete blood count, liver function tests, blood typing, and Coombs' test—to rule out other causes
2. Indirect bilirubin levels—elevated

MEDICAL MANAGEMENT

Medical management is largely supportive. Prevention of neonatal hyperbilirubinemia should always be attempted by initiating feedings as soon as possible after birth. Bilirubin levels should be monitored, and the infant will be placed under phototherapy as the blood level dictates. All other causes of hyperbilirubinemia should be ruled out at this time. Other causes include Rh incompatibility, hemolytic disease, and biliary atresia. Infants at high risk for developing hyperbilirubinemia, such as premature infants and those with hypoxia and acidosis, may be placed under phototherapy before developing a significantly elevated bilirubin level.

NURSING ASSESSMENT

1. Assess skin color for progression of jaundice by applying pressure over bony prominence, which causes blanching and allows yellow color to become more evident.
2. Assess hydration status.
3. Assess nutritional intake.
4. Assess temperature control when under phototherapy.
5. Assess bowel elimination pattern.

NURSING DIAGNOSES

- Fluid volume, Risk for deficient
- Fluid volume, Deficient
- Nutrition: less than body requirements, Imbalanced
- Constipation
- Parenting, Risk for impaired

NURSING INTERVENTIONS

1. Introduce feedings as soon as possible after birth as preventive measure.
2. Monitor hydration status.
3. During phototherapy do the following:
   a. Shield infant's eyes with eye patches; remove every 3 to 4 hours and assess eyes for drainage or irritation.
   b. Place infant nude under light, but cover testes when positioning supine.
   c. Change body position frequently.
   d. Monitor body temperature.
   e. Turn down phototherapy lights during blood sampling, since they can produce falsely low bilirubin level.
4. Administer glycerin suppository as needed to facilitate elimination of direct bilirubin in stool.
5. Promote bonding by encouraging parent to hold and feed infant while under phototherapy.

🏠 Discharge Planning and Home Care

1. Provide parent education regarding nutritional and hydration needs.
2. Instruct family in use of home phototherapy system.
3. Instruct family to obtain follow-up bilirubin level measurements.

CLIENT OUTCOMES

1. Infant's jaundice and bilirubin levels will decrease.
2. Infant will not sustain injury from phototherapy lights.
3. Infant will remain well hydrated.

REFERENCES

Ip S et al: An evidence-based review of important issues concerning neonatal hyperbilirubinemia, *Pediatrics* 114: e130-e153 (serial online): www.pediatrics.org/cgi/content/full/114/1/e130. Accessed January 4, 2006.

James SR et al: *Nursing care of children: principles and practice*, ed 3, Philadelphia, 2007, WB Saunders.

Porter ML, Dennis RL: Hyperbilirubinemia in the term newborn, *Am Fam Physician* 64: 599, 2002.

39

Hypertension

PATHOPHYSIOLOGY

Hypertension in the pediatric client is described as blood pressure that is persistently between the 90th and 95th percentiles. Table 39-1 identifies guidelines (based on age and sex) for suspect blood pressure values. A variety of mechanisms are associated with hypertension. The renin-angiotensin-aldosterone system maintains fluid volume and vascular tone through the production of angiotensin II (a vasoconstrictor) and the stimulation of aldosterone production (for sodium retention). The sympathetic nervous system affects peripheral vascular resistance, cardiac output, and renin release, influencing the regulation of blood pressure.

Hypertension is classified as primary or secondary. Primary hypertension can be ascribed to no identifiable cause, whereas secondary hypertension is attributable to a structural abnormality or to an underlying disease (renal, cardiovascular, endocrine, central nervous system, or collagenous). A variety of factors have been identified as contributing to hypertension, including diet (high in calories, saturated fats, and sodium), contraceptive use, positive family history, obesity, and minimal physical exercise. Children generally manifest no overt symptoms. If symptomatic, the disease may be quite severe. Prognosis is variable, depending on the age of onset and response to treatment.

Problems evident in adults may have originated during the first or second decade of life. The earlier the onset, the more severe the disease will be.

TABLE 39-1
Approximate Guidelines for Suspect Blood Pressure

	Age (years)	Blood Pressure (mm Hg)
Supine Position—Lowest of Three Readings		
Boys and girls	3–5	110/70
	6–9	>120/75
	10–14	>130/80
Seated Position—Average of Second and Third Readings		
Girls	14–18	>125/80
Boys	14	>130/75
	15	>130/80
	16–18	>135/85

Modified from Gilles S, Kagan B: *Current pediatric therapy*, ed 13, Philadelphia, 1990, WB Saunders.

INCIDENCE

1. Incidence is increased among children in lower socioeconomic groups.
2. Incidence is increased among African-American adolescents.
3. Incidence rates vary from 0.6% to 20.5% (depends on methodology used).
4. Noncompliance with treatment occurs among more than 50% of affected children; compliance improves when the child is dependent on the parent.
5. Males are affected more often than females.
6. In individuals 2 to 18 years of age, 45% to 100% of cases of hypertension are attributed to primary hypertension.
7. Of children with primary hypertension, 25% have a positive family history of the disorder.
8. Overall, 1% to 2% of children and 11% to 12% of adolescents are affected.
9. Hypertension is most often associated with coarctation of the aorta or renal disease.

CLINICAL MANIFESTATIONS

1. Severe headaches
2. Blurred vision, symptoms of increased intracranial pressure

3. Marked irritability
4. Nosebleeds
5. Dizziness
6. Fatigue
7. Nervousness
8. Anorexia, failure to thrive, weight loss
9. Focal or generalized seizures
10. Severe back and/or abdominal pain
11. Papilledema
12. Retinal hemorrhage or exudate
13. Left ventricular hypertrophy
14. Altered renal function

COMPLICATIONS

1. Ischemic (coronary) heart disease
2. Side effects associated with use of antihypertensives (e.g., postexercise syncope, depression, and dizziness)
3. Altered renal function

LABORATORY AND DIAGNOSTIC TESTS

1. Urinalysis, urine culture—to assess for renal cause
2. Serum electrolyte levels—to assess for renal and metabolic status
3. Complete blood count—to assess for infection, fluid overload
4. Creatinine, blood urea nitrogen levels—to assess for renal cause
5. Serum cholesterol level—higher than 250 mg/100 ml
6. Serum triglyceride level—increased
7. Lipoprotein electrophoresis—elevated lipoprotein levels
8. Electrocardiogram—left ventricular hypertrophy
9. Chest radiographic study—left ventricular hypertrophy
10. Rapid-sequence intravenous pyelogram—to assess activation of renin-angiotensin system
11. Plasma renin activity study—to assess activation of renin-angiotensin system
12. Excretory venogram—to detect renal and renovascular abnormalities

13. Arteriogram—to detect renal and renovascular abnormalities
14. Radionuclide studies—to detect renal and renovascular abnormalities

MEDICAL MANAGEMENT

The aim of controlling hypertension is to reduce the associated risk of cardiovascular and renal complications. The step approach to treatment for the pediatric client is to educate the child and family on the importance of prevention. Non-pharmacologic interventions such as diet adjustment, exercise, and weight control should be the first approach when possible. The goal of antihypertensive therapy is to maintain pressure below the 90th percentile using the least amount and number of drugs. Medications should be started one at a time using a diuretic, beta-blocker, or calcium antagonist. Keeping the medication schedule as simple as possible helps to promote compliance.

NURSING ASSESSMENT

1. See the Cardiac and Renal Assessment sections in Appendix A.
2. Assess neurologic status.
3. Assess nutritional history.

NURSING DIAGNOSES

- Tissue perfusion, Ineffective
- Cardiac output, Decreased
- Knowledge, Deficient

NURSING INTERVENTIONS

1. Monitor child's clinical status and assess for changes.
   a. Blood pressure
   b. Neurologic status
   c. Presence of bleeding
   d. Blurred vision
   e. Renal function
2. Monitor child's therapeutic and untoward response to administered medications.
3. Monitor and encourage child's nutritional intake.

a. Administer diet restricted in sodium, fats, and calories.
b. Reinforce dietary information and management plan provided by dietitian.
c. Include family members in teaching.

🏠 Discharge Planning and Home Care

Instruct child and family about management of hypertension:
1. Explanation of hypertension
2. Medications
3. Dietary restrictions and weight control
4. Use of oral contraceptives
5. Salt intake
6. Exercise
7. Smoking

CLIENT OUTCOMES

1. Child will remain normotensive.
2. Child and family will understand follow-up needs.
3. Child will remain compliant with medication regimen and diet.

REFERENCES

Flynn JJ: Pharmacologic management of childhood hypertension: current status, future challenges, *Am J Hypertens* 15(2 pt 2):30S, 2002.

Friedman AL: Approach to the treatment of hypertension in children, *Heart Dis* 4(1):47, 2002.

Robinson RF et al: Secondary pediatric hypertension, *Pediatr Nephrol* 19 (12):1379, 2004.

Schell, KA: Evidence-based practice: Noninvasive blood pressure measurement in children, *Pediatr Nurs* 32(2):263, 2006.

Sorof J, Daniels S: Obesity hypertension in children: a problem of epidemic proportions, *Hypertension* 40(4):441, 2002.

40

Hypertrophic Pyloric Stenosis

PATHOPHYSIOLOGY

Hypertrophic pyloric stenosis is one of the more frequently occurring conditions requiring surgery within the first 6 months of life. Hypertrophy (increased size) and hyperplasia (increased mass) of the circular muscle of the pylorus cause obstruction at the pyloric sphincter. The circular muscle increases to as much as twice the normal thickness, and the pylorus lengthens, which results in severe narrowing of the lumen. In addition, the stomach dilates, and hypertrophy of the gastric antrum occurs. The cause is unknown, but multiple factors have been implicated, and evidence suggests that local innervation is involved. Immaturity of function and the absence of pyloric ganglion cells has been suggested. Hypertrophic pyloric stenosis may be associated with intestinal malrotation, esophageal or duodenal atresias, and anorectal anomalies. In addition, there is a genetic predisposition. In 1999, the Centers for Disease Control and Prevention (CDC) reported a possible link between the use of oral erythromycin in infants and hypertrophic pyloric stenosis. The CDC does not recommend that physicians stop prescribing erythromycin, just that they be aware of the possible risk. A study done in Denmark determined that the maternal use of macrolides such as erythromycin during breast feeding increased the risk of infantile hypertrophic pyloric stenosis.

INCIDENCE

1. Hypertrophic pyloric stenosis occurs in 1 to 4 cases per 1000 live births, usually 2 to 8 weeks after birth, with peak incidence within the first 3 to 5 weeks of life.
2. Hypertrophic pyloric stenosis is less common in African Americans and is rare in Asian individuals. It is most commonly seen in white children.
3. Male/female ratio is 5:1. This ratio is not observed as much in children of low birth weight (<2500 g) as in children of birth weight over 2500 g.
4. The disorder is more common in firstborn children.

CLINICAL MANIFESTATIONS

1. Nonbilious vomitus; may be blood-streaked (initial symptom)
2. Vomiting, usually occurring 30 to 60 minutes after feeding
3. Vomiting that becomes progressively more projectile, projecting up to 3 feet from the infant
4. Appears hungry; eagerness to be fed after vomiting
5. Vomiting of retained feeding with current feeding
6. Signs of dehydration (decreased tears, poor skin turgor, dark circles under eyes, sunken fontanelle)
7. Lethargy
8. Failure to gain weight or weight loss
9. Fewer and smaller stools
10. Distended upper abdomen after feeding
11. Irritability, crying
12. Visible left-to-right gastric peristaltic waves
13. Palpable firm, movable, olive-shaped mass in right upper quadrant

COMPLICATIONS

1. Gastrointestinal: jaundice—caused by deficiency of hepatic glucuronide transferase
2. Fluid, electrolytes, and acid/base balance: hypochloremic metabolic alkalosis (acute); severe dehydration (acute), with increased blood urea nitrogen levels

LABORATORY AND DIAGNOSTIC TESTS

Refer to Appendix D for normal values and/or ranges of laboratory and diagnostic tests.

1. Complete blood count—elevated hemoglobin and hematocrit, due to hemoconcentration—used to determine fluid balance, specifically dehydration status
2. Serum electrolyte levels—hypochloremia, hypernatremia, hypokalemia (may be masked by hemoconcentration from extracellular fluid depletion)—used to determine electrolyte levels, which may be imbalanced as a result of vomiting
3. Arterial blood gas values—used to determine acid/base balance, specifically metabolic alkalosis related to vomiting
4. Upper gastrointestinal barium studies—diagnostic; show delayed gastric emptying and narrowing of the pyloric channel (barium is aspirated through a nasogastric tube after the procedure to decrease risk of aspiration)
5. Abdominal ultrasonography—first-line diagnostic study. Used to visualize hypertrophy and hyperplagia of pyloric sphincter
6. Urine specific gravity—used to determine hydration status
7. Blood urea nitrogen (BUN)—elevated BUN can indicate dehydration from vomiting and inadequate fluid intake

MEDICAL AND SURGICAL MANAGEMENT

Before surgery, fluid and electrolyte abnormalities and acid-base imbalances are corrected with intravenous (IV) fluids and electrolyte replacement. Antibiotics may be administered prophylactically. If emesis is excessive, a nasogastric tube may be inserted for gastric decompression. An open pyloromyotomy, involving a small transverse abdominal incision or a periumbilical incision, down to the mucosa and fully across the pyloric length, is the standard surgical treatment for this disorder. Laparoscopic pyloromyotomy has also been found to be safe and successful for the correction of hypertrophic pyloric stenosis, resulting in shorter surgical time, more rapid postoperative feeding, and quicker discharge. General anesthesia is usually used; however, studies have demonstrated the advantages of spinal anesthesia over general anesthesia in infants undergoing pyloromyotomy, especially to decrease the risks of apnea and aspiration of stomach contents. Overall surgery is well tolerated with few complications.

NURSING ASSESSMENT

1. See the Gastrointestinal Assessment section in Appendix A.
2. Assess for signs and symptoms of dehydration.
3. Assess for signs and symptoms of electrolyte imbalances.
4. Assess child's response to oral intake.
5. Assess child's response to pain.
6. Assess wound for drainage and infection.
7. Assess child and family coping.

NURSING DIAGNOSES

- Fluid volume, Deficient
- Nutrition: less than body requirements, Imbalanced
- Pain, Acute
- Infection, Risk for
- Knowledge, Deficient
- Sleep pattern, Disturbed
- Coping, Ineffective
- Therapeutic regimen management, Ineffective

NURSING INTERVENTIONS

Preoperative Care

1. Promote and maintain fluid and electrolyte balance.
   a. Maintain patent IV route for administration of ordered fluids at specified rate.
   b. Maintain patent nasogastric (NG) tube, if present.
   c. Maintain nothing-by-mouth status.
   d. Connect NG tube to low continuous suction to prevent distention and vomiting and to decrease risk of aspiration.
   e. Replace NG output with IV fluids as ordered.
   f. Perform gastric lavage with normal saline through NG tube until fluid is clear (preoperative preparation).
   g. Strictly monitor input and output by weighing diapers (including number and characteristics of stools, NG drainage, and amount of emesis).

    h. Record urine specific gravity every 8 hours.

    i. Record weight daily.

    j. Monitor for signs and symptoms of dehydration (vital signs, mucous membranes, fontanelle status/ urine output).

2. Monitor and report laboratory results.
3. Monitor for signs of fluid and electrolyte imbalances.

    a. Hypochloremia (hyperexcitability of the nervous sysytem and muscles, tetany, twitching, slowed respirations and hypotension)

    b. Hypernatremia (restlessness, thirst, flushed skin, dry mucous membranes and tongue)

    c. Hypokalemia (vertigo, hypotension, nausea, vomiting, diarrhea, muscle weakness, cardiac arrhythmias)

4. Prepare parents preoperatively for child's upcoming surgery (see the Preparation for Procedures or Surgery section in Appendix F).

Postoperative Care

1. Promote and maintain fluid and electrolyte balance.

    a. Maintain patent IV route for administration of ordered fluids at specified rate.

    b. Strictly monitor intake and output.

    c. Monitor for signs of dehydration (vital signs, mucous membranes, fontanelle status, urine output).

    d. Maintain patent NG tube, if present.

2. Monitor child's response to oral intake. (Traditionally, feedings have been reintroduced slowly, but recent studies indicate that ad lib feedings postoperatively are beneficial and result in earlier discharge from the hospital.)

    a. Initiate fluids by mouth 4 to 6 hours postoperatively; assess response.

    b. Provide small, frequent feedings (15 to 20 ml per feeding) as tolerated.

    c. Begin with clear liquids (glucose and electrolytes); increase to full-strength formula as tolerated.

    d. Feed infant in upright position.

    e. Observe for signs of vomiting and hematemesis (may delay feedings by mouth for 48 hours).

    f. Monitor for weight gain.

3. Provide nonpharmacologic and pharmacologic pain relief measures as indicated (see Appendix I).
   a. Monitor for signs of pain—crying, irritability, stretching, back arching, increased motor activity.
   b. Assess child's therapeutic and untoward reactions to medications.
   c. Avoid pressure on incision by not lifting infant's legs during diaper changes.
4. Monitor and maintain integrity of incisional site.
   a. Assess for signs of infection—redness, drainage, inflammation, warmth to touch, fever
   b. Perform incision site care per institution protocols
5. Provide psychosocial support (see the Supportive Care section in Appendix F).

🏠 Discharge Planning and Home Care

1. Instruct parents to monitor child's response to feedings and to observe for untoward symptoms.
   a. Persistent vomiting
   b. Signs of infection
   c. Weight loss
2. Instruct parents about care of incisional site.
3. Provide follow-up support and management for parents.
   a. Name and phone number of primary physician
   b. Phone number of clinic
   c. Name and phone number of clinical nurse specialist and primary nurse

CLIENT OUTCOMES

1. Child will retain feedings.
2. Child will be adequately hydrated and have normal electrolyte balance.
3. Child will have appropriate weight gain.
4. Child will experience no complications, such as infection.
5. Child will obtain pain relief.
6. Parents will demonstrate understanding of infant's or child's condition, possible complications, and home care requirements.

REFERENCES

Ball JW, Bindler RC: *Child health nursing: Partnering with children and families,* Upper Saddle River, NJ, 2006, Pearson Prentice-Hall.

Bianca S et al: Sex ratio imbalance and birth weight in newborns with isolated hypertrophic pyloric stenosis, *J Obstet Gynaecol* 23(1):43, 2003.

Morash D: An interdisciplinary project that changed practice in feeding methods after pyloromyotomy, *Pediatr Nurs* 28(2):113, 2002.

Morbidity and Mortality Weekly Report: Hypertrophic Pyloric Stenosis in Infants Following Pertussis Prophylaxis with Erythromycin–Knoxville, Tennessee, 1999, *MMWR Weekly* (serial online): www.cdc.gov/mmwr/preview/mmwrhtml/mm4849a1.htm. Accessed January 23, 2007.

Somri M et al: The effectiveness and safety of spinal anaesthesia in the pyloromyotomy procedure, *Paediatr Anaesth* 13(1):32, 2003.

Sorenson H et al: Risk of infantile hypertrophic pyloric stenosis after maternal postnatal use of macrolides, *Scand J Infect Dis* 35(2):104, 2003.

41

Idiopathic
Thrombocytopenic Purpura

PATHOPHYSIOLOGY

Idiopathic thrombocytopenic purpura (ITP) is one of the most common acquired, noninherited bleeding disorders. ITP is a condition in which the number of circulating platelets is reduced in the presence of normal marrow. The thrombocytopenia results from an antibody-mediated or transient immune platelet destruction process. Generally, ITP is preceded by a vaguely defined febrile illness 1 to 6 weeks before onset of symptoms. On occasion, it may occur as a result of bone marrow suppression following chemotherapy. Clinical manifestations vary considerably. ITP can be classified into three types: acute, chronic, and recurrent (Box 41-1). Children are initially seen with the following symptoms: (1) fever, (2) bleeding, (3) petechiae, (4) purpura with thrombocytopenia, and (5) anemia. Prognosis is favorable, especially in children with the acute form.

INCIDENCE

1. The age range of peak incidence is 2 to 5 years.
2. Frequency is 4 to 8 cases in 100,000 children per year.
3. ITP affects males and females equally.
4. ITP occurs more commonly in white individuals.
5. Eighty percent of ITP in children is the acute type.
6. Incidence is seasonal—occurrence is more frequent in winter and spring.

BOX 41-1

Types of Idiopathic Thrombocytopenic Purpura

Acute
- Child is initially seen with thrombocytopenia.
- Platelet count returns to normal within 6 months of diagnosis (spontaneous remission).
- Subsequent relapses are not seen.

Chronic
- Thrombocytopenia persists longer than 6 months after diagnosis.
- Onset is insidious.
- Platelet count remains below normal throughout disease.
- This form is seen primarily in adults.

Recurrent
- Individual is initially seen with thrombocytopenia.
- Repeated relapses occur.

7. Of affected children, 50% to 85% have a viral illness before onset of ITP.
8. Of affected children, 10% to 25% develop the chronic form of ITP.

CLINICAL MANIFESTATIONS

1. Prodromal phase—fatigue, fever, and abdominal pain
2. Spontaneous appearance on skin of petechiae and ecchymoses
3. Easy bruising
4. Epistaxis (initial symptom in one third of children)
5. Menorrhagia
6. Hematuria (infrequent)
7. Bleeding from oral cavity (infrequent)
8. Melena (infrequent)

COMPLICATIONS

1. Relapse
2. Central nervous system hemorrhage (less than 1% of affected individuals)

LABORATORY AND DIAGNOSTIC TESTS

1. Platelet count—decreased to less than 40,000/mm^3 and often less than 20,000/mm^3
2. Complete blood count—anemia results from inability of red blood cells to use iron
3. Bone marrow aspiration—increased megakaryocytes
4. White blood cell count—mild to moderate leukocytosis; mild eosinophilia
5. Platelet antibody tests—done when diagnosis is questionable
6. Tissue biopsy of skin and gingiva—diagnostic
7. Antinuclear antibody test—to rule out systemic lupus erythematosus
8. Slit-lamp examinations—to screen for uveitis
9. Renal biopsy—to diagnose renal involvement
10. Chest radiographic study and pulmonary function test—diagnostic for pulmonary manifestations (effusion, interstitial pulmonary fibrosis)

MEDICAL MANAGEMENT

The goal of treatment in ITP is the reduction of antibody production and platelet destruction, and elevation and maintenance of the platelet count. Corticosteroids are often used as the initial therapy for ITP. If the child does not respond to the corticosteroid regimens, intravenous immune globulin (IVIG) is administered. IVIG stimulates a rapid rise in platelet count within 24 hours of administration. Immunosuppressants (vincristine and cyclophosphamide) may be used in difficult cases. A splenectomy may be performed if ITP lasts longer than 1 year or the child is older than 5 years of age.

NURSING ASSESSMENT

1. See the Hematologic Assessment section in Appendix A.
2. Determine location of purpuric areas.
3. Determine sites of bleeding.

NURSING DIAGNOSES

- Tissue integrity, Impaired
- Tissue perfusion, Ineffective

- Injury, Risk for
- Fatigue
- Diversional activity, Deficient
- Knowledge, Deficient

NURSING INTERVENTIONS

1. Monitor child's clinical status.
   a. Vital signs—monitored every 2 hours (during acute phase)
   b. Bleeding sites
   c. Level of activity
   d. Purpuric area
   e. Areas susceptible to bruising and skin breakdown
2. Monitor for and prevent infection.
   a. Screen contacts with child.
   b. Institute clean techniques when in contact with child.
   c. Monitor for signs of infection (pulmonary, systemic, localized).
   d. Administer medications.
3. Monitor child's response to blood product transfusions (whole blood, packed cells, platelets).
4. Monitor child's therapeutic and untoward response to administration of medications.
   a. Antibiotics
   b. Antipyretics (avoid aspirin)
   c. Iron preparations
   d. Immunosuppressives
5. Promote rest and conservation of child's energy.
   a. Maintain complete bed rest during acute stages.
   b. Assess child's response to activity as means of assessing tolerance and progression.
6. Provide diversional and age-appropriate activities for child during periods of limited activities (see Appendix F).
7. Provide age-appropriate explanations before procedures, treatments, and surgery, if splenectomy is indicated (see the Preparation for Procedures or Surgery section in Appendix F).

🏠 Discharge Planning and Home Care

1. Provide parents and child with instructions about administration of medications.
   a. Time and route of administration
   b. Monitoring for untoward effects
2. Instruct parents and child to monitor for signs and symptoms of thrombocytopenia and report immediately (i.e., petechiae, ecchymosis, blood in urine or stool, and headache).
3. Instruct parents to monitor child's activities.
   a. Encourage quiet activities; have child avoid contact sports until platelet level returns to normal.
   b. Balance rest and activity periods; increase activity as tolerated.
4. Instruct parents to avoid contact by child with persons who have infections, especially upper respiratory tract infections.
5. Instruct parents to avoid use of over-the-counter medications that may affect clotting (i.e., antihistamines, aspirin, other nonsteroidal antiinflammatory drugs).

CLIENT OUTCOMES

1. Child's platelet count will return to normal between relapses.
2. Child will be free of complications of the disease.
3. Child will not demonstrate signs and symptoms of infection.
4. Child and family will verbalize knowledge of treatment regimen.

REFERENCES

Behrman RE, Kiegman R, Jenson HB: *Nelson textbook of pediatrics*, ed 17, Philadelphia, 2004, WB Saunders.

Curry H: Bleeding disorder basics, *Pediatr Nurs* 30(5):402, 2005.

Noonan N: Immune thrombocytic purpura, *J Soc Pediatr Nurs* 3(2):82, 1998.

42

Imperforate Anus

PATHOPHYSIOLOGY

The congenital malformation known as imperforate anus (anorectal agenesis) involves the anus, the rectum, or the junction between the two. There are two classifications of imperforate anus, related to the placement of the distal end of the colon (the rectum). In high lesions, the rectum ends above the puborectalis sling, the main muscle complex responsible for sphincter control and fecal continence. In low lesions, the rectum has traversed the puborectalis sling, with an abnormal location in the perineum. Affected infants can be expected to have rectal continence after repair.

Along with the imperforate anus, the following may also occur:

1. In girls, a fistula may be present between the rectum and the vagina.
2. In boys, a fistula may be present between the rectum and the urinary tract at the scrotum.

The appearance of the defect varies, depending on its severity. A less-involved imperforate anus appears as a deep anal dimple and exhibits strong muscular reaction to pinprick, which indicates innervation of that area. More severe involvement is initially seen as a flat perineum with no dimple and poor muscular response to pinprick, a result of defective perineal innervation and muscle formation. A highly involved defect includes other anomalies as well (Table 42-1). The infant may initially be seen with poorly developed labia, undescended testicles, or ambiguous genitalia. Outcomes are favorable after definitive surgery is performed.

TABLE 42-1
Associated Anomalies

Type	Incidence (%)*
Esophageal atresia	10–13
Intestinal atresia	4
Intestinal malrotation	4
Cardiovascular defects	12–22
Skeletal deformities (spina bifida, agenesis of sacrum)	6
Genitourinary anomalies (renal agenesis, hypospadias, epispadias)	20–54

*Approximate percentages.

INCIDENCE

1. Congenital anomalies of the anus and rectum are relatively common. Minor anomalies occur in approximately 1 per 500 live births; major anomalies occur in 1 per 5000 live births.
2. Most studies report a male preponderance of 55% to 65%. High anomalies occur more often in males, whereas low lesions occur more often in females.
3. Of affected infants, 20% to 75% have an associated anomaly, with genitourinary (GU) tract malformations found most frequently (20% to 54%), tracheoesophageal fistula occurring in 10% of infants, and cardiovascular malformations in 12% to 22%.
4. The associated anomalies are usually the cause of death.
5. There are no reported racial differences in disease incidence or severity of disease.

CLINICAL MANIFESTATIONS

1. Physical examination showing absent external anal opening, flat perineum with a short sacrum
2. Failure to pass meconium within first 24 hours after birth
3. Caregiver inability to locate anus to take infant's rectal temperature

4. Passage of meconium through fistula or misplaced anus
5. Gradual distention and signs of bowel obstruction if no fistula present

COMPLICATIONS

1. Renal and GU: hyperchloremic acidosis, continuing urinary tract infection, urethral damage (result of surgical procedure), problems or delays associated with toilet training
2. Gastrointestinal: constipation, eversion of anal mucosa, stenosis (result of contraction of scar from anastomosis), impactions and constipation (result of sigmoid dilation), problems or delays associated with toilet training, incontinence (result of anal stenosis or impaction), prolapse of anorectal mucosa (results in persistent seepage and incontinence), recurrent fistulas (result of tension in surgical site and infection)

LABORATORY AND DIAGNOSTIC TESTS

1. Visual and digital rectal examination is generally diagnostic.
2. If a fistula is present, urine may be examined for meconium epithelial cells.
3. Radiographic study after infant kept in knee-chest position for approximately 30 minutes. May demonstrate air collected in the blind-ending rectum at or near the perineum; may be misleading if the rectum is filled with meconium, which prevents air from reaching the end of the rectal pouch.
4. Ultrasonography may be helpful in locating the rectal pouch.
5. Cloacal anomalies deserve special attention. Hydrocolpos and bladder outlet obstructions can confound conventional radiographic evaluation. For these patients, voiding cystourethrography and vaginography are necessary to define the malformation.
6. A distal colostogram accurately defines the type of lesion and the usual rectal fistula.

SURGICAL MANAGEMENT

Surgical therapy in the newborn varies with the severity of the defect. The higher the lesion, the more complicated the corrective surgical procedure. The decision to perform an anoplasty in the newborn period or to delay the repair and perform a colostomy is based on the infant's physical examination findings, the appearance of the perineum, and any changes that occur over the first 24 hours of life. Operating early and in a single stage is potentially beneficial for the infant. However, a more conservative approach is warranted in low birth weight babies and those with associated cardiac or respiratory conditions. Anoplasty is recommended for both males and females with rectoperineal fistulas. Imperforate anus without fistula, rectal atresia, rectovesical fistula, and rectovaginal fistula requires a colostomy. A colostomy is performed a few days after birth. The definitive surgery, a perineal anoplasty (an abdominal-perineal pull-through procedure), is generally delayed 3 to 12 months. This delay allows the pelvis to enlarge and the musculature to develop. It also enables the infant to gain weight and attain satisfactory nutritional status. Low lesions are corrected by pulling the rectal pouch through the sphincter to the opening on the anal skin. Fistulas, if present, are closed. Membranous defects require only minimal surgical treatment. The membrane is punctured with a hemostat or scalpel.

In most instances, correction of the imperforate anus requires a two-stage surgical approach. For mild to moderate defects, the prognosis is favorable. The defect can be repaired, and normal peristalsis and continence can be obtained. More serious defects are usually associated with other anomalies, which complicate the surgical outcomes.

NURSING ASSESSMENT

1. See the Gastrointestinal Assessment section in Appendix A.
2. Assess nutritional status.

NURSING DIAGNOSES

- Fluid volume, Risk for deficient
- Nutrition: less than body requirements, Imbalanced
- Tissue integrity, Impaired
- Infection, Risk for
- Pain
- Home maintenance, Impaired

NURSING INTERVENTIONS
Preoperative Care
1. Monitor infant's condition before surgery.
   a. Measure abdominal girth (assess for abdominal distention).
   b. Monitor vital signs every 4 hours.
   c. Monitor for bowel complications (perforation and enterocolitis).
   d. Monitor fluid and electrolyte balance (intake and output, nasogastric [NG] drainage).
2. Prepare infant for surgery.
   a. Monitor infant's response to evacuation of bowel.
   b. Using NG tube, decompress stomach.
   c. Using catheter, decompress bladder.
   d. Provide only clear liquids for 24 to 48 hours before surgery.
   e. Monitor infant's response to antibiotics (e.g., neomycin) used to sterilize bowel.
3. Prepare infant for procedures and surgeries.

Postoperative Care
1. Monitor infant's response to surgery.
   a. Vital signs
   b. Intake and output—report discrepancies
   c. Surgical site—bleeding, intactness, signs of infection
2. Monitor for signs and symptoms of complications.
   a. Urinary tract infection
   b. Hyperchloremic acidosis
   c. Decreased urinary output
   d. Constipation
   e. Obstruction
   f. Bleeding
3. Promote and maintain fluid and electrolyte balance.
   a. Record intake per route (intravenous, NG, oral).
   b. Record output per route (urine and stool, NG drainage, emesis, Penrose drain).
   c. Assess hydration status (signs of dehydration, electrolyte imbalance).

4. Provide dressing care; maintain integrity of surgical site (depends on type of surgery).
   a. Monitor dilation of anus.
   b. Monitor endorectal pull-through incision (made over anal dimple and colon directly through to muscle cuff) for mucosal prolapse.
   c. Do not take rectal temperatures, give rectal medications, or perform rectal examinations.
   d. Keep anus clean and dry.
   e. Apply zinc oxide for skin lesions and irritation surrounding surgical site.
   f. Avoid tension on suture line; position infant on side or abdomen.
5. Promote adequate nutritional intake.
   a. Monitor bowel sounds; begin feeding fluids when bowel sounds are heard.
   b. Advance to full diet as tolerated.
6. Protect infant from infection.
   a. Provide Foley catheter care.
   b. Change dressing and note drainage.
   c. Monitor incisional site for drainage, redness, inflammation.
   d. Clean anal area frequently to prevent fecal contamination.
   e. Perform pulmonary toilet every 2 to 4 hours.
   f. Change infant's position every 2 hours.
   g. Monitor for signs of systemic infection or local abscess.
7. Promote functioning and maintain patency of colostomy.
8. Promote comfort and minimize pain.
   a. Provide sitz bath (initiate 1 week after surgery).
   b. Apply zinc oxide to excoriated and irritated areas of skin.
   c. Provide position of comfort.
   d. Use distractions (play activities).
   e. Monitor child's response to medication.

🏠 Discharge Planning and Home Care

1. Encourage parents to express concerns about outcomes of surgery.

2. Refer to specific institutional procedures for information distributed to parents about home care.
3. Instruct parents on signs of intestinal obstruction, poor tolerance of feedings, and impaired healing processes.
4. Instruct parents about follow-up techniques to promote optimal surgical outcomes.
   a. Colostomy care
   b. Dilation of anus
   c. Sitz baths
5. Instruct parents that, as children age, psychologic counseling should be part of follow-up care. Twenty nine percent of affected children experience some behavioral problems.

CLIENT OUTCOMES

1. Infant's gastrointestinal function will return to normal.
2. Infant will continue to grow at a steady pace.
3. Parents will verbalize understanding of home care and follow-up needs.

REFERENCES

Beals DA: *Imperforate anus* (website): www.emedicine.com. Accessed March 24, 2006.

Funakosi S et al: Psychosocial liaison-consultation for the children who have undergone repair of imperforate anus and Hirschsprung disease, *J Pediatr Surg* 40(7):1156, 2005.

Levitt MA, Pena A: Outcomes from the correction of anorectal malformations, *Clin Opin Pediatr* 17(3):394, 2005.

Magnuson DK, Parry RL, Chwals WJ: Selected Abdominal Gastrointestinal Anomalies. In: Martin RJ, Fanaroff AA, Walsh MC, editors: *Neonatal-perinatal medicine,* ed 8, St. Louis, 2006, Mosby.

Pena A, Levitt MA: Imperforate anus and cloacal malformations. In: Ashcraft KW, Holcomb GW, Murphy JP, editors: *Pediatric surgery,* ed 4, Philadelphia, 2005, WB Saunders.

Zderic SA: Developmental abnormalities of the genitourinary system. In: Taeusch HW, Ballard RA, and Gleason CA, editors. *Avery's diseases of the newborn,* ed 8, Philadelphia, 2005, WB Saunders.

43

Inflammatory Bowel Disease

PATHOPHYSIOLOGY

Ulcerative colitis (UC) and Crohn's disease (CD) are two major idiopathic inflammatory bowel disease (IBD) in children, with 15% falling in the indeterminate IBD category. They share many common characteristics such as diarrhea, pain, fever, and blood loss. The etiologies of both diseases are unknown, although recent research has focused on genetic (IBD disease gene on chromosome 16 [CARD15]), immunologic, dietary, and infectious causes. Some research implicates the presence in IBD of specific infectious agents such as *Bacteroides fragilis, Mycobacterium paratuberculosis,* paramyxoviruses, and *Listeria monocytogenes; Campylobacter jejuni, Salmonella, Shigella, Yersinia,* and *Eschericia coli* have also been associated with relapses of IBD. The single greatest risk factor for IBD is a positive family history (found in 15% to 30% of IBD patients). To date, there is no indication that emotional factors are the primary cause. The goal of therapy includes control of inflammation and associated signs and symptoms, improving nutritional status to allow optimal growth and sexual maturation, and good quality of life—both emotionally and physically.

An association between ankylosing spondylitis and the histocompatibility of human leukocyte antigen (HLA-B27) and inflammatory bowel disease is a possibility. Ulcerative colitis and Crohn's disease have similar initial signs, including diarrhea, rectal bleeding, abdominal pain, fever, malaise, anorexia, weight loss, and anemia. Children may initially be seen with vague symptoms such as growth failure, anorexia, fever, and joint pains with or without gastrointestinal symptoms.

Both conditions are characterized by remissions and exacerbations. Extracolonic manifestations such as joint problems, hepatobiliary conditions, skin rashes, and eye irritation can occur. Although the peak incidence of inflammatory bowel disease is between 15 and 25 years of age, 15% of all cases occur at age 15 years and younger. Prognosis is dependent on the following factors: (1) age at onset and rapidity of onset; (2) response to medical treatment; and (3) extent of involvement.

Ulcerative colitis is a recurrent inflammatory and ulcerative disease affecting primarily the large intestine. Lesions are continuous and involve the superficial mucosa, causing vascular congestion, capillary dilation, edema, hemorrhage, and ulceration. Muscular hypertrophy and deposition of fibrous tissue and fat result, which gives the bowel a "lead pipe" appearance because of narrowing of the bowel itself.

Crohn's disease is an inflammatory and ulcerative disease affecting any part of the alimentary tract from the mouth to the anus. Rectal pain and bleeding from fissures and fistulas occurs in 25% of CD patients. Of CD patients, 10% have proctitis, and 70% of these patients will develop more extensive disease. The CD affects the deep walls of the bowel. The lesions are discontinuous, resulting in a "skipping" effect, with the diseased portions of the bowel separated by normal tissue. Fissures, fistulas, and thickened intestinal walls result. Granulomas occur in approximately 50% of cases.

INCIDENCE

1. Annual incidence of UC and CD is 4 to 10 cases in 100,000 children; 2 to 14 cases occur in 100,000 in the general population. IBD affects male and female equally.
2. Ulcerative colitis represents more than half of the 20,000 to 25,000 newly diagnosed cases of IBD each year.
3. Age range of peak incidence is 15 to 25 years.
4. White individuals are affected more often than African-American individuals; IBD not seen in third-world countries.
5. A high preponderance of cases occur in American Jews.
6. Of those with ulcerative colitis, 29% have a family history of the disease.

7. Of those with Crohn's disease, 35% have a family history of the disease.

CLINICAL MANIFESTATIONS
Ulcerative Colitis

1. Frequent, bloody stools (number of stools varies from 4 to 24)—major symptom
2. Pain relief after defecation
3. Rectal bleeding, pain
4. Anorexia, pallor, and fatigue
5. Fever
6. Tachycardia
7. Peritoneal irritation
8. Electrolyte imbalance
9. Ten- to 20-pound weight loss over 2 months
10. Anemia, leukocytosis, increased erythrocyte sedimentation rate
11. Extraintestinal symptoms—skin rashes, arthritis
12. Flatulence
13. Severe pain, abdominal rigidity, distention
14. Growth retardation

Crohn's Disease

1. Diarrhea, occult blood
2. Cramping abdominal pain, aggravated by eating
3. Pain in right lower quadrant of abdomen, with or without palpable mass
4. Growth retardation
5. Weight loss
6. Abscess formation
7. Spiking fever
8. Leukocytosis
9. Perianal disease—fistula and fissures
10. Nutritional deficiencies—malnutrition, electrolyte imbalances
11. Amenorrhea, delay in sexual maturation
12. Cachexia
13. Finger clubbing
14. Arthritis

COMPLICATIONS
Ulcerative Colitis
1. Predisposition to cancer—20% increase in risk with each decade after first 10 years
2. Toxic megacolon
3. Hemorrhage
4. Sepsis

Crohn's Disease
1. Perforation
2. Toxic megacolon
3. Hemorrhage
4. Liver abscess and liver disease
5. Ureteral obstruction
6. Retroperitonitis
7. Erythema nodosum
8. Strictures
9. Fistulas

Surgical Complications
1. Necrosis of colostomy (caused by inadequate blood supply)
2. Stricture formation
3. Retraction of stoma
4. Prolapsed stoma
5. Herniation
6. Bleeding
7. Intestinal obstruction
8. Wound infection
9. Peritonitis
10. Spillover of stool
11. Constipation bordering on obstruction
12. Nephrolithiasis
13. Fistula (if multiple fistulas or extensive undermining of subcutaneous tissue occurs, stoma must be excised and located elsewhere)

LABORATORY AND DIAGNOSTIC TESTS

1. Complete blood count—anemia
2. White blood cell count—increased with inflammation
3. Erythrocyte sedimentation rate—increased with inflammation
4. Hematocrit—decreased because of blood loss
5. Serum electrolyte levels—decreased potassium
6. Serum protein level—decreased proteins
7. Stool culture—for presence of infectious organisms
8. Hematest of stool—for presence of blood in stool
9. D-Xylulose absorption blood and urine test—to measure intestinal absorption when there are fatty stools
10. Sigmoidoscopy—to evaluate mucosa, rectum, sigmoid colon directly
11. Colonoscopy—to evaluate colon directly
12. Upper gastrointestinal tract radiographic series with small bowel follow-through—differential diagnosis
13. Barium enema—differential diagnosis
14. Biopsy—to determine type of inflammatory bowel disease; tissue specimens taken from several sites

MEDICAL AND SURGICAL MANAGEMENT
Ulcerative Colitis

Medical management is the primary treatment of ulcerative colitis and centers around drug therapy and nutritional support. Antidiarrheal preparations may be used along with antiinflammatory (nonabsorbable salicylate derivatives [mesalamine] and corticosteroid) agents to control or suppress the inflammatory process. Immunosuppressants (such as azathioprine [Imuran]) are often used in advanced cases. Analgesics and narcotics may also be given for pain. Dietary modifications may be needed when diarrhea, fistulas, or lactose intolerance is present. Therapy depends on the severity of the illness. If the illness is severe, the child may require intravenous (IV) hyperalimentation, administration of corticosteroids, and close observation for electrolyte imbalances, acidosis, anemia, and intestinal perforation. Surgical intervention is eventually needed in 25% of cases (uncontrolled hemorrhage, toxic megacolon, unrelenting pain and diarrhea, and others) and provides a cure.

Crohn's Disease

Pharmacologic interventions for Crohn's disease are similar to those for ulcerative colitis, with the addition of antibiotics to eradicate inflammatory bacterial agents. Metronidazole (Flagyl) is used in treating CD in patients with perianal involvement. Disease tends to recur when the drug is discontinued. It also suggests that this medication (metronidazole) may be effective in treating CD of the colon. Because there is no known cure for this disease, the treatment goals are to reduce bowel inflammation, correct nutritional deficiencies, and provide relief of symptoms. Nutritional support may include dietary modifications, vitamins, oral supplements, or hyperalimentation. Up to 70% of children with Crohn's disease require surgery because of failure of medical management, intestinal fistulas or obstruction, and growth failure. The relapse rate 6 years after surgery is 60%. A recurrence is likely within 2 years, usually at the site of anastomosis.

Appropriate dietary support is imperative. A high-protein, high-carbohydrate, and low-fiber diet with normal amounts of fat is recommended, as well as daily vitamin, iron, and zinc supplements. Restrictive or bland diets result in poor intake and are often counterproductive.

Ileostomy

Ileostomy is performed to treat inflammatory bowel disease after medical therapeutic procedures have been unsuccessful. Ileostomy involves removal of the diseased portion of the bowel (small intestine), with the ileum used to form a stoma on the abdominal wall for bowel evacuation. A variety of surgical procedures may be used, depending on the extent and location of the affected portion of the bowel. An ileostomy with subtotal or total colectomy is performed on children who are malnourished and have moderate to severe rectal disease.

Colostomy

Permanent or temporary colostomies are performed for a variety of conditions. Permanent colostomies are performed for children with severe cases of Crohn's disease. The sigmoid colostomy is most frequently performed. Most often, temporary colostomies (e.g., transverse loop and double-barrel colostomies) are performed in children. In all types of colostomy, an intact portion of the colon is brought through an abdominal incision and is sutured to the abdominal wall to form a stoma.

Surgical Outcomes

The surgery should result in amelioration of symptoms associated with the primary disease. The child is left with an abdominal stoma through which bowel contents are emptied into an attached appliance or into an abdominal pouch (Koch pouch). Although the child does not live with a normally functioning bowel after surgery, most children do well. If the child or adolescent or the parent learns to care properly for the colostomy or ileostomy, a life filled with educational, social, and athletic activities can be expected.

NURSING ASSESSMENT

1. See the Gastrointestinal Assessment section in Appendix A.
2. Assess for abdominal distention, bowel sounds, tenderness and pain, and abdominal girth.

NURSING DIAGNOSES

- Diarrhea
- Pain
- Tissue integrity, Impaired
- Nutrition: less than body requirements, Imbalanced
- Infection, Risk for
- Fluid volume, Risk for deficient
- Body image, Disturbed
- Knowledge, Deficient
- Home maintenance, Impaired
- Injury, Risk for

NURSING INTERVENTIONS

1. Promote and maintain proper hydration status.
   a. Record input and output.
   b. Record weight daily.
   c. Assess for signs of dehydration.
   d. Promote oral intake when appropriate.
   e. Monitor administration of elemental feedings or hyper-alimentation.
2. Provide comfort and pain relief measures as indicated.
   a. Maintain bed rest during acute episode (decreased activity results in decreased peristalsis, diarrhea, pain).
   b. Provide diversional activities.
   c. Change child's position every 2 hours.
   d. Assess intensity, type, time, and pattern of occurrence of pain, and child's response to pain relief measures.
   e. Monitor child's response to analgesics and narcotics.
   f. Provide uninterrupted rest periods.
3. Promote skin integrity.
   a. For perineal care, apply A&D ointment or petroleum jelly to perineal area to prevent skin irritation or breakdown.
   b. Apply body moisturizers liberally.
   c. Provide sitz bath 3 times per day (for perianal or rectal fistulas or fissures).
   d. Provide foam mattress to prevent pressure sores.
   e. Change child's position every 2 hours.
4. Promote and support optimal nutritional status.
   a. Compile dietary history, including food allergies.
   b. Monitor tolerance to food, noting type and amount.
   c. Monitor response to elemental feedings.
   d. Monitor response to low-residue, bland, high-protein, high-calorie diet.
   e. Monitor for signs of electrolyte imbalances (hypotension, tachycardia, oliguria, atonic muscles, general sense of confusion).
   f. Restrict intake of greasy, spicy, and lactose-containing foods.
   g. Monitor administration of hyperalimentation; observe child's or adolescent's response.

      i.　Maintain sterility of central line.
     ii.　Accurately record input and output.
    iii.　Obtain weight daily.
    iv.　Monitor urinary specific gravity.
     v.　Check urinary glucose and acetone.
    vi.　Monitor electrolyte balance (especially blood glucose).

5. Monitor child's response to and untoward side effects of medications.
6. Monitor for, prevent, or report signs of potential or actual complications.
   a. Fistulas or fissures
   b. Hemorrhage
   c. Intestinal obstruction
   d. Liver abscess
   e. Ureteral obstruction
   f. Retroperitonitis
   g. Perforations
   h. Enterocolitis

Preoperative Care

Prepare infant, child, or adolescent physically for surgery.

1. Monitor infant's or child's response to enemas, laxatives, stool softeners (to evacuate bowel preoperatively).
2. Monitor infant's or child's response to decompression of stomach and bowel (nasogastric [NG] tube and rectal tube).
3. Provide nothing by mouth for 12 hours before surgery.
4. Insert Foley catheter to decompress bladder.
5. Administer antibiotics to sterilize bowel.
6. Monitor vital signs every 4 hours.
7. Monitor for bowel complications (perforation, toxic megacolon, or enterocolitis).
8. Demonstrate use of appliances.

Postoperative Care

1. Monitor child's response to surgery.
   a. Vital signs
   b. Intake and output (report any discrepancy)
   c. Dressing (amount of drainage, intactness)

2. Monitor for signs and symptoms of complications.
   a. Stoma complications (prolapse, bleeding, excessive diarrhea, ribbonlike stools, failure to pass stool, flatus)
   b. Intestinal obstruction or constipation
   c. Prolapse of proximal segment
   d. Bleeding
   e. Increased stooling
   f. Infection
3. Promote return of peristalsis.
   a. Maintain patency of NG tube.
   b. Check functioning of suction machine.
   c. Irrigate with normal saline solution every 4 hours and as needed.
   d. Check for placement of NG tube; auscultate and aspirate contents.
4. Promote and maintain fluid and electrolyte balance.
   a. Record intake per route (IV, NG, oral).
   b. Record output per route (urine, stool, NG drainage, emesis, stoma).
   c. Monitor for signs and symptoms of electrolyte imbalance.
   d. Consult with physician about disparities in input and output.
5. Alleviate or minimize pain and discomfort.
   a. Maintain position of comfort.
   b. Monitor child's response to administration of medications.
   c. Provide oral care (mouth can become dry with NG tube in place).
6. Provide stoma and skin care to promote healing and to prevent complications.
   a. Inspect stoma every 4 hours for retraction, prolapse, or protrusion greater than 2 cm.
   b. Check for bleeding at stoma site.
   c. Check for obstruction (enlarged, pale, and edematous stoma).
7. Provide ostomy care (refer to institutional manual for specific technical and institutional procedure).

   a. Care of appliance
   b. Skin care
   c. Prevention of complications
      i. Skin can become irritated by digestive enzymes.
      ii. Match adhesive to stoma size.
      iii. Apply protective cream to exposed area.
8. Protect child from infection.
   a. Provide Foley catheter care per hospital protocol.
   b. Change dressing as needed (perianal and colostomy).
   c. Monitor incision site.
   d. Refer to institutional procedure manual for care related to specific procedure.
   e. Perform pulmonary toilet every 2 to 4 hours.
   f. Change child's position every 2 hours (prevents atelectasis).
   g. Monitor for signs of systemic infection and local abscess.
9. Facilitate development of realistic adaptive body image.
   a. Encourage expression of feelings regarding stoma, outcome of surgery.
   b. Encourage socialization through peer support groups.
   c. Refer to community organizations.
   d. Provide active problem solving for concerns such as apparel and sexual activity.
10. Encourage socialization with peers as means to cope with impact of disease.
11. Modify chronic sick role behavior by promoting socialization and normal daily activities.
12. Encourage expression of fears of body mutilation.

🏠 Discharge Planning and Home Care

1. Instruct child, parents, and family about ostomy.
2. Instruct child or adolescent and parents to monitor for and report signs of complications.
   a. Mechanical obstruction
   b. Peritonitis or wound infection
3. Instruct child or adolescent and parents about administration of total parenteral nutrition or NG feedings.
4. Initiate referral to school nurse and teacher to promote continuity of care.

    a. Observations of child's response to condition

    b. Observations of untoward effects of medications and complications

    c. Observation of social interactions with peers and conduct in school

5. Refer to community organizations and other resources (Box 43-1).

CLIENT OUTCOMES

1. Child will have stable gastrointestinal function.
2. Child will have positive adaptation to psychosocial aspects of disease and/or surgery.
3. Child and family will understand home care and follow-up needs.

BOX 43-1
Resources

- Crohn's and Colitis Foundation of America
  386 Park Ave. S., 17th Floor
  New York, NY 10016-8804
  Phone: 800-932-2423
  Fax: 212-779-4098
  Website: www.ccfa.org
- United Ostomy Association, Inc.
  36 Executive Park
  Suite 120
  Irvine, CA 92714-6744
  Phone: 949-660-8624
- Managing Your Child's Crohn's Disease and Ulcerative Colitis
  Keith J. Benkov and Harland S. Winter
  New York, 1996, Master Media

REFERENCES

Baron M: Crohn's disease in children, *Am J Nurs* 102(10):26, 2002.

Behrman RE, Kiegman RM, Jenson HB: *Nelson textbook of pediatrics*, ed 17, Philadelphia, 2004, WB Saunders.

Centers for Disease Control, National Center for Chronic Disease Prevention and Health Promotion: *BMI for Children and Teens* (website): www.cdc.gov/nccdphp/dnpa/bmi/childrens_BMI/about_childrens_BMI.htm. Accessed April 21, 2006.

Hay WW et al: *Current pediatric diagnosis and treatment,* ed 17, New York, 2005, McGraw-Hill.

O'Brien ZS, Schudder LE: *Pediatric nurse practitioner review and resource manual,* ed 2, Maryland, 2005, American Nurses Credentialing Center–Institute for Credentialing Innovation.

Wong DL et al: *Maternal child nursing care,* ed 3, St. Louis, 2006, Mosby.

44

❖

Intellectual Disability

PATHOPHYSIOLOGY

Intellectual disability (the term that is gaining widespread usage in replacing the term *mental retardation*) is foremost amongst the developmental disabilities in terms of its prevalence. The term *intellectual disability* refers to significant limitations in cognitive and adaptive functioning. This is a cognitive disability manifested during childhood (before age 18 years) that is characterized by below-normal intellectual functioning (intelligence quotient [IQ] is approximately 2 standard deviations below the norm, in the range of 70 to 75 or below) with other limitations in at least two adaptive areas of functioning: speech and language, self-care skills, home living, social skills, use of community resources, self-direction, health and safety, functional academics, leisure, and work. Newer definitions of intellectual disability adopt a functional or ecologic approach rather than applying the terminology formerly used to describe levels of mental retardation, such as mild, moderate, severe, and profound. Refer to Box 44-1 and Box 44-2 for diagnostic criteria for mental retardation (currently still in use by some organizations). Many advocates promote the use of newer designations—cognitive disability, intellectual disability, and learning disability—rather than the term mental retardation.

Causes of intellectual disability can be classified as prenatal, perinatal, and postnatal. Prenatal causes include chromosomal disorders (trisomy 21 [Down syndrome], fragile X syndrome), syndrome disorders (Duchenne's muscular dystrophy, neurofibromatosis [type 1]), and inborn errors of metabolism (phenylketonuria [PKU]). Perinatal causes can be categorized as

BOX 44-1

Diagnostic Criteria for Mental Retardation

1. Significantly subaverage intellectual functioning: an intelligence quotient (IQ) of approximately 70 or below on an individually administered IQ test (for infants, a clinical judgment of significantly subaverage intellectual functioning)

2. Concurrent deficits or impairments in present adaptive functioning (i.e., the person's effectiveness in meeting the standards expected for his or her age by his or her cultural group) in at least two of the following areas: communication, self-care, home living, social and interpersonal skills, use of community resources, self-direction, functional academic skills, work, leisure, health, and safety

3. The onset is before age 18 years:
   Code based on degree of severity reflecting level of intellectual impairment:

   - **317** Mild mental retardation: IQ level 50–55 to approximately 70
   - **318.0** Moderate mental retardation: IQ level 35–40 to 50–55
   - **318.1** Severe mental retardation: IQ level 20–25 to 35–40
   - **318.2** Profound mental retardation: IQ level below 20 or 25
   - **319** Mental retardation, severity unspecified: when there is strong presumption of mental retardation but the person's intelligence is untestable by standard tests

From American Psychiatric Association: *Diagnostic and statistical manual of mental disorders,* ed 4, text revision (DSM-IV-TR), Washington, DC, 2000, The Association.

those related to intrauterine problems such as abruptio placentae, maternal diabetes, and premature labor, and those related to neonatal conditions, including meningitis and intracranial hemorrhage. Postnatal causes include conditions resulting from head injuries, infections, and demyelinating and degenerative disorders. Fragile X syndrome, Down syndrome, and fetal alcohol syndrome (FAS) account for one third of the cases of intellectual disability. The occurrence of associated problems such as cerebral palsy, sensory impairments, psychiatric disorders, attention deficit hyperactivity deficit (ADHD), and seizure disorders

BOX 44-2
Operational Definition of Mental Retardation

Mental retardation is characterized both by a significantly below-average score on a test of mental ability or intelligence and by limitations in the ability to function in areas of daily life, such as communication, self-care, and getting along in social situations and school activities. Mental retardation is sometimes referred to as a cognitive or intellectual disability.

Children with mental retardation can and do learn new skills, but they develop more slowly than children with average intelligence and adaptive skills. There are different degrees of mental retardation, ranging from mild to profound. A person's level of mental retardation can be defined by their intelligence quotient (IQ), or by the types and amount of support they need.

From Centers for Disease Control and Prevention: Mental Retardation, *Developmental Disabilities* (serial online): www.cdc.gov/ncbddd/dd/ddmr.htm. Accessed on June 10, 2007.

is more likely correlated with the more severe levels of intellectual disability. Diagnosis is established early in childhood. In a few instances, intellectual disability can be prevented as demonstrated with fetal alcohol syndrome by encouraging women not to injest alcohol during pregnancy. Children born with metabolic conditions such as PKU and congenital hypothyroidism can be medically treated to prevent the consequences of nontreatment resulting in intellectual disability. Long-term prognosis is determined ultimately by the extent to which the individual can function independently in the community (i.e., employment, independent living, social skills).

INCIDENCE

1. More than 85% of persons with intellectual disability have an IQ that classifies them in the mild level (IQ between 50 and 70).
2. Prevalence rate is 1% for children between the ages of 3 years to 10 years.

3. More than 600,000 children and youth ages 6 to 21 years are estimated to have intellectual disability.
4. One of every 10 children in special education has some variation of intellectual disability.
5. Intellectual disability is more common in older children (6 to 10 years) than in younger children (3 to 5 years).
6. Male/female ratio is 1.5:1. Incidence is higher in lower socioeconomic groups.
7. Prevalence rate is higher in African Americans than in whites.
8. Risk of recurrence in families is as follows:
   a. Child with moderate to severe intellectual disability of unknown origin: 3% to 9%
   b. Child with FAS and mother who continues to drink: 30% to 50%
   c. Child with Down syndrome (trisomy): less than 1%
   d. Child with Down syndrome (translocation): higher than 10%
9. Nearly 18% of infants with very low birth weight have severe disabilities.
10. Approximately 500,000 youths have an intellectual disability.
11. The high school dropout rate for students with disabilities is 25% to 30%.
12. The unemployment rate for persons with intellectual disabilities is estimated to be between 66% and 75%.
13. Lifetime costs for all individuals born with an intellectual disability in 2000 are anticipated to reach $51.2 billion, amounting to more than $1 million per person.

CLINICAL MANIFESTATIONS

1. Cognitive impairments
2. Delayed expressive and receptive language skills
3. Failure to achieve major developmental milestones
4. Head circumference above or below normal range
5. Possible delayed growth
6. Possible abnormal muscle tone
7. Possible dysmorphic features
8. Delayed gross and fine motor development

COMPLICATIONS

1. Cerebral palsy
2. Seizure disorder
3. Behavioral and/or psychiatric problems
4. Communication deficits
5. Constipation (caused by decreased intestinal motility secondary to anticonvulsant medications, insufficient intake of fiber and fluids)
6. Associated congenital anomalies such as esophageal malformation, small bowel obstruction, and cardiac defects
7. Thyroid dysfunction
8. Sensory impairments
9. Orthopedic problems such as foot deformities, scoliosis
10. Feeding difficulties

LABORATORY AND DIAGNOSTIC TESTS

1. Cognitive and developmental assessment tests, including the following:
   a. Stanford-Binet IV for individuals ages 2 years to 23 years—used to assess mild retardation.
   b. Wechsler Preschool and Primary Scale of Intelligence—Revised (WPPSI-R) for children ages 3 years to 7 years, 3 months; contains 12 subscales measuring verbal and performance domains.
   c. Wechsler Intelligence Scale for Children—Third Edition (WISC-III) for children ages 6 years to 16 years, 11 months; contains 12 subscales that yield three IQ scores: verbal IQ, performance IQ, and full-scale IQ.
   d. Wechsler Adult Intelligence Scale—Revised (WAIS-R) for youth and adults ages 16 years to 74 years, 11months; composed of Verbal and Performances Scales containing 11 subscales.
   e. Cognitive Assessment System for children ages 5 years to 17 years.
   f. Kaufman Assessment Battery for Children (K-ABC) for children ages 2.5 years to 12.5 years.
   g. Bayley Scales of Infant Development for infants ages 2 months to 36 months; composed of three scales: Mental scale, Motor scale, and Behavior Rating scale.

    h. Leiter International Performance Scale—Revised (Leiter-R) for nonverbal individuals ages 2 years to 21 years—to assess intelligence.

    i. Universal Nonverbal Intelligence Test (UNIT) for children ages 5 years to 17 years, 11 months.

    j. Differential Ability Scales (DAS), composed of a battery of tests that can be used with three age groups: lower preschool (2.5 years to 3 years, 5 months); upper preschool (3.5 years to 5 years, 11 months) and school-age (6 years to 17 years, 11 months)—measures cognition and achievement; can be used with children ages 3.5 years and older who have significant delays.

    k. McCarthy Scales—used with children ages 2.5 years to 8.5 years who have learning problems; composed of 6 scales (Verbal, Perceptual-Performance, Quantitative, Memory, Motor, General Cognitive).

2. Measurements of adaptive behaviors

    a. Vineland Adaptive Behavior Scales for children from birth to 19 years—used to assess social competence in children and youth with and without disabilities; three forms available: Survey Form, Expanded Form, Classroom Edition.

    b. Adaptive Behavior Assessment System for children 5 years and older, adults.

    c. American Association of Mental Retardation (AAMR) Adaptive Behavior Scales (ABS) for children ages 3 years to 21 years—measures adaptive and survival skills; two versions exist: School and Community (ABS-S:2), Residential and Community (ABS-RC:2).

3. Other laboratory and diagnostic tests (see Table 44-1)

MEDICAL MANAGEMENT

Medical management will be highly dependent on the health care needs of the child or youth and the specific diagnosis associated with the child or youth's intellectual disability. The goal of medical care is to promote the child's or youth's optimal health status and prevent complications and secondary conditions by providing primary and specialty health care. Another important goal of care is to ensure that the child or youth and

TABLE 44-1
Hypotheses and Strategies for Assessing Etiologic Risk Factors

Hypothesis	Possible Evaluation Strategies
Prenatal Onset	
Chromosomal disorder	Extended physical examination Referral to clinical geneticist Chromosomal and DNA analysis
Syndrome disorder	Extended family history and examination of relatives Extended physical examination Referral to clinical geneticist
Inborn error of metabolism	Newborn screening using tandem mass spectrometry Analysis of amino acids in blood, urine, and/or cerebrospinal fluid Analysis of organic acids in urine Measurement of blood levels of lactate, pyruvate, very long chain fatty acids, free and total carnitine, and acylcarnitines Measurement of arterial ammonia and gases Assays of specific enzymes in cultured skin fibroblasts Biopsies of specific tissue for light and electron microscopy and biochemical analysis
Cerebral dysgenesis	Neuroimaging (computed tomography or magnetic resonance imaging)
Social, behavioral, and environmental risk factors	Intrauterine and postnatal growth assessment Placental pathologic analysis Detailed social history of parents Medical history and examination of mother

Continued

TABLE 44-1
Hypotheses and Strategies for Assessing Etiologic Risk Factors—cont'd

Hypothesis	Possible Evaluation Strategies
	Toxicologic screening of mother at prenatal visits and of child at birth
	Referral to clinical geneticist
Perinatal Onset	
Intrapartum and neonatal disorders	Review of maternal records (prenatal care, labor, and delivery)
	Review of birth and neonatal records
Postnatal Onset	
Head injury	Detailed medical history
	Skull radiography and neuroimaging
Brain infection	Detailed medical history
	Cerebrospinal fluid analysis
Demyelinating disorders	Neuroimaging
	Cerebrospinal fluid analysis
Degenerative disorders	Neuroimaging
	Specific DNA studies for genetic disorders
	Assays of specific enzymes in blood or cultured skin fibroblasts
	Biopsies of specific tissue for light and electron microscopy and biochemical analysis
	Referral to clinical geneticist or neurologist
Seizure disorders	Electroencephalography
	Referral to clinical neurologist
Toxic-metabolic disorders	See "Inborn error of metabolism" in Prenatal Onset category of table
	Toxicologic studies

TABLE 44-1
Hypotheses and Strategies for Assessing Etiologic Risk Factors—cont'd

Hypothesis	Possible Evaluation Strategies
Malnutrition	Lead and heavy metal assays
	Body measurements
	Detailed nutritional history
Environmental and social disadvantage	Detailed social history
	History of abuse or neglect
	Psychologic evaluation
	Observation in new environment
Educational inadequacy	Early referral and intervention records
	Review of educational records

From American Association on Mental Retardation: *Mental retardation: definition, classification, and systems of supports,* ed 10, Washington, DC, 2002, The Association.

primary caretakers receive the instruction needed for the development of self-care skills to manage health, personal, and disability needs on a daily and long-term basis. As the section on complications and secondary conditions demonstrates, the child or youth may have a number of secondary conditions and diagnoses that significantly affect their overall health status, such as seizure disorders, cardiac problems, and psychiatric problems. Given the array of health needs, some of the following medications may be prescribed for a child or youth with intellectual disability:

a. Psychotropic medications (e.g., thioridazine [Mellaril], haloperidol [Haldol]) for youth with self-injurious behaviors

b. Psychostimulants for youth who demonstrate attention-deficit/hyperactivity disorder (e.g., methylphenidate [Ritalin])

c. Antidepressants (e.g., fluoxetine [Prozac])

d. Medications for aggressive behaviors (e.g., carbamazepine [Tegretol])

For medical management to be effective, it must be coordinated with the interdisciplinary team of professionals who use a framework of care based on the principles of being coordinated, culturally sensitive, comprehensive, family-centered, asset-oriented, and community-based.

NURSING ASSESSMENT

The assessment process is comprehensive in scope and based on the dimensions of biophysical, psychosocial, behavioral, and educational needs. Assessment consists of comprehensive evaluation of deficits and strengths related to the following adaptive skills: communication, self-care, social interactions, use of community resources, self-direction, maintenance of health and safety, functional academics, development of leisure and recreational skills, and work. Assessment considers the influence of the child's cultural and linguistic background, interests, and preferences.

Physical assessment includes measurement of growth (height and weight identified on growth charts) and evaluation for current infections, current status of congenital problems, thyroid functioning, dental care, auditory and visual acuity, nutritional and feeding problems, and orthopedic problems. Physical assessment also involves monitoring for secondary conditions associated with specific diagnoses, such as monitoring for hypothyroidism and depression in those with Down syndrome (for information on Down syndrome, see Chapter 21).

NURSING DIAGNOSES

- Self-care deficit, Bathing/hygiene
- Self-care deficit, Dressing/grooming
- Self-care deficit, Feeding
- Self-care deficit, Toileting
- Therapeutic regimen management, Ineffective
- Communication, Impaired verbal
- Nutrition: less than body requirements, Imbalanced
- Grieving, Anticipatory
- Family processes, Interrupted
- Bowel incontinence
- Urinary elimination, Impaired
- Caregiver role strain

NURSING INTERVENTIONS
Infants, Toddlers, and Preschoolers

1. Refer to early intervention program for development of individualized family service plan (IFSP) that is family centered, culturally sensitive, and developmental appropriate (infants from birth to 3 years) or, if child, to community service coordinator/individualized education plan (IEP) coordinator (see Appendix G) providing opportunities for developmental learning (older than 3 years of age) (Appendix B).
   a. Fine motor development
   b. Gross motor development
   c. Sensory development
   d. Cognitive development
   e. Language development
   f. Psychosocial development
   g. Moral and faith development
2. Refer family to family resource centers and parent information centers that serve parents of children from birth to age 3 who are enrolled in early intervention programs to assist with family support needs, respite care, and sibling needs.
3. Collaborate with other professionals and disability specialists to formulate interdisciplinary plan of care that incorporates lifespan approach with periodic evaluations and assessments of current needs.
4. Serve as health care resource and consultant to child's disability service coordinator or care manager to ensure child receives comprehensive, accessible, community-based health care provided in inclusive settings.
5. Assist family in obtaining access to care services such as assistive technology, health insurance coverage, dental care, therapy services, income assistance, employment training, advocacy services, and job placement.
6. Refer to other sections in text for specific plans of care for associated special health care needs and health problems.
7. Families are educated about their children's rights and protections and are supported/encouraged to adovcate on behalf of their children.

8. See the Discharge Planning and Home Care section in this chapter for long-term care.
9. Refer to Box 44-3 for support areas and representative support activities for nursing care needs of children and their families.

School-Aged Children

1. Collaborate with other professionals and disability specialists to formulate interdisciplinary plan of care that incorporates life-span approach with periodic evaluations and assessments of current needs.
2. Encourage family with child-rearing practices that support child's acquisition of skills related to communication skills, personal care, social interactions, household tasks, and health care self care.
3. Collaborate with members of the special education team in IEP development on identifying health-related needs that affect academic performance and adaptive functioning and to ensure that the child's educational program is provided in an inclusive enrivonment.
4. Collaborate with disability service coordinator or case manager to ensure that ongoing health-related needs associated with long-term disability management and primary care needs are addressed and that health care is community-based, appropriate, accessible, comprehensive, and provided in inclusive settings.
5. Assist family in obtaining access to care services such as health insurance coverage, dental care, therapy services, after-school programs, recreational programs, advocacy services, and social skills and mobility training.
6. Parents are encouraged to learn and advocate for their children's rights and protections and to foster the development of their children's advocacy.
7. Refer parents to family support services, such as parent-to-parent support to assist them in coping with the needs of their children with an intellectual disability and challenges of living with a child with an intellectual disability.
8. Refer to the Discharge Planning and Home Care section in this chapter.

BOX 44-3
Support Areas and Representative Support Activities

Human Development Activities

- Providing physical development opportunities related to eye-hand coordination, fine motor skills, and gross motor activities
- Providing cognitive development opportunities related to coordinating sensory experiences, representing the world with words and images, reasoning logically about concrete events, and reasoning in more realistic and logical ways
- Providing social-emotional developmental activities related to trust, autonomy, initiative, mastery, and identity

Teaching and Education Activities

- Interacting with trainers or teachers and fellow trainees or students
- Participating in training or educational decisions
- Learning and using problems-solving strategies
- Operating technology for learning
- Accessing training or educational settings
- Learning and using functional academics (e.g., reading signs, counting change)
- Learning and using health and physical education skills
- Learning and using self-determination skills
- Receiving transitional services

Home Living Activities

- Using the restroom and/or toilet
- Laundering and taking care of clothes
- Preparing and eating food
- Housekeeping and cleaning
- Dressing
- Bathing and taking care of personal hygiene and grooming needs
- Operating home appliances and technology
- Participating in leisure activities within the home

Community Living Activities

- Using transportation
- Participating in recreation or leisure activities in the community
- Using services in the community
- Going to visit friends and family

Continued

BOX 44-3

Support Areas and Representative Support Activities—cont'd

- Participating in preferred community activities (e.g., church, volunteer work)
- Shopping and purchasing goods

Employment Activities

- Accessing or receiving job or task accommodations
- Learning and using specific job skills
- Interacting with coworkers
- Interacting with supervisors or coaches
- Completing work-related tasks with acceptable speed and quality
- Changing job assignments
- Accessing and obtaining crisis intervention and assistance
- Accessing employee assistance services

Health and Safety Activities

- Accessing and obtaining therapy services
- Taking medications
- Avoiding health and safety hazards
- Receiving home health care
- Ambulating and moving about
- Communicating with health-care providers
- Accessing emergency services
- Maintaining a nutritious diet
- Maintaining physical health
- Maintaining mental health and emotional well-being
- Following rules and laws
- Receiving respiratory care, feeding, skin care, seizure management, ostomy care, and other services for exceptional medical needs

Behavioral Activities

- Learning specific skills or behaviors
- Learning or making appropriate decisions
- Accessing and obtaining mental health treatments
- Making choices and taking initiatives
- Incorporating personal preferences into daily activities
- Learning or using self-management strategies
- Controlling anger and aggression
- Increasing adaptive skills and behaviors

BOX 44-3
Support Areas and Representative Support Activities—cont'd

Social Activities
- Socializing within the family
- Participating in recreation or leisure activities
- Making appropriate sexuality decisions
- Socializing outside the family
- Making and keeping friends
- Associating and dissociating from people
- Communicating with others about personal needs
- Using appropriate social skills
- Engaging in loving and intimate relationships
- Offering assistance and assisting others

Protection and Advocacy Activities
- Advocating for self and others
- Managing money and personal finances
- Protecting self from exploitation
- Exercising legal rights and responsibilities
- Belonging to and participating in self-advocacy or support organizations
- Obtaining legal services
- Making suitable choices and decisions
- Using banks and cashing checks

From American Association on Mental Retardation: *Mental retardation: definition, classification, and systems of supports*, ed 10, Washington, DC, 2002, The Association.

9. Refer to Box 44-3 for support areas and representative support activities for nursing care needs of school-aged children and their families.

Adolescents
1. Collaborate with other professionals and disability specialists to formulate interdisciplinary plan of care that incorporates life-span approach with periodic evaluations and assessments of current needs.
2. Refer to other sections in text for special health care needs and health problems.
3. Collaborate with members of the IEP team in IEP transition planning to identify health-related needs that affect academic performance and adaptive functioning,

acquisition of community living skills, access to sex education, and work-based instruction and on-the-job training; and promote inclusive approaches in the IEP.

4. Encourage family with child-rearing practices that support child's acquisition of skills related to communication skills, personal care, sexuality, social interactions, and household tasks (remember, the child will have a number of options as to what his or her life goals are).

5. Coordinate with health care transition specialist to ensure that health insurance coverage continues when pediatric eligibility terminates, to transfer individual from pediatric to adult health care specialty and primary care professionals, and to ensure learning of health self-care skills.

6. Collaborate with disability service coordinator or case manager to ensure that ongoing health-related needs associated with long-term disability management and primary care needs are addressed.

7. Assist youth and family with transition access to care services such as health insurance coverage, dental care, therapy services, postsecondary training and education, employment training and placement, income assistance, rehabilitation services, recreational and leisure services, social and advocacy groups, and community living and mobility training (use of transportation).

8. Refer to family support services to assist family members in "letting go" of their adolescent in transition and to support him or her during the process.

9. Youth are encouraged to participate as fully as possible in decision making affecting their lives, and realize that they are fully informed of their legal rights and protections.

10. Refer to the Discharge Planning and Home Care section in this chapter.

11. Refer to Box 44-3 for support areas and representative support activities for nursing care needs of youth and young adults.

🏠 Discharge Planning and Home Care

1. Refer child and family to agencies and professionals who can provide specialized health care services related to well-child

and well-adolescent care and dental care and hygiene; health care provided must be appropriate to needs, community-based, accessible, and comprehensive.

2. Refer family to community resources for genetic counseling, financial assistance, adaptive equipment supply, and family support services.
3. Collaborate with families as needed in developing and implementing behavior treatment plan.
4. Facilitate learning of appropriate social, community, communication, community safety, healthy sexuality and stranger avoidance skills, and development of peer relationships and leisure and recreational interests.
5. Facilitate child's inclusion into early intervention and educational programs, recreational programs, and community settings.
6. Coordinate services with members of infant, child, or youth's interdisciplinary team in early intervention (IFSP) or educational (IEP) settings. Refer to Appendix G.
7. Ensure that if the appointment of guardian is necessary, the individual is fully informed about the child or youth's health-related needs.
8. Ensure that children and youth with intellectual disabilities participate in decision making as fully as possible and are informed of their rights and protections.

CLIENT OUTCOMES

1. Child or youth and family will express overall satisfaction as measured by quality-of-life indicators.
2. Family and child or youth will cope with challenges of living with disability.
3. Family will be adept in accessing community resources.
4. Child or youth will demonstrate autonomy, self-determination, and self-advocacy behaviors.
5. Youth will graduate from high school or obtain a high school certificate.
6. Youth will have acquired school-based work experience as precursor for adult employment.

7. Child or youth will have participated in inclusive school and community-based activities.
8. Child or youth will have age-appropriate social relationships with peers with and without disabilities.
9. Youth will have access to sex education enabling healthy sexuality, responsible sexual expression, and protection from sexual exploitation and abuse.

REFERENCES

American Association on Mental Retardation, The ARC: *Mental retardation: definition, classification, and systems of supports*, ed 10, Washington, DC, 2002, The Association.

American Association on Mental Retardation, The ARC: *Definition of mental retardation* (website): www.aamr.org/Policies/pdf/definitionofMR.pdf. Accessed July 2, 2006.

American Association on Mental Retardation, The ARC: *Frequently asked questions about mental retardation* (website): www.aamr.org/Policies/pdf/Whaismr.pdf. Accessed July 2, 2006.

American Association on Mental Retardation, The ARC: *Advocacy* (website): www.aamr.org/Policies/pos_ advocacy.shtml. Accessed July 2, 2006.

American Association on Mental Retardation, The ARC: *Early intervention* (website): www.aamr.org/Policies/pos_early_intervention.shtml. Accessed July 2, 2006.

American Association on Mental Retardation, The ARC: *Family support* (website): www.aamr.org/Policies/pos_fam_ support.shtml. Accessed July 2, 2006.

American Association on Mental Retardation, The ARC: *Guardianship* (website): www.aamr.org/Policies/pos_guardianship.shtml. Accessed July 2, 2006.

American Association on Mental Retardation, The ARC: *Health Care* (website): www.aamr.org/Policies/pos_healthcare.shtml. Accessed July 2, 2006.

American Association on Mental Retardation, The ARC: *Inclusion* (website): www.aamr.org/Policies/pos_inclusion.shtml. Accessed July 2, 2006.

American Association on Mental Retardation, The ARC: *Education* (website): www.aamr.org/Policies/pos_education.shtml. Accessed July 2, 2006.

American Association on Mental Retardation, The ARC: *Self determination* (website): www.aamr.org/Policies/pos_self-determination.shtml. Accessed July 2, 2006.

American Association on Mental Retardation, The ARC: *Sexuality* (website): www.aamr.org/Policies/pos_sexuality.shtml. Accessed July 2, 2006.

American Psychiatric Association: *Diagnostic and statistical manual of mental disorders*, ed 4, text revision (DSM-IV-TR), Washington, DC, 2000, The Association.

Batshaw M: *Children with disabilities*, Baltimore, 1994, Paul H. Brookes.

Batshaw M: Mental retardation, *Pediatr Clin North Am* 40(3):507, 1993.

Betz C: Nurse's role in promoting health transitions for adolescents and young adults with developmental disabilities, *Nurs Clin North Am* 18:1, 2003.

Centers for Disease Control and Prevention: Economic costs associated with mental retardation, cerebral palsy, hearing loss, and vision impairment—United States, *MMWR Weekly* (serial online): www.cdc.gov/mmwr/preview/mmwrhtml/mm5303a4.htm. Accessed July 2, 2006.

Centers for Disease Control, National Center on Birth Defects and Developmental Disabilities: *Mental retardation* (website): www.cdc.gov/ncbddd/dd/ddmr.htm. Accessed February 22, 2006.

National Dissemination Center for Children with Disabilities: *Mental retardation* (website): www.nichcy.org/pubs/factshe/fs8txt.htm. Accessed February 22, 2006.

45

Iron Deficiency Anemia

PATHOPHYSIOLOGY

Iron deficiency anemia is the most common anemia affecting children in North America. The full-term infant born of a well-nourished, nonanemic mother has sufficient iron stores until the birth weight is doubled, generally at 4 to 6 months. Iron deficiency anemia is generally not evident until 9 months of age. After that, iron must be available from the diet to meet the child's nutritional needs. If dietary iron intake is insufficient, iron deficiency anemia results. Most often, insufficient dietary iron intake results from inappropriately early introduction of solid foods (before age 4 to 6 months), discontinuation of iron-fortified infant formula or breast milk before age 1 year, and excessive consumption of cow's milk to the exclusion of iron-rich solids in the toddler. Also, the preterm infant, the infant with significant perinatal blood loss, and the infant born to a poorly nourished, iron-deficient mother may have inadequate iron stores. Such an infant would be at a significantly higher risk for iron deficiency anemia before age 6 months. Maternal iron deficiency may cause low birth weight and preterm delivery.

Iron deficiency anemia may also result from chronic blood loss. In the infant, this may be due to chronic intestinal bleeding caused by the heat-labile protein in cow's milk. In children of all ages, the loss of as little as 1 to 7 ml of blood daily through the gastrointestinal tract may lead to iron deficiency anemia. Other causes of iron deficiency anemia include nutritional deficiencies such as folate (vitamin B_{12}) deficiency, sickle cell anemia, thalassemia major, infections, and chronic inflammation. In teenaged girls, iron deficiency anemia may also be due to excessive menstrual flow.

INCIDENCE

1. Of infants 12 to 36 months of age, 3% have iron deficiency anemia.
2. Of infants 12 to 36 months of age, 9% are iron deficient.
3. Incidence of iron deficiency and iron deficiency anemia among adolescent girls is 11% to 17%.
4. The age range of peak incidence for iron deficiency anemia is 12 to 18 months.
5. Prevalence rates of iron deficiency are higher among children living at or below the poverty level and among African-American and Mexican-American children.
6. Of infants fed only non–iron-fortified formula or cow's milk, 20% to 40% are at higher risk for iron deficiency by age 9 to 12 months.
7. Of breast-fed infants, 15% to 25% are at higher risk for iron deficiency by age 9 to 12 months.
8. The leading cause of anemia in infants and children in the United States is iron deficiency. There was a significant increase in iron deficiency anemia in the United States in the 1990s.
9. Iron deficiency is the most common nutritional deficiency in the world. It is estimated that 20% to 25% of infants worlwide are affected by iron deficiency anemia.

CLINICAL MANIFESTATIONS

1. Conjunctival pallor (hemoglobin [Hb] 6 to 10 g/dl)
2. Palmar crease pallor (Hb below 8 g/dl)
3. Irritability and anorexia (Hb 5 g/dl or below)
4. Tachycardia, systolic murmur
5. Pica
6. Lethargy, increased need for sleep
7. Lack of interest in toys or play activities

COMPLICATIONS

1. Growth and development: developmental delays (birth to 5 years of age), decreased attention span, decreased social

interactions, decreased performance on developmental tests

2. Muskuloskeletal: poor muscular development (long-term)
3. Gastrointestinal: contribution to lead poisoning (decreased iron enables gastrointestinal tract to absorb heavy metals more easily)
4. Nervous system: increased incidence of cerebral vascular accident in infants and children
5. Hearing: decreased ability to process information

LABORATORY AND DIAGNOSTIC TESTS

Refer to Appendix F for normal values and/or ranges of laboratory and diagnostic tests.

No single test is acceptable for detecting or diagnosing iron deficiency.

1. Hb concentration (before treatment)—decreased (one of most common tests used); indicates concentration of iron-containing protein Hb in circulating red blood cells
2. Hematocrit—decreased (one of most common tests used); indicates proportion of whole blood occupied by red blood cells
3. Mean corpuscular volume and mean corpuscular hemoglobin concentration—decreased, yielding microcytic, hypochromic anemia or small, pale red blood cells
4. Red blood cell distribution width (cutoff: 14%)
5. Erythrocyte protoporphyrin concentration—1 to 2 years: 80 mcg/dl of red blood cells
6. Transferrin saturation—younger than 6 months: 15 mcg/L or less
7. Serum ferritin concentration—less than 16%
8. Reticulocyte count (during treatment)—increase within 3 to 5 days of initiating iron therapy indicates positive therapeutic response
9. Hb concentration (with treatment)—return to normal value within 4 to 8 weeks indicates adequate iron and nutritional support

MEDICAL MANAGEMENT

Treatment efforts are directed toward prevention and intervention. Prevention includes encouraging parents to feed the infant only breast milk until the infant is between 4 to 6 months of age, to eat foods that are iron-rich, and to take iron-fortified prenatal vitamins (supplementation with approximately 1 mg/kg of iron per day). Iron supplementation should begin when infants are switched to regular milk. Therapy to treat iron deficiency anemia consists of a medication regimen.

1. By 6 months of age, breast-fed infants should receive 1 mg/kg of iron drops per day.
2. For breast-fed infants who were born prematurely or had low birth weight, 2 to 4 mg/kg (maximum of 15 mg) of iron drops daily is recommended starting at 1 month and continuing until 12 months of age.
3. Up to 12 months of age, only breast milk or iron-fortified infant formula should be used for liquid portion of nutrients.
4. Between 1 and 5 years of age, children should not consume more than 24 ounces of soy, goat's, or cow's milk daily.
5. Between 4 and 6 months of age, infants should have two or more daily servings of iron-fortified cereal.
6. By 6 months of age, child should have daily feeding of foods rich in vitamin C to improve iron absorption.

Iron is administered by mouth. All iron forms are equally effective (ferrous sulfate, ferrous fumarate, ferrous succinate, ferrous gluconate). Vitamin C must be administered simultaneously with iron (ascorbic acid increases iron absorption). Iron is best absorbed when taken 1 hour before a meal. Iron therapy should continue for a minimum of 6 weeks after the anemia is corrected to replenish iron stores. Injectable iron is seldom used unless small bowel malabsorption disease is present.

Adolescent girls should be encouraged to eat foods rich in iron. Other prevention strategies include comprehensive screening for, diagnosis of, and treatment of iron deficiency.

NURSING ASSESSMENT

1. See the Cardiovascular Assessment section in Appendix A.
2. Assess child's response to iron therapy.

3. Assess child's activity level.
4. Assess child's developmental level (see Appendix B).

NURSING DIAGNOSES

- Activity intolerance
- Nutrition: less than body requirements, Imbalanced
- Fatigue
- Growth and development, Delayed
- Therapeutic regimen management, Ineffective

NURSING INTERVENTIONS

1. Encourage rest periods and naps.
2. Encourage developmentally appropriate play activities as tolerated.
3. Monitor child's therapeutic and untoward effects from iron therapy.
   a. Side effects (e.g., tooth discoloration) are infrequent with oral therapy.
   b. Instruct about measures to prevent tooth discoloration.
      i. Take iron with fluids, preferably orange juice.
      ii. Rinse mouth after taking medication.
   c. Encourage increased fiber and water intake to minimize constipating effects of iron.
   d. For severe iron-induced constipation, consider lowering iron dose but extending length of treatment.
4. Instruct parents about appropriate nutritional intake (see Medical Management section in this chapter).
   a. Reduce child's milk intake.
   b. Increase intake of meat and appropriate protein substitutes.
   c. Encourage inclusion of whole grains and green leafy vegetables in diet.
5. Gather information about dietary history and eating behaviors.
   a. Assess for factors contributing to nutritional deficiency—psychosocial, behavioral, and nutritional.

  b. Plan with parents acceptable approach toward dietary habits.
  c. Refer to nutritionist for intensive evaluation and treatment.
6. Encourage breast-feeding, because breast milk iron is well absorbed.
7. Make referrals to physical and occupational therapy as needed.
8. Make referrals to psychologist or mental health specialist for cognitive and developmental testing as needed.

🏠 Discharge Planning and Home Care

1. Instruct about administering iron therapy (see item 2 under Nursing Interventions).
2. Instruct about meal planning and nutritional intake (see item 4 under Nursing Interventions).
3. Instruct about need for follow-up screenings and treatment approaches.
4. Instruct about outpatient physical and occupational therapy as needed.
5. Instruct about the need for cognitive and developmental follow-up as needed.

CLIENT OUTCOMES

1. Child's skin color will improve.
2. Child's pattern of growth will improve (as indicated on growth chart).
3. Child's activity level will be appropriate for age.
4. Parents will demonstrate understanding of home treatment regimen (i.e., medication administration, diet with appropriate iron-rich foods).

REFERENCES

Baptist EC, Castillo SF: Cow's milk–induced iron deficiency anemia as a cause of childhood stroke, *Clin Pediatr* (Phila) 41(7):533, 2002.

Centers for Disease Control and Prevention: Iron deficiency—United States, 1999–2000, *JAMA* 288(17):2114, 2002.

Eden AN: The prevention of toddler iron deficiency, *Arch Pediatr Adolesc Med* 156(5):519, 2002.

Halterman JS et al: Iron deficiency and cognitive achievement among school-aged children and adolescents in the United States, *Pediatrics* 107(6):1381, 2001.

Lozoff B et al: Behavioral and developmental effects of preventing iron-deficiency anemia in healthy full-term infants, *Pediatrics* 112(4):846, 2003.

Saloojee H, Pettifor JM: Iron deficiency and impaired child development, *BMJ* 323(7326):1377, 2001.

46

❖

Juvenile Rheumatoid Arthritis

PATHOPHYSIOLOGY

Juvenile rheumatoid arthritis (JRA) is a chronic autoimmune disease that begins before 16 years of age. It is the most common rheumatic disease in children and is a leading cause of short- and long-term disability. It is also a major cause of eye disease leading to blindness. Although its exact etiology is unknown, it is immune-mediated, with abnormal cytokine production in the inflammatory pathway (increased tumor necrosis factor, interleukin-1 and interleukin-6). There are also genetic predispositions, as well as environmental triggers such as infection, trauma, or stress. JRA causes chronic inflammation of the synovium with joint effusion, which can result in eventual erosion and destruction of the articular cartilage. If the process persists long enough, adhesions between the joint surfaces and ankylosis of the joints develop.

The diagnosis is based on the following criteria defined by the American College of Rheumatology:

1. The age at onset must be less than 16 years.
2. Objective evidence of arthritis must be present (defined as swelling or effusion, or presence of two or more of the following: limitation of range of motion, tenderness or pain on motion, and increased heat) in one or more joints.
3. The duration of the disease is 6 weeks or longer.
4. The onset type is defined by the type of disease in the first 6 months:
   a. Polyarthritis: five or more inflamed joints

   b. Oligoarthritis (pauciarticular disease): fewer than five inflamed joints
   c. Systemic-onset: arthritis with characteristic fever
5. Other forms of juvenile arthritis must be excluded.
   Common characteristics of JRA include morning stiffness, joint pain, limping gait, fatigue, anorexia, anemia, and weight loss.

INCIDENCE

1. JRA is twice as common in girls.
2. The incidence of JRA varies from 2 to 20 in 100,000 per year. Prevalence is about 1 per 1000 children.
3. Age ranges of peak incidence are 1 to 3 years and 8 to 11 years.
4. Subtype frequencies are systemic, 10%; polyarticular, 30%; and pauciarticular, 60%.
5. Overall, 0.8% of JRA appears in sibling pairs.
6. JRA is half as common in African Americans.

CLINICAL MANIFESTATIONS
Systemic JRA

1. Systemic JRA is characterized by persistent, intermittent (quotidian) fever: daily or twice-daily temperature elevations to 102.2° F (39° C) or higher, with rapid return to normal temperature between fever spikes. The fever is usually present in the late afternoon to evening. It almost always occurs with the rheumatoid rash.
2. The rheumatoid rash is described as salmon-pink erythematous macules on the trunk and extremities.
   The rash is migratory and in 5% of cases is reported to be pruritic.
3. Arthritis may not occur until weeks or months after the onset of the symptoms.
4. It affects 10% of all JRA patients, with peak onset from 1 to 5 years of age.
5. The arthritis pattern may be pauciarticular (one to four joints affected) or polyarticular (five or more joints affected). Those children with polyarthritis have a tendency for erosions and a poorer prognosis.

6. Extraarticular symptoms are present, including hepatosplenomegaly, lymphadenopathy, pericarditis, and pleuritis.

Polyarticular JRA

1. Arthritis is present in five or more joints in the first 6 months of disease.
2. Peak age of onset is between ages 1 and 4 years, and between 6 and 12 years.
3. Systemic manifestations include low-grade fever, fatigue, anorexia, growth failure, and weight loss.
4. Morning stiffness, gelling or stiffness after inactivity, joint pain, and sluggishness with movement are characteristic.
5. Joint involvement is generally symmetric and usually involves the large joints of the knees, the wrists, the elbows, and the ankles. The small joints of the hands and the feet may also be affected.
6. The cervical spine and the temporomandibular joints are often involved.
7. If the temporomandibular joint is involved, impaired biting, shortness of the mandible, and micrognathia may result.
8. Those with onset in late childhood or adolescence who are rheumatoid factor–positive tend to have a more severe disease course than those who are rheumatoid factor–negative.
9. Rheumatoid nodules occur in 5% to 10% of children with JRA, but are most often seen in those with polyarticular disease who are rheumatoid factor–positive. The typical rheumatoid nodule is firm, movable, and nontender. They usually occur below the elbow or at other pressure points.

Pauciarticular JRA

1. Arthritis is present in one to four joints in the first 6 months of disease.
2. Pauciarticular-onset JRA primarily affects girls, aged 2 to 4 years.
3. The joints most commonly affected are the knees and the ankles.

4. The affected joints are swollen and warm, but usually not painful or tender.
5. Uveitis (15% to 20% of cases) is insidious and often asymptomatic.
6. Disease course is variable. After the first 6 months, 5% to 10% develop a polyarticular disease course.

COMPLICATIONS

1. Uveitis is intraocular inflammation of the iris and the ciliary body, found in 15% to 20% of children with pauciarticular-onset JRA, in 5% of those with polyarticular-onset JRA, and rarely in children with systemic-onset JRA. At increased risk for development of uveitis are girls with pauciarticular-onset disease. Those with a positive antinuclear antibody are at even higher risk. The onset is usually insidious and asymptomatic; however, approximately half of children have some symptoms (pain, redness, headache, photophobia, change in vision) later in the disease course. If not diagnosed early, the disease can result in cataracts, glaucoma, visual loss, and blindness. If the disease is detected early, the prognosis is improved. In about half of all patients with uveitis, it occurs before the arthritis is diagnosed, at the time of diagnosis or soon after. In 70% to 80% of children, the uveitis is bilateral.
2. Flexion contractures
3. Growth disturbances, including leg length discrepancy and micrognathia
4. Valgus deformity, cervical spine ankylosis
5. Wrist fusion
6. Cardiopulmonary complications and other systemic complications
7. Severe anemia and malnutrition
8. Renal, bone marrow, gastrointestinal, and liver toxicity to drugs
9. Macrophage activation syndrome is a rare but severe complication of systemic JRA leading to severe morbidity and sometimes death. The syndrome is characterized by rapid development of fever, hepatosplenomegaly, lymphadenopathy, and liver failure with encephalopathy,

purpura, bruising, and mucosal bleeding. A bone marrow aspiration showing active phagocytosis of red cells and white cells by macrophages and histiocytes confirms the diagnosis.
10. Osteopenia and osteoporosis

LABORATORY AND DIAGNOSTIC TESTS

There are no laboratory tests that yield the juvenile rheumatoid arthritis diagnosis. Lab testing is more supportive than diagnostic.

1. Erythrocyte sedimentation rate and C-reactive protein level—may be increased with inflammation. These are occasionally helpful in measuring disease activity and monitoring response to antiinflammatory medications. However, these values are often normal in JRA and do not necessarily correlate with response to medications.
2. Rheumatoid factor—present in only 15% of children with JRA (primarily those with polyarticular disease)
3. Antinuclear antibodies—primarily seen in pauciarticular JRA (in 40% of cases); reflect increased risk for uveitis
4. Complete blood count—leukocytosis is common with active disease, and can be very high (30,000 to 50,000/mm^3 in those with systemic-onset JRA); polymorphonuclear leukocytes predominate. The platelet count may be high in severe disease activity.
5. Complement levels (C3)—often increased with disease activity, acting as an acute phase protein
6. Immunoglobulin levels—correlate with disease activity
7. Synovial fluid analysis (cell count and culture)—to rule out other conditions, especially infection
8. Urinalysis—mild proteinuria may accompany increased fever, or may be related to medication side effects
9. Imaging studies such as plain film radiography, computed tomography (CT), high-resolution ultrasonography, radionucleotide imaging, and magnetic resonance imaging (MRI) are helpful in diagnosing arthritis and monitoring disease progression. Findings may include soft tissue swelling, epiphyseal overgrowth, marginal erosions, narrowing of cartilaginous space, joint subluxation, and bony fusion.

Dual-energy x-ray absorptiometry (DEXA) scan measures bone mineral density in order to diagnose osteopenia or osteoporosis.

MEDICAL MANAGEMENT

Treatment goals for JRA are to control pain; reduce the inflammatory process; preserve range of motion, and increase muscle strength and function; manage systemic complications; facilitate normal nutrition and growth; promote independence in activities of daily living; and maintain the child or adolescent's self-esteem and self-image in the face of a chronic illness. Drug therapy is used to reduce inflammation. JRA is treated earlier and more aggressively to decrease disability. Physical and occupational therapy and a regular daily program of exercise are essential to promote mobility and function. Heat is used to relieve joint pain and stiffness. The treatment plan also includes frequent slit-lamp microscopy examinations by an ophthalmologist according to specified guidelines (Table 46-1).

TABLE 46-1
Slit-Lamp Examination Guidelines

Type of JRA	ANA Test	Age at Diagnosis	Recommended Frequency of Slit-Lamp Examination
Pauciarticular or polyarticular	Positive	<7 years	Every 3–4 months for 7 years; then yearly
Pauciarticular or polyarticular	Negative	<7 years of age	Every 6 months for 7 years; then yearly
Pauciarticular or polyarticular	—	?7 years of age	Every 6 months for 4 years; then yearly
Systemic	—	—	Yearly

Modified from American Academy of Pediatrics, Section on Rheumatology and Section on Ophthalmology: Guidelines for ophthalmologic examinations in children with juvenile rheumatoid arthritis, *Pediatrics* 92(2):295, 1993.
ANA, Antinuclear antibodies; *JRA,* juvenile rheumatoid arthritis.

1. Nonsteroidal antiinflammatory drugs (NSAIDs) are used to control inflammation, fever, and pain. Aspirin and salicylates are no longer used as the first-choice NSAIDs because of the association with Reye's syndrome during influenza or varicella infection and the availability of other NSAIDs. Naproxen, ibuprofen, tolmetin, piroxicam, indomethacin, meloxicam, and diclofenac are common NSAIDs used in JRA. To be effective antiinflammatories, NSAIDs must be taken on a routine basis. If adequate effectiveness is not achieved after 2 to 3 months, an alternative NSAID can be tried. Many children require a second-line medication in addition to an NSAID to control disease activity.

2. Methotrexate is the initial second-line medication for the treatment of JRA. Given orally once a week in small doses, it has been markedly effective in the treatment of arthritis in children. It is also given subcutaneously once a week for higher dosages or in children with poor absorption or inadequate response.

3. Glucocorticoid drugs: systemic glucocorticoids (daily oral or intravenous pulse steroids) are used for uncontrolled or life-threatening systemic JRA or polyarticular disease that has been unresponsive to other therapies. They are also used as a temporary measure until the second-line drug is effective. Intraarticular steroid injections (triamcinolone hexacetonide) are indicated for the management of pauciarticular JRA that has not responded to NSAIDs, and for the management of polyarticular disease in which one or several joints have not responded to antiinflammatory drugs. These joint injections are generally done under anesthesia or conscious sedation.

4. Biologic response modifiers such as tumor necrosis factor (TNF) inhibitors have demonstrated much promise in the treatment of JRA. Etanercept has been approved for pediatric use as a subcutaneous injection given twice per week. It has become standard therapy for JRA that has not responded well to methotrexate. Infliximab, which is given as an infusion, is also being used for JRA treatment. Before starting biologic response modifiers, a negative skin reaction

to purified protein derivative (PPD) should be documented. These drugs should not be given while the child has a serious infection.

5. Other biological response modifiers: Anakinra, an IL-1 receptor inhibitor, is used as a once daily subcutaneous injection in systemic-onset JRA. Thalidomide has also been recommended for treatment of systemic-onset JRA.

6. Slower-acting antirheumatic drugs or disease-modifying antirheumatic drugs can be added to the medical treatment program for children who have an inadequate response to the NSAID, methotrexate, and a TNF blocker. These include hydroxychloroquine, sulfasalazine, parenteral gold compounds, and penicillamine.

7. Intravenous immunoglobulin is sometimes used in severe, progressive systemic and polyarticular disease.

8. Cytotoxic and immunosuppressive drugs (azathioprine, cyclophosphamide, and cyclosporin) are used occasionally in children with JRA who have life-threatening complications, major steroid toxicity, or severe progressive, erosive disease. Cyclosporin has been found to be beneficial in treatment of the macrophage activation syndrome seen in systemic JRA.

9. Autologous stem cell transplantation is an experimental treatment that is being evaluated in a small number of children. It is very risky and is associated with a high death rate.

NURSING ASSESSMENT

1. See the Musculoskeletal Assessment section in Appendix A.
2. Assess for pain.
3. Assess ability to perform activities of daily living.
4. Assess growth and development.

NURSING DIAGNOSES

- Pain
- Mobility, Impaired physical
- Self-care deficit, Bathing/hygiene
- Self-care deficit, Dressing/grooming
- Self-care deficit, Feeding

- Social interaction, Impaired
- Family processes, Interrupted

NURSING INTERVENTIONS

1. Provide pain relief measures as necessary.
   a. Tub bath or shower for joint stiffness
   b. Heating pad or ice packs applied to affected areas
   c. Whirlpool bath, paraffin bath, or hot packs for pain and stiffness
   d. Footed pajamas or sleeping bag
   e. Heated water bed or electric blanket
   f. Crutches, walker, or other device to avoid full-weight bearing
2. Promote joint mobility, maintain strength, and prevent deformity of joints.
   a. Encourage compliance with physical therapy and occupational therapy exercises (range of motion and/or passive range of motion).
   b. Encourage participation in physical activity and exercise, e.g. swimming, creative dance, bicycle riding, or walking.
   c. Avoid excessive strain on affected joints.
   d. Instruct to avoid activities that place total body weight on affected non–weight-bearing joints (cartwheels, chin-ups, handstands, aerobics, contact sports, roller skating).
   e. Encourage use of splints to prevent flexion contractures.
   f. Encourage compliance with prone and active gluteal exercise with hip involvement.
   g. Provide cast with knee in severe flexion.
   h. Provide cervical collar for neck pain.
3. Collaborate with physical therapist and/or occupational therapist to devise methods that will promote independent functioning.
   a. Use splints as needed.
   b. Make modifications to utensils for easier grasp, and recommend adaptive devises.
   c. Select clothes that are convenient to put on (Velcro fasteners).
   d. Elevate toilet seat.

4. Monitor growth and development pattern.
   a. Educate family about side effects of corticosteroid therapy, and refer to dietitian as needed.
   b. Encourage age-appropriate activities that will conserve energy and promote development of perceptual skills and coordination.
5. Assist child with intervention strategies for common school problems.
   a. Instruct family to meet with school personnel to discuss child's diagnosis and make classroom modifications.
   b. Instruct child to change position or stretch every 20 minutes to prevent stiffness.
   c. Have child use "fat" pens or pencils, or felt-tip pens, for writing.
   d. Recommend extra set of schoolbooks to keep at home.
   e. Suggest use of computer for reports, tape recorder for note taking, and oral tests.
   f. Suggest allowance of extra time between classes.
   g. Recommend allowance of extra time for completion of assignments and tests.
   h. Encourage rest period in the middle of the day if child is experiencing fatigue.
   i. Plan schedule with less demanding subjects in the morning.
   j. Encourage participation in activities with other children.
   k. Recommend modifications to physical education program so that student can participate as tolerated.
   l. Assist family and school personnel in developing individualized education plan (IEP) addressing modifications of school activities and special needs.
   m. Refer adolescent to vocational rehabilitation to assist with career planning (eleventh and twelfth grades).
6. Provide education and support to child and family to maximize coping with a chronic and sometimes disabling disease.
   a. Encourage participation in support groups with other JRA-affected children and their families. Refer family to Arthritis Foundation and American Juvenile Arthritis

Organization (see Box 46-1). Provide information to family about camps for children with arthritis.

b. Assist family in identifying Internet websites that provide accurate and up-to-date information about JRA, such as www.arthritis.org for the Arthritis Foundation.

c. Monitor child's therapeutic response and adverse reactions to medications.

d. Prepare child preoperatively for procedures and surgeries as indicated, which may include the following:
   i. Arthrocentesis
   ii. Arthroscopy
   iii. Soft tissue surgery
   iv. Osteotomy
   v. Total knee or hip replacement

e. Provide emotional support to child and family as indicated during hospitalization.

f. Provide education and guidance to child and family regarding unconventional or unproven therapies.

g. Assist adolescent or young adult with transition to adult medical providers.

Discharge Planning and Home Care

1. Instruct child and family about follow-up appointments.
   a. Name and phone number of physician and appropriate health care team members
   b. Date, time, and purpose of follow-up appointments

2. Instruct child and family to observe response to medications and notify physician of adverse reactions.

3. Reinforce information given about JRA, and encourage compliance with treatment plan.

4. Monitor compliance with consultation referrals.

CLIENT OUTCOMES

1. Child will exhibit no signs or symptoms of discomfort and will be able to move with minimal discomfort.

2. Child will be able to perform activities of daily living and participate in age-appropriate activities with minimal fatigue.

3. Child and family will demonstrate understanding of home treatment plan, including medications and home exercise program.

BOX 46-1

Resources

- www.pedrheumonlinejournal.org. The *Pediatric Rheumatology Online Journal* is a refereed publication developed for the international pediatric rheumatology community.
- www.goldscout.com. This is the pediatric rheumatology webpage developed by Thomas Lehman, MD (pediatric rheumatologist).
- www.arthritis.org. This is the official website for the Arthritis Foundation. The address for the national office is Arthritis Foundation, 1330 Peachtree Street, Atlanta, GA 30309 (404-872-7100). The American Juvenile Arthritis Organization (AJAO) is a council of the Arthritis Foundation, available online at www.arthritis.org/communities/juvenile_arthritis/about_ajao.asp. The Arthritis Foundation publishes *Kids Get Arthritis Too,* which includes articles on current topics, research reviews, "Ask the Experts" and "Kids Ask Kids" question sections, professional and patient interviews, and news. It can be ordered online or by phone 1-800-933-0032.

REFERENCES

American Academy of Pediatrics, Section on Rheumatology and Section on Ophthalmology: Guidelines for ophthalmologic examinations in children with juvenile rheumatoid arthritis, *Pediatrics* 92(2):295, 1993.

Calmak A, Nalan B: Juvenile rheumatoid arthritis: physical therapy and rehabilitation, *South Med J* 98(2):212, 2005.

Cassidy JT et al: *Textbook of pediatric rheumatology,* ed 5, Philadelphia, 2005, WB Saunders.

Feldman DE et al: Factors associated with the use of complementary and alternative medicine in juvenile idiopathic arthritis, *Arthritis Rheum* 51(4):527, 2004.

Lehman TJA: It's not just growing pains: A guide to childhood muscle, bone and joint pain, rheumatic diseases, and the latest treatments, Oxford, 2004, Oxford Press.

Mason TG, Reed AM: Update in juvenile rheumatoid arthritis, *Arthritis Rheum* 53(5):796, 2005.

Miller-Hoover S: Juvenile idiopathic arthritis: why do I have to hurt so much? *J Infusion Nurs* 28(6):385, 2005.

47

❖

Kawasaki Disease

PATHOPHYSIOLOGY

Kawasaki disease is an acute, self-limited vasculitic syndrome affecting infants and young children. Kawasaki disease is distinguished by marked immune system activation that contributes to the injury of small- and medium-sized blood vessels, with a predilection for the coronary arteries. Also known as mucocutaneous lymph node syndrome, Kawasaki disease affects multiple body systems and can have life-threatening cardiovascular consequences, including thrombosis of coronary arteries, coronary artery aneurysms, and coronary stenosis. Researchers speculate that Kawasaki disease has an infectious cause; however, the specific etiology remains unknown. The disease occurs in three phases; acute febrile, subacute, and late or convalescent. Diagnosis, which is sometimes confusing, has been based on strict adherence to clinical criteria. However, a substantial subset of children present with illnesses that do not completely fulfill the diagnostic criteria and are associated with the coronary diseases similar to that of the typical Kawasaki disease. These cases are labeled "atypical Kawasaki disease." Initial treatment focuses on reducing the vascular inflammatory process. With early recognition and treatment, prognosis is excellent. The long-term prognosis for children with coronary artery abnormalities who survive the disease is unknown, but recent surveys suggest that the sequelae of Kawasaki disease are likely important causes of ischemic heart disease in young adults.

INCIDENCE

1. Of all children with diagnosed Kawasaki disease, 80% are 5 years of age or younger, with toddlers most commonly affected (50% are younger than 2 years of age).

2. In the United States the peak age for being diagnosed with Kawasaki disease is 18 months.

3. Adults, adolescents, and children less than 6 months of age are rarely affected.

4. Outbreaks of Kawasaki disease are more common in the late winter and early spring but can be seen at any time during the year.

5. Annual incidence in the United States is 5.6 per 100,000 individuals as compared to 67 per 100,000 individuals in Japan.

6. The incidence is higher in boys than in girls (1.5:1). Boys have a higher ratio of fatalities due to Kawasaki disease.

7. The disease occurs in all races but has a higher predilection for Japanese children, followed by Asian and Pacific Islanders, African Americans, Hispanics and, finally, is at its lowest incidence in whites.

8. Kawasaki disease occurs more often in twins and siblings than in the general population.

9. No evidence exists to suggest that Kawasaki disease is spread by person-to-person contact.

10. The increased rates of occurrence in family members suggest there may be a genetic predisposition to Kawasaki disease.

11. Of untreated children with Kawasaki disease, 15% to 20% develop coronary artery aneurysms.

12. Of those children treated with intravenous gamma globulin (IVIG) in the acute phase of the disease, fewer than 5% develop coronary artery abnormalities.

CLINICAL MANIFESTATIONS

Acute Febrile Phase (0 to 19 Days)

For Kawasaki disease to be diagnosed, the child must have a fever for 5 days and four of the following acute phase criteria:

1. Fever is abrupt in onset, typically high (39° to 40° C), spiking, and remittent. If left untreated, the fever may

persist for 11 days on the average. The fever is present in 95% of children with Kawasaki disease.

2. Bulbar conjunctivitis is seen in the first few days of the illness, occurring shortly after the first fever. It is usually painless and not associated with exudate or edema.

3. Oropharyngeal manifestations include changes in the mouth and lips including erythema, dryness, fissuring, peeling, cracking, and bleeding of the lips; a "strawberry tongue"; and diffuse erythema of the oropharyngeal mucosa (nonexudative and nonulcerative).

4. Extremity changes include swelling and induration of the hands and feet, erythema of the palms and soles, and painful extremities; often, children no longer bear weight. The skin becomes shiny and stretched in appearance.

5. Erythematous body rash usually appears within 5 days of fever and may take many forms. Most commonly the rash is a nonspecific, diffuse, maculopapular eruption. The rash is most extensive to the trunk but can involve the face and extremities. The rash in the perineal area is accentuated, and early desquamation may occur.

6. Cervical lymphadenopathy is the least common of the criteria; it is usually unilateral and located in the anterior cervical triangle. The enlarged node is usually greater than 1.5 cm in diameter, nonfluctuant, and nontender.

7. Cardiac abnormalities include myocarditis, arrhythmias, hyperdynamic precordium, tachycardia, gallop rhythm, depressed myocardial contractility, mitral regurgitation, and coronary artery abnormalities.

Subacute Phase (12 to 25 Days)

1. Arthritis frequently includes multiple joints, most commonly large weight-bearing joints

2. Decrease in fever

3. Thick desquamation of the extremities, starting at the tip of the digits and progressing proximally

4. Panvasculitis of coronary arteries and formation of aneurysms; inflammation and thrombosis may lead to stenosis or obstruction

Convalescent Phase (6 to 8 Weeks)

1. Subsidence of the signs of illness
2. Appearance of deep linear transverse grooves across the fingernails and toenails (Beau's lines), which may progress to complete shedding of the nails
3. Abnormal laboratory values begin returning to normal
4. Normalization of personality, irritability, appetite, and energy level

COMPLICATIONS

1. Cardiac: myocardial infarction (the most common cause of death in Kawasaki disease), coronary artery aneurysms, coronary thromboses, congestive heart failure
2. Gastrointestinal: hydrops of the gallbladder (resolves spontaneously)
3. Pulmonary: pleural effusion, pneumonitis, pulmonary nodules
4. Neurologic: facial nerve palsy, hearing loss

LABORATORY AND DIAGNOSTIC TESTS

Refer to Appendix D for normal values and/or ranges of laboratory and diagnostic tests.

There are no specific diagnostic tests for Kawasaki disease; however, several abnormalities have been identified.

1. Electrocardiogram (ECG)—to assess electrical conduction of the myocardium
   a. Flat, depressed ST segment
   b. Flat, inverted T wave
   c. Conduction disturbances
2. Echocardiogram—to assess cardiac enlargement, contractility of ventricles, and coronary aneurysms
3. Complete blood count—to assess for suggestive indices of Kawasaki disease
   a. Leukocytosis with neutrophilia
   b. Mild anemia with normocytic red cell indices
   c. Thrombocytosis: usually seen by third week of illness; elevation may persist for 3 months after onset

4. Acute phase reactant elevation—to assess inflammatory processes
   a. Erythrocyte sedimentation rate
   b. C-reactive protein level
5. Liver function studies—to assess involvement of liver function
   a. Serum transaminase levels
   b. Mild hyperbilirubinemia
   c. Hypoalbuminemia
6. Serum lactic dehydrogenase level (LDH)—elevated during acute febrile phase and decreased during convalescent phase (LDH levels are nonspecific, but elevation is an early indicator of cellular death in the myocardium)
7. Immunoglobulin E and immunoglobulin M—to assess immune response during illness; elevation is observed during acute febrile phase and decreased during convalescent phase
8. Complement levels (C3 and C4)—to assess immune response; is increased in the first several weeks of the illness
9. Urinalysis may reveal a sterile pyuria
10. Cerebrospinal fluid may reveal aseptic meningitis with a predominance of mononuclear cells with normal protein and glucose

MEDICAL MANAGEMENT

Initial therapy is aimed at reducing the vascular inflammatory process and preventing thrombosis by inhibiting platelet aggregation. IVIG has made a tremendous difference to the treatment of Kawasaki disease. If given within 10 days from the onset of symptoms, IVIG significantly shortens the disease duration and minimizes complications. IVIG is given as a 2 g/kg infusion delivered over 10 to 12 hours, ideally within the first 7 days of the illness. The mechanism of action of IVIG is unknown, but it appears to have an antiinflammatory effect, which decreases the inflammation of the coronary arteries and speeds the resolution of the fever. IVIG may be repeated at the same dose for a second infusion if the fever persists longer than 36 hours after the first infusion.

Aspirin therapy has been used for years in Kawasaki disease. Aspirin is used in the acute phase for its antiinflammatory effect as well as for its antithrombotic effect. The dosing is divided into two different phases. During the initial phase, aspirin is given at 80 to 100 mg/kg/day in four divided doses. High-dose aspirin should be initiated as soon as Kawasaki disease is suspected and given until the child remains afebrile for 48 to 72 hours. After the resolution of the fever, the dose of aspirin is decreased to 3 to 5 mg/kg/day in a single daily dose for 6 to 8 weeks. After 6 to 8 weeks, if the echocardiogram is normal, the aspirin is discontinued. If the echocardiogram reveals coronary artery abnormalities, low-dose aspirin therapy (3 to 5 mg/kg/day) is continued indefinitely.

The use of corticosteroids is controversial, but may be used in children refractory to IVIG therapy. Warfarin (Coumadin) is sometimes used in children who have developed giant aneurysms. The international normalized ratio (INR) should be maintained between 2 to 2.5 while the child receives warfarin. Furosemide (Lasix) may be used in patients with congestive heart failure. Plasma exchange has been reported to be effective in treatment-refractory children in uncontrolled clinical trials.

NURSING ASSESSMENT

1. See the Cardiovascular Assessment section in Appendix A.
2. Assess skin for color, moisture, texture, turgor, rashes, lesions, and integrity.
3. Assess for clinical criteria of Kawasaki disease.
4. Assess for febrile seizures.
5. Assess adequacy of hydration.
6. Assess pain with age-appropriate pain scale.
7. Assess for allergic reaction to IVIG administration.

NURSING DIAGNOSES

- Fluid volume, Deficient
- Oral mucous membrane, Impaired
- Skin integrity, Impaired
- Hyperthermia
- Cardiac output, Decreased
- Injury, Risk for
- Pain
- Nutrition: less than body requirements, Imbalanced

- Mobility, Impaired physical
- Anxiety
- Therapeutic regimen management, Ineffective family

NURSING INTERVENTIONS

1. Monitor child's clinical status.
   a. Rectal temperature
   b. Skin integrity, mucous membranes, and anterior fontanelle
   c. Intake and output (should be strictly recorded), daily weights
   d. Stool output
   e. Erythematous body rash
   f. Vital signs
   g. Pain
   h. Edema
2. Institute measures to lower fever.
   a. Medicate with antipyretics; monitor child's response to medications.
   b. Provide tepid sponge baths for high temperatures that are not responding to antipyretics.
   c. Offer cool fluids.
   d. Assess which fluids (such as popsicles and gelatin) child prefers, and provide as tolerated.
   e. Maintain seizure precautions, because 3% to 5% of children between 6 months and 3 years of age may develop seizures when they have fevers even as low as 101.8° F (38.8° C).
   f. Explain unusual nature of fever to parents in terms of its intermittent pattern, duration, and resistance to antipyretics; anticipatory guidance will prevent parental anxiety about fever.
3. Monitor child for cardiac complications.
   a. Use cardiac monitor as ordered during acute and subacute phases; report arrhythmias to health care provider.
   b. Explain purpose of ECG and echocardiogram, and aberrations caused by child's movement to parents and child.
   c. Allow child to change his or her own electrodes during daily bath.

    d. Assess perfusion, vital signs, and level of consciousness for any changes and report to health care provider.

4. Monitor for untoward signs and symptoms (hypotension, diaphoresis, nausea and vomiting, chills) during IVIG administration, and stop infusion until symptoms have subsided. Keep epinephrine available to treat anaphylaxis.

5. Monitor for signs of bleeding due to aspirin or anticoagulant therapy.

6. Provide comfort measures for child.
   a. Perform oral hygiene frequently.
   b. Apply petroleum jelly to lips.
   c. Avoid soaps, ointments, and lotions on skin; keep skin clean, dry, and exposed to air.
   d. Cool, moist compresses may be applied to itching areas.
   e. Provide sheepskin for child to lie on.
   f. Discourage scratching by means of diversional activities; for young children, soft, loose mittens may be helpful.
   g. Encourage bed rest and elevation of extremities until swelling has subsided.
   h. Teach parents how to hold and comfort child who has IV line and electrodes in place.
   i. Keep stimulation to a minimum.
   j. Explain to parents that tactile stimulation may be irritating but soothing voice may provide security.
   k. Provide dim lights.
   l. Provide quiet music.
   m. Allow child to have comfort toy from home.

7. Provide for and promote child's nutrition.
   a. Provide comfort measures for mouth (see item 6).
   b. Begin with bland foods in small amounts.
   c. Ask parents about child's favorite foods, and provide if possible.
   d. Avoid hot, spicy foods.
   e. Offer high-calorie liquids.
   f. Avoid caffeinated beverages.

8. Prevent contractions related to imposed restrictions and range of motion (ROM) limitations.
   a. Perform passive ROM exercises gently on edematous extremities during child's bed rest; teach parents how to do these exercises, and explain their importance.

   b. When child is able, use active ROM exercises, making them into game for child.

   c. Place IV lines in position that allows maximal movement.

9. Alleviate anxiety caused by invasive procedures for diagnostic tests and by pain, new environment, strange people, knowledge deficit, and age-related fears (refer to Appendixes B and F).

   a. Provide play therapy during all phases of illness and for each new procedure (e.g., ECGs, needle-related); base therapy on child's developmental level (refer to Appendixes B and F).

   b. Explain each procedure at child's and parents' cognitive levels.

   c. Suggest ways for parents to support their child during hospitalization and procedures (e.g., holding child during or after procedures).

   d. Consult parents and child about preferences among "quiet" toys and activities during acute phase of illness; encourage parents and volunteers to play with child, allowing for rest periods and then passive participation.

   e. Explain meaning of presence of swollen lymph nodes to parents.

🏠 Discharge Planning and Home Care

Instruct about long-term management.

1. Instruct parents and child, in developmentally appropriate manner, about importance of follow-up care including ECGs, echocardiograms, and chest radiographic studies (two thirds of coronary aneurysms regress within 1 year).

2. Instruct parents verbally and with written reinforcement about signs and symptoms of cardiac complications (i.e., aneurysms and coronary thromboses); tell them to contact health care provider immediately if child has any of these signs and symptoms.

3. Instruct parents about importance of anticoagulant therapy such as aspirin and about side effects to watch for; explain to parents why some children with Kawasaki disease may need to undergo coronary artery bypass grafting.

4. Instruct parents about importance of good nutrition and adequate fluid intake.
5. Stress importance of adequate rest.
6. Educate parents about delaying administration of live virus vaccines (such as measles, varicella) for 11 months after child receives IVIG.
7. Avoid high-impact sports or activities while on anticoagulant therapy.
8. Instruct parents to have child checked for cardiovascular factors every 5 years.
9. Instruct parents to seek medical care immediately for flulike symptoms while on aspirin therapy.

CLIENT OUTCOMES

1. Child's temperature will return to normal.
2. Changes in skin will resolve.
3. Child will walk without joint pain.
4. Child will remain hemodynamically stable.
5. Child will remain free of nosocomial infections.
6. Child will resume age-appropriate activities.
7. Child will feel a sense of mastery about the illness experience.

REFERENCES

Nasr I, Tometzki AJP, Schofield OM: Kawasaki disease: An update, *Clin Exper Dermatol* 26:6, 2001.

Newburger JW et al: Diagnosis, treatment, and long-term management of Kawasaki disease: A statement for health professionals from the committtee on rheumatic fever, endocarditis, and Kawasaki disease council on cardiovascular disease in the young, American Heart Association, *Pediatrics* 114(6):1708, 2004.

Shulman S: Kawasaki disease. In: Feigen RD et al, editors: *Textbook of pediatric infectious disease*, ed 5, Philadelphia, 2004, WB Saunders.

Shulman ST, Rowley AH: Advances in Kawasaki disease, *Eur J Pediatr* 163: 285, 2004.

Yamamoto LG: Kawasaki disease, *Pediatr Emerg Care* 19(6):422, 2003.

48

Learning Disabilities

PATHOPHYSIOLOGY

Learning disabilities are a group of neurologic disorders that affect an individual's ability to store, process, and produce information. Learning disabilities significantly interfere with educational achievement and performance, and they create a gap between one's capabilities and performance. Impairment may be in the area of reading, writing, spelling, or mathematical functions. The most commonly identified learning disability is reading disability. Intelligence is generally average or above average in these children. However, academic achievement is markedly below what is expected given the person's intellect, age, and educational opportunities.

Etiologic factors associated with learning disabilities include genetic predisposition, perinatal and birth injuries, and medical conditions occurring in infancy or childhood, such as head injury, malnutrition, or poisoning. Late effects of cranial irradiation, as well as alcohol or tobacco use during pregnancy, have also been known to contribute to learning disabilities. Mental retardation, emotional or behavioral disorders, and autism are not learning disabilities. Environmental, socioeconomic, and cultural disadvantages do not produce learning disabilities. Learning disabilities can be categorized into several types: reading disorder, mathematics disorder, disorder of written expression, and learning disorder not otherwise specified (Box 48-1).

Reading disorders, mathematics disorders, and disorders of written expression can be specifically tested for in the school setting using individualized standardized tests. The child with

BOX 48-1

Learning Disabilities: DSM-IV Criteria

Reading Disorder DSM-IV Criteria

A. Reading achievement, as measured by individually administered standardized tests of reading accuracy or comprehension, is substantially below that expected given the person's chronologic age, measured intelligence, and age-appropriate education.

B. The disturbance in criterion A significantly interferes with academic achievement or activities of daily living that require reading skills.

C. If a sensory deficit is present, the reading difficulties are in excess of those usually associated with it.

Mathematics Disorder DSM-IV Criteria

A. Mathematical ability, as measured by individually administered standardized tests, is substantially below that expected given the person's chronologic age, measured intelligence, and age-appropriate education.

B. The disturbance in criterion A significantly interferes with academic achievement or activities of daily living that require mathematical ability.

C. If a sensory deficit is present, the difficulties in mathematical ability are in excess of those usually associated with it.

Disorder of Written Expression DSM-IV Criteria

A. Writing skills, as measured by individually administered standardized tests (or functional assessments of writing skills), are substantially below those expected given the person's chronologic age, measured intelligence, and age-appropriate education.

B. The disturbance in criterion A significantly interferes with academic achievement or activities of daily living that require the composition of written texts (e.g., writing grammatically correct sentences and organized paragraphs).

C. If a sensory deficit is present, the difficulties in writing skills are in excess of those usually associated with it.

Learning Disorder Not Otherwise Specified

There are no specific criteria for this form of learning disability. The student's difficulties with academic achievement are associated with learning problems in the three areas of achievement: reading, mathematics, and written expression.

From American Psychiatric Association: *Diagnostic and statistical manual of mental disorders*, ed 4, text revision (DSM-IV-TR), Washington, DC, 2000, The Association.

such disorders will score substantially below what is expected based upon chronologic age and measured intelligence.

Many states will quantify this "gap" between where the child is performing and where the child is expected to perform, and will use this quantification as criteria that will make a child eligible for special education services. The learning disorder not otherwise specified has no written criteria, but the student is performing significantly below age and/or intelligence level in reading, mathematics, and written expression.

Learning difficulties become apparent in the early years of elementary school (kindergarten through third grade). It is estimated that between 25% and 50% of children with learning disabilities have other problems that interfere with their school performance. These associated conditions are attention-deficit/hyperactivity disorder (ADHD), memory problems, emotional and behavioral problems, and problems with social skills. Once a child is assessed for learning disabilities and qualifies for special education services based upon the gap between performance and ability, the school staff works with the parent to develop an individualized educational plan (IEP). The IEP, which is signed by school staff and parents, will include present levels of function, goals and objectives, and time allotted for services on a weekly or monthly basis. The IEP is reviewed annually, and every 3 years the testing process is repeated to determine if the child's eligibility has changed.

Children with learning disabilities may also have speech and language disorders. The speech and language disorders often fall into general categories of receptive language, expressive language, and articulation. These are considered more as developmental disorders and not true learning disabilities. A child who has an IEP for learning disabilities may also receive services for speech and language disorders that are included on the same IEP.

INCIDENCE

1. Approximately 5% of students in public schools in the United States are identified as having a learning disorder, but up to 20% of the school-aged population may actually have a learning disorder.

2. Approximately 17.5% of public school students are estimated to have problems learning to read.
3. Among children 6 to 12 years of age, specific learning disorders are the most prevalent disability.
4. More than 50% of children receiving special education have specific learning disorders.
5. The high school drop-out rate for students with learning disabilities is 1.5 times higher than that for students in general education.
6. Of students with reading problems, 60% to 80% are male.
7. Male/female prevalence ratio for learning disorders is 4:1 to 5:1.
8. Reading disability accounts for approximately 80% of all learning disabilities.

CLINICAL MANIFESTATIONS
1. Difficulties with reading, writing, and/or mathematics
2. Deficits in school performance
3. School failure
4. Disruptive behaviors in classroom
5. Social skills deficits
6. Problems in relationships with peers and family members

COMPLICATIONS
1. Social skills deficits
2. Low self-esteem
3. Emotional and behavioral problems (e.g., conduct disorder, depression)
4. ADHD

LABORATORY AND DIAGNOSTIC TESTS
The more severe the learning disability, the earlier the disability will be detected.
1. Intelligence testing that is sensitive to child's ethnic and cultural background, used to determine intelligence based upon standardized tests (e.g., Wechsler Intelligence Scale for Children, ed 3; Woodcock-Johnson Psycho-Educational Battery—Revised: Tests of Cognitive Ability)

2. Tests of language and memory function, used to test language skills based upon standardized tests (e.g., Test of Awareness of Language Segments, Rapid Automatized Naming Test)
3. Measurements of visual-perceptual skills, used to assess for visual motor learning disabilities and self-concept (e.g., Bender Visual Motor Gestalt Test, Goodenough-Harris Drawing Test)
4. Standardized reading tests, used to test current reading level (e.g., Stanford Diagnostic Reading Test, Gray Oral Reading Test—Revised)
5. Standardized math tests, used to assess current level of math skills on a standardized test (e.g., Key Math—Revised)
6. Standardized written expression tests, used to test written skills on a standardized test (e.g., Test of Written Spelling, ed 2)
7. Classroom observation and behavioral assessment

MEDICAL MANAGEMENT

The medical management of the child with a learning disability involves coordination with a community-based interdisciplinary team. Special education specialists, general education teachers and counselors, transition specialists, school nurses, job developers, and rehabilitation specialists, including the medical team (child psychiatrists and pediatricians), work with the family to address the child's long-term needs. Medications may be used to treat associated problems such as ADHD and emotional problems that affect the child's ability to learn.

NURSING ASSESSMENT

1. Assess child's need for instructional assistance in health care settings and for adherence to treatment regimen.
2. Review interdisciplinary assessments and evaluations.
3. Assess visual and auditory acuity.

NURSING DIAGNOSES

- Thought processes, Disturbed
- Sensory perception, Disturbed
- Self-esteem, Chronic low

- Knowledge, Deficient
- Social interaction, Impaired

NURSING INTERVENTIONS

1. Consult with IEP specialists and educators in adapting strategies in health care settings.
2. Adapt instructional approaches, procedural explanations, and preprocedural preparations to be sensitive to child's learning disability.
3. Coordinate with special education members of child's team in formulating child's IEP as it pertains to child's health care needs.
4. Facilitate coordination and implementation of child's IEP while hospitalized.

🏠 Discharge Planning and Home Care

1. Coordinate services with members of IEP team and integrate with health care instruction and development of instructional materials.
2. Develop individualized health care plan (IHP). IHP may be written separately by school nurse or integrated as part of IEP–individualized family service plan.
3. Integrate IEP objectives and strategies into child's health care plan in school setting (refer to Appendix G).
4. Refer to community-based services and support services (see Appendix G).
5. Incorporate adaptations of learning style into discharge teaching.
6. Refer to counseling and/or therapy services—individual, family, or group.
7. Refer to social skills training group.
8. Provide opportunities for social skills training.

CLIENT OUTCOMES

1. Child will achieve annual IEP goals and objectives.
2. Child will express positive comments about him- or herself.
3. Child will engage in positive social interactions with peers and family members.

REFERENCES

American Psychiatric Association: *Diagnostic and statistical manual of mental disorders*, ed 4, text revision (DSM-IV-TR), Washington, DC, 2000, The Association.

House AE: *DSM-IV Diagnosis in the schools*, New York, 2002, Guilford Press.

Ldonline: *IDEA update* (website): www.ldonline.org/article.php?id=)&loc=109. Accessed January 14, 2006.

National Center for Learning Disabilities: *LD at a glance fact sheet* (website): www.ncld.org/LDInfoZone/InfoZone_FactSheet_LD_QuickLook.pdf. Accessed January 14, 2006.

National Dissemination Center for Children with Disabilities: *Fact sheet #7, 2004* (website): www.nichcy.org/pubs/factshe/fs7txt.htm. Accessed January 14, 2006.

Selekman J: Learning disabilities: A diagnosis ignored by nurses, *Pediatr Nurs* 28 (6):630, 2002.

Silver L: *Doctor to Doctor: Information on learning disabilities for pediatricians and other physicians* (website): www.ldaamerica.us/aboutld/professionals/doctor_to_doctor.asp. Accessed January 14, 2006.

49

Leukemia, Childhood

PATHOPHYSIOLOGY

Leukemia is a cancer of the hematapoietic tissues that produce white blood cells (leukocytes). In normal blood cell development, the undifferentiated puripotent stem cells in the bone marrow proliferate and differentiate into one of two cell lines: myeloid or lymphoid cells. Myeloid cells differentiate and mature into red blood cells, monocytes, granulocytes, and platelets. Lymphoid cells differentiate and mature into T and B cells. In leukemia, normal hematopoiesis is interrupted, and the cells are unable to differentiate and mature into the various functioning white cells. In acute leukemias of childhood, the leukemic cells infiltrate the bone marrow, displacing the normal cellular elements and resulting in anemia, thrombocytopenia, and leukopenia. Leukemic cells may also infiltrate lymph nodes, the spleen, the liver, bones, and the central nervous system (CNS), as well as the reproductive organs. Leukemic infiltrates of the skin called chloromas or granulocytic sarcomas are found in some affected children.

The classification of childhood leukemia is based on the predominant cell line that is affected. Acute lymphocytic leukemia (ALL) affects the lymphoid cell lines and is classified into acute T- and B-cell leukemia subtypes. Acute myelogenous leukemia (AML) affects any of the myeloid cell lines, such as in acute monoblastic, myeloblastic, promyelocytic, and myelocytic leukemias. Chronic leukemia is more commonly seen in adults; less than 5% of leukemia in children is chronic (chronic myleogneous leukemia and chronic lymphocytic leukemia). Acute leukemia is a rapidly progressing disease involving mostly immature, undifferentiated cells, as opposed to the chronic leukemias, which are more insidious in onset.

INCIDENCE
Acute Lymphocytic Leukemia (ALL)

1. Leukemia is the most common type of childhood cancer and accounts for approximately one fourth of all childhood cancers.
2. ALL accounts for 75% to 80% of all cases of childhood leukemia.
3. Highest incidence is in children between the ages of 2 and 5 years, with peak between 2 and 3 years of age.
4. ALL is most common in males and whites.
5. Females have a better prognosis overall than males.
6. For acute lymphocytic leukemia, 5-year survival rates exceed 80%, which is a dramatic improvement for a disease that was virtually incurable in the 1960s.
7. African Americans have less frequent remissions and a lower median survival rate.
8. Risk of the disease increases for children with Down syndrome.

Acute Myelogenous Leukemia (AML)

1. AML incidence is constant from birth to 10 years and then peaks slightly in adolescence.
2. Leukemia in infancy is more commonly AML than ALL.
3. AML accounts for 20% to 25% of all cases of childhood leukemia, and the ratio of ALL to AML incidence is 1:4.
4. Boys and girls are equally affected by the disease.
5. It is more difficult to induce remission in children with AML than in those with ALL (70% remission rate).
6. Five-year survival rates have increased from less than 5% in the 1970s to 43% today as a result of treatment intensification, bone marrow transplantation, and enhanced supportive care.
7. Risk of the disease increases for children with congenital conditions such as Down syndrome.

CLINICAL MANIFESTATIONS

ALL

1. Evidence of anemia, bleeding, and/or infections due to bone marrow infiltration
   a. Fever, chills, cough, malaise
   b. Fatigue, pallor, dizziness, tachycardia, dyspnea
   c. Petechiae, bruising, bleeding gums, epistaxis and/or hemorrhage
   d. Bone and/or joint pain, limping, arthralgias, refusal to walk
   e. Lymphadenopathy
2. Electrolyte imbalance secondary to rapid cell turnover and tumor lysis
   a. Muscle twitching, weakness, or cramping
   b. Numbness, tingling, paresthesias
   c. Cardiac arrythmias, tachycardia
   d. Weight gain, decreased urine output, renal failure
3. Gastrointestinal (GI) effects of hepatosplenomegaly
   a. Vague abdominal pain
   b. Early satiety and feeling of fullness
   c. Weight loss
   d. Palpable enlargement of liver and spleen, abdominal distention
4. CNS involvement
   a. Neck pain and stiffness
   b. Headache
   c. Irritability, photophobia
   d. Lethargy, somnolence
   e. Nausea and vomiting
   f. Papilledema and photophobia
   g. Cranial nerve palsies, especially of III to VII
   h. Visual disturbances, ptosis
   i. Learning difficulties

AML

1. Same clinical manifestations as in children with ALL (see previous section)
2. Gingival hypertrophy

3. Leukemia cutis—bluish/purple nontender skin nodules
4. Chloromas (tumors of AML blasts): orbital or spinal most common

COMPLICATIONS
ALL

1. CNS: increased intracranial pressure, seizures secondary to meningeal infiltration; muscle cramping and weakness due to electrolyte imbalance; stroke secondary to high white blood count, causing hyperviscosity of blood and cerebral vessels
2. Head, ears, eyes, nose, and throat (HEENT): recurrent sore throats and ear infections secondary to immunosuppression; bleeding gums and gingiva due to low platelet count; lymphadenopathy due to disease process
3. Skin: pallor, leukemia cutis, petechiae, bruising
4. Cardiovascular: tachycardia and cardiac failure secondary to profound anemia; fever, hypotension, septic shock secondary to infection/immunosuppression
5. Pulmonary: mediastinal mass causing respiratory compromise (T-cell ALL)
6. GI: abdominal distention due to hepatosplenomegaly; typhlitis secondary to immune suppression; GI bleeding due to low platelet count
7. Genitourinary: testicular swelling and pain secondary to leukemic infiltration
8. Musculoskeletal: bone pain due to bone marrow infiltration of leukemia

AML

1. Same complications as ALL (see previous section)
2. HEENT: orbital chloromas; gingival hypertrophy, bleeding gums
3. CNS: paresis secondary to spinal cord chloroma; intracranial bleed secondary to disseminated intravascular coagulation (DIC); most common in acute promyleocytic leukemia

LABORATORY AND DIAGNOSTIC TESTS

1. Complete blood count—children with white blood cell (WBC) count of less than 10,000/mm^3 at time of diagnosis have best prognosis; WBC count of more than 50,000/mm^3 is an unfavorable prognostic sign in children of any age. Low hemoglobin level and hematocrit indicate anemia. Low platelet count indicates potential for bleeding.

2. Lumbar puncture—to assess CNS involvement

3. Chest radiographic study—to assess for presence of a mediastinal mass

4. Bone marrow aspiration study—to determine the morphologic appearance, structure, and percentage of leukemic cells present in the bone marrow. A finding of greater than 25% blast cells confirms the diagnosis of leukemia.

5. Immunophenotyping of bone marrow cells—to determine the cell lineage and stage of differentiation of the cells

6. Cytogenetic testing of bone marrow cells—to assess for any abnormalities in the number of chromosomes (ploidy) and presence of changes in the chromosome structure of the leukemic cells, such as translocations. This testing provides important information for the risk classification of the leukemia and helps to assign the patient to an appropriate therapy. Hyperdiploidy is considered a good prognostic indicator in that hypodiploidy is a high-risk feature.

7. PT, PTT, fibrinogen—to assess for clotting defects or the presence of DIC

8. Metabolic profile to include blood urea nitrogen (BUN), creatinine, potassium, calcium, phosphorus, and uric acid—to assess for tumor lysis syndrome. The rapid release of intracellular metabolites from the leukemic cells when destroyed by chemotherapy can cause significant electrolyte imbalance and renal compromise.

9. Serum lactate dehydrogenase (LDH)—used as an indicator of rapid cell turnover/destruction

10. Echocardiogram, electrocardiogram (ECG)—to assess cardiac function before the initiation of therapy that may affect heart contractility

MEDICAL MANAGEMENT

Chemotherapy protocols vary according to the type and risk category of the leukemia. Age of patient, white cell count at diagnosis, cell type of leukemia, presence of cytogenetic abnormalities, and response to induction therapy all determine the risk category and intensity of treatment the child will receive. Chemotherapeutic agents are administered to prevent cancer cells from dividing and metastasizing. The mix of chemotherapeutic agents used in the protocols to treat leukemia is effective because they attack rapidly dividing cells in the different phases of cell division, optimizing cell kill. It is also because of this action on the normal rapidly dividing cells (such as in the bone marrow, the mucous membranes, and hair follicles) as well as on the leukemia cells that most of the side effects from therapy are seen.

The process of inducing remission in children with leukemia consists of three phases: induction, consolidation, and maintenance therapy, with CNS sanctuary therapy included and essential to each phase. During the induction phase (lasting for approximately 4 to 6 weeks), the child receives a variety of chemotherapeutic agents to induce remission from disease. Remission is considered to occur when there is no evidence of leukemia cells in peripheral blood, there are less than 5% blasts in the bone marrow and no evidence of CNS disease, and all cell lines have recovered from the induction therapy. Intensification therapy, known as consolidation, follows induction and is designed to strengthen the remission achieved in induction and to further reduce the leukemic burden before the emergence of drug resistance. The duration of consolidation and the intensity and choice of agents vary. Maintenance therapy is administered following consolidation and is designed to provide a sustained continuation therapy to eliminate all residual leukemic cells. Chemotherapy treatment protocols are approximately 2 to 3 years in duration for ALL and 6 to 9 months for AML. AML patients receive induction and consolidation therapy only. Chemotherapy agents used to treat childhood leukemias include but are not limited to steroids, vincristine, asparaginase, methotrexate, mercaptopurine, cytarabine, cyclophosphamide, etoposide, mitoxantrone, and daunorubicin. Other important supportive care drugs used during chemotherapy include allopurinol, leucovorin, and mesna.

Prednisone and Dexamethasone

Prednisone and dexamethasone (Decadron) have a direct lytic action on leukemia cells. They also inhibit tumor proliferation by blocking naturally occurring substances that stimulate tumor growth. Decadron is more commonly used in current therapies for leukemia since studies suggest it may be more efficient in crossing the blood-brain barrier. Dexamethasone is also used with antiemetics in acute cases of nausea to potentiate the effect of the antiemetic, increasing its ability to penetrate to the chemoreceptor zone of the brain. Possible side effects are the following:

1. Fluid and electrolyte disturbances—sodium retention, fluid retention, congestive heart failure in susceptible clients, potassium loss, hypertension
2. Musculoskeletal effects—bone pain, muscle weakness, osteoporosis, pathologic fracture of long bones, avascular necrosis of the hips in prolonged use
3. GI effects—gastritis and/or esophagitis, gastric ulceration, pancreatitis, abdominal distention, increased appetite, weight gain
4. Dermatologic effects—impaired wound healing, petechiae and ecchymoses, facial erythema, hirsutism, acne hypopigmentation or hyperpigmentation, striae with weight gain
5. Neurologic effects—leukoencephalopathy, raised intraocular pressure, convulsions, vertigo, headache, irritability, mood swings, psychosis
6. Endocrine effects—Cushing's syndrome, pituitary-adrenal axis suppression, manifestations of latent diabetes mellitus
7. Ophthalmic effects—posterior subcapsular cataracts
8. Metabolic effects—negative nitrogen balance resulting from protein catabolism
9. Immune suppression—elevated white blood cell count, increased risk of infection

Dosage is individualized based on child's body surface area and the treatment protocol and severity of the disease.

Children usually receive a month of steroid therapy during induction and later receive 1- to 2-week pulses at different phases of their therapy. It is an essential part of the therapy plan. Supportive care to treat the side effects of the steroid therapy is often needed. The drug is administered by mouth (PO), with food to decrease the GI upset and commonly in conjunction with an H_2 inhibitor to decrease the risk for gastritis. If the child is unable to take oral medications, the dose will be administered by intravenous (IV) route. It is added to intrathecal chemotherapy per protocol.

Vincristine (Oncovin)

Vincristine is an antineoplastic agent that inhibits cell division during metaphase. Possible side effects are the following:

1. Neuromuscular effects—peripheral neuropathy, paresthesias, numbness, loss of deep tendon reflexes, jaw pain, extraocular muscle paralysis, ptosis, vocal cord paralysis
2. Dermatologic effects—alopecia, tissue damage secondary to extravasation
3. GI effects—stomatitis, anorexia, nausea, vomiting, diarrhea, constipation, paralytic ileus
4. Hematologic—myelosuppression
5. Other effects—hypersensitivity, hyponatremia, syndrome of inappropriate antidiuretic hormone secretion (SIADH)

Refer to treatment protocol for dosage. Vincristine is administered by IV push, ideally via a central venous access device to reduce the risk of extravasation, which may cause severe tissue damage and necrosis. There must be a blood return before administration of drug. Prophylactic stool softeners are given to children receiving this drug. Dose modifications are required if evidence of significant peripheral neuropathy develops.

Asparaginase (Elspar)

Asparaginase decreases the level of asparagine (an amino acid necessary for tumor growth). It is used in the treatment of ALL. It is made from an *Escherichia coli* enzyme, and if a patient develops allergies to this enzyme, it is changed to another enzyme form called *Erwinia* asparaginase. Asparaginase is also used for the treatment of acute lymphocytic leukemia in a pegylated (slow-release) form called PEG-asparaginase. Possible side effects are the following:

1. Allergic manifestations—most serious side effects of asparaginase are the following:
   a. Chills and fever within 1 minute of administration
   b. Skin reactions
   c. Respiratory distress
   d. Hypotension
   e. Nausea and vomiting
   f. Anaphylaxis
2. Coagulopathy—low fibrinogen, thrombosis
3. Liver toxicity—jaundice, hypoalbuminemia, coagulation abnormalities
4. Pancreatitis—elevated amylase and/or lipase, hyperglycemia
5. Neurologic—rare cases of CNS ischemic attacks, somnolence, convulsions

Refer to treatment protocol for dosage. It is administered intramuscularly (IM). PEG-asparaginase is commonly split into two injections because of its volume.

Methotrexate (Amethopterin, MTX)

Methotrexate is classified as an antimetabolite. It interferes with folic acid metabolism. Folic acid is essential to the synthesis of the nucleoproteins required by rapidly multiplying cells. Methotrexate is used in the treatment of ALL.

Methotrexate is given in many different forms and used in all phases of ALL therapy. It can be given by the oral, IM, IV, or intrathecal routes. Vitamins containing folic acid must be avoided to prevent the metabolic block caused by methotrexate. Possible side effects are the following:

1. Skin reactions—generalized erythematous rash, urticaria, acne, pruritus, peeling, folliculitis
2. Alopecia
3. Oral and GI tract ulcerations
4. Fever and chills
5. Nausea and vomiting
6. Diarrhea
7. Bone marrow depression
8. Liver toxicity

9. Photosensitivity and/or hyperpigmentation
10. CNS deterioration: learning problems, seizures, somnolences, leukoencephalopathy
11. Renal toxicity with high doses

When intermediate- or high-dose methotrexate is given by IV route, a rescue agent called leucovorin is administered at timed intervals. Hydration and alkalinization fluids are run concurrently to prevent renal damage and to enable renal clearance of the methotrexate in a safe interval of time. Additional bone marrow-suppressive medications such as Bactrim are held when methotrexate is being administered. Patients are educated to avoid the sun and to wear sunblock when taking methotrexate, since even low doses can result in severe cases of sunburn with sun exposure.

Mercaptopurine (Purinethol, 6-MP)

Mercaptopurine interferes with the synthesis of nucleic acid, which is especially needed when cells are growing and multiplying rapidly. The primary effects of mercaptopurine occur in tissues with rapid cellular growth and a high rate of nucleic metabolism (e.g., bone marrow and gastric epithelium). Leukocyte, thrombocyte, and reticulocyte formation is reduced. The drug is used in the treatment of ALL and may be given by IV route or PO. Possible side effects are the following:

1. Anorexia
2. Nausea and vomiting
3. Diarrhea
4. Urticaria
5. Hyperbilirubinemia, liver fibrosis
6. Bone marrow depression

Refer to treatment protocol for dosage. When given orally, it is taken daily at least 2 hours after eating on an empty stomach.

Thioguanine (6-TG)

Thioguanine interferes with cell metabolism by inhibiting purine syntheses. It is given orally on a daily basis for 2-week periods in cycles of ALL therapy. Potential side effects include the following:

1. Myelosuppression
2. Anorexia, nausea, and vomiting

3. Diarrhea
4. Mucositis
5. Hepatic fibrosis, hyperbilirubinemia
6. Allergic reaction; urticaria; anaphylaxis (in rare instances)

Refer to the treatment protocol for specific dosage. Similar to oral mercaptopurine, this drug is given on an empty stomach 2 hours after the evening meal.

Cytarabine (ARA-C, Cytosine Arabinoside, Cytosar)

Cytarabine is a cell cycle–specific drug that inhibits cell development in the G1 to S phases of cell division. It is currently indicated for induction of remission in individuals with AML and ALL and is used in consolidation therapy for ALL. Cytarabine is a potent bone marrow suppressant and also has penetration into the CNS; therefore intrathecal chemotherapy is not given concurrently with this drug. Individuals receiving this drug must be under close medical supervision and, during induction therapy, should have leukocyte and platelet counts performed frequently. It is highly emetogenic at high doses. Possible side effects are the following:

1. Anorexia, nausea, and vomiting
2. Myelosuppression
3. Flulike symptoms: fever, chills, arthralgias
4. Rash
5. Conjunctivitis
6. Alopecia, stomatitis
7. Diarrhea
8. CNS: cerebellar dysfunction, encephalopathy, seizures, paresis, learning disabilities
9. Hepatotoxicity, veno-occlusive disease
10. Pneumonitis
11. Anaphylaxis
12. Gonadal dysfunction

Cytarabine may be given by IV, subcutaneous, or intrathecal route. It is a highly emetogenic drug and necessitates that antinausea medications be given before administration of the drug and continuously or at intervals afterward. Dexamethasone ophthalmic drops are administered every 2 to 3 hours with high-dose cytarabine and for 5 days following administration to reduce the risk of conjunctivitis. Tylenol is given for fevers related to the flulike symptoms associated with the drug, and care must be taken to monitor carefully for signs and symptoms of infection as a source of fever in an immune-suppressed child.

Cyclophosphamide (Cytoxan)

Cyclophosphamide is a nitrogen mustard derivative that acts as an alkylating agent by interfering with DNA replication and transcription of RNA in cell division. Cyclophosphamide is used in the treatment of ALL and AML. Possible side effects are the following:

1. Nausea and vomiting
2. Anorexia
3. Alopecia (occurs in at least 50% of individuals)
4. Leukopenia (decreased WBCs)
   a. Expected effect
   b. Ordinarily serves as guide to therapy
   c. Leaves child susceptible to bacterial infection
5. Sterile hemorrhagic cystitis (active mustard derivatives excreted in the urine cause bladder mucosal irritation and/or bladder fibrosis)
6. Liver dysfunction
7. Cardiotoxicity at high doses
8. Hyponatremia (due to SIADH) and hypokalemia
9. Pulmonary fibrosis
10. Gonadal suppression: sterility, ovarian fibrosis
11. Secondary malignancy

Cyclophosphamide is administered by IV route or PO. Administration of high doses of cyclophosphamide should be preceded by IV fluid administration to help irrigate the bladder, and a protective drug called mesna is often given at timed intervals with the cyclophosphamide since it binds to the breakdown products of cyclophosphamide in the bladder and reduces the risk of hemorrhagic cystitis. Children receiving cyclophosphamide should empty their bladder frequently, and it is ideally given during daytime hours to promote compliance with voiding and to prevent toxic metabolites accumulating in the bladder at night. Urine is monitored for hematuria, and additional fluids may be ordered if urine output decreases and evidence of blood in the urine appears.

Daunorubicin (Daunomycin, DNR)

Daunorubicin inhibits the synthesis of DNA. It is used to inhibit cell division in treatment of acute leukemias. It has antimitotic and immune-suppressive properties. Possible side effects are the following:

1. Sclerosing of vein (if given via peripheral IV)
2. Nausea and vomiting
3. Myelosuppression
4. Cardiac arrhythmia, cardiomyopathy (cumulative and dose-dependent, affecting contractility of cardiac muscle)
5. Elevated liver enzyme levels (elevated serum glutamate pyruvate transaminase [SGPT], elevated serum glutamic-oxaloacetic transaminase [SGOT])
6. Change in urine color to red
7. Radiation recall (skin erythema, rash, and exfoliation if given with radiation therapy)
8. Allergic reaction: anaphylaxis, rash
9. Alopecia, mucositis

Daunorubicin is administered via IV infusion or IV push.

Mitoxantrone (Novantrone)

Mitoxantrone interacts with DNA and inhibits the enzyme topoisomerase, causing cell lysis. It is used in the treatment of AML. It is administered via IV infusion and preferably via a central venous line, since it causes local ulceration and tissue necrosis if extravasation occurs. Potential side effects include the following:

1. Cardiac arrythmias, cardiomyopathy (dose-dependent)
2. Nausea and vomiting
3. Mucositis, diarrhea
4. Alopecia, rash, urticaria
5. Bone marrow suppression
6. Bluish-green urine and sclera (drug is bright blue)
7. Hepatotoxicity

This drug is not given if maximum cumulative doses of other cardiotoxic drugs have been given, and must be used with caution in patients who have received mediastinal or mantle radiation therapy or who have a cardiac condition.

Etoposide (VP-16, VePesid)

Etoposide is a plant alkaloid that inhibits DNA synthesis so that cells do not enter mitosis; it therefore prevents cell division. It is used in the treatment of AML and recurrent or refractory ALL. It is given by IV route and is available orally for use with other cancers. It is routinely given as a 1-hour infusion with careful monitoring of the patient during the infusion. Potential side effects include the following:

1. Nausea and vomiting
2. Myelosuppression
3. Alopecia
4. Diarrhea
5. Hypotension (during infusion)
6. Peripheral neuropathy, constipation
7. Skin rash, pruritus, urticaria
8. Anaphylaxis
9. Secondary malignancy

Blood pressure measurements are routinely monitored every 15 minutes during etoposide infusion. IV infusions must not be diluted to concentrations greater than 0.4 mg/ml since the drug becomes unstable.

Allopurinol (Zyloprim)

Allopurinol inhibits the production of uric acid by blocking the biochemical reactions that immediately precede uric acid formation. The result is a lowering of blood and urinary uric acid levels. The drug is given prophylactically to prevent tissue urate deposits or renal calculi in children with leukemia who are receiving chemotherapy that results in the elevation of serum uric acid levels. Allopurinol also inhibits the oxidation of mercaptopurine, so that smaller doses of mercaptopurine are required (one fourth to one third of the regular dose). Possible side effects are the following:

1. Occasional liver toxicity
2. Asymptomatic increase in SGOT and SGPT levels

Allopurinol is administered orally (it can be given by IV route during the induction phase if the child is unable to ingest the PO form). IV hydration is administered at least twice the maintenance amount and is given along with alkalinization therapy to prevent renal uropathy. Refer to treatment protocol for dosage.

Raspuricase (Elitek)

Raspuricase is a relatively new drug used in malignancies where there is a high tumor burden, such as acute leukemias and lymphomas. It converts uric acid to allantoin, an inactive and soluble metabolite readily excreted by the kidneys. It is administered by IV route before the first dose of chemotherapy and may be continued on a daily basis until the risk of tumor lysis and renal uropathy resolves. Raspuricase acts rapidly and works in the prevention and treatment of chemotherapy-induced hyperuricemia in children with leukemia who have a high cell turnover, to reduce the risk of an oncologic emergency and irreversible renal damage. Potential side effects include the following:

1. Skin rash
2. Anaphylaxis; allergic reaction is rare
3. Methemoglobinemia
4. Hemolotytic anemia in glucose-6-phosphate dehydrogenase (G6PD) deficiency
5. Headache, fever, rigors

NURSING ASSESSMENT

1. See the Cardiovascular Assessment, Respiratory Assessment, and Neurologic Assessment sections in Appendix A.
2. Assess child's reaction to chemotherapy.
3. Assess for signs and symptoms of infection.
4. Assess for signs and symptoms of bleeding.
5. Assess for signs and symptoms of anemia.
6. Assess for signs and symptoms of complications related to therapy: radiation somnolence, CNS symptoms, tumor lysis, renal uropathy.
7. Assess child's and family's understanding of diagnosis and therapy plan, and coping ability.

NURSING DIAGNOSES

- Activity intolerance
- Infection, Risk for
- Fluid volume, Risk for deficient due to bleeding
- Fluid volume, Excess
- Tissue integrity, Impaired
- Nutrition: less than body requirements, Imbalanced
- Injury, Risk for
- Body image, Disturbed
- Anxiety
- Cardiac output, Decreased
- Respiratory function, Risk for ineffective
- Fatigue
- Knowledge, Deficient
- Coping, Compromised family
- Pain, Acute
- Development, Risk for delayed
- Family processes, Interrupted
- Therapeutic regimen management, Ineffective

NURSING INTERVENTIONS

1. Monitor child for reactions to medications (Table 49-1).
2. Monitor for signs and symptoms of infection.
   a. Be aware that fever is most important sign of infection.
   b. Treat all children as if they are neutropenic until test results are obtained. Isolate from other patients and families, especially children with infectious diseases and particularly those with chickenpox or chickenpox exposure.
   c. Ensure that child wears mask if around other people and is severely neutropenic (WBC count lower than 500/mm^3).
   d. Be aware that if a child with acute leukemia is neutropenic, chemotherapy may be delayed unless in induction phase.
   e. Febrile, neutropenic patients will be hospitalized, cultured, and started on IV antibiotics immediately (more children with leukemia die from infection than from their disease).

Text continued on p. 410

TABLE 49-1
Nursing Interventions Related to the Child Undergoing Chemotherapy and Radiotherapy

Responses	Nursing Interventions
Diarrhea	Offer oral fluids frequently.
	Perform skin care to buttocks and perineal area.
	Apply barrier cream to prevent further skin breakdown.
	Monitor effectiveness of antidiarrheal medications.
	Avoid high-cellulose foods and fruit.
	Offer small, frequent feedings; include child's favorite foods if possible.
	Observe for signs of dehydration.
	Monitor IV infusions.
Anorexia	Monitor intake and output.
	Offer small, frequent feedings of any bland foods high in nutrients and calories.
	Consult with child and parents to develop meal plan that incorporates child's likes and dislikes.
	Maintain adequate fluid intake, using Popsicles, ice cream, gelatin, and noncarbonated beverages.
	Obtain weight daily.

Nausea and vomiting	Avoid noxious smells that may increase nausea and vomiting.
	Observe for dehydration.
	Monitor side effects of antiemetics (e.g., ondansetron [Zofran], granisetron [Kytril], promethazine HCI [Phenergan], diphenhydramine HCI [Benadryl]) and lorazepam [Ativan]).
Fluid retention	Monitor intake and output.
	Obtain weight daily.
	Evaluate for respiratory distress and edema.
	Provide frequent changes of position.
	Monitor side effects of diuretics.
Hyperuricemia	Monitor intake and output.
	Encourage fluid intake.
	Monitor IV hydration and alkalinization.
	Provide skin care to decrease itching.
	Monitor serum creatinine and uric acid levels.
	Monitor side effects of allopurinol.
	Monitor side effects of raspuricase.
Chills and fever	Monitor vital signs and frequency of symptoms.
	Evaluate source of symptoms (e.g., tumor or infection).

Continued

TABLE 49-1
Nursing Interventions Related to the Child Undergoing Chemotherapy and Radiotherapy—cont'd

Responses	Nursing Interventions
Stomatitis and mouth ulcers	Monitor side effects of antipyretics. Provide comfort measures such as blankets and tepid sponge baths. Provide antibacterial mouthwashes routinely. Administer pain medication to control mouth pain. Give topical mouthwashes such as Benadryl or Maalox to soothe the mucosal irritation. Avoid hard-bristled toothbrushes. Avoid glycerin swabs and alcohol-based mouthwashes. Avoid hard foods that require excessive chewing and foods that are acidic or spicy. Avoid hot foods.
Cardiotoxicity (doxorubicin and daunorubicin)	Monitor changes in ECG and vital signs. Observe for signs and symptoms of congestive heart failure.
Hemorrhagic cystitis	Encourage frequent voiding after drug administration (cyclophosphamide). Offer oral fluids in large amounts. Monitor IV fluids.

Alopecia

Encourage voiding before sleep.

Prepare child and family for hair loss.

Reassure child and family that hair loss is temporary.

Prepare child and family for hair regrowth that differs in color and texture from former hair.

Arrange for another child in same developmental stage to visit child and talk about the experience.

Suggest use of scarf, hat, or wig before hair loss as transition measure.

Pain

Evaluate child's verbal and nonverbal behavior for evidence of pain.

Note cultural factors affecting pain behavior.

Use age-appropriate terminology when asking child about pain experience.

Monitor vital signs.

Evaluate sleep patterns that may be altered by pain.

Monitor side effects of analgesics and narcotics.

Offer approaches to deal with pain such as hypnosis, biofeedback, relaxation techniques, imagery, distraction, cutaneous stimulation, and desensitization.

Leukopenia

Observe for signs and symptoms of infection and inflammation.

Monitor vital signs.

Continued

TABLE 49-1
Nursing Interventions Related to the Child Undergoing Chemotherapy and Radiotherapy—cont'd

Responses	Nursing Interventions
	Screen visitors for contagious diseases and infections.
	Monitor white blood cell count and differential.
	Ensure that good hygienic measures are maintained.
	Prevent breaks in skin integrity (e.g., keep nails short, prevent injuries).
Thrombocytopenia	Observe for signs and symptoms of bleeding (petechiae and/or hemorrhage).
	Monitor vital signs.
	Monitor platelet count.
	Prevent injury or trauma to body.
	Avoid taking temperature rectally.
	Avoid giving injections.
	Monitor platelet transfusions.
	Provide pressure on bleeding sites.
Anemia and/or fatigue	Evaluate signs and symptoms of anemia.
	Monitor complete blood count and differential.
	Provide for periods of rest and sleep.

	Encourage quiet play activities.
Increased risk of fractures	Avoid weight bearing on affected limb. Prevent accidents and injuries. Encourage nonambulatory play activities.
Delayed physical and sexual development	Provide anticipatory guidance to parents about child's growth retardation, skeletal deformities, and delayed sexual development. Discuss possibility of sterility with child and family.
Hypersensitivity to the medication, resulting in anaphylactic shock	Have available the following medications: hydrocortisone, epinephrine, and diphenhydramine (Benadryl). Observe for dyspnea, restlessness, and urticaria.
Phlebitis and necrosis of tissue, resulting from infiltration of IV infusion	Avoid administration of vesicant agents near a joint. Stop IV flow if infiltration is suspected. Tissue may be treated with drug-specific antidote and hydrocortisone. Apply warm compress to site (with some chemotherapy, compresses are not applied). Continue to observe site for signs of inflammation and necrosis. Grafting and surgical excision may be indicated if necrosis results.

ECG, Electrocardiogram; *IV,* intravenous; *PO,* by mouth.

   f. Children with AML will also need additional antimicrobial coverage if they develop fever since they are at an increased risk for *Streptococcus viridans* infection. They are also routinely prescribed antifungal prophylaxis throughout therapy because of the aggressive nature of their therapy.

3. Monitor for signs and symptoms of bleeding.
   a. Check skin for bruising and petechiae.
   b. Check for nosebleeds and bleeding gums.
   c. If injection is given, apply pressure to site for longer than usual (approximately 3 to 5 minutes) to ensure that bleeding has stopped. Check again later to be sure bleeding has not restarted.
   d. Avoid aspirin-containing products. Avoid all use of rectal thermometers, suppositories, or examination because of increased risk of bleeding.

4. Monitor for signs and symptoms of anemia.
   a. Assess for pallor of skin, sclera, palmar creases.
   b. Prevent patient from sudden changes in position, which may cause postural hypotension, dizziness.
   c. Promote rest to prevent dyspnea, tachycardia and cardiorespiratory compromise in presence of severe anemia.
   d. Monitor oxygen saturation and provide supplemental oxygen as needed.

5. Monitor for signs and symptoms of complications (refer to side-effects in the earlier Chemotherapy sections).
   a. CNS symptoms: these symptoms—headache, blurred or double vision, vomiting—can indicate CNS leukemic involvement.
   b. Respiratory symptoms: these symptoms—coughing, lung congestion, dyspnea—may indicate *Pneumocystis* or other respiratory infection.
   c. Tumor lysis: rapid cell lysis after chemotherapy in patients with a high tumor burden can affect blood chemistry results, causing increased uric acid, hyperkalemia, hyperphosphatemia, and hypocalcemia.

6. Monitor for concerns and anxiety about diagnosis of cancer and its related treatments; monitor for emotional responses such as anger, denial, and grief (see the Supportive Care section in Appendix F).

7. Support involvement in age-appropriate activities as tolerated.
   a. Contact with peers.
   b. School attendance in inclusive settings.
   c. Minimize intrusive effects (school absences) of treatment regimen and disease exacerbations by ensuring continuity with academic pursuits with the development and implementation of a 504 plan or individualized education plan (IEP) (refer to Appendix G).
   d. Participate in recreational and leisure activities.
   e. Participate in sports and physical activities.
8. Monitor disruptions in family functioning.
   a. Base all interventions on family's cultural, religious, educational, and socioeconomic background.
   b. Involve siblings as much as possible, because they have many concerns and feelings about changes in child and in family's functioning.
   c. Consider possibility that siblings feel self-blame and guilt.
   d. Encourage family unity by allowing 24-hour visitation privileges for all family members.

🏠 Discharge Planning and Home Care

The interventions identified for acute care management apply for long-term care as well.

CLIENT OUTCOMES

1. Child will achieve remission.
2. Child will be free of complications from the disease and from the side effects of treatment.
3. Child and family will learn to cope effectively with management of the disease.

REFERENCES

Baquiran DC: *Lippincott's cancer chemotherapy handbook*, ed 2, Philadelphia, 2001, Lippincott, Williams & Wilkins.

Barbour V: Long-term safety now priority in leukaemia therapy, *Lancet* 355 (9211):1247, 2000.

Bryant R: Managing side effects of childhood cancer treatment, *J Pediatr Nurs* 18(1):87, 2003.

Chessells JM: Recent advances in management of acute leukaemia, *Arch Dis Child* 82(6):438, 2000.

Colby-Graham MF, Chordas C: The childhood leukemias, *J Pediatr Nurs* 18 (1):87, 2003.

Friebert SE, Shurin SB: Acute lymphocytic leukemia. Part 1. ALL: Diagnosis and outlook, *Contemp Pediatr* 15(2):118, 1998.

Friebert SE, Shurin SB: Acute lymphocytic leukemia. Part 2. ALL: Treatment and beyond, *Contemp Pediatr* 15(3):39, 1998.

Golub TR, Arceci RJ: Acute myelogenous leukemia. In: Pizzo PA, Poplack DG: *Principles and practice of pediatric oncology*, ed 5, Philadelphia, 2004, Lippincott, Williams & Wilkins.

Greaves M: Childhood leukaemia, *BMJ* 324(7332):283, 2002.

Kanarek RC: Facing the challenge of childhood leukemia, *Am J Nurs* 98(7):42, 1998.

Kline NE: *The pediatric chemotherapy and biotherapy curriculum*, Glenview, IL, 2004, Association of Pediatric Oncology Nurses.

Margolin JF, Steuber CP, Poplack DG: Acute lymphoblastic leukemia. In Pizzo PA, Poplack DG: *Principles and practice of pediatric oncology*, ed 5, Philadelphia, 2004, Lippincott, Williams & Wilkins.

Smith MA, Gloeckler Ries LA: Childhood cancer: Incidence, survival and mortality. In: Pizzo PA, Poplack DG: *Principles and practice of pediatric oncology*, ed 5, Philadelphia, 2004, Lippincott, Williams & Wilkins.

Yeh CH: Adaptation in children with cancer: research with Roy's model, *Nurs Sci Q* 14(2):141, 2001.

50

Meningitis

PATHOPHYSIOLOGY

Meningitis is an acute inflammation of the meninges. The organisms responsible for bacterial meningitis invade the area either directly as a result of a traumatic injury or indirectly when they are transported from other sites in the body to the cerebrospinal fluid (CSF). A variety of agents can produce an inflammation of the meninges including bacteria, viruses, fungi, and chemical substances.

Since the introduction and widespread use of the *Haemophilus influenzae* type B (HIB) vaccine, this organism has been largely controlled in the developed world. The principal bacterial pathogen in children and adults is *Streptococcus pneumoniae*, followed by *Neisseria meningitidis*. In infants 0 to 3 months of age, the most common causes are group B *Streptococcus*, *Escherichia coli*, and *Listeria monocytogenes*.

Aseptic meningitis is usually caused by enteroviruses and affects young adults more often than children. Older children usually manifest a variety of nonspecific prodromal signs and flulike symptoms that last for 1 to 2 weeks. Although fatigue and weakness may persist for a number of weeks, sequelae are uncommon. The child is evaluated and treated until bacterial meningitis is ruled out. Viral meningitis usually requires only a brief hospitalization; supportive care at home is the primary intervention.

Otitis media, sinusitis, or respiratory tract infections may constitute the initial stage of infection. Newer technology, such as cochlear implants, may also lead to meningitis. Head injuries, penetrating wounds, and neurosurgery may also provide an opening into the meninges, leading to meningitis. In addition, a predisposition resulting from an immune deficiency increases the likelihood of occurrence of this disorder. Once the meninges are infected, the organisms are spread through the CSF to the brain and adjacent tissues.

Prognosis varies depending on the individual's age, the infecting organism, the speed with which antibiotic therapy is initiated, and the presence of complicating factors. Neonatal meningitis is associated with a high mortality rate and an increased incidence of neurologic sequelae. Meningococcal meningitis can also be rapidly fatal. In many affected individuals, bacterial meningitis can result in long-term behavioral changes, motor dysfunction, hearing loss, and cognitive changes such as perceptual deficits and learning disorders.

Ensuring vaccination with HIB vaccine during the infant and toddler years, and meningococcal vaccine during preteen years or before college entry can go a long way in prevention of meningitis. All children with cochlear implants should also receive pneumococcal vaccine to prevent meningitis caused by *S. pneumoniae*. Children with immune deficiencies are also recommended to have these vaccines.

INCIDENCE

1. Of all bacterial meningitis cases, 90% are in children younger than 5 years of age.
2. More males than females contract meningitis.
3. Age range of peak incidence is 6 to 12 months.
4. Age range with the highest rate of morbidity is birth to 4 years.
5. Meningitis occurs mostly during winter and early spring.
6. About 171,000 people worldwide die from bacterial meningitis yearly.

CLINICAL MANIFESTATIONS
Neonates

1. Subnormal temperature or low-grade fever
2. Pallor
3. Lethargy or somnolence
4. Irritability or fussiness
5. Poor feeding and/or sucking
6. Vomiting

7. Seizures
8. Poor tone or opisthotonic posturing
9. Diarrhea and/or vomiting
10. Bulging fontanelles

Infants and Young Children

1. Lethargy
2. Irritability
3. Pallor
4. Anorexia or poor feeding
5. Nausea and vomiting
6. Increased crying
7. Insistence on being held
8. Increased intracranial pressure
9. Increased head circumference
10. Bulging fontanelles
11. Seizures
12. "Sunset eyes"

Older Children

1. Headache
2. Fever
3. Vomiting
4. Irritability
5. Photophobia
6. Spinal and nuchal rigidity
7. Positive Kernig's sign
8. Positive Brudzinski's sign
9. Opisthotonic posturing
10. Petechiae (*H. influenzae* and meningococcal meningitis)
11. Septicemia
12. Shock
13. Disseminated intravascular coagulation (DIC)
14. Confusion
15. Seizures

COMPLICATIONS

1. Neurologic: subdural effusions (20% to 30% of cases), hydrocephalus, cerebral edema, chronic seizure disorder,

paresis of facial muscles, developmental delay or intellectual impairments
2. Sensory: deafness or hearing loss, blindness
3. Endocrine: increased secretion of antidiuretic hormone

LABORATORY AND DIAGNOSTIC TESTS

1. Lumbar puncture and culture of cerebrospinal fluid (CSF) with the following results:
   a. White blood cell count—increased to more than 100,000/mm^3
   b. Gram stain of CSF
   c. Glucose level—decreased (bacterial); normal (viral)
   d. Protein—high (bacterial, tubercular, congenital infections); slightly elevated (viral infections)
   e. Pressure—increased, higher than 50 mm Hg in noncrying infant and higher than 85 mm Hg in child
   f. Testing to identify causative organism—*N. meningitidis,* gram-positive organisms (streptococci, staphylococci, pneumococci, *H. influenzae*), or viral agents (coxsackievirus, echovirus)
   g. Lactic acid level—elevated (bacterial)
2. Serum glucose level—elevated
3. Complete blood count with differential, platelet count
4. Blood culture—to identify causative organism
5. Urine culture and urinalysis—to identify causative organism
6. Nasopharyngeal culture—to identify causative organism
7. Serum electrolyte levels—elevated if child is dehydrated; increased serum sodium (Na); decreased serum potassium (K)
8. Urine osmolarity—increased with increased secretion of antidiuretic hormone

MEDICAL MANAGEMENT

Meningitis is considered a medical emergency requiring early recognition and treatment to prevent neurologic damage. The child is placed in respiratory isolation for at least 24 hours after the initiation of therapy with intravenous (IV) antibiotics to which the causative organism is sensitive. Steroids may be administered as an adjunct to decrease the inflammatory process. Intravenous hydration therapy is instituted to correct electrolyte imbalances, in addition to providing hydration. With this fluid administration, the infused volume must be assessed frequently to prevent fluid overload complications such as cerebral edema. Frequent assessment of neurologic status is crucial. Treatment is then directed toward the identification and management of complications of the disease process. The most common complications are subdural effusion, DIC, and shock.

NURSING ASSESSMENT

1. See the section on Neurologic Assessment in Appendix A.
2. Assess hydration status; strictly record intake and output.
3. Assess for pain.
4. Assess for sensory deficits.

NURSING DIAGNOSES

- Sensory perception, Disturbed
- Fluid volume, Deficient
- Pain
- Injury, Risk for
- Knowledge, Deficient
- Infection, risk for

NURSING INTERVENTIONS

1. Monitor infant's or child's vital signs and neurologic status as often as every hour.
   a. Temperature, respiratory rate, apical pulse
   b. Level of consciousness
   c. Equality of pupil size, pupil reaction to light
   d. Movement of extremities
2. Monitor child's hydration status.
   a. Skin turgor
   b. Urinary output
   c. Urinary osmolarity
   d. Signs and symptoms of hyponatremia
   e. Urine specific gravity
   f. Intake and output
   g. Weight (daily measurement)
   h. Daily head circumference in infants.

3. Monitor child for seizure activity (see Chapter 69).
4. Institute isolation procedures with respiratory precautions to protect others from infectious contact; keep child in isolation for 24 hours after antibiotic therapy is started.
5. Monitor IV infusion and side effects of medications.
   a. Antibiotics
   b. Anticonvulsants
   c. Steroids
6. Provide comfort measures in environment that is quiet and has minimal stressful stimuli.
   a. Avoid bright lights and noise.
   b. Avoid excessive manipulation of child.
   c. Organize care into blocks of time, allowing for undisturbed blocks of time.
7. Position child with head of bed slightly elevated to decrease cerebral edema; monitor administration of fluids.
8. Reduce temperature through use of tepid sponge baths or antipyretics agents (acetaminophen, ibuprofen).
9. Provide emotional support when child undergoes lumbar puncture and other tests.
   a. Provide age-appropriate explanations before procedures.
   b. Restrain child to prevent occurrence of injury.
10. Provide emotional and other support to family.
    a. Provide and reinforce information about condition and hospitalization.
    b. Encourage expression of feelings of guilt and self-blame.
    c. Encourage use of preexisting support sources.
    d. Provide for physical comforts (e.g., sleeping arrangements, hygiene needs).
11. Provide age-appropriate diversional activities (see relevant section in Appendix F).

🏠 Discharge Planning and Home Care

1. Instruct parents about administration of medications and monitoring for side effects.

2. Instruct parents in monitoring for long-term complications and their signs and symptoms (learning disabilities and other educational difficulties).
3. Assess immunization status and recommend that parents consult child's primary care provider regarding needed immunizations.

CLIENT OUTCOMES

1. Child will return to normal central nervous system status or may control central nervous system symptoms.
2. Child will not experience neck and/or head pain.
3. Child will experience minimal (if any) academic or learning difficulties after recovery.

REFERENCES

Centers for Disease Control: *2006 Childhood Immunization Schedule* (website): www.cdc.gov/mmwr/preview/mmwrhtml/mm5451-Immunizationa1.htm. Accessed January 13, 2006.

Halket S et al: Long term follow up after meningitis in infancy: Behaviour of teenagers, *Arch Dis Child* 88(5):395, 2003.

Mandelco BL, Potts NL: Neurological alterations. In: Potts NL, Mandleco BL, editors: *Pediatric nursing: Caring for children and their families,* Clifton Park, NY, 2002, Delmar.

Medscape News Feature: Possible link between cochlear implants and bacterial meningitis, *Medscape* (serial online): www.medscape.com/viewarticle/439607. Accessed January 1, 2006.

Nigrovic LE, Kupperman N, Malley R: Development and validation of a multivariable predictive model to distinguish bacterial from aseptic meningitis in children in the post-Haemophilus influenza era, *Pediatrics* 110(4):712, 2002.

Porter V: Bacterial meningitis: A deadly but preventable disease, *Medscape* (serial online): www.medscape.com/viewarticle/481019. Accessed January 1, 2006.

Rusk J: Shift seen in burden of bacterial meningitis since 1998, *Infect Dis Child* 19(1):26, 2006.

Waknine Y: FDA warns of continuing meningitis risk in cochlear implant recipients, *Medscape* (serial online): www.medscape.com/viewarticle/523106. Accessed February 15, 2006.

51

Muscular Dystrophy

PATHOPHYSIOLOGY

The muscular dystrophies constitute a group of muscle diseases characterized by severe muscle weakness and atrophy, elevation of serum muscle enzyme levels, and destructive changes of muscle fibers. Affected muscles pseudohypertrophy, and the muscle tissue is replaced by connective tissue and fatty deposits. The traditional classification into Duchenne's muscular dystrophy (DMD), Becker's muscular dystrophy, limb-girdle dystrophies, and congenital dystrophies has become more precise with advances in genetics and the ability to identify specific defective proteins.

The most common form of muscular dystrophy (MD), Duchenne's, is a sex-linked recessive disorder, with mutation of the dystrophin gene and deficiency or absence of dystrophin in skeletal muscle. Onset of symptoms is between 3 to 5 years of age. It is characterized by progressive involvement of voluntary muscles: clumsy gait, lordotic posture, calf hypertrophy, and toe walking are early manifestations. Children with DMD rarely live beyond 20 years of age without mechanical ventilatory support.

Becker's MD is a sex-linked recessive disorder that involves a reduction in dystrophin, and it is the second most common form. Onset is between 5 and 15 years of age, with survival into the fourth or fifth decade.

Emery-Dreifuss muscular dystrophy (EDMD) has two genetic forms, an X-linked recessive form and a less common autosomal dominant one. EDMD is associated with mutations in emerin, a nuclear membrane protein. Symptoms begin within the first 2 decades of life. Muscle wasting of the biceps and triceps occurs and progresses to include pectoral and pelvic muscles. Typically early development of contractures and cardiac conducton defects occurs.

Limb-girdle muscular dystrophies may be autosomal dominant, autosomal recessive, or congenital. Diagnosis is made by identifying the missing protein with muscle biopsy. Symptoms are a slow onset of progressive muscle weakness; the age of onset varies.

Fascioscapulohumeral muscular dystrophy is the third most common type of MD; it usually begins in the second decade of life. It is an autosomal dominant disease. Muscle biopsy results vary. Clinical symptoms include the classic scapular winging as a result of early weakness of the scapular muscles.

INCIDENCE

1. DMD affects 1 of every 3000 boys (X-linked recessive). Rarely, girls can be affected.
2. DMD accounts for approximately 50% of all cases of muscular dystrophy.
3. Becker's MD affects boys and occurs in approximately 1 in 30,000 to 40,000 male births. Limb-girdle MD has approximately the same incidence.
4. Fascioscapulohumeral MD affects both sexes.
5. Approximately 30% of the sisters of boys with muscular dystrophy will be carriers, and one half of their male offspring will inherit the disease.
6. Learning disabilities and mild mental retardation are not uncommon in MD.
7. Female carriers of DMD are at risk of developing cardiomyopathy and require periodic cardiovascular screening.

CLINICAL MANIFESTATIONS

Symptoms are related to the voluntary muscles that are affected. The most frequently occurring symptoms are the following:

1. Weakness and poor balance
2. Difficulty climbing stairs
3. Waddling gait or toe walking

4. Gowers' sign (hands "climbing" up legs when arising from sitting position)
5. Difficulty running, clumsiness
6. Difficulty lifting arms above head owing to involvement of shoulder girdle muscles
7. Often, loss of ambulation by age 8 to 12 years (Duchenne's) or 40 years (Becker's)
8. Pseudohypertrophy, particularly of calf muscles, giving a hard, "woody" appearance
9. Occurrence of scoliosis after child becomes wheelchair dependent

COMPLICATIONS

1. Cardiac: cardiac decompensation, cardiomyopathy, arrythmias, heart failure
2. Pulmonary: pulmonary compromise, infections, pulmonary failure
3. Musculoskeletal: osteoporosis, contractures, scoliosis
4. Obesity
5. Depression
6. Cognitive delays and learning disabilities

LABORATORY AND DIAGNOSTIC TESTS

1. Creatine phosphokinase level—marked increase in early stages of disease
2. Genetic and protein studies, such as dystrophin deletion studies—identification of MD type
3. Muscle biopsy—diagnostic; indicates absence of dystrophin and gives evidence of severe destructive myopathy

MEDICAL MANAGEMENT

A comprehensive, interdisciplinary team approach is used in the long-term management of MD in children. Generally, an interdisciplinary approach with participation of specialists in neurology, orthopedics, physical and occupational therapy, psychology and/or social work, and nursing is used. In those with Duchenne's MD, spinal fusion is usually performed in early adolescence or when the curvature is between 30 to 50 degrees. Optimal timing for surgery is while lung function is satisfactory and before cardiomyopathy is severe enough to increase the risk of an arrythmia occurring under anesthesia.

Respiratory management requires periodic evaluation including pulmonary function studies, patient education, and decision making about what mechanical ventilatory support is desired. Typically, normal pulmonary function fails, resulting in ineffective cough, inadaquate nighttime ventilation, and then inadequate daytime and nighttime ventilation as the disease progresses. Appropriate mechanical support can prolong and improve quality of life. Cardiac evaluation should be done upon diagnosis and at least biannually starting at age 10 years or with presentation of symptoms. Some studies claim to show benefit from the use of steroids in the treatment of DMD, increasing muscle strength and function as well as prolonging pulmonary function. Controversy persists, however, and steroid use is not yet uniformly recommended. Ongoing research supports the use of gene and cell therapies, but this treatment is not considered ready for clinical practice.

NURSING ASSESSMENT

1. See the Musculoskeletal Assessment section in Appendix A.
2. Assess child's adherence to physical therapy regimen.
3. Assess child's and family's adherence to pulmonary regimen.
4. Assess child's level of self-care functioning.
5. Assess child's and family's level of coping (refer to Appendix F).
6. Assess child's and family's management of home treatment regimen. Assess home equipment needs.
7. Assess child's and family's need for information.
8. Consult with school nurse to assess for special accommodations needed at school (see Appendix G).

NURSING DIAGNOSES

- Mobility, Impaired physical
- Growth and development, Delayed
- Constipation (related to decreased mobility)
- Gas exchange, Impaired
- Nutrition: more than body requirements, Risk for imbalanced
- Family processes, Interrupted

- Diversional activity, Deficient
- Self-care deficit, Bathing/hygiene
- Self-care deficit, Dressing/grooming
- Self-care deficit, Toileting
- Self-esteem, Chronic low
- Home maintenance, Impaired
- Knowledge, Deficient
- Therapeutic regimen management, Ineffective
- Caregiver role strain
- Grieving, Dysfunctional

NURSING INTERVENTIONS

1. Advise use of braces and splints as indicated to avoid contractures.
2. Advise consumption of high-fiber, low-fat diet with adequate water intake.
3. Advise use of breathing aids to assist in gas exchange.
4. Assist parents in expressing and working through feelings of guilt, resentment, and anger.
5. Encourage and support parents seeking genetic counseling and support in self-care and health maintainance.
6. Encourage parents and siblings to mourn (loss of "perfect" child) and to learn to cope.
7. Encourage participation in academic and peer support groups (see Appendixes F and G).
8. Advise importance of avoidance of secondhand smoke, routine immunizations, and annual influenza immunization.

🏠 Discharge Planning and Home Care

1. Promote optimal muscular functioning.
   a. Reinforce physical therapy exercise regimen.
   b. Discourage inactivity; encourage moderate activity with frequent rest periods.
2. Promote self-care activities as means of enhancing child's sense of independence and self-sufficiency.
   a. Investigate and recommend use of adaptive devices as appropriate.

b. Provide recommendations for home adaptations (e.g., grab bars, overhead slings, raised toilets, ramps, alternating pressure mattresses).

c. Recommend use of adaptive equipment as necessary (e.g., braces to prevent slumping and to facilitate standing so as to prevent contractures).

d. Facilitate acquisition of durable medical equipment such as wheelchair, hospital bed, lifting devices, and respiratory support equipment as needed.

3. Encourage parents, in collaboration with child, to select realistic goals for achievement and living.
4. Provide support for child and family as they cope with disease.
   a. Refer to social worker or psychologist.
   b. Refer to Muscular Dystrophy Association (www.mda.org).
   c. Refer to parent support group.
   d. Refer to peer support group.
5. Provide information about and make referrals to available educational resources (see Appendix G).
   a. Refer parents to educational specialist.
   b. Promote child's full inclusion in school.
6. Provide information and assess long-term care needs pertaining to the following:
   a. Scoliosis
   b. Pulmonary and cardiac problems
   c. Contractures, especially of hips, knees, and ankles
   d. Genetic transmission
   e. End of life planning including respiratory support and palliative care options as disease progresses (Appendix H)

CLIENT OUTCOMES

1. Child will maintain optimal physical mobility.
2. Child will maintain optimal cardiopulmonary function.
3. Child will maintain inclusion in social, educational, and recreational activities as able.
4. Child and family will make informed decisions about treatment and management of the disease including respiratory support, end of life issues, and advance directive.
5. Child and family will express feelings as disease progresses.

REFERENCES

American Thoracic Society: Respiratory care of the patient with Duchenne muscular dystrophy: ATS consensus statement, *Amer J Respir Crit Care Med* 170(4):456, 2004.

Biggar W, Douglas MD: Duchenne muscular dystrophy, *Pediatr Rev* 27(3):83, 2006.

Klitzner T et al: Cardiovascular health supervision for individulas affected by Duchenne or Becker muscular dystrophy, *Pediatrics* 116(6):1569, 2005.

Moxley RT III et al: Practice parameter: Corticosteroid treatment of Duchenne dystrophy: Report of the quality standards, Subcommittee of the American Academy of Neurology and the Practice Committee of the Child Neurology Society, *Neurology* 64(13):13, 2005.

Nolan MA et al: Cardiac assessment in childhood carriers of Duchenne and Becker muscular dystrophies, *Neuromusc Disorders* 13(2):129, 2003.

Robinson L, Linden M: Muscle disorders. In: Robinson, L. (Ed). *Clinical genetics handbook,* ed 2, Boston, 1993, Blackwell Scientific.

Sritippayawan S et al: Initiation of home mechanical ventilation in children with neuromuscular diseases, *J Pediatr* 142(2):481, 2003.

Tidball J, Wehling-Henricks M: Evolving therapeutic strategies for Duchenne muscular dystrophy: Targeting downstream events, *Pediatr Res* 56(6):831, 2004.

52

Necrotizing Enterocolitis

PATHOPHYSIOLOGY

Necrotizing enterocolitis (NEC) is the most common acquired gastrointestinal (GI) disease among sick newborns and is the single most common surgical emergency among newborns. It is a spectrum of illness that varies from a mild, self-limiting process to a severe disorder characterized by inflammation and diffuse or patchy necrosis in the mucosal and submucosal layers of the intestine. The cause of NEC has been the focus of research for over 30 years; although many theories have been proposed, however, the pathogenesis remains elusive and controversial. Most researchers agree that, regardless of the initiating event(s), the pathogenesis of NEC is multifactorial. At present, the etiology is thought to involve three major pathologic mechanisms occurring in combination to create a favorable disease environment: ischemic injury to the bowel, bacterial colonization of the bowel, and the presence of a substrate such as formula.

The hypoxic or ischemic injury causes a reduced blood flow to the bowel. Birth asphyxia, umbilical artery cannulation, persistence of a patent ductus arteriosus, respiratory distress syndrome, maternal cocaine abuse, and/or exchange transfusion may be the initiating factor(s). Intestinal hypoperfusion damages the intestinal mucosa, and the mucosal cells lining the bowel stop secreting protective enzymes. Bacteria, whose proliferation is aided by enteral feedings (substrate), invade the damaged intestinal mucosa. Bacterial invasion results in further intestinal damage because of the release of bacterial toxins and hydrogen gas. The gas initially dissects into the serosal and submucosal layers of the bowel (pneumatosis intestinalis).

The gas may also rupture through the bowel into the mesenteric vascular bed, where it can be distributed to the venous system of the liver (portal venous air). The bacterial toxins in combination with ischemia result in necrosis. Full-thickness bowel necrosis results in perforation, with the resulting release of free air into the peritoneal cavity (pneumoperitoneum) and peritonitis. This chain of events is considered a surgical emergency.

INCIDENCE

The incidence of NEC varies considerably from nursery to nursery, both within a given geographic region and from region to region. These estimates may not accurately reflect the true incidence because of inconsistencies in definitions and in reporting of cases that are complicated by other confounding variables such as prematurity.

1. NEC occurs in 1% to 8% of all infants admitted to neonatal intensive care units.
2. NEC occurs in 6% to 10% of neonates with birth weights of less than 1500 g.
3. Seventy to 90% of cases occur in high-risk low birth weight infants.
4. Of infants who develop NEC, 10% to 25% are full-term. Many of these infants have specific risk factors such as asphyxia, intrauterine growth retardation (IUGR), umbilical vessel catheters, anatomic GI malformations, polycythemia, or other medical problems.
5. NEC is the third leading cause of neonatal death, with an overall mortality rate of 20% to 40%.
6. Extremely low birth weight infants (1000 grams) are particularly vulnerable, with reported mortality rates of 40% to 100%.
7. Mortality rates for term versus preterm infants are reported as 4.7% and 11.9%, respectively.
8. Of those who survive, approximately 23% experience long-term sequelae related to the GI tract.
9. There is a slightly increased prevalence in male infants.
10. In some studies, higher NEC rates are seen in African-American than in white or Hispanic neonates.

CLINICAL MANIFESTATIONS

The onset of NEC occurs most commonly between days 3 and 12 of life, but it can occur as early as the first 24 hours of life or as late as 90 days of age. The disease is characterized by a broad range of signs and symptoms that reflect the differences in severity, complications, and mortality of the disease. Typically, suspected NEC (stage I) consists of nonspecific clinical findings that represent physiologic instability and may resemble the findings of other common conditions in premature infants. These include the following:

1. Temperature instability
2. Lethargy
3. Recurrent apnea and bradycardia
4. Hypoglycemia
5. Poor peripheral perfusion
6. Increased pregavage gastric residuals
7. Feeding intolerance
8. Emesis (that may or may not be bilious)
9. Mild abdominal distention
10. Guaiac-positive stools

Proven NEC (stage II) consists of the aforementioned nonspecific clinical findings plus the following:

1. Severe abdominal distention
2. Abdominal tenderness
3. Grossly bloody stools
4. Palpable bowel loops
5. Edema of abdominal wall
6. Possible absence of bowel sounds

Advanced NEC (stage III) occurs when the infant becomes acutely ill with peritonitis and/or radiographic evidence of intestinal perforation. Associated signs and symptoms include the following:

1. Deterioration of vital signs
2. Evidence of septic shock
3. Edema and erythema of abdominal wall
4. Right lower quadrant abdominal mass
5. Acidosis (metabolic and/or respiratory)
6. Disseminated intravascular coagulation

COMPLICATIONS

1. Immediate complications include the following:
   a. Cardiac: patent ductus arteriosus, shock
   b. Respiratory: respiratory failure (91%)
   c. GI: perforation, hepatic failure (15%)
   d. Renal: renal failure (85%)
   e. Hematologic: sepsis (9%), anemia, disseminated intra-
      vascular coagulation, thrombocytopenia
2. Long-term complications include the following:
   a. Neurologic: neurodevelopmental sequelae (15% to 33%)
   b. GI: stricture (10% to 35%), short bowel syndrome (9%
      to 23%), recurrent NEC (4% to 6%), complications from
      total parenteral nutrition (TPN) (15%), malabsorption
      (23%), anastomotic leak, cholestasis, enterocolic fistula
      (2%), atresia

LABORATORY AND DIAGNOSTIC TESTS

1. Laboratory results that reflect signs of sepsis include the
   following:
   a. Complete blood count with differential
      i. Leukopenia (total white blood cell [WBC] count
         below 6000/mm^3)
      ii. Elevated WBCs with increased band count
      iii. Thrombocytopenia (platelet count above 50,000/
         mm^3)—50% of infants with proven NEC have
         platelet counts <50,000/mm^3
      iv. Absolute neutrophil count less than 1500 cells/mm^3
   b. Serum electrolyte imbalance
      i. Hyponatremia
      ii. Hyperkalemia
      iii. Acidosis: metabolic; low serum bicarbonate
         (<20 meq)
   c. Arterial blood gases
      i. Hypoxia
      ii. Acidosis: respiratory
      iii. Hypercapnea
   d. Cultures: positive results of blood, stool, or urine cultures

2. Radiologic findings are the cornerstone for confirming the diagnosis of NEC. The standard anteroposterior and left lateral decubitus (or cross-table lateral) radiographs may show any or all of the following:
   a. Focal, nonspecific gaseous distention of bowel loops
   b. Thickening of bowel wall from edema
   c. Pneumatosis intestinalis (bubbles of subserosal air in bowel wall)
   d. Persistently dilated bowel loop
   e. Portal venous air
   f. Pneumoperitoneum (free abdominal air)
3. Other diagnostic studies are emerging that may be of diagnostic benefit, particularly in the early stages of NEC. These include the following:
   a. Portal vein ultrasonography—detects microbubbles in the portal vein before they can be identified on plain radiograph
   b. Abdominal ultrasonography—recent data suggest that ultrasonographic assessment of major splanchnic vasculature can help in the differential diagnosis of NEC from other more benign and emergent disorders
   c. Upper GI series with metrizamide contrast—detects pneumatosis before it is identified on plain radiograph
   d. Paracentesis—a positive finding with at least 0.5 ml of brownish fluid that contains bacteria on Gram staining is highly specific for intestinal necrosis

MEDICAL MANAGEMENT

In the absence of intestinal necrosis or perforation, aggressive medical management is the treatment of choice. Medical management is based on three general principles: (1) rest the bowel, (2) prevent continuing injury, and (3) correct or modify the systemic responses. Enteral feedings are discontinued, the GI tract is decompressed by low intermittent suction, and fluid and electrolyte imbalances are corrected. Intravenous antibiotic therapy directed against enteric flora is started; respiratory support, including intubation and ventilation, is often required; and efforts to support blood pressure and adequate perfusion to the bowel prevent continuing injury and help to correct systemic responses. Abdominal radiographs are obtained every 6 to 8 hours to monitor progression of the disease or detect perforation.

Although many infants can be treated successfully with medication and bowel rest, 25% to 50% require surgery. Indications for surgical intervention differ from institution to institution. A hallmark of successful surgical therapy is the anticipation of impending intestinal necrosis before perforation occurs to prevent gross peritoneal contamination. Evidence of progressive deterioration and ongoing necrosis is noted in worsening metabolic acidosis, respiratory failure, thrombocytopenia, oliguria, shock, and increasing abdominal wall distention. Indications for immediate surgical intervention are (1) pneumoperitoneum, (2) presence of portal venous air, (3) abdominal wall erythema or edema, and (4) intestinal gangrene (positive results on test of abdominal paracentesis specimen).

The principles of surgical management include (1) intestinal decompression, (2) careful examination of bowel with resection of perforated or unquestionably necrotic tissue, (3) preservation of as much bowel as possible, (4) preservation of the ileocecal valve if possible, and (5) preservation of bowel of questionable viability, with creation of a stoma proximal to this bowel. Marginally viable bowel may not be removed during the initial procedure; rather, resection may be deferred, with a follow-up second-look operation carried out in 24 to 48 hours to reassess bowel viability.

The type of surgical procedure required depends on the extent of bowel necrosis. If a short segment of necrotic bowel is present, a primary anastomosis may be adequate. Extensive necrosis or necrosis in a variety of areas may necessitate resection and placement of an enterostomy. If an extensive amount of necrotic bowel is resected, the infant may be left with an insufficient length of bowel for digestion, which causes malabsorption, failure to thrive, and short bowel syndrome.

The timing of stoma closure is somewhat arbitrary. If the infant is thriving on enteral feedings and is gaining weight, the stoma is usually closed at 3 to 5 months. A very proximal stoma that necessitates TPN or one that causes serious fluid and electrolyte problems should be closed sooner, usually after 4 to 6 weeks. If a stricture is found, it is resected during the procedure to close the stoma, and complete intestinal continuity is reestablished.

NURSING ASSESSMENT

1. See the Cardiovascular Assessment, Respiratory Assessment, and Gastrointestinal Assessment sections in Appendix A.
2. Assess hydration status.
3. Assess infant's temperature.
4. Assess postoperative pain.
5. Assess family coping strategies.

NURSING DIAGNOSES

- Infection, Risk for
- Fluid volume, Risk for deficient
- Nutrition: less than body requirements, Imbalanced
- Tissue perfusion, Ineffective
- Pain
- Parenting, Risk for impaired

NURSING INTERVENTIONS

1. Monitor cardiac and respiratory status (may need to monitor as often as every hour during acute phase of disease).
2. Observe and report signs of change in cardiac status.
3. Observe and report signs of change in respiratory status.
4. Administer antibiotics as ordered.
5. Promote and maintain adequate body temperature.
6. Assess and maintain optimal hydration status.
    a. Ensure adequate intake of fluids (100% to 150% of maintenance level).
    b. Monitor urine output (1 to 2 ml/kg/hr).
    c. Monitor orogastric tube drainage.
    d. Maintain nothing-by-mouth (NPO) status.
7. Administer pain medications as ordered.
8. Promote process of attachment between parents and infant.

9. Provide developmentally appropriate stimulation activities (see relevant section in Appendix F).

Preoperative Care

1. Monitor infant's condition before surgery.
   a. Measure abdominal girth (assess for increasing abdominal distention).
   b. Monitor vital signs every 1 to 2 hours.
   c. Monitor for GI complications (perforation).
   d. Monitor fluid and electrolyte status (intake and output, orogastric tube drainage).
   e. Arrange for radiologic examination every 6 to 8 hours.
2. Prepare infant for surgery by obtaining assessment data.
   a. Complete blood count, urinalysis, serum glucose level, blood urea nitrogen level
   b. Baseline electrolyte levels
   c. Blood coagulation testing
   d. Type and cross-match of blood
3. Prepare parents for infant's surgery.
   a. Provide information regarding disease process.
   b. Allow parents to express feelings.
   c. Emphasize that surgery will not immediately cure infant and that critical postoperative period is not unusual.

Postoperative Care

1. Monitor infant's response to surgery.
   a. Vital signs
   b. Intake and output—report discrepancies
   c. Surgical site—bleeding, intactness, signs of infection
2. Monitor for and report signs and symptoms of complications.
   a. Increased need for respiratory support
   b. Decreased urinary output
   c. Bleeding
3. Promote and maintain fluid and electrolyte balance.
   a. Record parenteral intake accurately.
   b. Record output per route (urine, orogastric tube drainage, stoma drainage).

   c. Assess hydration status (signs of dehydration, electrolyte imbalance).
4. Provide dressing care; maintain integrity of surgical site and stoma area.
5. Protect infant from infection.
   a. Monitor incision for drainage, redness, and inflammation.
   b. Administer antibiotics as ordered.
6. Promote comfort and minimize pain.
   a. Provide position of comfort using blanket rolls or positioning mattress.
   b. Cluster care.
   c. Monitor infant's response to nonpharmacologic comfort measures (swaddling, containment).
   d. Monitor infant's response to pain medications.
7. Provide emotional support to parents during infant's hospitalization.
   a. Encourage parental expression of feelings.
   b. Provide reinforcement of parents' caregiving activities.
   c. Encourage parents to call and visit as often as possible.

🏠 Discharge Planning and Home Care

1. Encourage parents to express concerns about outcomes of surgery.
2. Refer to specific institutional procedures for information to be distributed to parents about home care.
3. Instruct parents regarding signs of intestinal obstruction, strictures, poor tolerance of feedings, and impaired healing processes.
4. Instruct parents about follow-up techniques to promote optimal surgical outcomes.
   a. Ostomy care
   b. Central line care (if on long-term TPN)
5. Provide family with name of physician to contact for medical or health care follow-up.

CLIENT OUTCOMES

1. Infant will return to normal GI function.
2. Infant's growth will continue at steady pace following growth chart parameters.
3. Parents will verbalize understanding of home care and follow-up needs.

REFERENCES

Berseth CL, Poenaru D: Necrotizing enterocolitis and short bowel syndrome. In: Taeusch HW, Ballard RA, and Gleason CA, editors: *Avery's diseases of the newborn*, ed 8, Philadelphia, 2005, WB Saunders.

Henry MC, Moss RL: Current issues in the management of necrotizing enterocolitis, *Semin Perinatol* 28(3):221, 2004.

Maayan-Metzger A et al: Necrotizing enterocolitis in full-term infants: Case control study and review of the literature, *J Perinatol* 24(8):494, 2004.

Pierro A, Hall N: Surgical treatment of infants with necrotizing enterocolitis, *Semin Neonatol* 8(3):223, 2003.

Reber KM, Nankervis CA: Necrotizing enterocolitis: Preventative strategies, *Clin Perinatol* 31(1):157, 2004.

Salhab WA et al: Necrotizing enterocolitis and neurodevelopmental outcome in extremely low birth weight infants <1000 grams, *J Perinatol* 24(9):531, 2004.

St Peter SD, Ostlie DJ: Necrotizing enterocolitis. In: Ashcraft KW et al, editors: *Pediatric surgery*, ed 4, Philadelphia, 2005, WB Saunders.

Thigpen JL, Kenner C: Assessment and management of the gastrointestinal system. In: Kenner C et al, editors: *Comprehensive neonatal nursing*, ed 3, St. Louis, 2003, WB Saunders.

53

❖

Nephrotic Syndrome

PATHOPHYSIOLOGY

Nephrotic syndrome is the clinical state in which the glomerular membrane has an increased permeability to plasma proteins. This leads to severe edema, proteinuria, and hypoalbuminemia. The loss of protein from the vascular space causes decreased plasma osmotic pressure and increased hydrostatic pressure, resulting in the accumulation of fluids in interstitial spaces and the abdominal cavity. The decrease in vascular fluid volume stimulates the renin-angiotensin system, resulting in secretion of antidiuretic hormone (ADH) and aldosterone. Tubular resorption of sodium (Na^+) and water is increased, expanding the intravascular volume. This fluid retention leads to increased edema as retained fluid shifts into the interstitial space. Coagulation and venous thrombosis may occur as a result of decreased vascular volume, which causes hemoconcentration and urinary loss of coagulation proteins. Loss of immunoglobulins through the glomerular membrane can lead to increased susceptibility to infection. Hyperlipidemia is believed to occur because of increased synthesis of lipoproteins in response to low plasma oncotic pressure.

Nephrotic syndrome is the pathologic outcome of various factors that alter glomerular permeability. The causes of nephrotic syndrome can be categorized into primary (idiopathic) and secondary (Box 53-1). Primary nephrotic syndrome is divided into three histologic groups: minimal-change nephrotic syndrome (MCNS), focal segmental glomerulosclerosis (FSGS), and membranous neuropathy (rare in children). Based on clinical classification, the syndrome types differ according to the course of the disease, treatment, and prognosis. It is considered a chronic

BOX 53-1
Causes of Nephrotic Syndrome

Primary

- Minimal-change nephrotic syndrome (MCNS)—most common type
- Focal segmental glomerulosclerosis (FSGS)—10% to 15% of pediatric nephrotic syndrome
- Glomerular disease
- Immunoglobulin A (IgA) neuropathy
- Systemic lupus erythematosus
- Finnish type of congenital nephrotic syndrome
- Genetic and congenital disorders
- Metabolic disorders
- Various syndromes
- Sickle cell disease

Secondary

- Infection (bacterial, hepatitis, human immunodeficiency virus [HIV], malaria, syphilis, toxoplasmosis)
- Medications
- Radiocontrast dye
- Vascular disease
- Heredity diseases
- Heavy metals
- Cancer
- Allergic nephrosis

illness because of the occurrence of relapses. Many children will have five or more relapses over the course of the disease. A child is considered to have frequently relapsing nephrotic syndrome if there are two or more relapses within the first 6 months and/or four or more relapses within a 12-month period. The frequency of relapse decreases over time and becomes relatively rare by adolescence.

INCIDENCE

1. The prevalence of idiopathic nephrotic syndrome is approximately 16 per 100,000.

2. Idiopathic nephrotic syndrome can occur at any age. Most often, it first manifests in children between ages 2 and 6 years.
3. Of all cases of nephrotic syndrome in children, 80% are MCNS. Incidence is slightly greater in males.
4. The mortality and prognosis of children with nephrotic syndrome vary with the disorder's etiology and severity, the extent of renal damage, the child's age and underlying condition, and response to treatment.
5. Nephrotic syndrome mortality and prognosis can range from complete recovery to causing end-stage renal disease (ESRD).
6. Children with MCNS tend to have a good prognosis.
7. Prognosis is more likely to be poor in children who do not respond to treatment and/or with some of the less common types of nephrotic syndrome such as FSGS.

CLINICAL MANIFESTATIONS

Although the child's symptoms will vary with different disease processes, the most common symptoms associated with nephrotic syndrome are the following:
1. Decreased urine output with dark, frothy urine
2. Edema (may be severe)
   a. Most commonly seen as facial, periorbital, abdominal, and/or genital and in the extremities.
   b. Often facial and/or periorbital edema is most severe in the morning when the child wakes. As the child is upright throughout the day, edema may shift to the abdomen, the genitals, and the extremities.
   c. Respiratory difficulty, abdominal pain, anorexia, and diarrhea may occur due to abdominal distention.
3. Pallor
4. Fatigue and activity intolerance
5. Abnormal laboratory test values

COMPLICATIONS

1. Fluid/electrolyte balance: intravascular volume depletion (hypovolemia), respiratory compromise (related to fluid

retention and abdominal distention), skin breakdown (from severe edema, poor healing)

2. Cardiovascular: hypercoagulability (venous thrombosis)
3. Immune: infection (especially cellulitis, peritonitis, pneumonia, septicemia)
4. Multiple body systems: untoward side effects of medications, growth failure, and muscle wasting (long-term)

LABORATORY AND DIAGNOSTIC TESTS

Nephrotic syndrome is generally diagnosed based on clinical presentation and laboratory test results.

Refer to Appendix D for laboratory and diagnostic values.

1. Urinalysis, urine dipstick—to detect protein and blood in the urine.
   a. Proteinuria (urinary protein loss)
   b. Hematuria (may be microscopic)
2. Urinary protein/creatinine ratio—calculated to monitor persistent proteinuria; best if first void of the morning is used; more accurate than 24-hour urine protein collection
   a. Normal value <0.5
   b. Values of >2 mg protein/mg creatinine are associated with nephrotic syndrome
3. Serum chemistry, lipid panel—to assess electrolytes, serum protein, renal function, lipids
   a. Serum electrolytes—vary with individual disease states and treatments
   b. Blood urea nitrogen and creatinine—may be increased if renal impairment has occurred
   c. Serum albumin—decreased, related to protein loss
   d. Serum cholesterol and triglycerides—increased and related to increased lipoprotein synthesis
4. Complete blood count—to monitor for hemoconcentration and infection
   a. Hemoglobin, hematocrit, and platelets—increased (related to hemoconcentration)
   b. White blood cell count—may be increased if infection is present

5. Renal biopsy—is done to determine the glomerular status, type of nephrotic syndrome, response to medical management, and disease course, most often used for patients who are steroid resistant and/or steroid dependent. Microscopic evaluation shows abnormal appearance of basement membranes.

MEDICAL MANAGEMENT

Medical management will vary according to the type of nephrotic syndrome and as new data are available regarding the efficacy of various treatments. Corticosteroids (prednisone, prednisolone) are traditionally administered daily until remission is achieved (cessation of urinary protein loss). Corticosteroids are usually tapered off by administering on alternate days and/or with decreasing doses. Children with MCNS tend to respond quickly to steroid therapy. Approximately 75% achieve remission by 2 weeks and 95% by 8 weeks. Only about 20% of children with FSGS achieve remission by 8 weeks. Relapses may be treated with additional courses of corticosteroids. For children who fail to achieve remission after 8 weeks of steroids, they are often deemed "steroid resistant." Immunosuppressive therapy (alkylating agents [cyclophosphamide, chlorambucil], cyclosporine, or levamisole) may be used to stimulate remission in children with steroid-resistant nephrotic syndrome and/or to decrease the frequency of relapses. Dietary sodium restriction (no added salt) is used to reduce edema. A high protein diet and/or intravenous albumin infusion are used for protein replacement and to restore fluid balance.

Diuretic therapy may be needed to treat severe edema (i.e., when severe fluid retention interferes with respiration and/or causes skin breakdown). Diuretics should be used with caution to prevent intravascular volume depletion, thrombus formation, and/or electrolyte imbalances. Electrolyte replacement is administered as needed. Antibiotics may be administered to prevent or treat infection. Pain (related to edema and invasive therapy) may be treated with medications and nonpharmacologic approaches (see Appendix I). Anticoagulants may be used to prevent or treat thrombosis. Antihypertensives (i.e., angiotensin-converting enzyme [ACE] inhibitors) may be used as needed to control blood pressure and decrease urinary protein losses.

NURSING ASSESSMENT

1. Assess for signs and symptoms of fluid volume excess.
   a. Local edema: periorbital, facial, external genitalia, and/or extremities
   b. Abdominal edema (ascites): clothing that feels or appears to be "too tight," increased abdominal girth, abdominal distention with taut and shiny skin (severe edema)
   c. Anasarca (severe, generalized edema)
   d. Weight gain
   e. Decreased urine output
   f. Dark, frothy urine
   g. Pulmonary congestion, increased respiratory effort, pleural effusions, pulmonary edema
2. Assess for signs of electrolyte imbalance.
   a. Assess for signs of hypokalemia.
      i. Cardiovascular: arrhythmias, flattened T waves, decreased ST segment, widened QRS, increased PR interval, gallop rhythm, increased or decreased heart rate, hypotension
      ii. Central nervous system (CNS) and musculoskeletal: apathy, drowsiness, muscle weakness, muscle cramping, hyporeflexia
   b. Assess for signs of hyponatremia (related to diuresis).
      i. CNS: apathy, weakness, dizziness, lethargy, encephalopathy, seizures
      ii. Cardiovascular: hypotension
      iii. Gastrointestinal (GI): nausea, abdominal cramping
   c. Assess for signs of hypernatremia (related to hemoconcentration)
      i. CNS: disorientation, muscle twitching, lethargy, irritability
      ii. GI: intense thirst, dry membranes, nausea, and vomiting
      iii. Other: dry, flushed skin; increased temperature; oliguria

3. Assess protein loss and nutritional status.
   a. Monitor serum protein and urine lab tests.
   b. Assess appetite and nutritional intake.
   c. Assess nails for signs of prolonged hypoalbuminemia (white [Muehrcke's] lines parallel to the lanula).
   d. Assess for pallor.
   e. Assess for irritability, weakness, and fatigue.
4. Assess for side effects from medication administration.
   a. Steroids: cushingoid features, hyperglycemia, infection, hypertension, obesity, GI bleeding, growth retardation, bone demineralization, cataracts
   b. Alkylating or cytotoxic agents: leukopenia, infection, GI discomfort, GI bleeding, alopecia, impaired growth, gonadal dysfunction and/or sterility (long-term effect)
   c. Diuretics: intravascular volume depletion, thrombus formation, electrolyte imbalance
   d. Antihypertensives: hypotension, dizziness
   e. Anticoagulants: bleeding (GI, nose bleeds, oozing from puncture sites, etc.)
5. Assess for signs of decreased cardiovascular functioning (hypotension, hypertension, shock, congestive heart failure, cardiac arrhythmias, fluid volume deficit).
   a. Blood pressure (hypotension or hypertension)
   b. Heart rate and rhythm (tachycardia, arrhythmias)
   c. Distal perfusion (pulses, capillary refill, temperature, color)
   d. Left ventricular hypertrophy (arrhythmias, increased heart size, decreased output)
6. Assess for signs of orthopnea, pulmonary congestion, and/or pulmonary infection.
   a. Respiratory rate and pattern (tachypnea, irregular pattern)
   b. Use of accessory muscles (retractions, shoulder shrugging) and nasal flaring
   c. Need to sit upright or to have the head of the bed elevated
   d. Abnormal breath sounds (rales, ronchi, decreased breath sounds in lower lobes)
   e. Abnormal chest x-ray

     f. Cyanosis, decreased oxygen saturations

     g. Respiratory acidosis

  7. Assess for signs of infection.

     a. Fever

     b. Increased white blood cell count

     c. Positive cultures (pulmonary secretions, urine, blood, other body fluids)

     d. Signs of cellulitis: local swelling, redness, tenderness

     e. Signs of pneumonia (see above)

     f. Signs of peritonitis: red, tender abdomen

     g. Septicemia, septic shock

  8. Assess for skin breakdown from severe edema.

  9. Assess child's comfort level and ability to tolerate activity. Address child's and family's concerns and fears related to disease and altered body image.

10. Assess child's and family's coping response to illness.

     a. Assess family functioning related to child's irritability and mood swings.

     b. Assess coping related to altered body image from severe edema and pallor.

     c. Assess child's and family's response to bed rest and activity limitation.

NURSING DIAGNOSES

- Fluid volume, Excess; Fluid volume, Risk for deficient (related to diuresis and/or vascular loss)
- Imbalanced nutrition: less than body requirements
- Breathing pattern, Ineffective
- Impaired skin integrity, Risk for
- Infection, Risk for
- Pain
- Comfort, Impaired
- Fatigue; Activity intolerance
- Knowledge, Deficient
- Ineffective Coping
- Disturbed Body Image

NURSING INTERVENTIONS

1. Monitor and maintain fluid balance.
   a. Assess hydration status frequently.
   b. Monitor ascites by monitoring abdominal girth.
   c. Closely monitor edematous areas; report changes as indicated.
   d. Measure and record daily weights; report changes as indicated.
   e. Record accurate input and output.
   f. Administer diuretics if ordered; assess effectiveness; closely monitor for side effects.
   g. Replace fluids lost as a result of interstitial fluid shifts.
   h. Administer albumin if ordered to increase vascular volume and serum protein.
   i. Monitor type of fluids and administration rate to avoid fluid overload and cerebral edema while maintaining adequate vascular volume.
   j. Promote bed rest as needed during periods of severe edema and periods of rapid weight loss during periods of diuresis.
2. Monitor electrolytes on an ongoing basis. Administer measures to correct electrolyte imbalance as indicated.
3. Encourage and support nutritional intake and proper nutritional status.
   a. Continually monitor appetite and nutritional intake.
   b. Complete calorie counts and nutritional screens as indicated.
   c. Provide diet high in calories and protein.
   d. Decrease sodium intake (avoid high-sodium foods, no added salt diet).
   e. Avoid extreme salt restrictions or extremely high-protein foods since these may be undesirable to children and/or lead to paradoxic problems.
   f. Allow the child as many dietary choices as possible; provide child's favorite foods as allowed.
   g. Offer food in small quantities and in an attractive manner.

    h. Support family in providing a calm, relaxed atmosphere during mealtimes (avoid high-pressure feeding or disruptive events).

    i. Consider intravenous (IV), nasogastric, or nasojejunal feedings if patient is unable to maintain proper nutritional status.

    j. Collaborate with clinical nutritionist as indicated.

4. Assess adequacy of ventilation and promptly implement airway stabilization methods as indicated; encourage patient to cough and deep breathe (refer to Nursing Assessment in this chapter for signs of respiratory distress).

5. Maintain skin integrity and prevent infection.

    a. Practice good handwashing, use of alcohol based agents, and aseptic technique.

    b. Provide skin care, eye care, and perianal care on an ongoing basis.

    c. Reposition and turn patient frequently; prevent pressure ulceration with pressure relief/reduction surfaces; avoid hard objects (tubing, cables) under patient.

    d. Avoid restrictive clothing, armbands, and tape.

    e. Place on pressure-relief surface as needed if there is severe edema and/or skin breakdown.

    f. Maintain sterility of all invasive lines, and perform dressing changes and site care as needed and on schedule.

    g. Monitor for signs of infection and implement appropriate interventions as indicated.

6. Monitor for pain and provide pain relief measures as needed (see Appendix I).

    a. Assist child to find comfortable positions; reposition frequently.

    b. Administer analgesics as needed.

    c. Use nonpharmacologic pain relief methods as appropriate.

    d. Continually reevaluate the effectiveness of pain relief measures.

7. Provide emotional support to child and family (see Appendix F).

    a. Coping and managing the disease

    b. Dealing with changes with bodily appearance and function

🏠 Discharge Planning and Home Care

1. Provide child and parents with developmentally appropriate verbal and written instruction regarding home management of the following:
   a. Disease process: expected clinical progress and signs of relapse
   b. Medications: dose, route, schedule, side effects, complications
   c. Nutrition: high-protein, low-salt diet guidelines
   d. Prevention of infection: avoid live virus vaccination and other conditions that may lead to infection while on high-dose steroids or receiving immunosuppressive therapy
   e. Skin care: assess for breakdown; prevent breakdown
   f. Pain management: nonpharmacologic pain measures and analgesic agents
   g. Activity: limitations as needed, promote return to normal activity level as symptoms resolve
   h. Follow-up care as indicated

CLIENT OUTCOMES

1. Child will maintain fluid/electrolyte and acid/base balances within appropriate limits.
2. Child will have optimal nutrition, growth, and development.
3. Child and family will adhere to treatment regimen, and complications will not occur.
4. Child will maintain optimal comfort level and coping with illness.
5. Child will resume activities of daily living.

REFERENCES

ANNA Pediatric Nephrology Special Interest Group: *Pediatric nephrotic syndrome fact sheet* (website): www.annanurse.org/download/reference/practice/pns.fact.pdf. Accessed February 7, 2007.

Broome L: Treating pediatric nephrotic syndrome: A clinical challenge, *Nephrol Nurs J* 30(6):662, 2003.

Eddy A, Symons JM: Nephrotic syndrome in childhood, *Lancet* 362(9):384, 2003.

Luxner KL: *Delmar's pediatric nursing care plans,* ed 3, Clifton Park, NY, 2005, Delmar Thompson Learning.

Moses S: *Family practice notebook: Urine protein to creatinine ratio* (website): www.fpnotebook.com/URO72.htm. Accessed May 4, 2006.

54

Neuroblastoma

PATHOPHYSIOLOGY

Neuroblastomas are soft, solid tumors originating from neural crest cells that are precursors of the adrenal medulla and sympathetic nervous system. Neuroblastomas can occur wherever sympathetic nervous tissue is found. The majority of tumors are usually in the abdomen, either in the adrenal gland or the sympathetic ganglia. Less common primary sites include the paraspinal area of the thorax, the neck, and the pelvis. Neuroblastomas often impinge on adjacent tissues and organs and can metastasize to the lymph nodes, bone, bone marrow, and/or subcutaneous tissue. Researchers are studying genetic mutations in the neuroblastoma cells as they seek to identify the etiology of neuroblastoma.

INCIDENCE

1. Neuroblastoma is the most common extracranial solid tumor of childhood and the most common neoplasm of infants.
2. It is the second most common type of childhood tumor.
3. Approximately 650 new cases are diagnosed each year in the United States.
4. The estimated incidence is 1 in 7000 births.
5. Neuroblastoma most commonly occurs in children between birth through the fourth year of life.
6. The unique phenomenon of spontaneous tumor regression and maturation into benign forms may allow many cases of neuroblastoma to go undetected.
7. Survival rates are 90% in low-risk patients, 70% to 90% in intermediate-risk patients, and 30% in high-risk patients

(see Medical and Surgical Management section in this chapter).

CLINICAL MANIFESTATIONS

1. Symptoms related to abdominal mass
   a. Firm, irregular abdominal mass that crosses midline
   b. Altered bowel and/or bladder function
   c. Vascular compression with edema of lower extremities
   d. Back pain, weakness of lower extremities
   e. Sensory loss
   f. Loss of sphincter control
2. Symptoms related to neck or thoracic mass
   a. Cervical and supraclavicular lymphadenopathy
   b. Congestion and edema of face
   c. Respiratory dysfunction and/or distress
   d. Ecchymotic orbital proptosis
   e. Horner's syndrome (unilateral ptosis, myosis, and anhidrosis)
3. Symptoms related to metastasis to bone and/or bone marrow
   a. Fatigue
   b. Pain
   c. Fever
   d. Limp
4. Symptoms related to catecholamine secretion
   a. Hypertension
   b. Sweating
   c. Flushing
   d. Irritability

COMPLICATIONS

1. At diagnosis: Depending on the location of the tumor, neuromuscular complications can include lower-extremity weakness or paralysis. A hematologic complication is metastasis to lymph nodes, bone, and bone marrow.
2. During treatment: Adverse events from chemotherapy, radiation therapy, and/or surgery can be life-threatening. These can include infection and organ toxicities.

LABORATORY AND DIAGNOSTIC TESTS

1. Complete blood count—to detect anemia caused by many secondary factors (e.g., hemorrhage, disseminated intravascular coagulation)
2. Urinary levels of catecholamines (vanillylmandelic acid and homovanillic acid)—tumor markers that are elevated owing to overproduction by tumor cells or defective storage within tumor cells
3. Ferritin level—increase correlates with poorer prognosis
4. Neuron-specific enolase level—elevated owing to correlation with amount of active neuronal tissue
5. Bilateral bone marrow aspiration and biopsies—to reveal marrow involvement, confirm diagnosis, and allow staging
6. Chest radiographic study—to delineate primary thoracic neuroblastoma and vertebral and paravertebral involvement
7. Computed tomography and magnetic resonance imaging—to determine extent of disease
8. Bone scan—to assess for metastasis
9. Metaiodobenzylguanidine (MIBG) scan—to assess involvement of bone and tissue. An MIBG scan provides a scintigraphic image of neuroendocrine tumors.
10. Tumor biopsy—for pathologist to examine tumor tissue and provide diagnosis. Biology studies provide information on which risk category is based. These studies include the following elements:
    a. *MYCN* status (a proto-oncogene)—nonamplified (favorable) versus amplified (unfavorable)
    b. Shimada histopathology—favorable versus unfavorable
    c. DNA index—hyperdiploid (>1) (favorable) versus diploid (1) (unfavorable)

MEDICAL AND SURGICAL MANAGEMENT

The international staging system for neuroblastoma (INSS) standardizes definitions and categorizes disease according to radiographic and surgical findings, plus bone marrow status. Localized tumors are divided into stages 1, 2A, and 2B depending on the extent of tumor excision and the status of regional lymph nodes. In stage 3, the tumor crosses the vertical midline of the body (marked by the spine) and cannot be removed surgically, or the tumor is restricted to one side of the body but there are lymph nodes on the opposite side of the body that are positive for cancer. The patient with stage 4 neuroblastoma has had the disease spread to distant lymph nodes, bone, bone marrow, liver, skin, and/or other organs. Stage 4S is a unique stage; the "S" stands for "special." These tumors often spontaneously regress without any treatment. The child with stage 4S must be less than 12 months of age and have a localized primary tumor that has spread only to the skin, the liver, or the bone marrow.

The Children's Oncology Group, the pediatric cancer cooperative study group in North America, is investigating a system for assigning patients to treatment according to one of three risk groups, low, intermediate, or high. The risk is based on the child's INSS stage, age, *MYCN* status, Shimada histology, and DNA ploidy.

Children with a low-risk tumor are generally treated with surgical resection. Stage 2 low-risk tumors are treated with chemotherapy only if less than 50% of the tumor has been removed. In the other low-risk children, chemotherapy is recommended only for life-threatening symptoms that cannot be relieved by safe surgical resection of the tumor. Chemotherapy agents include carboplatin, cyclophosphamide, doxorubicin, and etoposide, given in moderate doses. The treatment of children with low-risk 4S neuroblastoma is determined by the child's symptoms.

Intermediate-risk tumors are treated with moderate doses of carboplatin, cyclophosphamide, doxorubicin, and etoposide given for 12 to 24 weeks. Surgical resection may be done before starting chemotherapy, or, if surgery cannot be performed safely, it may be delayed until the completion of chemotherapy.

Children who are in the high-risk group are treated aggressively with high doses of combination chemotherapy. Agents used include cyclophosphamide, ifosfamide, cisplatin, carboplatin, vincristine, doxorubicin, and etoposide. After the primary tumor has been shrunk with induction chemotherapy, surgical resection is performed. Children are then treated with myeloablative chemotherapy and stem cell rescue (i.e., bone marrow and/or peripheral blood stem cell transplantation). Radiation treatment is given to the primary tumor site. Some children may also receive radiation to sites of metastasis. After recovery, children are treated with the biologic modifier oral 13-cis-retinoic acid for 6 months. Current research is investigating the use of purged peripheral blood stem cells for use in the stem cell rescue procedure. Immunologic interventions that are currently being studied use monoclonal antibodies to the GD2 ganglioside, an antigen expressed on the surface of neuroblastoma cells.

NURSING ASSESSMENT

1. Refer to Appendix A for system-specific assessments.
2. Be aware that physical assessment depends on tumor site and related system. Palpation of tumor site should be avoided.
3. Be aware that assessment of the child with neuroblastoma should encompass all aspects of medical treatment, including chemotherapy, surgery, radiation, and stem cell transplantation.
4. Assess child for verbal and nonverbal expressions of pain (see Appendix I).
5. Assess child and family's coping responses.
6. Assess child's level of development (see Appendix B).

NURSING DIAGNOSES

- Anxiety
- Infection, Risk for
- Pain, Acute
- Gas exchange, Impaired
- Fatigue
- Fluid volume, Excess
- Fluid volume, Deficient
- Mobility, Impaired physical
- Nutrition, less than body requirements, Imbalanced
- Therapeutic regimen management, Ineffective
- Growth and development, Delayed

- Knowledge, Deficient re cancer and its treatment
- Family processes, Interrupted

NURSING INTERVENTIONS
Surgical Phase

1. Prepare child for clinical staging procedures with age-appropriate approach (see the Preparation for Procedures or the Surgery section in Appendix F).
2. Monitor for signs of infection including fever, chills, lethargy, erythema, and/or drainage at central line site and/or surgical site.
3. Monitor respiratory function including respiratory rate and effort, lung auscultation, and oxygen saturation.
4. Provide fluid and electrolyte management including the following: monitor intake and output (I&O), monitor electrolytes, replace drainage and electrolytes per order, assess chemistries, assess skin turgor and mucous membranes, and assess for edema.
5. Provide pain management (refer to Appendix I).

Chemotherapy and/or Radiation Phase

1. Assess tumor site using observation and inspection; palpation is contraindicated.
2. Minimize side effects of multiagent chemotherapy and radiation therapy. Refer to Table 49-1 in chapter on leukemia: Nursing Interventions Related to the Child Undergoing Chemotherapy and Radiotherapy.
3. Observe for medication or transfusion reactions.
4. Assess integrity of skin and mucous membranes.
5. Monitor for signs of infection including fever, chills, lethargy, erythema, and/or drainage at central line site.
6. Monitor physical and emotional growth and development of child (see Appendix F).
7. Teach parents about medications their child is receiving (see Appendixes B and E).
8. Refer child and/or siblings to child life specialist.
9. Assess for pain using age-appropriate technique (see Appendix I).

10. Provide pain management (see Appendix I).

🏠 Discharge Planning and Home Care

Instruct parents about home care management:

1. Signs of infection and guidelines on when to seek medical attention.
2. Postoperative wound care after tumor excision including assessment of wound site, cleansing site, and changing dressing.
3. Care of child's central venous access device, including site care, dressing change, flushing, cap change, and emergency care.
4. Adherence with treatment and medical appointments.
5. Facilitate understanding of the action of the medications and monitoring of their untoward effects.
6. Ensure the child's nutritional needs are met including use of home enteral nutrition.
7. Observe for potential behavioral changes in child and/or siblings following hospitalization and during long-term management of the child's medical needs. Direct families in activities to support ongoing growth and development.
8. Refer family to social services for support and resource utilization (see Appendix G).

CLIENT OUTCOMES

1. Child and family will demonstrate ability to cope with life-threatening illness.
2. Child will be free of infection.
3. Child and family will understand home care and long-term follow-up needs.
4. Child will progress in achieving developmental milestones.
5. Child will maintain/exceed body mass index (BMI) baseline status.
6. Child will be free of pain.
7. Child will resume prehospital and/or pretreatment levels of activity.

REFERENCES

Brodeur GM, Maris JM: Neuroblastoma. In: Pizzo PA, Poplack DG, editors: *Principles and practice of pediatric oncology,* ed 5, Philadelphia, 2006, Lippincott, Williams & Wilkins.

Curesearch: *Neuroblastoma* (website): www.curesearch.org/for%5Fparents%5Fand
%5Ffamilies/newlydiagnosed/article.aspx?ArticleId=145&StageID=1&TopicId
=1&Level,=1. Accessed March 9, 2006.

Dadd G: Neuroblastoma. In: Baggott CR et al, editors: *Nursing care of children
and adolescents with cancer,* ed 3, Philadelphia, 2002, WB Saunders.

Duffey-Lind E: Neuroblastoma. In: Kline NE, editor: *Essentials of pediatric
oncology nursing: A core curriculum,* ed 2, Glenview, IL, 2004, Association
of Pediatric Oncology Nurses.

Kline NE, Sevier N: Solid tumors in children, *J Pediatr Nurs* 18(2):96, 2003.

National Cancer Institute: *Neuroblastoma (PDQ) Health Professional Version*
(website): www.cancer.gov/cancertopics/pdq/treatment/neuroblastoma/
HealthProfessional/page1. Accessed March 9, 2006.

55

❖

Newborn Screening for Genetic Disorders

PATHOPHYSIOLOGY

Infants born with inborn errors of metabolism lack an enzyme essential in the body's biochemical reactions, or have deficient amounts of it. All ingested food is broken down into fats, proteins, carbohydrates, vitamins, and minerals, and is then metabolized by enzymes. An enzyme deficiency, as seen with inborn errors of metabolism, prevents the usual chain of biochemical reactions, referred to as the metabolic pathway, from occurring properly. Instead, abnormal chains of metabolic substances are formed owing to a deficiency in the key, normally present enzyme, which can cause a number of untoward outcomes, as observed with inborn errors of metabolism. Box 55-1 presents numerous genetic disorders that are enzyme deficiencies. Most of these enzyme deficiencies are inherited as autosomal recessive traits; others (rarely) are transmitted as sex-linked or mitochondrial disorders.

Metabolic disorders in the newborn are not necessarily identified in the hospital, because the clinical manifestations may not become evident until weeks or even months later. Clinical manifestations can be specific or general, depending on the disorder. Metabolic disorders have been categorized into three types: (1) those that are "silent" or slowly manifest symptoms, such as phenylketonuria (PKU), and that if not treated early can result in mental retardation; (2) those such as urea cycle disorders or organic acidemias that manifest as an acute metabolic crisis shortly after birth (a few days), in which the

BOX 55-1

Inborn Errors of Metabolism

- Disorders of carbohydrate metabolism
- Disorders of galactose metabolism
- Disorders of fructose metabolism
- Carbohydrate malabsorption in the intestinal brush border
- Glycogen storage diseases
- Disorders of amino acid metabolism
- Disorders of histidine metabolism
- Amino acid transport disorders
- Urea cycle disorders
- Branched-chain amino acid and keto acid disorders
- Organic acidemias: disorders of propionate and methylmalonate metabolism
- Disorders of pyruvate dehydrogenase complex
- Disorders of pyruvate carboxylase complex
- Pyruvate kinase and glucose-6-phosphatase deficiencies
- Disorders of lipid metabolism
- Familial hyperlipoproteinemia: familial lipoprotein lipase deficiency
- Familial cholesterolemia
- Disorders of lysosomal enzyme
- Gangliosidoses
- Disorders of purine metabolism

Adapted from Theorell C, Degenhardt M: Assessment and management of metabolic dysfunction. In: Kenner C et al, editors: *Comprehensive neonatal nursing: a physiologic perspective*, ed 2, Philadelphia, 1998, WB Saunders.

infant demonstrates symptoms of respiratory distress, vomiting, and lethargy leading to coma, and which can be life threatening if not identified and treated; and (3) those that cause progressive neurologic disorders, such as Tay-Sachs disease. It is important that these disorders be detected and treated as soon as possible to prevent or minimize serious outcomes of developmental delays, learning disabilities, attention-deficit/hyperactivity disorder, or mental retardation. Widespread screening exists for the following inborn errors of metabolism: (1) PKU, (2) congenital hypothyroidism, (3) galactosemia, (4) maple syrup urine disease, and (5) congenital adrenal hyperplasia. Note that PKU, congenital hypothyroidism, and

BOX 55-2
Newborn Screening Programs

Newborn screening is a general term for a nationwide program, governed by individual states, that uses a simple blood test called tandem mass spectrometry to screen for three categories of disorders: inborn errors of metabolism (e.g., PKU; galactosemia; maple syrup urine disease [MSUD]); hemoglobinopathies (e.g., sickle cell disease [see Chapter 71]; and hemophilia [see Chapter 32]); and endocrinopathies (e.g., congenital hypothyroidism; congenital adrenal hyperplasia; and cystic fibrosis (see Chapter 17). There are over 100 different tests that newborns could be screened with. A complete listing of the tests that are required by each state can be found at www.genes-r-us.uthscsa.edu/nbsdisorders.pdf. A list of resources is included at the end of this chapter for families who may wish to have optional testing done. This chapter focuses primarily on inborn errors of metabolism since sickle cell disease, hemophilia, and cystic fibrosis are covered elsewhere in this book. Newborn screening guidelines are available from the Health Resources and Services Administration of the U.S. Department of Health and Human Services, under the title "U.S. Newborn Screening System Guidelines II: Follow-Up of Children, Diagnosis, Management, and Evaluation: Statement of the Council of Regional Networks for Genetic Services (CORN)" (available from www.ask.hrsa.gov/detail.cfm?id=MCHN011).

galactosemia are the only three newborn screening tests required by all states (Box 55-2).

In the future, gene-based therapy may offer promising options to correct the deficiency of the enzyme or substrate. Risk factors associated with inborn errors of metabolism include past family history of unexplained neonatal and/or sibling deaths, consanguinity, multiple spontaneous abortions, psychomotor difficulties in family members, and symptoms in previous children associated with metabolic diseases, such as metabolic acidosis, ataxia, and hypoglycemia.

INCIDENCE

1. Incidence is fewer than 1 in 10,000 births.
2. Of pregnancy losses, 60% are caused by genetic problems.

3. Of infant mortality, 20% to 30% are due to genetic defects, the leading cause of infant mortality.
4. Between 30% and 50% of postneonatal infant deaths are due to congenital anomalies.
5. Genetic defects are the fourth leading cause of diminished life span.
6. In most infants, autosomal recessive conditions will be identified by 1 month of age.
7. Incidence for certain disorders (e.g., sickle cell disease, Tay-Sachs disease, cystic fibrosis) is higher among specific ethnic groups.

CLINICAL MANIFESTATIONS

A number of presenting symptoms are linked with inborn errors of metabolism. Symptoms may be generalized, or manifestations may be specific. Clinical manifestations associated with selected disorders may include one or more of the following:

1. Neuromuscular dysfunction
2. Cerebral, cognitive, and/or developmental dysfunction
3. Respiratory dysfunction
4. Cardiovascular dysfunction
5. Immunologic or hematologic disturbances
6. Gastrointestinal and/or hepatic dysfunction
7. Genitourinary disturbances
8. Fluid-electrolyte imbalance
9. Integumentary system effects
10. Musculoskeletal abnormalities

COMPLICATIONS

Complications will vary depending on when the enzyme deficiency was identified and treated.

1. Developmental disabilities (the most common are movement or neuromuscular disorders and mental retardation)
2. Irreversible brain damage
3. Coma
4. Congenital heart defects
5. Hepatic failure

LABORATORY AND DIAGNOSTIC TESTS

1. Initial newborn screen—to screen for genetic disorders (see Box 55-3)
2. Listed here are the laboratory tests most commonly used in addition to the initial newborn screen for the diagnosis of inborn errors of metabolism. Selection of tests will depend on the clinical presentation and severity of symptoms (refer to Appendix D for normal ranges).
   a. Serum glucose level
   b. Blood gas values
   c. Serum ammonia level
   d. Complete blood count with differential

BOX 55-3
Newborn Screening Test

Tandem mass spectrometry is abbreviated MS/MS and commonly but erroneously referred to simply as "the PKU test". Blood is collected from the infant's heel and evenly blotted into five circular areas outlined on a special filter paper. The filter paper is allowed to dry immediately after the blood specimen is collected, before sending it to the state health department to be analyzed. The filter paper is attached to an information sheet used by individual states to track documentation and reporting of the results for the newborn from whom the specimen was drawn.

Timing of Screen for Term and Well Newborns:
- Before any blood transfusion
- At 3 to 5 days of life or just before discharge, whichever comes first
- If screened before 24 hours of age, repeat screen is required at 3 to 5 days of age

Timing of Screen for Preterm or Sick Newborns:
- Before any blood transfusion
- At 3 to 7 days of life, or at the time of discharge, whichever comes first; and a repeat screen at 14 days of age
- If screened before 24 hours of age, repeat screen is required at 7-14 days of age

   e. Coagulation studies

   f. Serum electrolyte levels

   g. Blood urea nitrogen assay

   h. Serum creatinine level

   i. Plasma ammonia level

   j. Serum anion gap

   k. Plasma and cerebrospinal fluid lactate levels

   l. Urine test for glucose, ketones, phenylpyruvic acid, toxic substances

  m. Urine level of reducing substances

  n. Urine level of organic acids

  o. Magnetic resonance imaging

  p. Computed tomography

  q. Electroencephalography

  r. Nerve conduction velocity studies

  s. Electromyography

3. In the event of infant death, the following tests should be performed to rule out undiagnosed inborn errors of metabolism as the cause of death:

   a. Skin sample analysis for enzymes and culture of fibroblasts

   b. Needle biopsy of kidney, liver, muscle, and brain

MEDICAL MANAGEMENT

The first priority of medical therapy is to treat the infant who has life-threatening symptoms such as acute metabolic encephalopathy, with the goal of stabilizing the infant. Other acute episodes of illness the infant may experience involve metabolic acidosis, electrolyte disturbances, respiratory distress, intractable seizures, and sepsis. These critical problems require aggressive medical treatment such as exchange transfusion, venovenous hemofiltration, peritoneal dialysis, hemodialysis, and assisted ventilation. The goal of this phase of critical care is stabilization of the infant and prevention of complications.

The approaches to long-term treatment to manage enzyme disorders can be described in the following general terms. Dietary substances creating the toxic substrate, such as phenylalanine, are restricted or excluded from the diet. An enzyme replacement can be given for enzyme deficiencies, similar to thyroid replacement for hypothyroidism. An alternative metabolic pathway can be stimulated that circumvents the blocked metabolic pathway. Clinical status can be improved with the administration of high doses of vitamins (e.g., pyridoxine, biotin, vitamin B_{12}). Enzyme therapy that involves replacing the deficient enzyme with a synthetic product is another treatment option. Depending on the diagnosis, a specific management plan for treatment will be instituted. Treatment plans will vary according to the particular syndrome and include nutritional therapy, such as administration of commercially prepared synthetic formulas; dietary supplementation; and, in some instances, invasive treatments such as splenectomy. Depending on the enzyme involved, bone marrow transplantation, liver transplantation, and gene therapy may be used to correct the metabolic disorder. Early detection and treatment are key to preventing or ameliorating the long-term effects of enzyme deficiencies.

NURSING ASSESSMENT

The purpose of the nursing assessment of the child with an inborn error of metabolism varies depending on the circumstances. During the diagnostic period, nursing assessment is focused on stabilization of the infant's condition, diagnosis of the metabolic disorder, and initiation of the long-term treatment plan. Once the acute phase subsides, nursing assessment is directed to monitoring the child's growth and development, the response to treatment, long-term effects, and family management of the child's ongoing and long-term treatment plan. The assessment information listed below addresses the long-term components of care. Assessment parameters for the acute phase can be found in other chapters pertaining to the infant's presenting symptoms, such as apnea or renal failure.

Ongoing nursing assessment of the child includes obtaining the nursing history and family pedigree (genogram); this includes gathering information on the family history of children with hypoglycemia, acute encephalopathy, metabolic acidosis, and psychomotor difficulties. Information is obtained on the mother's pregnancy history, such as spontaneous abortions, previous pregnancies, and unexplained neonatal deaths.

1. Assess for dysmorphic features, including evaluation of the following:
   a. Shape of head; presence of microcephaly (small for size), macrocephaly (large for size), or hydrocephaly (due to increase in cerebrospinal fluid)
   b. Shape and placement of ears
   c. Face—spacing of features, symmetry, signs of weakness or paralysis
   d. Eyes—level, spacing between eyes, color of iris, lens, epicanthal folds, cataracts, retinal changes
   e. Appearance of neck
   f. Shape of nose
   g. Shape and contour of lips, size of jaw, tongue size
   h. Hair distribution
2. Assess integumentary system.
   a. Skin pigmentation
   b. Ear tag
   c. Hairy patch at base of spine
3. Assess musculoskeletal system.
   a. Poor muscle tone
   b. Size of chest
   c. Extremities, including webbing of fingers, and finger and toe length
4. Assess for neurologic signs and symptoms.
   a. Altered level of consciousness
   b. Lethargy
   c. Deficient motor skills
   d. Abnormal reflexes (hypotonia)
   e. Poor sucking
   f. Seizures
5. Assess for other anomalies (not listed earlier).
6. Assess for signs of infection (fever, increased white blood cell count, septic shock).
7. Assess for skin breakdown from pruritus, malnutrition, edema, and decreased ability to heal.

8. Assess for malnutrition (lethargy, weakness, poor feeding, decreased appetite, vomiting, failure to gain weight, inadequate caloric intake).
9. Assess child's comfort level (see Appendix I).
10. Assess coping responses and child's level of activity, and provide therapeutic environment for child.
    a. Encourage child and parents to express feelings of concern about child's condition.
    b. Provide developmentally appropriate information and reinforce data provided to child and parents (see the Preparation for Procedures or Surgery section in Appendix B and Appendix F).
11. Assess family's ability to manage child's long-term care and to access community-based services, and provide supportive measures as indicated (see Appendix G).
12. Assess for developmental delay, achievement of growth and development milestones, and age at which milestones are achieved (see Appendix B).

NURSING DIAGNOSES

- Injury, Risk for
- Body temperature, Risk for imbalanced
- Intracranial adaptive capacity, Decreased
- Tissue perfusion, Ineffective
- Gas exchange, Impaired
- Respiratory function, Risk for ineffective
- Fluid volume, Excess
- Nutrition: less than body requirements, Imbalanced
- Infection, Risk for
- Family processes, Interrupted
- Growth and development, Delayed
- Therapeutic regimen management, Ineffective
- Caregiver role strain

NURSING INTERVENTIONS
Care During Acute Phase

1. Monitor clinical status and immediately report any changes.
    a. Early signs of encephalopathy:

      i. Poor feeding
     ii. Vomiting
    iii. Lethargy
    iv. Irritability
     v. Abnormal muscle tone

  b. Other symptoms to report immediately:
      i. Apnea episodes
     ii. Drowsiness
    iii. Hiccups
    iv. Myoclonus
     v. Bulging fontanelles
    vi. Change in level of consciousness

2. Maintain cardiorespiratory stability.
  a. Establish infant's baseline respiratory and cardiac values and monitor for changes (see Appendix A).
     i. Monitor depth, symmetry, and rhythm of respirations.
    ii. Monitor rate and quality of heart sounds, murmurs.
  b. Monitor responsiveness to medical interventions.
  c. Monitor trends in oxygenation through oximetry and/or transcutaneous monitoring; monitor correlation between environment, positioning, and transcutaneous monitoring readings.
  d. Monitor arterial blood gas values and laboratory data.
  e. Monitor blood pressure and fluctuations with activity and treatments.
  f. Monitor action and side effects of medications.
  g. Coordinate delivery of routine care and procedures, and cluster care as appropriate.
  h. Suction as needed.
  i. Administer sedative and analgesics as needed.

3. Monitor neurologic status with serial measures.
  a. Report any deterioration or questionable findings; intervention may be required on emergency basis.
  b. Monitor level of consciousness.
     i. General appearance
    ii. Arousability
    iii. Orientation
    iv. Lethargy, reaction to sound, touch, and bright colors

    c. Monitor vital signs.
      i. Respiratory pattern
      ii. Blood pressure
      iii. Heart rate
      iv. Temperature
    d. Check pupils (pupils equal, react to light, accommodate).
    e. Monitor reaction to pain (see Appendix I).
    f. Check head circumference (check fontanelles).
    g. Use Glasgow Coma Scale (see the Neurologic Assessment section in Appendix A).
    h. Provide calm, quiet environment.
4. Monitor and maintain appropriate fluid, nutrient, and caloric intake.
    a. Maintain intravenous access as needed.
    b. Administer feedings via most appropriate route for medical status.
    c. Record weight daily and length and head circumference weekly.
    d. Monitor and record intake and output (including blood products, urine, and stool); check pH and specific gravity.
5. Assess for signs of infection and implement preventive measures.
    a. Practice good handwashing and aseptic technique.
    b. Perform care for all invasive catheters and lines according to institutional procedures.
    c. Adhere to institutional policy for isolation procedures as indicated.

Ongoing and Long-Term Care

1. Monitor for adequate caloric intake and growth over time.
    a. Monitor for weight gain of approximately 20 to 30 g/day (see Appendix E).
    b. Monitor infant's ability to maintain adequate oral intake. (Infants who are tachypneic and have increased work of breathing may not be able to take food orally because of compromise of airway and risk of aspiration.)

    c. Monitor for increased oxygen requirements during and immediately after oral feedings; provide increased oxygen as needed.

    d. Provide supplementation to oral feedings through gavage or gastrostomy tube feedings.

       i. Ensure proper placement of gastrostomy and gavage feeding tubes.

       ii. Monitor for adverse response to feedings.

       iii. Provide oral stimulation with feedings.

2. Promote growth and development by integrating play and positive stimulation into care routine (see Appendix B).

    a. Provide opportunities for developmentally appropriate visual, auditory, tactile, and kinesthetic stimulation when infant is alert and stable.

    b. Integrate pattern and routine into care, including undisturbed nighttime sleep and predictable daytime activities.

    c. Monitor infant's response to caregiving and developmental activities.

    d. Assess for increased oxygen requirements during and immediately following activity.

    e. Assess for patterns of response to activities and caregivers.

    f. Develop list of likes, dislikes, and comfort measures from assessed patterns of response.

    g. Decrease environmental and caregiver stimulation during periods of agitation and/or stress.

3. Facilitate integration of infant into his or her family.

    a. Assist parents in recognizing infant's responses to activity.

    b. Teach parents how they can best interact with and provide care for their child.

    c. Facilitate parents' confidence in caring for their child.

    d. Promote visitation and caregiving by other key family members, including siblings, as soon as appropriate.

4. Refer family to genetic specialists, because genetic counseling is advisable in view of genetic factor(s) associated with inborn errors of metabolism. If parents are planning

for additional children, they may benefit from information about heritable nature of this child's condition.

  a. Carefully record family history, prior reproductive history of couple, and so on (may be very helpful to genetic specialists).

  b. Follow up with family after referral to genetic specialist.

  c. Answer any additional questions; clarify misconceptions.

  d. Reinforce information.

⌂ Discharge Planning and Home Care

1. Evaluate readiness for discharge. Factors to assess include the following:
   a. Stable cardiorespiratory and neurologic status
   b. Adequate nutritional intake and growth
   c. Stable medication needs
   d. Medical treatment plan that is realistic for home
      i. Parents or other caregivers can provide needed care.
      ii. Needed home equipment and monitoring are provided.
      iii. Parents have necessary social and/or financial support.
      iv. Provision is made for respite or home nursing needs.
2. Provide discharge instruction for parents covering the following:
   a. Explanation of genetic disorder
   b. Information on how to monitor for signs of respiratory distress and other medical problems
   c. Individualized feeding needs
   d. Well-baby needs
   e. Guidelines on when to call doctor
   f. Method of performing cardiopulmonary resuscitation
   g. Use of home equipment and monitoring devices
   h. Method of administering medications and monitoring for their effects
   i. Infection prevention
   j. Importance of smoke-free environment
   k. Appropriate developmental activities

l. Recognition of infant's stress and interaction cues
m. Available community resources and support services
(e.g., early intervention) (see Appendix G) (Box 55-4)

3. Provide follow-up to monitor ongoing cardiorespiratory,
neurologic, nutritional, developmental, and other
specialized needs.

BOX 55-4
RESOURCES

(Non-Profit)

- March of Dimes Birth Defects Foundation
  1275 Mamaroneck Avenue
  White Plains, NY 10605
  888-MODIMES or 914-428-7100
  www.modimes.org
- National Newborn Screening and Genetics Resource Center
  1912 W. Anderson Lane, Suite 210
  Austin, TX 78757
  512-454-6419
  genes-r-us.uthscsa.edu
- Save Babies Through Screening Foundation
  4 Manor View Circle
  Malvern, PA 19355-1622
  888-454-3383
  www.savebabies.org

(For-Profit)

- Baylor Medical Center
  800-4Baylor (800-422-9567)
  www.bhcs.com/MedicalSpecialties/MetabolicDisease
- Pediatrix Screening
  P.O. Box 219
  Bridgeville, PA 15017
  866-463-6436
  www.pediatrixscreening.com
- University of Colorado Health Sciences Center at Fitzsimons
  Biochemical Genetics Laboratory
  Mail Stop 8313, P.O. Box 6511
  Aurora, CO 80045-0511
  303-724-3826
  www.uchsc.edu/newbornscreening/contact.htm

a. Help parents make first follow-up appointments; provide written documentation of appointment times.

b. Reinforce and reiterate information provided from genetic evaluation and counseling.

c. Make referral for in-home nursing visits or care based on needs of infant and family.

4. Refer as needed for counseling and other support resources.

a. Refer to counseling professionals.

b. Refer to parent support groups.

c. Refer to community-based family resource centers (see Appendix G).

d. Refer to Internet resources, family support websites.

CLIENT OUTCOMES

1. Infant will have stable physiologic functioning.
2. Infant will reach maximum potential for growth and development.
3. Parents will be competent in care of their child.

REFERENCES

American Academy of Pediatrics, Committee on Bioethics: Ethical issues with genetic testing in pediatrics, *AAP Policy* (serial online): http://aappolicy. aappublications.org/cgi/reprint/pediatrics;107/6/1451.pdf. Accessed May 7, 2006.

Banta-Wright SA, Steiner RD: Tandem mass spectrometry in newborn screening: A primer for neonatal and perinatal nurses, *J Perinat Neonatal Nurs* 18(1):41, 2004.

Bryant KG et al: A primer on newborn screening, *Adv Neonatal Care* 4(5):306, 2004.

Department of Health and Human Services, Centers for Disease Control and Prevention: *Quality assurance and proficiency testing for newborn screening* (website): www.cdc.gov/nceh/dls/newborn_screening.htm. Accessed May 8, 2006.

Health Resources and Services Administration of the U.S. Department of Health and Human Services: *U.S. Newborn screening system guidelines II: Follow-up of children, diagnosis, management, and evaluation: Statement of the Council of Regional Networks for Genetic Services (CORN)* (website): www.ask.hrsa. gov/detail.cfm?id=MCHN011). Accessed May 9, 2006.

National Newborn Screening and Genetics Resources Center: *National newborn screening status report* (website): http://genes-r-us.uthscsa.edu/nbsdisorders. pdf. Accessed May 8, 2006.

Theorell C, Degenhardt M: Assessment and management of the metabolic system. In: Kenner C et al, editors. *Comprehensive neonatal nursing: a physiologic perspective,* ed 3, Philadelphia, 2003, WB Saunders.

56

❖

Non-Hodgkin's Lymphoma

PATHOPHYSIOLOGY

Non-Hodgkin's lymphoma (NHL) is a highly malignant neoplasm of the lymphatic system and lymphoid tissue. As is the case with most childhood neoplasms, the cause of NHL has not been identified. Several factors including viral infections, immunodeficiency, chromosomal aberration, chronic immunostimulation, and environmental exposure have been implicated in precipitating malignant lymphomas.

Childhood NHL tends to have a rapid onset and is characterized by aggressive, widespread disease that generally shows a quick response to treatment. Common sites of involvement include the intraabdominal, mediastinal, peripheral nodal, and nasopharyngeal areas. Common extralymphoid sites include bone, skin, bone marrow, testes, kidneys, intracranial, and the central nervous system (CNS).

Because several classification systems for NHL have been proposed, categorization remains complex. NHL can be divided into three types: (1) lymphoblastic, (2) small non-cleaved cell, and (3) large cell. Favorable prognosis is indicated by the following:

1. Involvement is confined to one lymph node and possibly area surrounding it OR involvement is found in two or more lymph nodes either above or below the diaphragm (Stage 1).
2. Found in an area of one organ outside the lymph system OR located in localized group of lymph nodes with extension into a nearby organ (Stage 11).
3. No lymphoma is found outside the lymph system.

4. Normal LDH levels
5. Extent to which the individual is active

INCIDENCE

1. Malignant lymphomas are the third most common malignancy in children under 15.
2. NHL occurs from infancy through adolescence, with a peak incidence between ages 7 and 11 years.
3. Males are affected more often than females, in a 3:1 ratio.
4. NHL constitutes 55% to 60% of all lymphomas.
5. The overall 5-year survival rate is greater than 80%.

CLINICAL MANIFESTATIONS
Intraabdominal Involvement

1. Possible symptoms mimicking appendicitis (pain, right lower quadrant tenderness)
2. Intussusception
3. Ovarian, pelvic, retroperitoneal masses
4. Ascites
5. Vomiting
6. Diarrhea
7. Weight loss

Mediastinal Involvement

1. Pleural effusion
2. Tracheal compression
3. Superior vena cava syndrome
4. Coughing, wheezing, dyspnea, respiratory distress
5. Edema of upper extremities
6. Mental status changes

Primary Nasal, Paranasal, Oral, and Pharyngeal Involvement

1. Nasal congestion
2. Rhinorrhea
3. Epistaxis
4. Headache
5. Proptosis
6. Irritability
7. Weight loss

COMPLICATIONS

Metabolic: The major complication is tumor lysis syndrome (as a result of treatment), which can cause major metabolic and electrolyte dysfunctions. The following electrolyte disturbances will be evident early on with this complication, without apparent clinical symptoms: (1) hyperuricemia, (2) hyperkalemia, (3) hyperphosphatemia and (4) hypocalcemia. The child may experience nausea and vomiting, cloudy urine, shortness of breath, and lethargy. The child's condition can progress to renal failure, cardiac arrhythmias, and seizures.

LABORATORY AND DIAGNOSTIC TESTS

1. Bone marrow biopsy—to identify malignant cells with bone marrow involvement
2. Lumbar puncture—to determine presence of malignant cells in CNS
3. Complete blood count—diagnostic for bone marrow dysfunction; may show elevated white blood cell count, decreased hemoglobin level, hematocrit, and platelet count (see Appendix D for normal ranges)
4. Liver and kidney function tests—liver function test values may be elevated with liver involvement; kidney function test values may be elevated with kidney involvement (see Appendix D for normal ranges)
5. Lactate dehydrogenase level—elevated owing to tumor lysis (see Appendix D for normal range)
6. Serum uric acid level—elevated owing to cellular tumor load (see Appendix D for normal range)
7. Epstein-Barr virus test—positive result has been associated with NHL
8. Bone scan—to determine the presence of metastases in the bone
9. Chest radiograph—to determine the presence of metatases in the lung
10. Computed tomography and magnetic resonance imaging—to determine the presence of metastases in other areas of the body (refer to Chapters 81 and 91)

MEDICAL MANAGEMENT

Current therapy for NHL is based on the stage of the disease, the immunophenotype, and the histopathologic findings. Treatment for NHL is multiagent chemotherapy to eradicate the disease and to prevent further dissemination. Chemotherapy regimens have become more effective, therefore the use of radiation therapy in treating NHL has decreased. In children with NHL, surgery is used only for diagnostic purposes.

The following medication regimens may be used:
1. Stage I or II (excellent prognosis)
   a. Vincristine—inhibits cell division at metaphase
   b. Cyclophosphamide—blocks DNA, RNA, and protein synthesis
   c. Prednisone—used in conjunction with antineoplastic agents
   d. Anthracycline or methotrexate may also be used
2. Stage III or IV (lymphoblastic)
   a. Vincristine—inhibits cell division at metaphase
   b. Prednisone—used in conjunction with antineoplastic agents
   c. Asparaginase—inhibits DNA, RNA, and protein synthesis
   d. Anthracycline—inhibits DNA replication and/or RNA transcription
   e. Methotrexate—inhibits folate metabolism
   f. Cytosine arabinoside—arrests cellular metaphase
   g. Cyclophosphamide—blocks DNA, RNA, and protein synthesis
   h. May or may not use intrathecal drugs
3. Stage III or IV (Burkitt type; small, noncleaved)
   a. Cyclophosphamide—blocks DNA, RNA, and protein synthesis
   b. Methotrexate or doxorubicin—inhibits folate metabolism, inhibits DNA replication and/or RNA transcription
   c. Prednisone—used in conjunction with antineoplastic agents
   d. Vincristine—inhibits cell division at metaphase
   e. May use intrathecal therapy

4. Stage III or IV (large cell)
   a. Methotrexate—inhibits folate metabolism
   b. Cytarabine—arrests cellular metaphase
   c. Prednisone—used in conjunction with antineoplastic agents
   d. Cyclophosphamide—blocks DNA, RNA, and protein synthesis
   e. Vincristine—inhibits cell division at metaphase
   f. Doxorubicin—inhibits DNA replication and/or RNA transcription
   g. Etoposide—arrests the S or G phase of cellular metabolism
   h. Ifosfamide—inhibits DNA replication
   i. Intrathecal methotrexate and cytarabine

NURSING ASSESSMENT

1. Assess child's physiologic status (see Appendix A).
   a. Signs and symptoms of NHL
   b. Involvement of other body systems (e.g., gastrointestinal, respiratory)
   c. Adverse effects of treatment
   d. Signs and symptoms of tumor lysis syndrome (hypocalcemia, hyperphosphatemia, hyperkalemia, hyperuricemia)
2. Assess child and family for psychosocial needs:
   a. Knowledge of disease and treatment regimen
   b. Body image
   c. Family structure
   d. Family stressors
   e. Coping mechanisms
   f. Support systems
3. Assess child's level of development (see Appendix B).

NURSING DIAGNOSES

- Injury, Risk for
- Fluid volume, Excess
- Pain

- Nutrition: less than body requirements, Imbalanced
- Anxiety
- Activity intolerance, Risk for
- Therapeutic regimen management, Ineffective
- Coping, Ineffective
- Coping, Compromised family

NURSING INTERVENTIONS
Diagnosis and Staging Phase

1. Provide preprocedural education to child and family (see the Preparation for Procedures or Surgery section in Appendix F).
2. Prepare child for diagnostic procedures with age-appropriate approach (see the Preparation for Procedures or Surgery section in Appendix F).
3. Observe for signs and symptoms of systems involvement.
   a. Respiratory distress
   b. Superior vena cava syndrome
   c. CNS changes
4. Refer to child life specialist as appropriate for preprocedural preparation.
5. Assist and support child in collection of laboratory specimens.
6. Provide anticipatory guidance and family crisis intervention.

Treatment Phase

1. Monitor cardiorespiratory status.
2. Prepare for treatment-induced emergencies.
   a. Metabolic crises
   b. Hematologic crises
   c. Space-occupying tumors
3. Administer chemotherapeutic agents (see the Medical Management section in this chapter).
4. Assess for signs of extravasation.
   a. Cell lysis
   b. Tissue sloughing
5. Minimize side effects of chemotherapy.
   a. Bone marrow suppression

    b. Nausea and vomiting

    c. Anorexia and weight loss

    d. Oral mucositis

    e. Pain

6. Monitor for signs and symptoms of infection.
7. Monitor for signs and symptoms of relapse.
   a. CNS changes
   b. Infection
   c. Tumor recurrence
   d. Leukemic conversion
8. Provide ongoing emotional support to child and family (see the Preparation for Procedures or Surgery section in Appendix F).
9. Refer to child life specialist for continued coping strategies.
10. Provide ongoing education about treatment and medications.
11. Refer family to social services for support and resource utilization.
12. Monitor for tumor lysis syndrome.

🏠 Discharge Planning and Home Care

Instruct child and parents about home care management:

1. Signs of infection and when to seek medical attention
2. Care of child's central venous access device including site care, dressing change, flushing, and emergency care
3. Medication administration (provide written information)
4. Importance of compliance with treatment and medical procedures
5. Proper nutrition for optimal weight gain and health maintenance
6. School attendance and/or activity restrictions
7. Signs and symptoms of relapse
8. Potential behavioral changes in child and/or siblings
9. Access to support services, such as parent support groups (see Supportive Care section in Appendix F and Appendix G)

CLIENT OUTCOMES

1. Child and family will demonstrate ability to cope with life-threatening illness.
2. Child will be free of infection.
3. Child and family will understand home care and long-term follow-up needs.

REFERENCES

American Cancer Society: *How is Non-Hodgkin Lymphoma Staged?* (website): www.cancer.org/docroot/CRI/content/CRI_2_4_3X_How_is_non-Hodgkins_lymphoma_staged_32.asp?rnav=cri. Accessed February 19, 2007.

Baggott CR et al: *Nursing care of children and adolescents with cancer,* ed 3, Philadelphia, 2002, WB Saunders.

Buyulpamukcu M et al: Renal involvement of non-Hodgkin's lymphoma and its prognostic effect in childhood, *Nephron Clin Pract,* 100(3):c86, 2005.

Hafner JW et al: Childhood primary parotid non-Hodgkin's lymphoma with direct intracranial extension: A case report, *Ear Nose Throat J,* 83(12):828, 2004.

Young G et al: Recognition of common childhood malignancies, *Am Fam Physician* 61(7):2144, 2000.

57

Osteogenic Sarcoma

PATHOPHYSIOLOGY

Osteogenic sarcoma, also known as osteosarcoma, is a tumor found in the diaphysis of a long bone (femur, radius, ulna, proximal humerus, or ilium). It also can affect the flat bones, which include the head, the pelvis, and the spine. The most common sites of occurrence are the femur and the knee, followed in order by the tibia, the humerus, the pelvis, the jaw, the fibula, and the ribs. The clinical course takes the following sequence: (1) the normal bone is destroyed and is replaced by tumor cells, which results in osteoid tissue and bone; (2) growth penetrates the cortex and extends beyond it (radiating spindles of bone are characteristic of this process); and (3) the tumor extends through the bone marrow cavity. Metastasis occurs through veins and involves the lungs first.

INCIDENCE

1. Osteogenic sarcoma is the most common bone tumor in children and accounts for 60% of malignant bone tumors in children under 15 years of age.
2. It occurs most commonly during the adolescent growth period and in young adulthood.
3. It is uncommon before age 10 years.
4. Age range of peak incidence is 10 to 15 years.
5. More males than females are affected.
6. Surgery and chemotherapy can extend the overall survival rates from 65% to 75%.
7. Two thirds of those with nonmetastatic osteogenic sarcoma will be long-term survivors after treatment with surgery and chemotherapy.

CLINICAL MANIFESTATIONS

Symptoms are gradual in onset. The child may have symptoms for 6 to 9 months before treatment is sought. Children often present with a history of a minor injury while participating in sports. The symptoms are as follows:

1. Local pain during activity and more severe pain with passage of time (most common symptom)
2. Limping or gait variation
3. Limitation of joint motion
4. Joint tenderness
5. Local edema

COMPLICATIONS

Complications of Amputation are the Following:

1. Reactive hyperemia—reddened skin, particularly at pressure points; subsides as keratoma layer forms
2. Contact dermatitis—most often caused by contact with prosthetic materials (e.g., polyester resins, chrome)
3. Infections—including fungal and pyogenic infections (e.g., furuncles)
4. Epidermal cysts—evident at points of friction at or near brim of socket; most often caused by ill-fitting prosthesis
5. Stump edema syndrome—consisting of worsening reactive hyperemia, which results in oozing and capillary rupture
6. Terminal bone overgrowth
7. Bony spurs—developing at corners or margins of amputation as a result of periosteal irritation
8. Neuroma—a nerve tissue tumor
9. Phantom limb—feelings of pain and sensation in the amputated limb
10. Stump scarring—caused by inguinal weight bearing and increased shearing force at stump-socket interface

Additional Complications for Limb Salvage are the Following:

1. Nonunion of the bones
2. Stress fracture through the grafted bone

Long-term Complications

Pathologic fractures occur with larger lesions and many times are the initial symptoms seen.

LABORATORY AND DIAGNOSTIC TESTS

1. Serum alkaline phosphatase levels—confirms diagnosis; elevated because of osteoid production (see Appendix D, for normal range)
2. Tissue biopsy—reveals presence of malignant cells
3. Anteroposterior lateral radiographic studies—detect presence of soft tissue mass associated with destructive bone lesion, and calcification
4. Skeletal bone scan—detects presence of metastatic bone lesions
5. Computed tomography and magnetic resonance imaging—determines extent of disease and metastasis

MEDICAL AND SURGICAL MANAGEMENT

An important component of treatment of osteogenic sarcoma is surgery. Osteogenic sarcoma is resistant to radiation therapy; therefore, the most important prognostic factor is the ability of the physician to resect the tumor. Chemotherapy may be used before and after surgery. Type of surgery is determined by the age of the child and tumor size and location. It may be either an amputation or a limb salvage. Because of the availability of new chemotherapy regimens and complex reconstruction surgeries, amputation is no longer the surgery of choice. Minimally invasive surgery for diagnosis and treatment of solid tumor in children, such as osteogenic sarcoma, has become the preferred surgery. Both procedures are performed to excise the tumor and obtain a biopsy specimen for diagnosis. Following surgery, routine postoperative care is provided as described in the Nursing Interventions section in this chapter, in addition to monitoring complications following surgery as identified in the section on Complications.

Chemotherapy may be given before surgery in an attempt to promote the success of the surgery by first decreasing the tumor size. Preoperative tumor response to chemotherapy has been found to be very important in the prognosis of patients with nonmetastatic osteogenic sarcoma. Both intravenous and intraarterial chemotherapy may be given preoperatively.

After surgery, chemotherapy is given. The chemotherapy regimens contain various combinations of the following: methotrexate, doxorubicin, bleomycin, cyclophosphamide, cisplatin, and ifosfamide. When methotrexate infusion is given, leucovorin calcium is given afterward to reverse the action of the methotrexate and decrease its toxicity. The dosage of leucovorin calcium is equivalent to the amount of methotrexate administered. Allopurinol is also given with chemotherapy to decrease the level of uric acid, which is a by-product of chemotherapy.

NURSING ASSESSMENT

1. Assess child's and family's emotional response to upcoming surgery and need for information.
2. Assess postoperatively for signs and symptoms of impending complications, such as signs of infection and swelling at stump or surgical site.
3. Assess for wound drainage and signs and symptoms of infection.
4. Assess child's response to chemotherapy.
5. Assess continually the child's and family's coping.
6. Assess child's and family's ability to manage home treatment regimen.
7. Assess child's and family's use of community resources (Appendix G).
8. Refer to Musculoskeletal Assessment section in Appendix A.

NURSING DIAGNOSES

- Infection, Risk for
- Tissue integrity, Impaired
- Mobility, Impaired physical
- Injury, Risk for
- Pain
- Body image, Disturbed
- Fluid volume, Excess
- Therapeutic regimen management, Ineffective

- Coping, Ineffective
- Family processes, Interrupted
- Growth and development, Delayed
- Caregiver role strain, Risk for

NURSING INTERVENTIONS
Preoperative Care
1. Prepare operative site according to hospital procedure.
2. Encourage use of exercises to strengthen muscles.
3. Provide emotional support to child and parents.
   a. Provide active listening to concerns.
   b. Encourage expression of feelings of loss.
   c. Provide anticipatory information about emotional responses to surgery.
4. Provide preoperative information to decrease anxiety about unknown aspects (see the Preparation for Procedures or Surgery section in Appendix F).
5. Prepare child before laboratory and diagnostic testing.
   a. Complete blood count (CBC) (see the Preparation for Procedures or Surgery section in Appendix F)
   b. Urinalysis
   c. Bone scan
   d. Radiographic studies
   e. Type and cross-match of blood

Postoperative Care
1. Monitor for signs of complications and report immediately (see the Complications section in this chapter).
2. Observe and monitor for signs of hemorrhage every hour for 24 hours, then every 4 hours.
3. Promote patency and healing of surgical site (after amputation).
   a. Apply pressure dressing (figure eight) to stump.
   b. Institute range of motion exercises according to physical therapist's orders.
   c. Reinforce exercise program with physical therapist.
   d. Cleanse stump and socket every day with soap and water; dry thoroughly.

    e. Avoid use of skin lotions (can cause maculation and superficial infection).

4. Position child correctly to prevent deformities (after amputation).
    a. Trendelenburg's position
    b. Pillow beneath knee for 24 hours to decrease edema
    c. After 24 hours, no pillow beneath knee (causes flexion of knee)
    d. Prone position for several hours every day (to prevent hip flexion and contracture)

5. Monitor for pain; administer pain medication (refer to Appendix I).

6. Promote use of and adaptation to prosthetic device (after amputation).
    a. Perform prosthetic fitting immediately after surgery, because this promotes stump maturation, early ambulation, and resumption of normal activities.
    b. Encourage expression of feelings about having a disability.
    c. Explain restrictions on activities.

7. Monitor administration of chemotherapy.
    a. Provide adequate hydration (hydrate 12 hours before infusion of chemotherapy).
    b. Record intake and output hourly.
    c. Measure specific gravity to assess hydration.
    d. Monitor urine pH and Hematest results (majority of medication is excreted in urine in the first 24 hours); urine must be alkaline, or its precipitates in kidney will cause tubular necrosis.
    e. Assist with collection of specimens for blood chemistry analysis, CBC, and platelet count.
    f. Assist with collection of urine for urinalysis.

8. Monitor for child's or adolescent's untoward and therapeutic responses to chemotherapy.
    a. Observe for oral and gastrointestinal tract ulcerations and report to MD.
    b. Note presence of diarrhea.
    c. Observe for symptoms of ulcerative stomatitis (hemorrhagic enteritis and death can occur).

   d. Observe child for skin reactions that include urticaria, rashes.
   e. Observe for symptoms and signs of cystitis—inflammation of urinary tract.
   f. Institute supportive measures (i.e., antiemetics, dietary modifications) as ordered for presence of nausea and vomiting.
9. Minimize negative consequences of chemotherapy.
   a. Provide good mouth care.
   b. If the child or youth is smoking, urge him or her to stop.
   c. Advise child or adolescent to stay out of sun (methotrexate can cause skin blotches).
   d. Push fluids.
   e. Administer antiemetics.
   f. Provide bland, soft diet.
   g. Elevate head of bed.
   h. Teach self-hypnosis and relaxation techniques.
10. Monitor for complications.
   a. Pneumothorax (symptoms: shortness of breath, dyspnea, chest pain)
   b. Depression of hematologic values 10 days after methotrexate administration
   c. Renal toxicity—dysuria, oliguria (monitor intake and output)
11. Provide emotional support to parents and child (see the Preparation for Procedures or Surgery section in Appendix F).

🏠 Discharge Planning and Home Care
Chemotherapy Regimen

1. Instruct parents and child or adolescent about home care management.
   a. Take leucovorin calcium on time (wake up child if necessary).
   b. Take antiemetic for nausea and vomiting.
   c. Drink increased amount of fluids (2 qt per day); milk tends to increase mucous secretions.

d. Check pH of urine.

e. Recommend staying out of sun.

2. Refer to community resources for follow-up (see Appendix G).

Postoperative Care

1. Instruct child and parents about stump care or surgical site care.

2. Provide reinforcement information about physical therapy regimen.

3. Refer to school nurse and clinic and advise them about child's status (refer to the Special Education section in Appendix G).

4. Explore compliance potential by asking about following items:

a. Means of transportation

b. Resources for child care

c. Finances

d. Level of motivation

e. The youth's and family's understanding of need for long-term follow-up every 3 to 4 months until growth is complete

CLIENT OUTCOMES

1. Child will achieve remission.

2. Side effects of chemotherapy experienced by child will be minimized.

3. Child and family will adhere to home treatment regimen and outpatient physical therapy regimen as prescribed.

REFERENCES

Alcoser P, Rodgers C: Treatment strategies in childhood cancer, *J Pediatr Nurs* 18(2):103, 2003.

Baggott CR et al, editors: *Nursing care of children and adolescents with cancer,* ed 3, Philadelphia, 2002, WB Saunders.

Bryant R: Managing side effects of childhood cancer treatment, *J Pediatr Nurs* 18(2):113, 2003.

Papagelopoulos PJ et al: Current concepts in the evaluation and treatment of osteosarcoma, *Orthopedics* 23(8):858, 2000.

Sailhamer E et al: Minimally invasive surgery for pediatirc solid neoplams, *Am Surgeon* 69(7):566, 2003.

Trueworthy RC: Malignant bone tumors presenting as musculoskeletal pain, *Pediatr Ann* 31(6):355, 2002.

Wilkins RM et al: Superior survival in treatment of primary nonmetastatic pediatric osteogemic sarcoma of the extremity, *Ann Surg Oncol* 10(5):498, 2003.

Wittig JC et al: Osteosarcoma: a multidisciplinary approach to diagnosis and treatment, *Am Fam Physician* 65(6):1123, 2002.

58

Osteomyelitis

PATHOPHYSIOLOGY

Osteomyelitis is an infection of the bone that can occur in any bone in the body. The most common locations are the femur and the tibia. The humerus and the hip are rarely affected. The skull is a common location in infants. Usually a predisposing condition such as poor nutrition or poor hygiene exists.

Bacterial emboli reach the small arteries in the metaphysis, where circulation is sluggish. An abscess forms and replaces bone, causing increased pressure and secondary necrosis. This abscess eventually can rupture into the subperiosteal space. The infection spreads beneath the periosteum, thrombosing vessels and causing increased necrosis. The cycle of impaired circulation is thus established. A sinus can form and extend the infection to the skin. Extension to a joint results in septic arthritis. The condition can become chronic and thus quite resistant to therapy, often necessitating involved surgical intervention. The epiphysis is usually spared because it has a separate circulation.

There are several classsifications of osteomyelitis. One classification is by the duration of the disease: acute or chronic. Acute osteomyelitis is considered to occur over several days or weeks, and the chronic form is considered to be a long-standing infection. A second classification is by the source of the infection. The first is the hematogenous route, referring to circumstances when the infection originates from a bacteremia or by seeding through the bloodstream. This is the more common route, and sources include furuncles, skin abrasions, upper respiratory tract infections, otitis media, abscessed teeth, and pyelonephritis. The second is the contiguous route, where the infection originates in the nearby tissue as in the following: contamination from penetrating wounds, open fractures, or surgical wounds, or secondary extension through an abscess, burn, or wound. The third route is the presence of systemic disease or vascular insufficiency that causes the infection.

INCIDENCE

1. The highest incidence of osteomyelitis is found in 5- to 14-year-olds.
2. Osteomyelitis is twice as common in males as in females.
3. In the United States, 1 in 5000 children under age 13 will have osteomyelitis.

CLINICAL MANIFESTATIONS

1. Pain of abrupt onset—point tenderness above bone and swelling and warmth over bone
2. Fever
3. Possible dehydration
4. Unwillingness to move limb or bear weight
5. Holding of extremity in semiflexed position (muscle spasm)
6. Irritability
7. Poor appetite
8. Local signs of inflammation and infection (warmth, erythema, drainage, decreased range of motion)
9. Lethargy

COMPLICATIONS

Musculoskeletal: pathologic fractures, septic arthritis

LABORATORY AND DIAGNOSTIC TESTS

See Appendix D for normal values and ranges of laboratory and diagnostic tests.

1. Complete blood count—marked leukocytosis, indicates presence of infection
2. Erythrocyte sedimentation rate—elevated, indicates presence of infection
3. Blood culture and sensitivity test—positive culture in 50% of cases; common causative organisms vary with age and

other factors; determine causative organism and preferred antibiotic

   a. All ages—staphylococci, primarily *Staphylococcus aureus*
   b. Young children—*Haemophilus influenzae*
   c. Neonates—coliforms *(Escherichia coli)*
   d. Sickle cell anemia—*Salmonella* organisms
   e. Foot—*Pseudomonas* organisms

4. Radiographic studies—findings are normal in first 10 to 12 days until bone destruction occurs (soft tissue swelling is evident early)
5. Computed tomography or magnetic resonance imaging—shows bone involvement
6. Bone scan—is often positive early for inflammation
7. Direct needle aspiration or biopsy—confirms diagnosis and provides site specimen for culture (best method for diagnosis)

MEDICAL AND SURGICAL MANAGEMENT

Intravenous antibiotics are begun after blood has been drawn for culture. Antibiotics are administered for a minimum of 4 weeks but usually for 6 weeks, depending on duration of symptoms, response to treatment, and sensitivity of the organism. Intravenous antibiotics may be administered on an outpatient basis or at home, or the child may be given oral antibiotics to complete the course at home to decrease costs. The type of antibiotic used to treat osteomyelitis depends on the results of culture and sensitivity testing. Bed rest may be prescribed, and the affected extremity is usually immobilized with a cast or splint. Surgery may be performed to drain the area and remove necrotic bone. During surgery, polyethylene tubes are placed in the bone—one for instilling an antibiotic solution (usually the upper tube) and the other for drainage. Local débridement may be performed to remove the source of infection and cleanse the area.

NURSING ASSESSMENT

1. See the Musculoskeletal Assessment section in Appendix A.
2. Assess pain for location, duration, intensity, description (refer to Appendix I).

3. Assess nutritional status for adequacy of caloric intake, as well as intake of protein and fluids.

NURSING DIAGNOSES

- Infection, Risk for
- Hyperthermia
- Pain
- Tissue perfusion, Ineffective
- Nutrition: less than body requirements, Imbalanced
- Therapeutic regimen management, Ineffective

NURSING INTERVENTIONS

1. Immobilize extremity to facilitate healing and prevent complications.
   a. Apply splint, bivalved cast, or complete cast with window.
   b. Allow no weight bearing (high risk of pathologic fracture).
      i. Use gurney or wheelchair; elevate extremity slightly.
      ii. Use active range of motion exercises on unaffected extremity after inflammation subsides.
2. Monitor for signs of infection and alterations in thermoregulation.
   a. Increased temperature (institute cooling measures)
   b. Signs of inflammation
   c. Drainage or musty odor with cast
3. Provide cast care.
   a. Monitor skin temperature; casting creates concern for thermoregulation in young infants and children.
   b. Monitor color, heat, sweating, tenderness, capillary refill, and motion of digits.
   c. Keep cast clean and dry.
   d. Perform child and family teaching (e.g., about placing nothing inside cast).
   e. Consult physician regarding use of diphenhydramine (Benadryl) for itching.
4. Use contact precautions if any drainage occurs. Refer to institutional procedures manual for isolation techniques.

5. Monitor child's response to antibiotic irrigation of site (up to 6 weeks).
   a. For first 3 days, expect blood, debris, and pus (have tendency to clog tubes).
      i. Reversing flow direction of tubes at intervals can prevent blockage; do so with physician consultation only.
      ii. Physician may elect to irrigate with heparin and saline solution if blockage occurs.
      iii. Use prescribed suction (usually low suction).
   b. If tubes are functioning properly, wound and dressing should remain dry.
   c. Maintain records of instillation and output (clarity, color, and volume of drainage); often up to 1000 ml/day is instilled.
   d. When tubes are removed, usually instillation tube (upper) is removed first, with drainage tube left until no further drainage occurs.
   e. Sudden pain at site of irrigation may indicate blockage of drainage tube.
6. Monitor child's response to medications.
   a. Antibiotics
   b. Antipyretics
   c. Sedatives
   d. Antihistamines
7. Provide pain relief measures (see Appendix I).
   a. Allow comfortable position.
   b. Support affected limb on pillows.
   c. Use care in turning and moving child.
   d. Monitor child's response to analgesia and sedation as necessary.
8. Promote adequate nutritional intake.
   a. Promote high-caloric intake (juices, gelatin, Popsicles).
   b. Initially appetite is poor; appetite usually returns when acute symptoms subside.
9. Provide age-appropriate diversional activities (see the relevant section in Appendix F).
10. Provide emotional support to parents (see the Supportive Care section in Appendix F).

🏠 Discharge Planning and Home Care

1. Instruct parents about elements of rehabilitation (see Appendix F).
   a. Risk of fracture
   b. Necessity for hospitalization
   c. Necessity for operations
2. Instruct parents about administration of antibiotics. Home referral may be made (e.g., percutaneous intravenous central catheter lines may be inserted).
   a. Therapeutic responses
   b. Side effects—because many antibiotics used have negative renal, audiologic, and hepatic effects, these systems must be monitored closely during therapy (intravenous medication may be prescribed if treatment is longer than 3 weeks)

CLIENT OUTCOMES

1. Child will be free of infection.
2. Child will be free of disease complications.
3. Child and family will learn to adhere to home treatment regimen.

REFERENCES

Auh JS, Binns HJ, Katz B: Retrospective assessment of subacute or chronic osteomyelitis in children and young adults, *Clin Pediatr* 43(6):549, 2004.

Branom RN: Is this wound infected? *Crit Care Nurs Q* 25(1):55, 2002.

Carek P et al: Diagnosis and management of osteomyelitis, *Am Fam Physician* 63(12):2413, 2001.

Lazzarini L, Mader JT, Calhoun JH: Current concepts review: Osteolyelitis in long bones, *J Bone Joint Surg Am Vol* 86(10):2305, 2004.

Lew DP, Waldvogel FA: Osteomyelitis, *Lancet* 364(9431):369, 2004.

McCarthy JJ et al: Musculoskeletal infections in children: Basic treatment principles and recent advancements, *J Bone Joint Surg* 86(4):850, 2004.

59

Otitis Media

PATHOPHYSIOLOGY

Acute otitis media (AOM) is an inflammation of the middle ear. Children 6 years of age and younger are at particular risk for acute otitis media because their eustachian tubes are shorter and more horizontal, and lack the cartilaginous support found in older children and adults. This allows the eustachian tubes to collapse, which causes negative pressure in the middle ear. In turn, there is impaired drainage of middle ear fluid and possible reflux of pharyngeal secretions into this normally sterile area. The eustachian tubes of infants and children with cleft palate or Down syndrome are also wider, so they remain open; this allows bacteria to travel easily from the nasopharynx into the middle ear, and this further predisposes such children to infection. Acute otitis media is the most common infection for which antibacterial agents are prescribed for children in the United States. Among childhood diseases, it is second in prevalence only to the common cold, accounting for 1 in 3 pediatric sick visits in this country and over 13 million annual prescriptions. Growing concerns about the rising rates of antibacterial resistance have prompted changes in the medical management of uncomplicated AOM. Two types of otitis media are common in clinical pediatrics: acute otitis media and otitis media with effusion.

Acute Otitis Media

Acute otitis media is characterized by fluid in the middle ear with signs and symptoms of ear infection (bulging eardrum usually accompanied by pain, or perforated eardrum, often

496

with drainage of purulent matter). The pathogens most commonly associated with otitis media include *Streptococcus pneumoniae* (25% to 50% of cases), nontypeable *Haemophilus influenzae* (15% to 30% of cases), *Moraxella catarrhalis* (3% to 20% of cases), viruses, and certain anaerobes. In the neonate, gram-negative enteric organisms or *Staphylococcus aureus* may also be the causative organisms. Group A *Streptococcus* and *S. aureus* (2% to 3% combined) were less common causes of acute otitis media in the pediatric population during the 1990s. *Chlamydia pneumoniae* infections may also be seen, most frequently in children aged 8 to 16 months.

Otitis Media with Effusion

Otitis media with effusion is characterized by fluid in the middle ear without signs and symptoms of ear infection. No definitive causative agent has been identified, although otitis media with effusion is seen more commonly in children with allergies or viral upper respiratory infections, and in those recovering from acute otitis media.

INCIDENCE

1. Otitis media occurs most often in children between 3 months and 3 years of age; age ranges of peak incidence are 5 to 24 months and 4 to 6 years.
2. Of affected children, 70% have one episode by age 3 years, with one third having more than three episodes. The younger the child at the time of the first infection, the greater the chance of recurrent infections.
3. Boys have more ear infections than girls.
4. Children are more likely to experience repeated episodes if a parent and/or sibling also had ear infections.
5. Children with craniofacial conditions such as a cleft lip and/or palate and Down syndrome are also at greater risk. Of children with cleft palate, 50% have chronic otitis media before surgical correction.
6. Children placed in large group day care settings from an early age have greater exposure to all causative bacteria and viruses from other children.

Complications that may result include atrophy of the tympanic membrane, tympanosclerosis (scarring of the tympanic membrane), chronic perforation, and cholesteatoma.

Initial management of the child involves observation or treatment with antibiotic therapy (optional at this time). In most cases, otitis media with effusion resolves spontaneously within 3 months. Parents should be encouraged to avoid exposing their children to passive smoking as a means of controlling an environmental risk factor. Myringotomy is not recommended for initial management of otitis media with effusion in an otherwise healthy child.

After 3 months, if the child has hearing in the normal range, as indicated by a hearing threshold level of better than 20 dB in the better-hearing ear, the child is observed or treated with antibiotics (this remains optional at this time). In most cases, otitis media with effusion resolves spontaneously.

If the child has bilateral hearing deficits of 20 dB hearing threshold level or worse, the child is treated with antibiotic therapy or undergoes a bilateral myringotomy with tympanostomy tubes. Either one or both treatment approaches may be chosen to manage bilateral otitis media with effusion that has lasted a total of 3 months in an otherwise healthy child aged 1 to 3 years who has a bilateral hearing deficit.

Management strategies used after 4 to 6 months include a bilateral myringotomy with tympanostomy tubes to manage bilateral otitis media with effusion that has lasted a total of 4 to 6 months in an otherwise healthy child aged 1 to 3 years who has a bilateral hearing deficit.

NURSING ASSESSMENT

1. Assess for verbal and nonverbal pain behaviors.
2. Assess for elevated temperature (100° to 104° F).
3. Assess for enlarged lymph glands in neck area.
4. Assess nutritional status and adequacy of caloric fluid intake.
5. Assess for hearing loss.
6. Assess for speech loss and development.

NURSING DIAGNOSES

- Pain
- Comfort, Impaired
- Sensory perception, Disturbed
- Communication, Impaired verbal

NURSING INTERVENTIONS

Acute Otitis Media

1. Treat and instruct family to treat child with analgesics and/or antipyretics as needed for symptoms.
   a. Fever
   b. Ear pain
2. Offer small amounts of fluids frequently with cup or spoon if breast or bottle is refused, because sucking may cause increased ear pain in younger child.
   a. Nonnutritive (pacifier) sucking may be source of comfort to equalize pressure and/or relieve ear "popping" (chewing sugar-free gum may have same desired effect for older child).
   b. Caution parents against bottle-feeding or bottle-propping while child is lying down.
3. Be aware that increased fluid intake is vital to any child with fever or illness to prevent dehydration and promote healing.
4. Instruct family about safe and effective use of prescribed antibiotic.
5. Monitor and instruct family to observe for (and report) common allergic or adverse reactions to antibiotic therapy (e.g., diarrhea, nausea and vomiting, skin rash or urticaria). Serious dermatologic, hematologic, renal, hepatic, neurologic, endocrine, and/or cardiorespiratory reactions are rare.
6. Monitor and instruct family to observe for signs of complications with acute otitis.
   a. Ear drainage
   b. No improvement of signs and symptoms with treatment, especially after 48 hours of appropriate antibiotic therapy
   c. Stiff neck, severe fussiness and irritability (meningitis), dizziness with clumsiness or falling (labyrinthitis)

Otitis Media with Effusion

1. Educate family about course of disease and lack of definitive cause and treatment.
2. Support child and family if conductive hearing loss is present; reassure them that this is likely to resolve spontaneously.
3. If myringotomy is required, supply age-appropriate explanations of procedure to child and parents (see Appendix F).

Postoperative Care

Monitor child's response to surgical intervention (myringotomy with insertion of tympanostomy tubes).
1. Vital signs (increased temperature indicates infection)
2. Otorrhea from ears
3. Presence of bleeding
4. Pain (provide comfort measures and pain medications as needed—see Appendix I)
5. Hearing status
6. Speech development

🏠 Discharge Planning and Home Care

1. Instruct child and parents about maintaining patency of tympanostomy (e.g., when child is swimming or bathing, use ear plugs).
2. Instruct about limiting child's activities until fully recovered.
   a. Avoid rigorous activities.
   b. Provide frequent rest periods.
   c. Allow return to school after child receives medical approval.
3. Educate about importance of avoiding exposure of children to passive tobacco smoke; if household members or child care providers are unable to quit smoking, smoking should be done outdoors, away from child.
4. Inform parents there are no recommendations for complementary and alternative medicines such as acupuncture, herbal remedies, chiropractic treatments, and nutritional supplements in children.

CLIENT OUTCOMES

1. Child will be free of pain as demonstrated by verbal and nonverbal behaviors.
2. Child's activity level and appetite will return to normal.
3. Child will demonstrate no hearing loss.
4. Child will demonstrate no speech delay.
5. Family will be referred to educational resources on otitis media (Box 59-1).

BOX 59-1

Resources

- Agency for Healthcare Research and Quality (AHRQ)
  Publications Clearinghouse
  P.O. Box 8547
  Silver Spring, MD 20907-8547
  Website: www.ahcpr.gov
  Phone: 800-358-9295
  Toll-free TDD service (hearing impaired only): 888-586-6340
- American Academy of Pediatrics: www.aap.org
- American Medical Association and Nemours Foundation:
  Childhood infections: otitis media, Kidshealth (website): www.
  kidshealth.org. Accessed June 10, 2003.

REFERENCES

American Academy of Pediatrics and American Academy of Family Physicians: Diagnosis and management of acute otitis media, *Pediatrics* 113(5):1451, 2004.

Asch-Goodkin J: Acute otitis media: What the evidence says, *Contemp Pediatr* 19(suppl):4, 2002.

Takata GS et al: Evidence assessment of management of acute otitis media: I. The role of antibiotics in treatment of uncomplicated acute otitis media, *Pediatrics* 108(2):239, 2001.

60

❖

Overweight and Obesity in Childhood

PATHOPHYSIOLOGY

Today's rapid increase in overweight and obese children is considered a critical public health problem related to early-onset cardiovascular disease (CVD) morbidity and mortality. CVD is the number one cause of death of adults in Western society today and is a contributing factor to mortality worldwide.

The estimated annual health care costs attributed to obesity and some comorbid diseases in the United States are about $117 billion dollars. The complex interaction of factors surrounding obesity, behavior choices, environmental influences, and genetic predisposition affect all aspects of pediatric health care.

The World Health Organization (WHO) placed overweight in the list of top 10 health risks in the world, and the top 5 in developed nations. The American Heart Association (AHA) lists the significant long-term effects of childhood overweight and obesity to include cardiovascular disease, type 2 diabetes, metabolic and orthopedic abnormalities, asthma, sleep apnea and some cancers. Psychosocial consequences of adolescent obesity reported by the American College of Sports Medicine (ACSM) include social isolation, high-risk behavior (alcohol and drug use, and early sexual experimentation), low self-esteem, depression, and eating disorders.

The pathophysiology of overweight and obesity is described as an imbalance between energy intake and energy expenditure. The regulation of energy intake requires the body to differentiate short-term signals controlling hunger, food intake, and satiety from long-term signals reflecting energy stores and lean tissue. Overall, the function of food regulation and ingestion originates from signals in the brain and hormonal releases.

Adipose tissue development into adipocytes in the fetus begins midway to late in the third trimester and continues throughout life. Crucial periods of adipose tissue development can be affected by infant feeding practices, puberty, and other factors.

Additional research is required into the development and regulation of adipocyte number and volume. Intrauterine influences have been correlated with environmental factors and have emerged as an important area of research today. Epidemiologic investigation has identified a direct positive relationship between birth weight and body mass index (BMI) later in life.

Puberty and adolescence are marked by influential physiologic and psychologic changes in both boys and girls. In boys, fat-free mass increases, and body fat as a percentage of body weight decreases. In adolescent females, both fat and free mass increase, and fat-free mass as a percentage of body weight decreases. The influence of hormones on fat distribution is evident and is differentiated by sex. Adolescent fat stores are centralized, with increased amounts of subcutaneous and visceral fat in the abdominal regions in females, and even more so in males. Young females typically demonstrate fat deposits in the breasts, the hips, and the buttocks. Adolescence is a critical period of development in prevention of adult obesity and obesity-related comorbidities in both sexes.

BMI is a measurement tool defining the terms *overweight* and *obesity* in children and adults. BMI percentile calculations are based on the ratio dividing the weight (kilograms) by the height in meters squared, correlating with age and sex. Growth charts using BMI-for-ages 2 to 20 years by sex can be accessed at www.cdc.gov/growcharts. For children, a BMI between the 85th and 95th percentiles is considered overweight, and a BMI at or greater than the 95th percentile is considered obese. It is estimated that of adolescents with a BMI at or above the 95th percentile, approximately 50% will become obese adults.

Adiposity is another marker for determining at risk status for overweight and obesity and can be evaluated using the skin-fold test. Based on the compelling evidence of an obesity epidemic, The American Academy of Pediatrics (AAP) and the Institute of Medicine (IOM) recommend annual assessments of BMI as a strategy to affect the problem of childhood obesity (Box 60-1).

Biology (genetics) is the contributor to individual differences in weight and height, whereas trends in rapid weight gain are primarily attributed to changes in the environment and behavior factors. Modern lifestyles in the United States and developed countries demonstrate increased consumption of energy and decreased energy expenditure. Factors contributing to overconsumption of energy include availability and variety of good-tasting, inexpensive, energy-dense foods served in large portions. Factors related to a decrease in total energy expenditure include a marked decline in overall physical activity at school and in daily living, and increased sedentary leisure time spent watching television, surfing the Web, and playing video games.

A number of factors have been identified as contributing to childhood obesity. Genetic factors related to childhood obesity include maternal obesity, gestational diabetes, and genetics. Increased incidence of obesity in adolescents is related to adolescents who engage in high-risk behaviors because of peer pressure (smoking, ethanol use, and premature sexual experimentation). Social factors related to childhood obesity include lack of parental monitoring, single-parent families, educational level, and access to safe recreational facilities. Dietary factors associated with childhood obesity include reduced daily recommended dietary intake (RDA) of fruits and vegetables, absent or limited breast-feeding practices, high consumption of soft drinks, lack of family meals, dietary factors during infancy, meal preparation, and portion size.

Parental denial or lack of understanding related to overweight or obesity and associated psychosocial and physiologic health care disparities has been associated with childhood obesity. Parents and caregivers who have problems with health literacy and/or an inability to communicate effectively with

BOX 60-1

BMI for Children and Teens (sometimes referred to as "BMI-for-age.")

From Centers for Disease Control and Prevention

BMI is used differently with children than it is with adults.

In children and teens, body mass index is used to assess underweight, overweight, and risk for overweight. Children's body fatness changes over the years as they grow. Also, girls and boys differ in their body fatness as they mature. This is why BMI for children, also referred to as BMI-for-age, is sex- and age-specific. BMI-for-age is plotted on sex-specific growth charts. These charts are used for children and teens 2 to 20 years of age. For the 2000 Centers for Disease Control and Prevention (CDC) growth charts and additional information see Appendix E. Each of the CDC BMI-for-age sex-specific charts contains a series of curved lines indicating specific percentiles. Health care professionals use the following established percentile cutoff points to identify underweight and overweight in children.

Underweight	BMI-for-age <5th percentile
Normal	BMI-for-age from 5th percentile to <85th percentile
At risk of overweight	BMI-for-age from 85th percentile to <95th percentile
Overweight	BMI-for-age ≥95th percentile

Why is BMI-for-age a useful tool?

BMI-for-age is used for children and teens because of their rate of growth and development. Several things make it a useful tool:

- BMI-for-age provides a reference for adolescents that can be used beyond puberty.
- BMI-for-age in children and adolescents compares well to laboratory measures of body fat.
- BMI-for-age can be used to track body size throughout life.

For the 2000 CDC Growth Charts and additional information, visit the National Center for Health Statistics website: www.cdc.gov/growthcharts.

health care providers will have problems in managing their child's diet, lifestyle changes, and exercise routine to effectively deal with their child's obesity.

The public health challenge of preventive pediatric obesity is best addressed with early recognition of preventable and/or modifiable risk factors: diet, exercise, lifestyle, and parental education. Multidisciplinary strategies are needed from primary, secondary, and tertiary health care professionals to prevent, educate, treat, manage, and engage in research efforts to eradicate the epidemic of childhood obesity. The efforts of family, society, insurance companies, and policy makers are required to combat the challenges of childhood obesity threatening current and future generations.

INCIDENCE

1. The high incidence of overweight children 5 years of age and younger is a major health problem identified by the Centers for Disease Control (CDC) among all ethnic groups.
2. The ratio of overweight boys to girls is about 1:1, although there is ethnic variability.
3. The prevalence of obesity in Mexican-American males (42.8%) aged 5 to 19 years is greater than in African Americans (31.0%) or whites (29.2%).
4. Obesity in African-American females occurs at a rate of 40.1%, greater than that in Mexican Americans (36.6%) or whites (27%).
5. Of U.S. children ages 8 to 16 years, 20% are physically active fewer than 2 times a week.
6. Over the last 2 decades the incidence of overweight or obesity has increased by 50%.
7. Four or more hours of daily television watching is related to increased BMI.

CLINICAL MANIFESTATIONS

1. Children at risk for being overweight have BMI-for-age above the 85th percentile and below the 95th percentile.
2. Children who are considered obese have BMI-for-age and sex above the 95th percentile.

3. Hypertension
4. Hypercholesterolemia
5. Hyperlipidemia
6. Type 2 diabetes or insulin-resistant syndrome
7. Depression
8. Eating disorders

COMPLICATIONS

1. Cardiovascular disease: hypertension, elevated cholesterol and triglycerides, stroke
2. Cancer: breast, colon
3. Endocrine: diabetes Type 2, insulin-resistance syndrome
4. Gastrointestinal: gallbladder disease, colon cancer
5. Gynecologic: irregular menses, abnormal growth acceleration
6. Orthopedic: osteoporosis, growth plate abnormalities
7. Psychosocial: depression, low self-esteem, social isolation, eating disorders, suicide, behavior problem and syndromes, high-risk behavior (alcohol use, smoking, illicit drug use, early-onset sexual experimentation)
8. Respiratory: asthma, sleep apnea, snoring and other sleep-related disturbances
9. Increased risk for morbidities and early mortality in adulthood

LABORATORY AND DIAGNOSTIC TESTS

Refer to Appendix D for normal values and ranges of laboratory and diagnostic tests. The following are based on present and past medical history, physician preference, and health care coverage.

1. Annual BMI—recommended as the primary method to assess obesity in children and adolescents. BMI at or above 95th percentile is the clinical definition of obesity (Box 60-1).
2. Skinfold measurement—measurement involving skinfold thickness of the triceps. Clinicians must be proficient at using skin calipers if this test is to be accurately predictive. BMI and the skinfold measurements are equally predictive of the morbidity of obesity.

3. Sleep studies—gold standard is polysomnography assessing the electroencephalogram (EEG), electromyogram, electrooculogram, heart rate, respiratory rate, and behavior. It is performed to determine the presence of sleep disorders.

4. Pulmonary function test—to monitor children and adolescents with known respiratory disease and growth hormone deficiency, and to establish reduced physical activity as an etiology for obesity; in addition, evaluates fitness in patients with congenital heart diseases.

5. Diabetes management per hemoglobin A1C—to monitor blood glucose levels over a 5- to 6-week period; predicts a mean glucose level

6. Complete blood count—to evaluate the hemoglobin, hematocrit, white, red, and platelet cell counts, cell morphology

7. Lipid profile—to determine general baseline, and to assess for premature coronary artery disease, familial hypercholesterolemia, and rare but possible xanthomas

8. Hormone studies (luteinizing, follicle-stimulating or testosterone levels)—baseline studies to evaluate any potential growth, pituitary, or hormonal abnormality

9. Thyroid panel—associated with short stature or Cushing's or Turner's syndrome

10. Liver function—to assess for potential steatosis or steatohepatitis, which can be asymptomatic

11. Chemistry panel—to evaluate electrolyte imbalances

12. Electrocardiogram (ECG)—based on significant past and present medical history; used to assess for cardiac arrhythmias

13. Genetic evaluation—to determine if obesity is associated with physiologic, genetic, and/or psychologic history

MEDICAL MANAGEMENT

Medical management begins with complete physical examination including BMI and skinfold measurements. A complete psychosocial history is conducted including identification of high-risk behaviors. Laboratory and diagnostic tests are ordered to collect data that will contribute to the diagnostic work-up (refer to foregoing Laboratory and Diagnostic Tests section). Parents and child may be asked to complete a personal dietary and activity diary on the child to gather relevant information.

Based upon the comprehensive assessment, treatment modalities and referrals are initiated that can include dietary and weight management, exercise programs, and support groups. In addition, referrals are made as appropriate to a clinical psychologist, psychiatrist, and behavior modification programs such as Weight Watchers and Overeaters Anonymous. Consistent follow-up and monitoring is needed to provide ongoing support and treatment to ensure positive outcomes. Treatment modalities should accentuate long-term permanent changes, not rapid or short-term diet and activity programs.

Depending on the school district, the school may have weight management programs and educational programs related to nutrition and exercise. School nurses are integral members of the team managing the child's long-term management needs. School nurses perform annual BMI screening and identify at risk children and adolescents. Physical education teachers may be the professional who identifies a student in physical education class who has a BMI at or above the 85th percentile, and may refer the child to appropriate community-based resources and support groups.

NURSING ASSESSMENT

1. Obtain information on the child's present and past history and complaints.
   a. Past medical history (PMH) and significant family history
   b. Reproductive history as appropriate
   c. Psychosocial history (including potential: alcohol and drug use and sexual behaviors)
   d. Medication history
   e. Lifestyle (diet, level of activity and exercise)
2. Assess vital signs.
3. Calculate BMI.

4. Identify ethnicity and cultural beliefs.
5. Identify support systems (e.g., family, friends, teachers, health care).
6. Identify barriers to health promotion (access to health care, transportation, role models).
7. Make referrals as needed to social services, community clinics, interpreter services, and so forth.

NURSING DIAGNOSES

- Activity Intolerance
- Nutrition: More than body requirements, Imbalanced
- Health maintenance, Ineffective
- Parenting, Impaired, Risk for
- Coping, Ineffective
- Self esteem, Chronic low
- Therapeutic regimen management, Family, Ineffective
- Coping, Ineffective
- Self-esteem, Chronic low

NURSING INTERVENTIONS

1. Promote multidisciplinary approach in childhood obesity programs, including dietary changes, nutritional information, physical activity, behavior modification, parental involvement and education, and setting realistic goals.
2. Promote a positive, nonthreatening environment with parents and/or caregivers when discussing lifestyle changes, weight management, diet, and physical activity related to overweight or obesity.
3. Answer questions, reinforce information, and address parental and child's concerns related to child's problems with being overweight or obese.
4. Refer to appropriate community resources for childhood obesity.
5. Provide culturally appropriate education in schools and communities related to nutrition and regular physical activity based on dietary guidelines for Americans for individuals of all ages.
6. Refer to Box 60-2 for long-term advocacy interventions.

BOX 60-2
Long-Term Advocacy Interventions

- Educate health care providers about overweight and obesity risk factors across the life span.
- Support the efforts of pediatric health care providers to promote and eradicate childhood overweight and obesity.
- Encourage health care providers, parents, and community members to get involved at the local, state, and federal levels to promote healthy living and decrease the incidence of overweight and obesity in children and adolescents.
- Collaborate with school nurses to facilitate annual BMI screening and routine follow-up with students at risk for being overweight and with overweight and obese students.
- Collaborate with physical education teachers to identify students who have a BMI at or above the 85th percentile through physical education classes; consult with students in a nonthreatening manner and refer to school nurse for appropriate interventions or referrals.
- Educate expectant parents on the benefits and potential long-term effects of breast-feeding.
- Facilitate task forces in community hospitals and nursing programs in the fight against childhood obesity.
- Support private and public funding and research to endorse effective strategies in the prevention of overweight and obesity in children and adolescents.
- Provide culturally appropriate education in schools and communities related to nutrition and regular physical activity based on dietary guidelines for Americans for individuals of all ages.
- Support the study of the prevalence of overweight and obesity among ethnically diverse individuals, and according to sex, social-economic status, and age groups, to identify effective and culturally competent interventions.
- Provide access to interpreter services to promote school and community educational efforts related to primary, secondary, and tertiary prevention in the treatment of childhood obesity.
- Promote family education and empower parents through anticipatory guidance; help them to recognize the impact they have on their child's lifelong habits of nutrition, diet, and physical activity behavior(s).
- Use and refer parents to computer information resources promoting physical activity through the Obesity Education Initiative at www.nhlbi.nih.gov/about/oei/index.htm.

Continued

BOX 60-2
Long-Term Advocacy Interventions—cont'd

- Foster relationships with community agencies serving low-income families to develop programs and educational materials related to childhood obesity (refer to Appendix G).
- Support marketing research to promote healthy food choices and regular physical activity.

🏠 Discharge Planning and Home Care

1. Integrate the CDC nutrition and physical activity programs at www.cdc.gov/nccdphp/dnpa/programs/index.htm into long-term therapeutic home care program.
2. Establish partnerships with parent(s) in all stages of therapeutic plans related to overweight or obesity.
3. Promote and provide continuing information to parents and caregivers related to changes in regimen or special needs related to dietary and weight management programs.
4. Promote physical activity of at least 30 minutes a day, 4 to 5 days a week.
5. Recommend the Kids Walk to School program at www.cdc.gov/nccdphp/dnpa/kidswalk/resources.htm.

CLIENT OUTCOMES

1. Child or youth will maintain BMI below 85th percentile.
2. Parent(s) and child or adolescent will verbalize understanding of therapeutic regimen related to dietary and nutritional guidelines, and physical activity to decrease the incidence of overweight and obesity.
3. Professionals, families, and/or youth will access available health care resources to promote and limit the incidence of overweight and obese children and adolescents.
4. Interpreters will limit language and cultural barriers for individuals and/or family(s) in the promotion of healthy behaviors related to diet, nutrition, exercise, and health disparities in the prevention of overweight and obesity.
5. Parent or adolescent will verbalize age-appropriate understating of the long-term effects of breast-feeding and weight management.

6. Parent, child, and/or adolescent will verbalize understanding of the cardiovascular mortality and morbidity related to overweight and obesity.

REFERENCES

American Academy of Pediatrics: Policy statement. Committee of nutrition; prevention of pediatric overweight and obesity, *Pediatrics* 112(8):2, 2003.

CDC Center for Disease Control and Prevention: *Overweight and obesity* (website): www.cdc.gov/nccdphp/dnpa/obesity/index.htm. Accessed July 25, 2006.

Baker S et al: Overweight children and adolescents: A clinical report of the North American Society for Pediatric Gastroenterology, Hepatology and Nutrition, Daniels SR et al: Overweight in children and adolescents: pathophysiology, consequences, prevention and treatment, *Circulation* 111:1999, 2005.

Doak CM et al: The prevention of overweight and obesity in children and adolescents: A review of interventions and programmes, *Obesity Rev* 7:111, 2006.

Hill JO et al: Obesity and the environment: Where do we go from here? *Science* 299(5608):853, 2003.

National Institute for Health Care Management: Childhood obesity—advancing effective prevention and treatment: An overview for health professionals, *NIHCM Foundation* (serial online): www.nihcm.org/ChildObesityOverview.pdf. Accessed Feb. 19, 2007.

Snethen JA, Broome ME, Cashin SE: Effective weight loss for overweight children: A meta-analysis of intervention studies, *J Pediatr Nurs* 21(1):45, 2006.

Story MO, Tracy C: Building evidence for environmental and policy solutions to prevent childhood obesity: The healthy eating research program, *Am J Prev Med* 30(1):96, 2006.

61

Patent Ductus Arteriosus

PATHOPHYSIOLOGY

The ductus arteriosus is a large vessel that connects the main pulmonary trunk (or left pulmonary artery) with the descending aorta approximately 5 to 10 mm from the origin of the left subclavian artery. Patent ductus arteriosus (PDA) is the persistent patency of the ductus arteriosus after birth, which results in the shunting of blood directly from the aorta (higher pressure) into the pulmonary artery (lower pressure). This left-to-right shunting causes the recirculation of increased amounts of oxygenated blood in the lungs, which raises demands on the left side of the heart. The additional effort required of the left ventricle to meet this increased demand leads to progressive dilation and left atrial hypertension. The cumulative cardiac effects cause increased pressure in the pulmonary veins and capillaries, which results in pulmonary edema. The pulmonary edema leads to decreased diffusion of oxygen and hypoxia, with progressive constriction of the arterioles in the lungs. Pulmonary hypertension and failure of the right side of the heart ensue if the condition is not corrected through medical or surgical treatment. Most PDAs are a left-to-right shunting of blood, but right-to-left ductal shunting may occur with associated pulmonary disease, left-heart obstructive lesions, and coarctation of the aorta. Closure of the PDA depends primarily on the constrictor response of the ductus to the oxygen tension in the blood. Other factors affecting ductus closure include the action of prostaglandins, pulmonary and systemic vascular resistances, the size of the ductus, and the condition of the infant (premature or full-term). PDA occurs more frequently in premature infants; it is also less well tolerated in these infants, because their cardiac compensatory mechanisms are not as well developed and left-to-right shunts tend to be larger.

INCIDENCE

1. Precise incidence varies depending on gestational age and according to the means of diagnosing (clinical signs as opposed to echocardiography).
2. Approximately 5% to 10% of infants with PDAs have additional cardiac defects (coarctation of the aorta, ventricular septal defect, aortic stenosis).
3. PDA is present in 60% to 70% of infants with congenital rubella infection.
4. PDA occurs 2 to 3 times more often in girls than in boys.
5. PDA is found in approximately 45% of infants <1750 g; and in infants <1000 g, the incidence is 80%.

CLINICAL MANIFESTATIONS

The disorder may be manifest at birth, but usually it is first noticed on days 1 to 4 of life. Manifestations of PDA in premature infants are often clouded by other problems associated with prematurity (e.g., respiratory distress syndrome). Signs of ventricular overload are not apparent for 4 to 6 hours after birth. Infants with small PDAs may be asymptomatic; infants with large PDAs may manifest signs of congestive heart failure (CHF):

1. Persistent murmur (systolic, then continuous; heard best at left upper sternal border)
2. Hyperactive precordium (result of increased left ventricular stroke volume)
3. Prominent to bounding pulses
4. Wide pulse pressure (higher than 25 mm Hg)
5. Decreased mean arterial blood pressure
6. Tachypnea (respiratory rate higher than 70 breaths/min)
7. Increased ventricular requirement (associated with pulmonary problems)
8. Tachycardia (apical pulse higher than 170 beats/min); usually associated with congestive heart failure
9. Metabolic acidosis (may not be present)

COMPLICATIONS

1. Cardiovascular: arrhythmias (digitalis toxicity)
2. Respiratory: concurrent pulmonary disorder (e.g., respiratory distress syndrome or bronchopulmonary dysplasia), pulmonary hemorrhage
3. Gastrointestinal (GI): necrotizing enterocolitis, GI hemorrhage (decreased platelet count), failure to thrive, decreased blood flow to intestines with use of indomethacin
4. Renal: hyperkalemia (decreased urinary output), decreased blood flow to kidneys with indomethacin
5. Hematologic: sepsis secondary to impaired white blood cell motility with use of indomethacin

LABORATORY AND DIAGNOSTIC TESTS

1. Echocardiography—two-dimensional echocardiographic visualization of the ductus with Doppler measurements is sensitive and specific for identifying PDA; M-mode measurements of left atrial to aortic root ratio greater than 1.4:1 in full-term infants or greater than 1.0 in preterm infants (caused by increased left atrial volume as a result of left-to-right shunt)
2. Doppler color flow mapping—to evaluate blood flow and its direction
3. Chest radiographic study—prominent or enlarged left atrium and left ventricle (cardiomegaly); increased pulmonary vascular markings
4. Electrocardiography (ECG)—findings vary with degree of severity: no abnormality noted with small PDA; left ventricular hypertrophy is typically seen as tall R waves in V6 with large PDA, limited value in assessment
5. Cardiac catheterization—performed only when further evaluation of confusing echocardiographic or Doppler findings is needed or when additional defects are suspected to be present

MEDICAL AND SURGICAL MANAGEMENT

Interrupting the left-to-right flow of blood is the goal of management for the uncomplicated PDA. When the shunt is hemodynamically significant, conservative measures may be tried initially. Conservative management consists of fluid restriction and medications. Furosemide (Lasix) is used along with fluid restriction to promote diuresis and minimize the effects of cardiovascular overload. Fluid restriction alone is unlikely to cause PDA closure and, in combination with diuretics, may lead to electrolyte abnormalities and dehydration as well as caloric deprivation, which impairs growth.

Indomethacin (Indocin) may be used if fluid management and diuretics fail to significantly decrease the left-to-right ductal shunting. Indomethacin, a prostaglandin synthetase inhibitor, promotes closure of the ductus. It works best in newborns younger than 13 days old and has been shown to be effective as late as 1 month of age. Its side effects include transitory changes in renal function, increased incidence of occult blood loss via the GI tract, and inhibition of platelet function for 7 to 9 days. Prophylactic administration of indomethacin soon after birth in very premature infants has also been advocated to decrease the incidence of PDA, intraventricular hemorrhage, and mortality. However, uncertainty exists about routine early prophylactic use of indomethacin because of the possible negative effects of the drug on neonatal vasoregulation and cerebral blood flow. Contraindications for the use of indomethacin are as follows:

1. Blood urea nitrogen (BUN) levels higher than 30 mg/dl
2. Creatinine levels higher than 1.5 mg/dl to 2.0 mg/dl
3. Urine output of less than 0.6 ml/kg/hr over the preceding 8 hours
4. Platelet count lower than 50,000/mm^3, because it prolongs platelet activity
5. Active bleeding
6. Clinical or radiographic evidence of necrotizing enterocolitis
7. Sepsis, proven or strongly suspected

The more immature the ductus, the greater the chance of its reopening. In one study, 23% of infants who were delivered before 26 weeks of gestation demonstrated reopening; in contrast, only 9% of those delivered between 26 and 27 weeks demonstrated reopening if the ductus was found to be closed by echocardiography after treatment with indomethacin. Early treatment leads to a higher rate of permanent ductus closure. If the ductus reopens, a second course of indomethacin treatment may be used.

Ibuprofen is another prostaglandin synthetase inhibitor that has been shown to be equally effective in closing the ductus. It does not appear to reduce the mesenteric and renal blood flow as much as indomethacin and is associated with fewer renal side effects. There is less experience with the use of ibuprofen as compared to indomethacin. It has not been studied sufficiently in preterm infants of less than 27 weeks' gestation, and, to date, the intravenous product has not been readily available.

The use of digitalis is controversial and is contraindicated in premature infants. Digitalis is not useful because myocardial contractility is increased rather than reduced in infants with PDA. Digitalis increases the force of contraction of the heart, increases the stroke volume and cardiac output, and decreases cardiac venous pressures. It is used to treat CHF and selected cardiac arrhythmias. Using digoxin (digitalis) in combination with indomethacin may increase the infant's susceptibility to the toxic effects of digoxin.

Medical management also includes prophylactic administration of antibiotics to prevent bacterial endocarditis. In older children, there are no exercise restrictions if no evidence of pulmonary hypertension is present.

Increasing positive end expiratory pressure is helpful in managing infants with PDA. When end expiratory pressure is added, the degree of left-to-right shunting through the ductus is decreased; as a result, systemic blood flow increases.

A low hematocrit has been shown to aggravate left-to-right shunting by lowering the resistance of blood flow through the pulmonary vascular circulation. Increasing the hematocrit above 40% to 45% will decrease excessive shunting through the PDA and help systemic oxygenation when perfusion is limited. Conservative management therapies usually only delay the ultimate need for PDA closure.

Surgical Management

Surgery is indicated if the ductus arteriosus remains hemodynamically significant after indomethacin therapy or if indomethacin use is contraindicated. Surgical management consists of PDA ligation. Two major groups of children have been identified as requiring this surgery. The first includes infants with CHF, usually premature neonates who did not respond to indomethacin therapy. Children older than 6 months of age whose ductus did not close spontaneously (and who are at risk for pulmonary hypertension and subacute endocarditis) make up the second group. Both groups require a left thoracotomy incision. Bypass is unnecessary. Infants are usually at greater risk for complications, so the PDA is doubly ligated in a comparatively quick procedure. For older children, surgery is advised during their preschool years and is performed by dividing the ductus between clamps and suturing the ends closed. Coil closure of the PDA to plug the ductus during cardiac catheterization or video-assisted transthoracic endoscopic closure of the PDA can also be performed, but its use is limited by the size of the patient and the diameter of the PDA.

The hemodynamic results of PDA ligation are truly curative, in contrast to the palliative procedures of many heart surgeries. Closure decreases the pulmonary flow while increasing the systemic flow, creating normal hemodynamics. Unfortunately, if severe pulmonary hypertension existed before surgery, closure will not reverse this process.

After an infant's first birthday, the most common treatment for a PDA is occlusion at cardiac catheterization. Today the most common device used for PDA occlusion is a spring occluding coil. Coil occlusion is best suited to close PDAs with an internal diameter of less than 2.5 mm. If the PDA is larger, alternative techniques should be used.

NURSING ASSESSMENT

1. See the Cardiovascular Assessment and Respiratory Assessment sections in Appendix A.
2. Assess hydration status.
3. Assess child's temperature.
4. Assess postoperative pain.
5. Assess child and family coping strategies.

NURSING DIAGNOSES

- Cardiac output, Decreased
- Tissue perfusion, Ineffective
- Ventilation, Impaired spontaneous
- Fluid volume, Excess
- Thermoregulation, Ineffective
- Infection, Risk for
- Injury, Risk for
- Family processes, Interrupted

NURSING INTERVENTIONS

1. Monitor cardiac and respiratory status (may need to monitor as often as every hour during acute phase).
2. Observe and report signs of changes in cardiac status (color, vital signs, peripheral perfusion, level of consciousness, activity level, signs of CHF).
3. Observe and report signs of respiratory distress and changes in respiratory status.
4. Monitor and report responses to ventilator assistance.
5. Assess for and maintain optimal hydration status.
   a. Limit intake of fluids (65 to 100 ml/kg/day).
   b. Monitor urinary output.
   c. Observe for signs of fluid overload.
6. Promote and maintain optimal body temperature.
   a. Use radiant warmer.
   b. Keep child covered.
7. Monitor action and side effects of medications.
   a. Diuretics (e.g., furosemide)—decreases fluid overload, increases urinary output
   b. Indomethacin—inhibits prostaglandins, promotes closure of PDA
   c. Digitalis—increases contractility of heart (monitor serum levels)
8. Monitor response to and side effects of blood transfusions.
9. Promote process of attachment between parents and infant.
10. Provide developmentally appropriate stimulation activities (see the relevant section in Appendix F).

Preoperative Care

1. Allow parents to express feelings; despite its being relatively minor heart surgery, PDA repair is still overwhelming to parents.
2. Prepare child for surgery by obtaining assessment data.
   a. Complete blood count, urinalysis, serum glucose level, BUN level
   b. Baseline electrolyte levels
   c. Blood coagulation studies
   d. Type and cross-match of blood
   e. Chest radiographic study, ECG
3. Because older child is usually of preschool age, prepare him or her accordingly; do not tell child that surgery will make him or her "feel better," because child is usually asymptomatic.

Postoperative Care

1. Monitor child's or infant's cardiac status (see the Cardiovascular Assessment section in Appendix A).
   a. Vital signs (temperature, apical pulse, respiratory rate, blood pressure)
   b. Arterial blood pressure and central venous pressure
   c. Peripheral pulses—quality and intensity
   d. Capillary refill time
   e. Presence of ascites (rare)
   f. Arrhythmias
2. Monitor for and report signs and symptoms of complications.
   a. Atelectasis
   b. Bleeding
   c. Chylothorax
   d. Hemothorax
   e. Pneumothorax
   f. Phrenic nerve damage
   g. Recurrent laryngeal nerve damage
3. Treat chylothorax if present.
   a. Provide and monitor child's intake of medium-chain triglyceride diet.
   b. Monitor for signs of respiratory distress.

4. Provide intensive pulmonary toilet.
   a. Perform postural drainage and percussion.
   b. Change child's position every 2 hours.
   c. Encourage deep breathing and use of spirometer hourly.
   d. Encourage coughing; if child cannot cough, use suction.
5. Provide intensive pain control, because pain with thoracotomy incision is usually greater than that with median sternotomy.
6. Monitor child's response to medications.
   a. Diuretics
   b. Digitalis
7. Provide emotional support to infant or child during hospitalization.
   a. Use age-appropriate explanations before treatments.
   b. Encourage, through age-appropriate means, child's expression of fears and anxieties (e.g., verbal expression, play, drawings).
   c. Encourage parental expression of feelings.

🏠 Discharge Planning and Home Care

1. Instruct parents to observe for and report signs of cardiac or respiratory distress.
2. Instruct parents about administration of medications.
3. Provide parents with name of physician or nurse to contact for medical or health care follow-up.
4. Instruct parents about principles of infection control and well-child care (e.g., use of prophylactic medications before dental care).
5. Encourage and instruct parents about providing developmentally appropriate stimulation activities (see the relevant section in Appendix F).

CLIENT OUTCOMES

1. Adequate cardiac output will be achieved.
2. Respiratory compromise will be reduced.

REFERENCES

Clyman RI: Patent ductus arteriosus in the premature infant. In: Taeusch HW et al, editors: *Avery's diseases of the newborn,* ed 8, Philadelphia, 2005, WB Saunders.

Gomella TL: Patent ductus arteriosus. In: Gomella TL, editor: *Neonatology: Management, procedures, on-call problems, diseases and drugs,* ed 5, New York, 2004, Lange Medical Books/McGraw-Hill.

Jaillard S et al: Consequences of delayed surgical closure of patent ductus arteriosus in very premature infants, *Ann Thorac Surg* 81(1):231, 2006.

Lott JW: Assessment and management of the cardiovascular system. In: Kenner C et al, editors: *Comprehensive neonatal nursing,* ed 3, Philadelphia, 2003, WB Saunders.

Shah S, Ohlsson A: Ibuprofen for the prevention of patent ductus arteriosus in preterm and/or low birth weight infants, *Cochrane Database Syst Rev* 25(1): CD004213, 2006.

62

Pneumonia

PATHOPHYSIOLOGY

Pneumonia is an inflammation or infection of the pulmonary parenchyma. Pneumonia is attributable to one or more agents: viruses, bacteria (e.g., *Mycoplasma pneumoniae*, *Streptococcus pneumoniae*, *Staphylococcus aureus*), fungi, parasites, or aspirated foreign substances. The pattern of the illness depends on the following: (1) causative agent, (2) age of the child, (3) child's reaction, (4) extent of lesions, and (5) degree of bronchial obstruction. The clinical features of viral, mycoplasmal, and other bacterial pneumonias are listed in Box 62-1.

INCIDENCE

1. Pneumonia accounts for 10% to 15% of all respiratory infections, especially during the fall and winter months. The incidence in children younger than 5 years of age is 34 to 40 in 1000; in children 9 to 15 years of age, the incidence drops to 9 in 1000.
2. Viral pneumonia occurs more frequently than bacterial pneumonia, representing about 70% to 80% of all cases. Respiratory syncytial virus (RSV) accounts for 50% of all pneumonia cases.
3. Pneumonia is more severe and more common in infancy and early childhood.
   a. Neonatal causes: group B streptococci, gram-negative enteric bacteria, *Chlamydia trachomatis*
   b. Causes from 2 months to 3 years: usually viral, more frequent in fall and winter months, especially RSV (2 to 5 months)

BOX 62-1
Clinical Features of Bacterial, Viral, and Mycoplasmal Pneumonia

Bacterial Pneumonia

Chlamydia trachomatis, Chlamydia pneumoniae, staphylococcal, streptococcal (90% of bacterial cases), and pneumococcal pneumonia occur most frequently.

Initial Symptoms
Mild rhinitis
Anorexia
Listlessness

Progresses to Abrupt Onset
Acute onset of high fever
Toxic appearance
Productive cough, diminished breath sounds, rales on auscultation
Rapid and shallow respirations (50 to 80 breaths/min), dyspnea
Nasal flaring, retractions, expiratory grunt
Increased white blood cell count, predominantly PMNs
Younger than 2 years of age—vomiting and mild diarrhea
Older than 5 years of age—headache and chills, often complaint of chest and abdominal pain
Chest radiographic finding of lobar pneumonia

Viral Pneumonia

Causative viruses include RSV (usually in infants 2 to 5 months old), influenza virus, parainfluenza virus, adenovirus, and enterovirus.

Initial Symptoms
Cough, usually nonproductive
Rhinitis
Often other family members are ill with similar symptoms

Progresses to Insidious or Abrupt Onset
Range of symptoms—mild fever, slight cough, and malaise to high fever, severe cough, cyanosis and respiratory fatigue
Tachypnea, although infants with RSV infection may have apnea; retractions, nasal flaring
Scattered rales, rhonchi, wheezing
Normal or slight elevation in white blood cell count, with lymphs predominant

Continued

BOX 62-1

Clinical Features of Bacterial, Viral, and Mycoplasmal Pneumonia—cont'd

Chest radiographic finding of diffuse or focal lobar infiltrates; hyperinflation due to air trapping is common

Mycoplasmal Pneumonia (Most Common Type in Children Older Than 5 Years of Age)

Initial Symptoms

Low-grade fever

Chills

Pharyngitis

Headache and malaise

Anorexia

Progresses to the Following Symptoms

Persistent, nonproductive cough, usually for 3 to 4 weeks

Dry, hacking cough—blood-streaked sputum

Rhinitis

Rales, rash, and wheezing

Chest radiographic findings vary, interstitial infiltrates

Fatigue

---

   c. Causes over 3 years: usually *S. pneumoniae, S. aureus, and M. pneumoniae*

4. Of children with bacterial pneumonia, 25% to 75% have a concurrent viral infection.

CLINICAL MANIFESTATIONS

Major clinical signs include the following (see Box 62-1 for specific clinical manifestations):

1. Cough
2. Dyspnea
3. Tachypnea
4. Decreased or absent breath sounds
5. Retractions of chest wall: intercostal, substernal, diaphragmatic, or supraclavicular
6. Nasal flaring

7. Paroxysmal cough simulating pertussis (common in smaller children)
8. Abdominal pain (caused by irritation of diaphragm by adjacent infected lung)
9. Pale, dusky, or cyanotic appearance (usually late sign)
10. Older child does not appear ill

COMPLICATIONS

Respiratory: chronic interstitial pneumonia, chronic segmental or lobar atelectasis, airway damage, pleural effusion, pulmonary calcification, pulmonary fibrosis, obliterative bronchitis and bronchiolitis, and persistent atelectasis

LABORATORY AND DIAGNOSTIC TESTS

Refer to Appendix D for normal values and ranges of laboratory and diagnostic tests.

1. Pulse oximetry—to assess oxygen saturation in children with respiratory distress, significant tachypnea or pallor
2. Mucus/sputum sample—to rapidly test for RSV, influenza, adenovirus, and so on
3. Chest radiographic studies—to assess for air trapping, infiltrates, consolidation
4. Complete blood count with differential—to detect presence of respiratory infection
   a. Viral infection often reveals a normal or slightly elevated white blood cell (WBC) count with predominant lymphocytes
   b. Bacterial infection typically shows an increased WBC count with predominant polymorphonuclear cells (PMNs)
5. Blood culture and Gram stain—to identify causative agents
6. Tuberculin skin test—to rule out tuberculosis if child does not respond to treatment; uses purified protein derivative; is nonreactive in 10% of children with pulmonary tuberculosis (false negative result)
7. Gram stain and culture of sputum, if available—to rule out tuberculosis; usually done for children older than 10 years of age; if tuberculosis is suspected, morning gastric aspirate

   b. Side effects
   c. Child's response
2. Provide information to parents about measures for infection control and prevention.
   a. Avoid exposure to infectious contacts.
   b. Adhere to immunization schedule.
   c. Children will have period when they tire easily and need additional rest periods and frequent, small feedings.

CLIENT OUTCOMES

1. Child's respiratory rate, oxygen saturation, and arterial blood gas levels will be within age-acceptable parameters without use of supplemental oxygen.
2. Child will have adequate hydration.
3. Child's temperature will remain within normal range.
4. Child will participate in self-care activities with minimal to no complaints of breathing difficulty.

REFERENCES

Garzon LS, Wiles L: Management of respiratory syncytial virus with lower respiratory infection in infants and children, *AACN Clin Issues* 13(3):421, 2002.

Klig JE: Current challenges in lower respiratory infections in children, *Curr Opin Pediatr* 16(1):107, 2004.

Kline A: Pinpointing the cause of pediatric respiratory distress, *Nursing* 33 (9):59, 2003.

Ostapchuk M, Roberts DM, Haddy R: Community-acquired pneumonia in infants and children, *Am Fam Physician* 70(5):899, 2004.

63

Poisoning

PATHOPHYSIOLOGY

Poisoning is defined as exposure to a potentially toxic substance and can occur by ingestion, inhalation, or absorption through the skin. The most frequent substances for poison exposures in the child less than 6 years of age are those that are readily available in the environment such as cosmetics, plants, cleaning supplies, pain medication, and cough and cold remedies. Pharmaceuticals are involved in a significant number of the fatalities resulting from pediatric poisonings. Poison control centers, safety education, and child-resistant packaging for drugs and hazardous chemicals have contributed to prevention of poisoning in children.

Childhood lead poisoning occurs when lead is absorbed, primarily through the gastrointestinal tract, after ingestion of lead-contaminated substances. Lead-based paint is the most common source and serious cause of lead poisoning. Children are exposed to lead-based paint when they ingest the fine dust particles from lead-based paint, paint chips from the walls of old homes, or lead-contaminated soil. Less common sources of lead include ceramics, hobby materials, and imported canned foods. Lead is a component of several folk remedies used in Mexico (*azarcón* and *greta* for digestive problems), the Middle East (*farouk* rubbed on gums to help teething, *bint al zahib* used for colic), and Southeast Asia (*pay-loo-ah* for fever and rashes). A high incidence of lead poisoning is associated with pica.

Lead poisoning is the excessive accumulation of lead in the blood. The majority of children with lead poisoning are asymptomatic, and diagnosis is often made as a result of screening. A lead level of less than 10 mg/dl indicates no lead poisoning; lead levels of 10 to 14 mg/dl are considered borderline; and lead levels of 15 mg/dl or higher require some degree of intervention. Acute symptoms of lead poisoning are generally not evident until the lead level reaches 50 mg/dl or higher.

Excessive amounts of absorbed lead accumulate in the bones, soft tissue, and the blood. Soft tissue absorption is of great concern because it can result in central nervous system (CNS) toxicity and irreversible renal failure. Late signs of lead toxicity include coma, stupor, and seizures. Lead poisoning is considered chronic if the lead has been accumulated over a period longer than 3 months. Lead interferes with heme synthesis and has a toxic effect on the red blood cells; this results in a decrease in the number of red blood cells and the amount of hemoglobin in cells, which leads to anemia.

INCIDENCE

1. Children under 6 years of age are more likely to have unintentional exposure to poisons compared to adolescents and adults. Adolescents are at risk for poisoning exposures both intentional and unintentional—about half of the poisoning exposures are considered suicide attempts in the adolescents.
2. Most poisonings take place in the home; the most common location is the child's own residence, and the second most common is the grandparents' home.
3. Times of peak incidence are evenings at mealtimes, weekends, and holidays.
4. The peak age of incidence for poisoning is between 1 and 3 years, when a child is autonomous and exploring.
5. Lead poisoning peak incidence occurs between 1 and 2 years of age. Children between the ages of 6 months and 6 years who live in poorly maintained older housing are at highest risk.
6. In the United States, about 2% of children less than 6 years of age have blood lead levels of 10 mg/dl or more.

Declines in the incidence are attributed to the elimination of lead from paint, gasoline, and food cans.

CLINICAL MANIFESTATIONS

The manifestations of poisoning depend on the agent that is ingested. The following are some examples:

1. Nausea
2. Tachycardia or bradycardia
3. Salivation
4. Dilated pupils
5. Diarrhea
6. Metabolic acidosis
7. Hyperthermia or hypothermia
8. Seizures
9. Lethargy
10. Dry mouth
11. Stupor
12. Delirium
13. Coma

Lead poisoning is detected during routine screening of high-risk children because most children are asymptomatic until the lead levels are high. Symptoms that may be seen as lead levels rise include the following:

1. Gastrointestinal: anorexia, constipation or diarrhea, nausea, vomiting, abdominal pain, or colic
2. Neurologic: irritability and malaise. When lead poisoning is chronic, increased incidence of learning disorders, behavioral disorders, perceptual deficits, and hyperactivity with decreased attention span can be seen

COMPLICATIONS

1. Pulmonary: respiratory arrest, acute respiratory distress syndrome, tracheal corrosion if a caustic substance is ingested
2. Cardiovascular: shock, cardiac arrest, congestive heart failure
3. Gastrointestinal: liver failure, esophageal corrosion if a caustic substance is ingested

4. Renal failure
5. Neurologic: cerebral edema, convulsions

Complications of Lead Poisoning Include the Following:

1. Renal toxicity
2. Neurologic: Cerebral edema, persistent vomiting, irritability, clumsiness, ataxia, loss of developmental skills, severe and permanent brain damage (occurs in 80% of children who develop severe and acute encephalopathy)
3. Late signs: stupor, coma, seizures, hypertension, and death

LABORATORY AND DIAGNOSTIC TESTS

1. Blood toxicology screen
2. Urine toxicology screen
3. Blood levels of specific drug ingested (i.e., acetaminophen)
4. Blood gas analysis
5. Electrolyte levels
6. Tests for lead ingestion:
   a. Blood lead levels—to determine the extent of the exposure; levels are considered elevated if they are equal to or greater than 10 mg/dl. Elevated level in a capillary specimen must be verified using a venous specimen
   b. Complete blood count—used to assess for anemia and basophilic stippling
   c. Flat-plate radiographic study of abdomen—used to assess presence of lead; a positive result indicates recent ingestion of lead

MEDICAL MANAGEMENT

The first step in managing poisoning is to assess and support the airway, breathing, and circulation. The child is stabilized by providing oxygen and intravenous fluids and maintaining the airway with intubation if needed. Treatment of shock, congestive heart failure, cerebral edema, and convulsions occurs as needed. Acute poisoning management depends on the amount, toxicity, and time since ingestion or exposure to the poison. The poison may be eliminated from skin contact by removing clothing and liberally washing the contact area. With ocular exposure, eyes are rinsed with water or normal saline.

For ingestions, the use of ipecac syrup to induce vomiting is no longer recommended as a home treatment. While ipecac is considered a safe emetic, it does not completely remove the toxin and may cause continued vomiting, which leads to less tolerance of other orally administered poison treatments. Gastric lavage may be done to remove some poisons, and it may be helpful to send a gastric specimen to the laboratory for identification when the substance ingested is unknown. When the child is comatose, endotracheal intubation is performed before gastric lavage. Activated charcoal is given to bind to the poison in the gastrointestinal tract and is most effective when given soon after the poison has been ingested. Specific antidotes, such as acetylcysteine (Mucomyst) for significant acetaminophen ingestions or naloxone (Narcan) for narcotic ingestions, are used when appropriate.

The primary focus of medical care for lead poisoning is screening and decreasing primary exposure by removing lead sources from the child's environment. Screening includes assessing risk for lead poisoning at each physician's appointment. This assessment may be done by asking three risk-assessment questions:

1. Does your child live in or regularly visit a house or child care facility built before 1950?
2. Does your child live in or regularly visit a house or child care facility built before 1978 that is being remodeled or renovated or has been remodeled or renovated within the last 6 months?
3. Does your child have a sibling or playmate who has or did have lead poisoning?

Centers for Disease Control and Prevention (CDC) now recommends targeted screening of children at risk. All Medicaid- eligible children must be screened. State public health officials determine appropriate screening using local data related to blood lead levels and housing data from the census. Table 63-1 summarizes screening frequency, environmental evaluation, education, and medical management based on blood lead level.

TABLE 63-1
Lead Poisoning Screening and Intervention Guidelines

Blood Lead Level	Screening Frequency	Environmental Education	Inspection	Chelation Therapy
10-14 mcg/dl	Borderline; confirm test results within 1 month, and repeat in 3 months if still within range	Need to decrease lead exposure; importance of obtaining follow-up lead levels	—	—
15-19 mcg/dl	Confirm test results within 1 month; repeat again in 2 months	Sources of lead exposure, symptoms of poisoning, and nutritional counseling	Obtain environmental history; intervene if appropriate	—
20-44 mcg/dl	Confirm test within 1 week; if still within this range, a complete medical history is taken, and nutritional assessment and physical examination are performed	Sources of lead exposure, symptoms of poisoning, and nutritional counseling	Environment is evaluated; lead sources are identified and removed	Considered when child is symptomatic, and in some cases if lead level is >25 mg/dl

| 45-69 mcg/dl | Confirm test results within 48 hours; closely monitor levels for response to chelation therapy | Sources of lead exposure, symptoms of poisoning, nutritional counseling, and chelation therapy | Environment is evaluated; lead sources are identified and removed | Initiated for both symptomatic and asymptomatic cases |
| ≥70 mcg/dl | Confirm test results immediately, but do not wait for results to implement therapy | Sources of lead exposure, symptoms of poisoning, nutritional counseling, and chelation therapy | Environment is evaluated; child is not returned to environment until sources of lead are removed | A medical emergency; hospitalize for immediate intravenous chelation therapy |

When blood lead levels rise above 45 mg/dl, chelation therapy is indicated to reduce lead burden in the body. All drugs used for chelation bind to the lead, which facilitates removal of the lead via urine (and, with some drugs, also via stool) and depletes the amount of lead in the tissues. Before outpatient therapy is begun, the lead must be removed from the child's environment to prevent possible increased absorption of lead by the chelating drug. Children hospitalized for chelation therapy are not discharged until environmental lead is removed or alternative housing is available. The major chelating agents used for children include succimer and edetate calcium disodium. Chelation therapy is also administered to children who are symptomatic who have blood lead levels lower than 45 mg/dl.

The child admitted to hospital with symptoms of encephalopathy receives immediate intravenous chelation therapy. Lumbar punctures are to be avoided in these children whenever possible. Fluids and electrolyte levels are closely monitored. Fluids may be restricted to basal requirements plus adjustments for fluid losses such as in vomiting. Mannitol is used to decrease cerebral edema and intracranial pressure. Seizures are managed initially with diazepam, followed by long-term anticonvulsant therapy. Iron deficiency anemia must be treated in all affected children. Prognosis and residual effects are related to how high lead levels were and how long they were elevated. Learning disorders and behavioral problems may result from even low levels of lead.

NURSING ASSESSMENT

1. Take detailed history (agent ingested, dose, time of ingestion, underlying problems of child, age and weight of child, signs and symptoms present, treatment rendered).
2. Perform complete system-by-system assessment (see Appendix A).
3. Assess hydration and nutritional status for lead poisoning.
4. Assess home environment for lead source.
5. After child is stabilized and during well-child visits starting around 6 months of age, assess childproofing of home.

NURSING DIAGNOSES

- Injury, Risk for
- Anxiety
- Knowledge, Deficient
- Poisoning, Risk for
- Home maintenance, Impaired (related to lead poisoning)

NURSING INTERVENTIONS

1. Monitor child during decontamination procedures and until stable.
2. Provide emotional support to child and family (refer to the Supportive Care section in Appendix F).
3. Provide anticipatory guidance related to childproofing the home, especially regarding potential sources of poisoning.

Lead Poisoning Interventions

1. Monitor child's neurologic status and report changes in level of consciousness, seizure activity, headaches, projectile vomiting, bulging fontanelles, or abnormal pupillary responses.
2. Monitor child's vital signs and report increased apical pulse, decreased or increased blood pressure.
3. Monitor intake and output, and maintain fluid restrictions.
4. Monitor child's reaction to chelation therapy.
   a. Succimer
      i. Nausea, vomiting, diarrhea
      ii. Rash
      iii. Hypertension
      iv. Infection
   b. Edetate calcium disodium
      i. Decreased urine output
      ii. Decreased blood pressure (20 to 30 minutes after infusion)
      iii. Pain, erythema at infusion site
      iv. Symptoms of hypercalcemia
      v. Nausea, vomiting, anorexia
      vi. Numbness, tingling, myalgia, arthralgia

vii. Maintain fluid restrictions if lead encephalopathy is present.

5. Provide diet with regular meals rich in iron and calcium, low in fat.

🏠 Discharge Planning and Home Care

1. Teach parents about poison-proofing at home and poison management.
2. Make sure that all poisonous substances and medicines remain in their original containers, have child-resistant caps, and are out of reach of children.
3. Post poison control center number on telephone. The universal poison control center telephone number in the United States is 800-222-1222; the call will be routed to the local poison control center.
4. Syrup of ipecac is no longer routinely recommended for home use and, if present in the home, should be appropriately discarded.

Additional Lead Poisoning Instructions

1. Instruct parents to identify and remove lead hazards from environment(s) in which child spends considerable time before discharge. Refer to community agencies for environmental evaluation and lead removal, if appropriate.
   a. Have lead-containing paint removed from surfaces by trained personnel.
   b. Regularly wet-mop and wash surfaces.
2. Instruct parents to supervise child with pica more closely and encourage frequent handwashing.
3. Instruct and counsel parents about recommended follow-up services (see Table 63-1).
   a. Blood lead level is rechecked 7 to 21 days after chelation therapy to determine need to re-treat.
   b. Children who have had chelation therapy will be closely followed for a year or more.

    i. Those undergoing most types of chelation therapy will be seen every other week for 6 to 8 weeks, then monthly for 4 to 6 months.

    ii. Those who have had courses of edetate calcium disodium will be seen weekly for 4 to 6 weeks, then monthly for 12 months.

4. Provide education about lead poisoning.
   a. Symptoms of lead poisoning
   b. Sources of lead in environment and need to remove sources of lead to protect child
5. Encourage parents to take precautionary measures.
   a. Make sure child does not have access to peeling paint.
   b. Wash child's hands and face before he or she eats.
   c. Wash toys and pacifiers at least daily.

CLIENT OUTCOMES

1. Child will have minimal injuries related to poisoning.
2. Parents will express their fears and concerns.
3. Parents will understand child's developmental level as it relates to childproofing home and supervising child appropriately.
4. Child will return to lead-free environment.
5. Child and family will understand importance of follow-up.

REFERENCES

American Academy of Pediatrics Committee on Drugs: Acetaminophen toxicity in children, *Pediatrics* 108(4):1020, 2001.

American Academy of Pediatrics Committee on Injury, Violence and Poison Prevention: Policy statement: Poison treatment in the home, *Pediatrics* 112(5):1182, 2003.

American Academy of Pediatrics Committee on Environmental Health: Policy statement: Lead exposure in children: Prevention, detection, and management, *Pediatrics* 116(4):1036, 2005.

Centers for Disease Control National Center for Injury Prevention and Control: *Poisonings: Fact Sheet* (website): www.cdc.gov/ncipc/factsheets/poisoning.htm. Accessed April 30, 2006.

Centers for Disease Control and Prevention: Nonfatal, unintentional medication exposures among young children—United States, 2001-2003, *MMWR weekly* 55(01):1, 2006.

Manogura AS, Cobaugh DJ, and Members of the Guidelines for the Management of Poisonings Consensus Panel: Guideline on the use of ipecac syrup in the out-of-hospital management of ingested poisons, *Clin Toxicol* 1:1, 2005.

Wax PM et al: β-Blocker ingestion: An evidence-based consensus guideline for out-of-hospital management, *Clin Toxicol* 43:131, 2005.

64

Renal Failure: Acute

PATHOPHYSIOLOGY

Acute renal failure (ARF) is the abrupt reduction or cessation of renal function secondary to a sudden loss of functioning nephrons. The rapid loss of renal function leads to a reduction in the glomerular filtration rate (GFR). This causes a build-up of urea and creatinine, fluid-electrolyte imbalances, and other related problems. ARF occurs from a variety of causes (see Box 64-1). These causes are grouped into three categories: prerenal (hypoperfusion), intrarenal (intrinsic renal), and postrenal (obstructive). Acute prerenal failure results from decreased blood flow to the kidneys. Subsequent renal hypoxia causes cellular edema and injury and cell death. Acute intrarenal failure results from injury to the kidney tissue. Acute postrenal failure results from urinary outflow obstruction. ARF occurs suddenly and entails multiple problems and potentially threatening complications. Children with ARF and their families need ongoing support and education. ARF outcomes range from complete recovery to the development of chronic renal failure.

INCIDENCE

1. Incidence and prognosis vary according to age, etiology, associated problems, underlying condition, geographic location, and type of treatment.
2. ARF in infants and children is most frequently caused by prerenal failure (hypoperfusion).
3. ARF is a common complication of critical illness. ARF in critically ill patients has been associated with high mortality

BOX 64-1
Causes of Acute Renal Failure

Prerenal (Hypoperfusion)

- Severe hypovolemia and/or severe hypotension: severe dehydration, shock, cardiac failure, severe vascular fluid shifts and/or third-space losses, hemorrhage
- Pharmacologic effects: renal vasoconstriction, severe hypotension, impaired renal autoregulatory response owing to blocked prostaglandin production (nonsteroidal antiinflammatory drugs, cyclooxygenase inhibitors and angiotensin-converting enzymes)
- Renal artery thrombosis or renal artery trauma
- Cardiac arrest

Intrarenal (Intrinsic)

- Small renal vessels: embolism, hemolytic-uremic syndrome (HUS), thrombotic thrombocytopenic purpura, severe hypertension
- Glomerulus: glomerulonephritis, renal vasculitis
- Tubules: acute tubular necrosis from ischemia (sepsis, hypovolemia, hypotension) or toxins; obstruction from uric acid, calcium oxylate or other compounds
- Interstitium: interstitial nephritis, pyelonephritis, infiltration from tumors or other agents
- Congenital kidney abnormalities: polycystic kidney disease, renal dysplasia, bilateral agenisis, glomerular maturation arrest
- Nephrotoxic agents: chemotherapy, cyclosporine, antibiotics (aminoglycosides, penicillins, cephalosporins, sulfonamides, amphotericin), radiographic contrast dye, heavy metals (mercury), myoglobin, organic solvents, pesticides, arsenic (rat poisoning)

Postrenal (Obstruction)

- Ureteral obstruction: calculi, thrombosis
- Structural abnormalities: retropelvic stenosis, urethral structure, urethral valves, vesicoureteral reflux, ureterocele
- Tumors
- Neurogenic bladder

(>60%). When ARF is combined with multisystem organ failure, the risk of death is even higher.

CLINICAL MANIFESTATIONS

The clinical presentation of ARF will vary based on the underlying cause.

1. Azotemia is the cardinal sign for ARF, regardless of type. (In critically ill children, the precipitating disease process frequently overshadows clinical manifestations of ARF.)
2. Oliguria with fluid retention and edema
3. Electrolyte alterations
4. Acid-base imbalance
5. Hypertension
6. Central nervous system dysfunction
7. Anemia
8. Decreased urine output is frequently associated with ARF; patients with nonoliguric ARF may have normal or increased urine output.

COMPLICATIONS

1. Fluid balance complications: fluid overload, intravascular volume depletion from third-space losses, pulmonary edema, ascites causing respiratory difficulty
2. Electrolyte imbalances—arrhythmias, cardiac arrest, seizures
3. Cardiovascular: congestive heart failure, hypertension, hypotension, arrhythmias, shock, cardiac arrest
4. Respiratory: tachypnea, pulmonary edema, respiratory failure
5. Neurologic: altered level of consciousness, seizures, intracranial bleeding in neonates
6. Hematologic: anemia due to lack of erythropoietin and decreased blood cell production, bleeding (coagulopathies)
7. Infection can occur since the child is immunocompromised
8. Skin breakdown due to poor healing, malnutrition, pruritus
9. Malnutrition from decreased caloric intake, nausea, vomiting, diarrhea, and protein loss

LABORATORY AND DIAGNOSTIC TESTS

Refer to Appendix D for normal values and/or ranges of laboratory and diagnostic tests.

1. Blood tests: chemistry panel provides information related to levels of blood urea nitrogen (BUN), creatinine, serum

electrolytes (potassium, sodium, calcium, magnesium, and phosphorus), glucose, and protein (albumen, total protein), as well as acid-base status (bicarbonate). Complete blood count (CBC) provides data related to the hematocrit, hemoglobin, and platelets. Serum blood gas results (arterial, capillary, or venous) provide data related to blood pH and acid-base status. Common alterations of these laboratory results in patients with ARF are listed as follows:

a. BUN and serum creatinine—increased; related to impaired renal excretion of toxins

b. Serum sodium and calcium—decreased; sodium decreases because of hemodilution from fluid retention; calcium is inversely related to increased phosphorus

c. Serum potassium, magnesium, phosphorus—increased; related to altered renal filtration and/or decreased excretion

d. Serum pH and bicarbonate (HCO_3)—decreased; related to impaired renal excretion of acid causing metabolic acidosis

e. Hemoglobin, hematocrit, platelet count—decreased due to bleeding, hemolysis, hemodilution, decreased production and/or decreased life span of blood cells

f. Serum albumin—decreased due to decreased intake (nausea and vomiting are common with uremia), fluid shifts, and/or protein loss

g. Serum glucose—decreased, particularly in infants; related to decreased intake and/or stress, which initially increases serum glucose

h. Serum uric acid—increased; related to decreased renal excretion

i. Blood cultures—positive; related to systemic infection such as sepsis

2. Urine tests: urinalysis—to test for blood in the urine and for excretion of electrolytes; quantification of excreted electrolytes provides information related to renal function.

a. Urinalysis: RBCs and/or casts—indication of renal damage from various causes

b. Urine electrolytes, osmolality, and specific gravity—vary with disease process and stage of ARF

   c. Uric acid (24 hour)—decreased; related to decreased excretion with some types of renal disease

3. Electrocardiogram (ECG)—to assess changes associated with electrolyte imbalance and heart failure
4. Chest and abdominal x-ray studies—to assess for fluid retention, kidney presence and size
5. Ultrasonography—to determine kidney size, urinary tract obstruction, tumors, cysts
6. Renal Doppler blood flow—to determine if renal vascular disease is present
7. Radiographic imaging (intravenous pylography, radionuclide studies, renal arteriogram)—to examine for renal obstruction, blood flow, kidney structures, renal function

MEDICAL MANAGEMENT

Evaluation of the child's history, symptoms, and laboratory results assists with determining the cause of ARF and the appropriate treatment approach. One of the highest priorities is to stabilize the fluid and electrolyte status. This is done through strict intake-and-output monitoring and setting fluid limits as appropriate for each child's fluid needs. At times, fluid bolus and/or additional maintenance fluids may be needed to ensure adequate circulating volume to prevent further renal damage related to hypoperfusion. This should be done carefully to prevent overhydration. Electrolyte balance is managed by carefully monitoring serum levels, ensuring appropriate hydration, limiting potassium and phosphorus as needed, and infusing deficient electrolytes as appropriate. Severe hyperkalemia (>6 to 7 mEq/L) is a medical emergency requiring immediate action. This is done through rectal or nasogastric (NG) administration of sodium polystyrene sulfonate (kayaxalate), inhaled beta agonists, hemodialysis, and/or intravenous insulin and glucose, sodium bicarbonate, and/or calcium. Hyperphosphatemia can be treated with phosphate binders.

    Other important aspects of managing ARF include supporting cardiovascular function (avoid fluid overload, treat hypertension, and avoid hypotension), supporting respiratory function (providing oxygen and/or mechanical ventilation as needed), treating anemia (administering blood products and/or other medications for anemia and controlling bleeding), preventing infection (administering antibiotics and minimizing invasive procedures when possible), and supporting nutrition (administering parenteral nutrition and/or enteral feeds and ordering a low salt diet.

NURSING ASSESSMENT

1. Assess for signs and symptoms of fluid volume excess.
   a. Local edema (periorbital, facial, extremities, dependent edema, external genitalia swelling, facial edema) progressing to generalized edema
   b. Pulmonary congestion progressing to pulmonary edema
   c. Ascites (abdominal distention progressing to the extent that skin is taut and shiny over the abdomen)
   d. Intake greater than output
   e. Weight gain
2. Assess for signs of electrolyte imbalance. Frequently monitor serum electrolytes for range values.
   a. Hyperkalemia: levels above 6 mEq/L can lead to life-threatening arrhythmias (bradycardia, heart blocks, asystole and/or other arrhythmias), severe hemodynamic instability, and cardiorespiratory arrest.
      i. ECG: "tented" or peaked T waves, progressing to widening PR interval with flattening and then disappearance of the P wave, progressing to widened QRS, and finally leading to merging of QRST complex and cardiac arrest.
      ii. Other signs: muscle cramping, decreased muscle tone, abdominal pain, and neuromuscular irritability (twitching, tingling in lips or fingertips). Severe hyperkalemia can lead to muscle and/or respiratory paralysis.
   b. Hypocalcemia
      1. Central nervous system (CNS): tetany, anxiety, seizures
      2. Cardiovascular: hypotension
      3. Neuromuscular: Trousseau's sign, Chvostek's sign, muscle cramping

   c. Hyponatremia
      i. CNS: apathy, weakness, dizziness, lethargy, encephalopathy, seizures
      ii. Cardiovascular: hypotension
      iii. GI: nausea, abdominal cramping
   d. Hypermagnesemia
      i. CNS: depressed CNS, peripheral neuromuscular function, and deep tendon reflexes
      ii. Cardiovascular: hypotension, cardiac arrhythmias, depressed cardiac functioning
   e. Hyperphosphatemia
      i. Monitor serum magnesium levels
      ii. Usually asymptomatic until levels are very high (>10 mEq/L)

3. Assess for signs of uremia.
   a. CNS: lethargy, confusion, seizures
   b. Cardiovascular: hypotension
   c. GI: nausea, vomiting, anorexia

4. Assess for signs of decreased cardiovascular functioning (hypotension, hypertension, shock, congestive heart failure, cardiac arrhythmias, fluid volume deficit).
   a. Blood pressure (hypotension or hypertension)
   b. Central venous pressure (increased or decreased)
   c. Heart rate and rhythm (monitor for tachycardia and signs of arrhythmias related to hyperkalemia as described above)
   d. Distal perfusion (pulses, capillary refill, temperature, color)

5. Assess for signs of ineffective breathing pattern.
   a. Respiratory rate and pattern (tachypnea, abdominal breathing, shallow breathing, apnea)
   b. Use of accessory muscles (retractions, shoulder shrugging) and nasal flaring
   c. Grunting (infants)
   d. Cyanosis and/or decreased oxygen saturations
   e. Respiratory acidosis

6. Assess for signs of hematologic dysfunction (anemia, bleeding, thrombocytopenia, platelet dysfunction).

    a. Anemia: pallor, tachycardia, lethargy, weakness, short-
       ness of breath

    b. Bleeding: occult blood, intracranial hemorrhage, other
       signs of bleeding

    c. Laboratory: decreased hemoglobin and hematocrit,
       decreased platelet count, increased bleeding time

7. Assess for signs of infection (fever, increased white blood
cell count, septic shock).

8. Assess for signs of failure to thrive (FTT) and malnutrition
(lethargy, weakness, poor feeding, decreased appetite,
vomiting, failure to gain weight, inadequate caloric intake,
loss of developmental milestones).

9. Assess for skin breakdown.

10. Assess child's comfort level (refer to Appendix I).

11. Assess child's level of activity and developmental needs
(refer to Appendix B).

12. Assess child and family's coping response, caregiver roles,
knowledge level, and ability to manage the child's long-
term care.

NURSING DIAGNOSES

- Urinary elimination, Impaired
- Fluid volume, Excess
- Fluid volume, Risk for deficient
- Tissue perfusion, Ineffective
- Breathing pattern, Ineffective
- Intracranial adaptive capacity, Decreased
- Infection, Risk for
- Nutrition: less than body requirements, Imbalanced
- Skin integrity, Risk for impaired
- Comfort, Impaired
- Activity intolerance
- Coping, Risk for ineffective
- Development, Risk for delayed
- Caregiver role strain, Risk for
- Family processes, Interrupted
- Knowledge, Deficient

NURSING INTERVENTIONS

1. Monitor and maintain fluid balance.
   a. Frequently assess hydration status.
   b. Record accurate input and output.
   c. Monitor and record daily weights.
   d. Monitor type of fluids and administration rate.
      i. Maintain fluid limit, and avoid fluid overload. Avoid using excess fluids when administering medications and flushing lines.
      ii. Maintain circulating volume: replace fluids (vascular loss from excessive edema, aggressive dialysis), promptly correct hypotension, and carefully monitor fluid losses related to dialysis and other therapies.

(Note: Administration of diuretics and "renal dose" dopamine has not been shown to improve outcomes, and they are not routinely used with ARF.)

2. Monitor serum electrolytes and acid-base balance. Implement corrective measures as indicated.
3. Frequently reassess respiratory and cardiovascular status, supportive measures, and airway stabilization as indicated.
   a. Position child to open the airway.
   b. Administer oxygen and/or mechanical ventilation as needed.
   c. Provide cardiac support through medication administration and decreasing myocardial workload (i.e., sedation, assistance with ventilation, etc.) as needed.
4. Monitor neurologic functioning, and promptly report deterioration in status. Promptly respond to seizure activity.
5. Assess for signs of bleeding, and implement bleeding precautions (soft toothbrush, minimize needle sticks, avoid invasive procedures).
6. Monitor for signs of anemia, and implement corrective measures as indicated (blood transfusion, medication); use minimum volumes for blood draws.
7. Assess for signs of infection and implement preventive measures.
   a. Use proper handwashing techniques and/or antiseptic gel.

    b. Perform appropriate care for all invasive catheters and lines.

    c. Protect from infectious contacts.

  8. Assess for signs of malnutrition, and provide nutritional support.

    a. Administer parenteral nutrition as indicated.

    b. Assess tolerance of enteral feeds via oral, nasogastric, or nasojejunal route.

    c. Oral feedings: offer appetizing foods while implementing dietary restrictions.

    d. Monitor caloric intake.

    e. Collaborate with nutritionist as indicated.

  9. Monitor for signs of skin breakdown, and implement corrective measures:

    a. Turn frequently, avoid placing on hard surfaces (tubing, monitor cables, wrinkled sheets), and use pressure-relief surface with severe edema and/or skin breakdown.

    b. Perform frequent mouth and skin care.

    c. Administer medications for pruritus as needed.

10. Assess child's comfort level and implement pain control measures (see Appendix I).

11. Provide developmentally appropriate activity while ensuring adequate rest periods (refer to Appendix B).

12. Assess coping responses, and provide therapeutic environment for the child and family.

    a. Encourage child and parents to ventilate feelings and concerns.

    b. Assess knowledge base, provide developmentally appropriate teaching, and reinforce information provided to child and parents (see Appendix F).

13. Assess family's ability to manage their child's long-term care and provide supportive measures as indicated.

⌂ Discharge Planning and Home Care

If ARF has not resolved before discharge, provide child and parents with developmentally appropriate verbal and written instruction regarding home management of the following:

a. Disease process (include expected clinical process and signs of complications)
b. Medications (dose, route, schedule, side effects, and complications)
c. Nutrition and diet
d. Prevention of infection and skin care
e. Follow-up care

CLIENT OUTCOMES

1. Child's fluid-electrolyte and acid-base status will be within normal limits.
2. Child will not demonstrate signs and symptoms of complications related to ARF.
3. Child will demonstrate normal growth and development.
4. Child and family will demonstrate sense of mastery in dealing with disease process.

REFERENCES

Campbell D: How acute renal failure puts the brakes on kidney function, *Nursing2003,* 33(1):54, 2003.

Jamal A, Ramzan A: Renal and post-renal causes of acute renal failure in children, *J Coll Physicians Surg Pak* 14(7):411, 2004.

Kee JL: Laboratory and diagnostic tests with nursing implications, ed 7, Upper Saddle River, NJ, 2005, Prentice-Hall.

Needham E: Management of acute renal failure, *Am Fam Physicians* 72(9):1739, 2005.

Shigehiko U et al: Acute renal failure in critically ill patients: A multinational, multicenter study, *JAMA* 294(7):813, 2005.

Singri N, Ahayi SN, Levin ML: Acute renal failure, *JAMA* 289(6):747, 2003.

65

Renal Failure: Chronic

PATHOPHYSIOLOGY

Chronic renal failure (CRF) is most frequently a result of chronic kidney disease (CKD). The National Kidney Foundation's Kidney Disease Outcomes Quality Initiative has defined CKD as structural or functional abnormalities that persist for 3 months or longer. Pathologic abnormalities or other markers of kidney damage (abnormal blood or urine tests or imaging studies) are present, with either normal or decreased glomerular filtration rate (GFR). CKD also includes conditions in which the GFR is less than 60 mL/min/1.73 m^2 for 3 months or longer. Irreversible deterioration of renal function may occur over months to years.

CKD is classified into five stages. During stage 1, kidney damage is present, with normal or increased glomerular filtration rate (GFR). The focus of stage 1 is on diagnosis, treatment of associated conditions, and slowing the disease process. Stages 2, 3, and 4 represent a progressive decline in GFR. The focus of these stages is on monitoring and treating complications. Preparation for kidney replacement therapy (dialysis) occurs during stage 4. Stage 5 represents renal failure, when the GFR falls below 15 mL/min/1.73 m^2. During this stage, the loss of nephrons and renal function affects the kidney's ability to maintain normal physiologic functioning.

CRF is associated with a variety of biochemical dysfunctions. Sodium and fluid imbalances result from the kidney's inability to concentrate urine. Hyperkalemia results from decreased potassium secretion. Impaired resorption of bicarbonate and hydrogen ion retention lead to metabolic acidosis. Uremia occurs, with a build-up of blood urea, creatinine, and waste products.

Encephalopathy and neuropathy have been associated with the accumulation of uremic toxins. Poor appetite, nausea, and vomiting lead to malnutrition. Anemia results from impaired red blood cell (RBC) production, decreased RBC life span, an increased tendency to bleed (due to impaired platelet function), and poor nutrition. Bone demineralization and impaired growth result from secretion of parathyroid hormone, elevation of plasma phosphate (decreasing serum calcium), acidosis (causing calcium and phosphorus release into the bloodstream), impaired intestinal calcium absorption, and poor nutrition (related to dietary restrictions and other factors). Renal osteodystrophy (altered bone growth) is related to dysfunctional interactions between parathyroid hormone, calcium, phosphorus, and Vitamin D. Growth failure has been associated with growth hormone imbalance and other nutritional and metabolic factors. Altered sexual development has been associated with a variety of biochemical processes.

Causes of CRF are associated with a variety of congenital and acquired factors including the following:

1. Glomerular disease (e.g., pyelonephritis, glomerulonephritis, glomerulouropathy)
2. Obstructive uropathies (e.g., vesicoureteral reflux)
3. Renal hypoplasia or dysplasia
4. Inherited renal disorders (e.g., polycystic kidney disease, congenital nephrotic syndrome, Alport syndrome)
5. Vascular neuropathies (e.g., hemolytic-uremic syndrome [HUS], renal thrombosis)
6. Kidney loss or damage (e.g., severe renal trauma, Wilms' tumor)

INCIDENCE

1. The incidence of CRF in children has been increasing for many years. It is expected to rise in the future along with the increasing incidence of diabetes, hypertension, and obesity in the United States.
2. The exact incidence of CRF in children is difficult to quantify. It has been estimated at approximately 1:100,000. Incidence is highest in adolescents and males.

3. The most frequent causes (nearly 50%) of CRF in young children are related to congenital renal and urinary tract malformations (e.g., renal hypoplasia, renal dysplasia, obstructive uropathies, vesicoureteral reflux). Acute renal diseases such as glomerulonephritis, HUS, and pyelonephritis are the most frequent causes of acquired CRF in older children.

CLINICAL MANIFESTATIONS

Although the child's symptoms will vary with different disease processes, the most common symptoms associated with CRF are the following:

1. Fluid and electrolyte imbalance, leading to the following:
   a. Fluid overload
   b. Vascular volume depletion
2. Metabolic acidosis causing tachypnea and/or decreased serum bicarbonate
3. Blood cell functioning
4. Anemia, resulting in the following:
   a. Shortness of breath
   b. Pallor
   c. Tachycardia
   d. Fatigue
   e. Exercise intolerance
5. Uremic neurologic effects (neuropathy and encephalopathy), leading to the following:
   a. Itching (uremic frost skin deposits)
   b. Muscle cramps and weakness
   c. Slurred speech
   d. Paresthesia of the palms and/or soles
   e. Poor concentration and/or memory loss
   f. Drowsiness
   g. Seizures
   h. Elevated intracranial pressure (ICP) and/or coma
6. Renal osteodystrophy leading to the following:
   a. Abnormal bone growth patterns
   b. Small stature for age
   c. Bone deformities and fractures

7. Growth and development dysfunction leading to the following:
   a. Delayed sexual development
   b. Menstrual irregularities
   c. Malnutrition
   d. Muscle wasting
   e. Bone pain and/or activity intolerance
8. Psychosocial factors
   a. Anxiety
   b. Altered self image
   c. Depression
   d. Social isolation from peers
   e. Family stress

COMPLICATIONS

1. Cardiovascular: alteration in fluid and electrolytes, acid-base imbalance (metabolic acidosis), and anemia can lead to cardiac dysfunction, congestive heart failure, hypertension, left-ventricular hypertrophy, tachycardia, arrhythmias, cardiac arrest, and/or vascular volume depletion (with excessive fluid loss or removal). Fluid overload can lead to edema, oliguria, hypertension, and/or congestive heart failure. Conversely, polyuria, decreased fluid intake, and other factors causing vascular volume depletion can lead to dehydration, hypotension, and shock.
2. Electrolyte imbalances: hyperkalemia can lead to cardiac rhythm disturbances and myocardial dysfunction. Hypernatremia can lead to thirst, stupor, tachycardia, increased deep tendon reflexes, and/or decreased level of consciousness. Hypercalcemia and/or hyperphosphatemia can lead to muscle cramps, tetany, paresthesias, irritability, depression, and/or psychosis.
3. Respiratory: fluid overload can lead to pulmonary edema, increased work of breathing, and respiratory failure. Shortness of breath and exercise intolerance related to anemia can exacerbate respiratory compromise.
4. Neurologic: altered level of consciousness, increased ICP, seizures, and coma can result from the build-up of

toxins, fluid and electrolyte imbalance, and other metabolic factors.

5. Hematologic: bleeding and/or anemia—bruising, mouth sores, gastrointestinal bleeding, oozing from puncture sites, and other bleeding can occur related to hematologic dysfunction and/or prolonged bleeding time.

6. Infection: increased susceptibility, decreased ability to fight infection, and invasion of opportunistic organisms is related to invasive lines and procedures, skin breakdown, poor nutrition, and the need to administer antibiotics with caution (related to the kidneys' limited ability to metabolize and excrete).

7. Alteration in growth and bone: altered growth patterns, short stature, osseous deformities, dental defects, and mouth sores are related to poor nutrition, osteodystrophy, and/or other factors affecting bone growth and formation.

8. Psychosocial: living with a chronic disease, repeated hospitalizations, dealing with frequent and painful medical interventions, altered growth patterns, chronic stress, and other factors can lead to developmental delays, altered body image, behavioral issues, altered family functioning, anxiety, depression, and/or other psychosocial issues.

LABORATORY AND DIAGNOSTIC TESTS

1. Blood chemistry panel—provides information about common CRF-related alterations including blood urea nitrogen (BUN), creatinine, electrolytes (potassium, sodium, calcium, magnesium, and phosphorus), acid-base status (bicarbonate), glucose and protein (albumen, total protein)

   a. Blood urea nitrogen (BUN) and serum creatinine—increased due to impaired clearance; leads to the build-up of toxic wastes in the blood

   b. Serum potassium, magnesium, and phosphorus—increased; related to altered renal filtration and/or decreased excretion. Potassium can reach critical levels with CRF

   c. Serum sodium—increased due to hemodilution from fluid retention

   d. Serum calcium—decreased; related to hemodilution, calcium inversely related to increased phosphorus
   e. Bicarbonate (CO_2)—decreased; due to impaired renal excretion of acid causing metabolic acidosis
   f. Serum albumin and total protein—decreased; related to decreased intake, nausea and vomiting related to uremia, fluid shifts and/or urinary protein loss
   g. Serum glucose—is decreased particularly in infants; related to decreased intake and/or stress, which initially increases serum glucose
2. Complete blood count (CBC)—provides information related to alterations of the hematocrit, hemoglobin, and white blood cell (WBC) count associated with renal disease
   a. Hemoglobin, hematocrit, platelet count—decreased; related to bleeding, hemolysis, hemodilution, decreased production and/or decreased life span of blood cells, platelet dysfunction and white blood cell and platelet function
   b. WBC—normal, increased or decreased; related to presence of infection, impaired blood cell production, and white cell function
3. Serum uric acid—increased; related to decrease renal excretion
4. Serum blood gas results (arterial, capillary or venous) provide data related to oxygenation and acid-base status
   a. Serum pH and bicarbonate—decreased; related to metabolic acidosis
   b. Serum oxygen—normal, increased or decreased; related to effectiveness of breathing, and use of supplemental oxygen use
5. Cultures—should be obtained with signs of infection (i.e., fever; high or low WBC count; localized redness, odor, swelling and/or white or yellow drainage; cloudy urine, etc.)
   a. Blood cultures—positive with systemic bacterial infections such as sepsis
   b. Urine cultures—positive with the presence of urinary tract infection
   c. Wound cultures—positive with infected wounds or invasive lines

6. Urine tests—provide information related to alterations in excretion of electrolytes, urine osmolality, and urine specific gravity and presence of hematuria and/or proteinuria associated with renal disease
   a. Urinalysis—RBCs, protein and/or casts; indicates renal damage from various causes
   b. Urine electrolytes, osmolality, and specific gravity—varies with disease process
   c. Urine sodium (24-hour collection)—quantifies sodium secretion
   d. Uric acid (24-hour)—decreased; related to decreased excretion with some types of renal disease
7. Electrocardiogram (ECG)—to assess for ECG changes and/or arrhythmias
8. Chest and abdominal x-ray studies—to assess for fluid retention and kidney presence and size
9. Ultrasonography—to determine kidney size, urinary tract obstruction, tumors, cysts
10. Renal Doppler blood flow—to assess for renal vascular disease
11. Radiographic imaging: computed tomography (CT) scan, magnetic resonance imaging (MRI), intravenous pylography, radionuclide studies, renal arteriogram—to examine for renal obstruction, blood flow, kidney structures, renal function

MEDICAL MANAGEMENT

A primary goal is to stabilize the fluid volume and balance by limiting fluids, which is an important and ongoing aspect of CRF management. This is achieved through closely monitoring intake and output, monitoring weight gain patterns, administering fluid therapy to maintain adequate circulation and avoid volume overload, and removing excess fluids when needed. Maintaining electrolyte and glucose balances is critical. This is achieved by closely monitoring electrolytes, limiting potassium and sodium intake, and promptly correcting imbalances. If hyperkalemia is present, resin binding agents (Kayexalate), glucose and insulin, calcium gluconate, sodium bicarbonate, and/or dialysis may be needed. Calcium supplements, vitamin D, and phosphate binders may be helpful in maintaining calcium and phosphate balance. Glucose is administered when needed for hypoglycemia.

Supporting cardiovascular and respiratory function is important, particularly when complications are present. This is achieved by avoiding fluid overload while maintaining circulating volume, controlling hypertension (with antihypertensive medications and sodium restriction), and providing cardiovascular and respiratory support medications as needed (diuretics, inotropes, antiarrhythmic medications, oxygen). Other important aspects of CRF management include preventing and treating infections, nutritional support, management of anemia, and bleeding control. When CKD progresses to CRF, dialysis is often needed to prevent uremia. For children with severe CRF, renal transplantation may be an option.

NURSING ASSESSMENT

See Appendix A.

1. Assess for signs of fluid and electrolyte status.
   a. Urine amount, quality, intake-output balance, weight gain-loss patterns
   b. Signs of fluid overload
      i. Localized edema (periorbital, facial, external genitalia, extremities) progressing to generalized edema
      ii. Pulmonary congestion progressing to pulmonary edema and respiratory distress
      iii. Ascites with taut and shiny skin over the abdomen
      iv. Weight gain and decreased output
   c. Signs of hyperkalemia, hypocalcemia, hyponatremia, hypermagnesemia and hypoglycemia
2. Assess for signs of cardiovascular dysfunction (tachycardia, severe hypertension, delayed capillary refill, cool extremities, weak pulses, hypotension, cardiac arrhythmias).
3. Assess for signs of respiratory compromise (pulmonary edema, increased work of breathing and use of accessory muscles [retractions, nasal flaring, grunting], oxygen desaturation, respiratory acidosis).
4. Assess for signs of infection (fever, increased WBC count, positive cultures, shock).
5. Assess for signs of uremia.

    a. Neurologic: lethargy, confusion, tremors, muscle twitching, seizures

    b. Cardiovascular: hypertension, congestive heart failure

    c. Respiratory: pulmonary edema

    d. Gastrointestinal: nausea, vomiting, anorexia, bloody diarrhea, unpleasant breath odor

    e. Hematologic: anemia, thrombocytopenia, bruising, platelet dysfunction, increased bleeding time

    f. Skin: uremic frost, severe itching, mouth sores

6. Assess for signs of life-threatening complications: sepsis, shock, fluid overload, severe hypertension, heart failure, respiratory failure, severe electrolyte imbalance, severe acidosis, uncontrolled bleeding, coma, and seizures.

7. Assess for signs of malnutrition, growth retardation, and bone deformity.

8. Assess child's comfort level, activity level, and developmental level.

9. Assess child's coping response to long-term illness, alteration in development, treatment regimen, and possibility of renal transplant and/or death.

10. Assess family's ability to cope with their child's long-term needs and provide effective care.

NURSING DIAGNOSES

- Fluid volume, Risk for imbalanced (fluid volume excess, fluid volume deficient)
- Urinary elimination, Impaired
- Cardiac output, Decreased
- Tissue perfusion, Ineffective
- Airway clearance, Ineffective
- Tissue integrity, Impaired
- Injury, Risk for
- Infection, Risk for
- Nutrition: less than body requirements, Risk for imbalanced
- Activity intolerance, Risk for
- Growth and development, Delayed
- Comfort, Impaired
- Coping, Ineffective
- Social isolation

- Family processes, Interrupted
- Therapeutic regimen management, Ineffective

NURSING INTERVENTIONS

1. Monitor fluid-electrolyte and acid-base balance.
   a. Record accurate input and output; frequently reassess hydration status.
   b. Record frequent weights as ordered.
   c. Maintain fluid limit.
   d. Administer diuretics as needed; monitor response.
   e. Monitor serum electrolytes and glucose; implement corrective measures as indicated.
   f. Administer dialysis as ordered.
   g. Monitor acid-base balance; implement corrective measures as indicated.
   h. Teach patient and family about fluid limits and dietary electrolyte restrictions.
2. Support cardiovascular, pulmonary, and hematologic functioning.
   a. Monitor for fluid volume overload; administer diuretics and dialysis as ordered.
   b. Monitor for signs of dehydration (dry membranes, tachycardia, altered skin turgor and restlessness, leading to delayed capillary refill, weak pulses, cool extremities, lethargy, and hypotension); replace fluids as needed.
   c. Monitor for ECG changes related to electrolyte imbalance.
   d. Monitor vital signs, including blood pressure; administer antihypertensives as indicated.
   e. Administer erythropoietin (to promote red blood cell production) and iron supplements (to treat anemia) as indicated.
   f. Administer blood products as ordered; assess for transfusion reaction; use minimum volumes for blood draws.
   g. Assess adequacy of ventilation and promptly implement airway stabilization methods as indicated; encourage patient to cough and deep breathe.
   h. Promote periods of rest and sleep.

3. Maintain skin integrity and prevent infection.
   a. Provide daily bath, frequent mouth care, and skin care.
   b. Assist with turning and prevent pressure ulceration (pressure-relief and pressure-reduction surfaces; avoid lying on hard objects; avoid pressure on bony prominences).
   c. Use bleeding precautions (soft toothbrush; minimize needle sticks when possible).
   d. Avoid patient's contact with infectious visitors.
   e. Maintain sterility of all invasive lines; perform meticulous vascular access device dressing changes and site care.
   f. Monitor for signs of infection (fever, lethargy, nausea, vomiting, diarrhea, increased WBC count, wound infection), and begin antibiotic therapy promptly.
   g. Administer medications for pruritus.
4. Promote growth and nutrition (work with dietitian).
   a. Assist patient in finding appetizing choices in a low-potassium, low-sodium, low-phosphorus, high-calcium, high-protein diet.
   b. Monitor caloric intake.
   c. Monitor patient's growth status by assessing growth trends.
   d. Administer enteral or intravenous IV nutrition as needed (assess tolerance of feeds).
   e. Administer vitamins (including vitamin D), iron supplements, calcium supplements, and phosphate binders as indicated.
   f. Administer growth hormone as ordered.
5. Assess child's comfort level, and implement pain control measures (see Appendix I).
6. Assess coping responses, and provide psychosocial support for the child and family (see Appendix F).

🏠 Discharge Planning and Home Care

Assess the child's and family's understanding and ability to comprehend teaching. Promote the child's and parents' self-efficacy, self-confidence, and skill mastery related to the long-term management of CKD and CRF. Provide the child and the parents with developmentally appropriate verbal and written instruction (using appropriate language and reading level), demonstration, practice, and return demonstration of skills as indicated. Topics should include the following:

1. Disease process (include expected clinical progress and signs of complications)
2. Medications (dose, route, schedule, side effects, complications)
3. Nutrition (dietary restrictions and supplements)
4. Skin care and bleeding precautions
5. Prevention of infection and wound and/or line care as indicated (dressing change, site assessment, flushing, emergency care as needed)
6. Home or outpatient dialysis (peritoneal or hemodialysis) as indicated
7. Child's developmental needs—assist family to address the need for developmental support and activity despite the child's fatigue, exercise intolerance, altered body image, potential mood alterations, disruption in home and school routines (e.g., doctor's appointments, dialysis, frequent hospitalizations), and other factors affecting normal growth and development patterns (refer to Appendix B)
8. Multidisciplinary support services (e.g., case management, social services, psychology, clergy, support groups, school programs, outpatient therapy, home nursing, respite care)— assist families to manage the financial, emotional, physical, and spiritual burdens of having a child with a chronic and life-threatening medical condition (see Appendix G)
9. Follow-up care, monitoring, and long-term treatment

CLIENT OUTCOMES

1. Child will maintain fluid-electrolyte and acid-base balance within appropriate limits.
2. Child will be free of infection.
3. Child and family will adhere to treatment regimen without the occurrence of complications.
4. Child will have optimal growth and development.
5. Family will maintain optimal functioning.

REFERENCES

ANNA Pediatric Nephrology Special Interest Group: ESRD peritoneal dialysis fact sheet, *American Nephrology Nursing Association*, Pitman, New Jersey, 2005.

Chadha V, Warady BA: Epidemiology of pediatric chronic kidney disease, *Adv Chronic Kidney Dis* 12(4):343, 2005.

Cimete G: Stress factors and coping strategies of parents of children treated by hemodialysis: A qualitative study, *J Pediatr Nurs* 17(4):297, 2002.

Furth SL: Growth and nutrition in children with chronic kidney disease: *Adv Chronic Kidney Dis* 12(4):366, 2005.

Joint Commission on Accreditation of Healthcare Organizations: A report on national kidney disease guidelines and pediatric nursing measures, *Joint Commission Benchmark*: 7(1):8, 2005.

Miller D, MacDonald D: Management of pediatric patients with chronic kidney disease, *Pediatr Nurs* 32(2):128, 2006.

Sofer D: Chronic kidney disease: The emerging epidemic, *AJN* 103(12):23, 2003.

Thomas-Hawkins C, Zazworsky D: Self management of chronic kidney disease, *AJN* 105(10):40, 2005.

Wright E: Assessment and management of the child requiring chronic haemo-dialysis, *Paediatr Nurs* 16(7):37, 2004.

66

Respiratory Distress Syndrome

PATHOPHYSIOLOGY

Respiratory distress syndrome (RDS) results from the absence, deficiency, or alteration of the components of pulmonary surfactant. Surfactant, a lipoprotein complex, is an ingredient of the filmlike surface of each alveolus that prevents alveolar collapse. It is secreted from type II respiratory cells in the alveoli. When surfactant is inadequate, alveolar collapse occurs and hypoxia results. Pulmonary vascular constriction and decreased pulmonary perfusion then occur, which lead to progressive respiratory failure.

INCIDENCE

1. The incidence of RDS shows an inverse relationship to gestational age: the younger the infant, the greater the risk of RDS. However, the occurrence of RDS appears to be more dependent on lung maturity than on actual gestational age.
   a. Diagnosed in 60% of infants at less than 28 weeks' gestation, in 30% of infants born between 28 weeks and 34 weeks gestation; and 5% of infants born after 34 weeks' gestation
2. The severity of RDS is decreased in infants whose mothers received corticosteroids 24 to 48 hours before delivery. There appears to be an additive effect in improved lung function when antenatal steroid therapy is combined with postnatal surfactant administration.
3. RDS occurs twice as often in males as in females.

4. Incidence increases in full-term infants in the presence of certain factors:
   a. Diabetic mother who delivers at less than 38 weeks' gestation
   b. Cesarean delivery without labor
   c. Perinatal hypoxia

CLINICAL MANIFESTATIONS

The following symptoms are observed in the first 2 to 8 hours of life. Symptoms are progressive as atelectasis increases:
1. Tachypnea (more than 60 breaths/min)
2. Intercostal and sternal retractions
3. Audible expiratory grunting
4. Nasal flaring
5. Cyanosis as hypoxemia increases
6. Decreasing lung compliance (paradoxic seesaw respirations)
7. Systemic hypotension (peripheral pallor, edema, capillary filling delayed by more than 3 to 4 seconds)
8. Decreased urinary output
9. Decreased breath sounds with rales
10. Tachycardia as acidosis and hypoxemia progress

RDS is a self-limiting disease. Improvement is typically seen 48 to 72 hours after birth, when type II alveolar cell regeneration occurs and surfactant is produced. Presentation and duration of symptoms can be altered with surfactant replacement therapy.

COMPLICATIONS

1. Metabolic: acid-base imbalance
2. Pulmonary: air leaks (pneumothorax, pneumomediastinum, pneumopericardium, pneumoperitoneum, subcutaneous emphysema, pulmonary interstitial emphysema), pulmonary hemorrhage, chronic lung disease of infancy (in 5% to 10% of infants, see Chapter 13), apnea
3. Cardiovascular: systemic hypotension
4. Hematologic: anemia
5. Infection: pneumonia, septicemia—transplacental or nosocomial
6. Developmental: altered infant development and parenting behaviors

Complications Associated with Intubation

1. Endotracheal tube complications (displacement, dislodgement, occlusion, atelectasis after extubation, palatal grooves)
2. Tracheal lesions (erosion, granuloma, subglottic stenosis, necrotizing tracheobronchitis)

Complications Associated with Prematurity

1. Cardiovascular: patent ductus arteriosus, often associated with pulmonary hypertension, intraventricular hemorrhage, retinopathy of prematurity
2. Neurologic impairment

LABORATORY AND DIAGNOSTIC TESTS

1. Chest radiographic studies—to visualize lung and cardiac involvement
   a. Diffuse reticulogranular pattern in superimposed air bronchograms
   b. Central lung markings and heart border that are difficult to see; hypoinflated lungs
   c. Possible presence of cardiomegaly when other systems are also involved (infants of diabetic mothers, infants with hypoxia or congestive heart failure)
   d. Large thymic silhouette
   e. Whiteout (uniform granularity) in air bronchograms, indicating severe disease if present in first few hours
2. Arterial blood gas values—to determine the level of oxygen and carbon dioxide in the blood; hypoxemia with respiratory and/or metabolic acidosis
3. Complete blood count—to determine the cellular profile of the blood such as red blood cells, white blood cells, hemoglobin, hematocrit, and platelet count
4. Serum electrolytes, calcium, sodium (Na^+), potassium (K^+), glucose levels
5. Lecithin/sphingomyelin ratio and phosphatidylglycerol levels are beneficial in determining timing for labor induction or elective cesarean deliveries as a means of preventing RDS

MEDICAL MANAGEMENT

The goal of medical management is to improve oxygenation and maintain optimal lung volume. Stabilization of the infant's condition is indicated by laboratory values of arterial partial pressure of oxygen (Pao_2) of 50 to 80 mm Hg, arterial partial pressure of carbon dioxide ($Paco_2$) of 40 to 50, and pH of at least 7.25. This aim is achieved by the following: (1) treat the infant with warm, humidified oxygen; (2) replace surfactant via endotracheal tube (ET); and (3) provide continuous positive airway pressure via nasal prongs or ET tube to prevent volume loss during expiration or mechanical ventilation for severe hypoxemia (Pao_2 lower than 50 mm Hg) and/or hypercapnia ($Paco_2$ higher than 60 mm Hg). Transcutaneous monitoring and pulse oximetry are done to monitor the infant's response to oxygen supplementation and adjusted as necessary. Aerosol administration of bronchodilators is administered as needed, as is chest physiotherapy. Additional cardiorespiratory measures include high-frequency ventilation and nitric oxide.

Efforts are directed to maintaining temperature stabilization, and appropriate fluid, electrolyte, and nutritional intake are provided. Arterial blood gas levels, hemoglobin level and hematocrit, and bilirubin level are monitored closely to determine the infant's status. An arterial line is inserted for monitoring PaO_2 and blood sampling. Blood is transfused as needed to maintain hematocrit, for optimal oxygenation. Medications are administered as indicated. These medications include the following:

1. Diuretics to minimize interstitial edema
2. Sodium bicarbonate ($NaHCO_3$) or sodium acetate for metabolic acidosis
3. Antibiotics for associated infection
4. Analgesics for pain and irritability
5. Theophylline as a respiratory stimulant
6. Vasopressors (dopamine, dobutamine)
7. Corticosteroids to enhance lung maturity
8. Bronchodilators

Refer to Chapter 13 for management of ongoing problems.

NURSING ASSESSMENT

1. See the Respiratory Assessment section in Appendix A.
2. Assess child's cardiorespiratory status.
3. Assess child's oxygenation.
4. Assess child's hydration status.
5. Assess child's nutritional status.
6. Assess child's developmental level (see Appendix B).
7. Assess infant-family interaction.
8. Assess family's ability to cope with home care needs.

NURSING DIAGNOSES

- Gas exchange, Impaired
- Airway clearance, Ineffective
- Breathing pattern, Ineffective
- Nutrition: less than body requirements, Imbalanced
- Hypothermia
- Tissue perfusion, Ineffective
- Fluid volume, Excess
- Growth and development, Delayed
- Parenting, Impaired
- Therapeutic regimen management, Ineffective

NURSING INTERVENTIONS

1. Maintain cardiorespiratory stability.
   a. Monitor depth, symmetry, and rhythm of respirations.
   b. Monitor rate, quality, and murmurs of heart sounds.
   c. Assess responsiveness to medical interventions: mechanical ventilation, aerosol administration, and surfactant replacement therapy.
   d. Monitor Pao_2 through pulse oximetry and/or transcutaneous monitoring.
   e. Monitor arterial blood gases and laboratory data.
   f. Monitor blood pressure and fluctuations with activity and treatments.
   g. Administer medications as indicated.
2. Optimize oxygenation.
   a. Monitor correlation between environment, positioning, and transcutaneous monitoring readings.

    b. Coordinate delivery of routine care and procedures and cluster care as appropriate.

    c. Maintain ET or nasal prong position and patency.

    d. Suction as needed. Insert suction catheter only as far as end of ET tube.

    e. Administer sedatives and analgesics as needed.

    f. Maintain temperature stability through thermoregulation strategies.

3. Maintain appropriate fluid, nutrient, and caloric intake.

    a. Maintain intravenous access as needed.

    b. Administer feedings via most appropriate route for medical and developmental status.

    c. Record weight daily and length and head circumference weekly.

    d. Monitor and record intake and output (including blood products, urine, and stool); check pH and specific gravity.

4. Promote normal growth and development (see Appendix B).

    a. Maintain therapeutic environment with controlled handling and appropriate stimulation.

    b. Identify individual stress and interaction cues.

    c. Coordinate nursing care and procedures with tolerance level of infant.

    d. Facilitate parent-infant interaction by teaching parents infant cues and encouraging parents to hold infant, to participate in kangaroo care, and to provide some routine care for infant (e.g., feeding and bathing).

5. Incorporate other immediate family members (siblings) into infant's care as soon as appropriate.

🏠 Discharge Planning and Home Care

1. Monitor readiness for discharge (see Chapter 13).
2. Provide appropriate discharge instructions for parents (see Chapter 13).

CLIENT OUTCOMES

1. Infant will have optimal lung functioning, with gas exchange and oxygenation sufficient for tissue perfusion and growth.

2. Infant will meet growth and development parameters appropriate for corrected age.
3. Parents will be competent in care of their infant.

REFERENCES

American Lung Association: Respiratory distress syndrome of the newborn fact sheet, *American Lung Association* (serial online): www.lungusa.org/site/apps/s/content.asp?c=dvLUK9O0E&b=34706&ct=3052585. Accessed February 25, 2007.

Guillory C, Cabrera-Meza G: Approaches to the patient with respiratory disease. In: Weisman LE, Hansen TN, editors: *Contemporary diagnosis and management of neonatal respiratory diseases*, ed 3, Newtown, PA, 2003, Handbooks in Health Care.

Kenner C, Lott J, editors: *Comprehensive neonatal nursing: a physiologic perspective*, ed 3, Philadelphia, 2003, WB Saunders.

Merenstein G, Gardner S, editors: *Handbook of neonatal intensive care*, ed 6, St. Louis, 2006, Mosby.

U.S. National Library of Medicine, National Institutes of Health: Respiratory distress syndrome (RDS) in infants, *MedlinePlus* (serial online): www.nlm.nih.gov/medlineplus/ency/article/001563.htm. Accessed February 24, 2007.

Zukowsky K: Respiratory distress. In: Verklan MT, Walden M, editors: *Core curriculum for neonatal intensive care nursing*, ed 3, St. Louis, 2004, Elsevier.

67

Respiratory Tract Infections

PATHOPHYSIOLOGY

Respiratory tract infections are those caused by either a virus or bacterium in either the upper or lower respiratory tract. Viral infections are most common. Upper respiratory tract infection affects the trachea and larynx and is known as croup or laryngotracheobronchitis. It is caused by parainfluenza virus types I, II, or III, adenovirus, respiratory syncytial virus (RSV), or influenza virus types A or B. This infection leads to inflammation and edema of the laryngeal mucosa, followed by epithelial necrosis and shedding. Narrowing of the subglottic regions results in a characteristic barky cough, harsh voice, stridor, and retractions of the chest wall. Children are more susceptible to upper airway obstruction because the diameters of their supraglottic, glottic, and subglottic regions are small. Edema in these areas can lead to asynchronous chest and abdominal movement, fatigue, hypoxia, hypercapnia, and respiratory failure. Fever is usually present. Symptoms are almost always worse at night and show improvement during the day and, for 60% of children, resolve within 48 hours.

Lower respiratory tract infections are commonly known as bronchiolitis. This illness may be caused by RSV, parainfluenza, adenoviruses, rhinoviruses, enteroviruses, or human metapneumovirus. It is characterized by cough, nasal secretions, tachypnea, expiratory wheezing, and retractions because of inflammation of the small bronchi and smaller bronchioles. Edema of the mucous membranes lining the walls of the bronchioles along with cellular infiltrates and increased mucus production result in obstruction of the bronchioles. This causes hyperinflation of the affected areas, since expired air is trapped distally, resulting in hypoxemia. The obstructions do not occur uniformly throughout the lung. In addition, resistance to airflow increases. This leads to dyspnea, tachypnea, and lower tidal volumes, which may result in hypercarbia in severely affected individuals. Symptoms are more severe in infants because the diameter of the lumina of their bronchioles is smaller.

These viral illnesses are transmitted by respiratory secretions through close contact with infected individuals or contaminated surfaces or objects. The viruses can remain on surfaces for several hours and longer than 30 minutes on hands. Good handwashing is critical in preventing transmission.

INCIDENCE

1. Incidence is seasonal: infections of the upper respiratory tract are most common in late fall and early winter. Infections of the lower respiratory tract are most common in winter and spring.
2. RSV is present in 80% of respiratory tract infections.
3. Age range of occurrence is 3 months to 3 years; peak age of onset is 2 years of age.
4. Boys are more affected than girls.
5. Lower respiratory tract infections are the leading cause of hospitalization in infants under 1 year of age.
6. Mortality is increased with children who have other underlying pulmonary or cardiac conditions.

CLINICAL MANIFESTATIONS

1. Rhinorrhea and/or nasal congestion
2. Persistent barking cough that worsens
3. Hoarse cry
4. Stridor (progression of stridor is an indicator of the severity of the disease)
5. Increased respiratory rate
6. Retractions at rest, nasal flaring
7. Expiratory wheeze
8. Signs of respiratory failure (agitation, restlessness, listlessness, decrease in stridor and retractions without clinical improvement, and cyanosis)

9. Low-grade fever
10. Difficulty feeding or refusal to eat
11. Malaise and irritability

COMPLICATIONS

1. Pulmonary: atelectasis, apnea, respiratory failure requiring intubation and mechanical ventilation, pneumonia, and a possible link between RSV in infancy and the development of childhood asthma
2. Weight loss due to inability to eat and drink owing to increased respiratory effort
3. Secondary bacterial infection

LABORATORY AND DIAGNOSTIC TESTS

1. Rapid viral diagnostic techniques: enzyme-linked immunosorbent assay (ELISA) or rapid immunofluorescent antibody (IFA) from direct aspiration, swab, or nasal washings to isolate virus
2. Chest radiographic study—hyperinflation with air trapping and patchy atelectasis
3. Arterial blood gas values—to assess gas exchange
4. White blood cell count—normal or mild elevation
5. Electrolyte panel—to assess for dehydration

MEDICAL MANAGEMENT

Respiratory tract infections are usually managed at home with hydration, humidification, and rest. Progressive respiratory distress and apnea are indicators for hospitalization and possible admission to the intensive care unit. Supportive therapy includes humidified oxygen, pulmonary hygiene, intravenous (IV) fluids, and rest. Administration of bronchodilators, corticosteroids, and heliox (helium-oxygen mixture) is controversial. Antibiotics are not indicated unless diagnosis is confirmed by bacterial culture or secondary bacterial infection is detected. Pharmacologic intervention is approved as prophylaxis for children at high risk for RSV. Palivizumab (a monoclonal antibody) is given as intramuscular (IM) injections monthly for 5 months from November to March. It is indicated for infants born at 32 weeks' gestation or younger, those with chronic lung disease or congenital heart disease, and immunocompromised infants.

NURSING ASSESSMENT

1. See the Respiratory Assessment section in Appendix A.
2. Assess for signs and symptoms of dehydration.
3. Assess for fever.

NURSING DIAGNOSIS

- Airway clearance, Ineffective
- Breathing pattern, Ineffective
- Gas exchange, Impaired
- Fluid volume, Risk for deficient
- Nutrition: less than body requirements, Imbalanced
- Anxiety
- Knowledge, Deficient

NURSING INTERVENTIONS

1. Monitor respiratory status (including vital signs).
   a. Assess vital signs every 2 hours until stable, and then every 2 to 4 hours and as necessary.
   b. Assess for and report signs of increased respiratory distress and changes in respiratory status including hypoxemia (tachypnea, increased work of breathing, retractions).
   c. Perform cardiorespiratory monitoring.
   d. Monitor oxygen status with pulse oximetry (oxygen saturation <92% is an indicator of severe disease).
2. Monitor child's response to humidified oxygen therapy through hood, tent, or nasal cannula.
3. Promote respiratory function.
   a. Maintain a clear airway with use of bulb syringe or nasopharyngeal suction catheter.
   b. Place in semiprone or side-lying position, avoiding neck hyperextension.
   c. Promote opportunities for rest.
4. Monitor hydration status.
   a. Monitor intake, output, and urine specific gravity.
   b. Monitor weight.

   c. Monitor laboratory values.

   d. Assess for signs of dehydration: dry mucous membranes, decreased skin elasticity, decreased urine output, increased specific gravity, sunken fontanelle in infants, increased heart rate.

5. Assess child for untoward therapeutic response to medications if indicated.

6. Encourage intake of diet high in calories and protein.

   a. Serve favorite foods if possible.

   b. Encourage use of routine feeding practices (feeding times, meals with parents, etc.).

7. Encourage age-appropriate quiet play (see relevant section in Appendix B).

8. Alleviate or minimize child's and parents' anxiety during hospitalization (see Appendix F).

9. Provide consistent nursing care to promote trust and to alleviate anxiety.

🏠 Discharge Planning and Home Care

Instruct parents about the following for home care of child:

1. Use of humidifiers (may use moisture from hot shower)—cold vs. warm mist

2. Use of bulb syringe

3. Signs of secondary infection

4. Infection control and prevention measures

5. Provision of adequate fluid intake and small, frequent feedings

6. Need to keep immunization status current

CLIENT OUTCOMES

1. Child will maintain patent airway with easy respiratory effort.

2. Child will exhibit appropriate hydration status.

3. Child will exhibit no signs of anxiety or apprehension.

REFERENCES

Ball JW, Binder RC: *Clinical handbook for pediatric nursing*, Upper Saddle River, NJ, 2006, Pearson Education.

Bjornson CL, Johnson DW: Croup treatment update, *Pediatr Emerg Care* 21 (12):863, 2005.

Brown JC: The management of croup, *Brit Med Bull* 61(1):189, 2002.

Chaves-Bueno S et al: Respiratory syncytial virus: Old challenges and new approaches, *Pediatr Ann* 34(1):62, 2005.

Cherry J: State of the evidence for standard of care treatments for croup: are we where we need to be? *Pediatr Infect Dis J* 21(11):198, 2005.

Domachowske JB, Rosenberg HF: Advances in the treatment and prevention of severe viral bronchiolitis, *Pediatric Annals* 34(1):35, 2005.

Gupta VK, Cheifeta IM: Heliox administration in the pediatric intensive care unit: An evidence-based review, *Pediatr Crit Care Med* 6(2):204, 2005.

Pruitt B: Keeping respiratory syncytial virus at bay, *Nursing 2005* 35(11):62, 2005.

Vazquez D, Philotas R: Peds respiratory emergencies, *Adv for nurses (Florida Edition)* 5(20):17, 2004.

68

Scoliosis

PATHOPHYSIOLOGY

Scoliosis, a frequently occurring orthopedic problem, is the lateral curvature of the spine with a Cobb angle of more than 10 degrees accompanied by vertebral rotation. It can occur anywhere along the spine. Curvatures in the thoracic area are the most common, although curvatures of the cervical and lumbar areas are the most deforming. There are two basic forms of scoliosis: functional and structural. Functional scoliosis is secondary to a preexisting problem such as poor posture or unequal leg length. This form of scoliosis can be corrected through exercises or the use of shoe lifts. Structural scoliosis results from the congenital deformity of the spinal column. This condition often occurs in children with myelomeningocele and muscular dystrophy. Scoliosis is also seen in children with cerebral palsy and osteogenesis imperfecta. The structural form of scoliosis can be classified into three basic types: (1) infantile, which occurs during the first year of life (more than 20% of affected children have spontaneous resolution); (2) juvenile, which occurs between 5 and 6 years of age (bracing is used for management); and (3) adolescent, which is not evident until 11 years of age (when skeletal maturation occurs). Management of scoliosis may include nonsurgical and/or surgical methods. Most spinal curvatures do not progress more than 20%. The curvature is flexible initially and becomes rigid with age.

INCIDENCE

1. Familial tendency is noted in one third of diagnosed cases of children.

2. Male-female ratio of occurrence is 1:6.
3. Adolescent scoliosis is the most common form.

CLINICAL MANIFESTATIONS

1. Major symptoms:
   a. Localized lordosis
   b. Axial rotation
   c. Lateral curvature of the spine
2. Asymmetry of hips
3. Asymmetry of shoulders
4. Shortened trunk
5. Associated skin and soft tissue change
6. Patches of hair in sacral area
7. Unequal leg lengths
8. Asymmetric scapulae
9. Malalignment of trunk and pelvis
10. Asymmetry of flanks
11. Asymmetry of breasts

COMPLICATIONS

1. Urinary problems (most common)
2. Neurologic problems
3. Cardiopulmonary impairment

LABORATORY AND DIAGNOSTIC TESTS

Refer to Appendix D for normal values and/or ranges of laboratory and diagnostic tests.
1. Forward bending test, or Adam's position—to assess inequality of flank and ribs (screening test)
2. Cobb diagnostic method—to assess angle of curvature on radiographic studies
3. Anteroposterior and lateral radiographic studies of spine—to evaluate curvature of spine
4. Three-dimensional computed tomography—to assess for axial rotation of the spine
5. Magnetic resonance imaging—to assess for intraspinal pathology

Preoperative Tests

1. Complete blood count—to assess for anemia
2. Blood chemistry analysis—to assess for electrolyte imbalances
3. Type and cross-match for blood transfusions
4. Coagulation studies—to assess for deficiency in clotting factors
5. Radiography of skull—to assess for area of spinal curvature
6. Pulmonary function tests—to assess for pulmonary complications.
7. Arterial blood gas values—to assess for pulmonary complications

MEDICAL AND SURGICAL MANAGEMENT

Curves of less than 20 degrees require evaluation every 3 to 12 months. If the curve progresses, several corrective devices can be used to stop its progression. The Milwaukee brace is used for treatment of lateral curvature of 20 to 40 degrees; the brace consists of neck ring and pelvic girdle, and it must be worn 23 hours a day until curvature is corrected. The thoracolumbar-sacral orthosis (TLSO, or the Boston brace) is a molded plastic jacket that comes up to beneath the underarms and is worn 20 hours a day. A Cheneau orthosis can also be used. The Charleston bending brace is worn at night.

Surgical Management

A posterior spinal fusion is the treatment of choice for a spinal curvature greater than 40 degrees or for a curve that progressively worsens in spite of nonsurgical treatment. Spinal fusion provides a permanent method of halting the progressive worsening of the spinal curvature. Several different types of instrumentation are used to stabilize the spine internally, including the Harrington rod, the Luque rod (segmental spinal instrumentation), and Dwyer cables. Use of the Luque rod instrumentation is a more recent and preferred technique in the surgical correction of scoliosis. During the surgery, bone chips from the posterior iliac crest are positioned on top of the spine. External immobilization with the use of a body cast is then not needed, because greater internal immobilization is achieved with this technique.

Anterior thoracic discectomy procedures with endplate ablations and posterior spinal fusions are recommended for individuals with severe scoliosis. Video-assisted thoracoscopic surgery is used in some institutions to release the anterior spine of these individuals.

NURSING ASSESSMENT

1. See the Musculoskeletal Assessment section in Appendix A.
2. Assess for asymmetry of flank, ribs, scapulae, and hips.
3. Assess for malalignment of trunk and pelvis.

NURSING DIAGNOSES

- Knowledge, Deficient
- Anxiety
- Injury, Risk for
- Mobility, Impaired physical
- Gas exchange, Impaired
- Fluid volume, Risk for deficient
- Peripheral neurovascular dysfuntion, Risk for
- Therapeutic regimen management, Ineffective
- Body image, Disturbed

NURSING INTERVENTIONS

Preoperative Care

1. Prepare child or adolescent and family before preoperative and operative procedures for sequence of events and sensations that will be experienced.
   a. Refer to section on Laboratory and Diagnostic Tests.
2. Prepare child or adolescent for surgery (see the Preparation for Procedures or Surgery section in Appendix F).
3. Orient child or adolescent to intensive care unit and treatment procedures used postoperatively (e.g., blow gloves and spirometer).

Postoperative Care

1. Monitor for signs and symptoms of potential complications.
   a. Monitor arterial lines.

b. Monitor temperature, respirations, blood pressure, and pulse every 1 to 2 hours until stable, and then every 4 hours.

c. Auscultate breath sounds; report changes in respiratory status (increased respirations, increased congestion, color change, chest pain, dyspnea).

d. Monitor for spinal nerve trauma—observe lower extremities for warmth, sensation, movement, pulses, and pain.

e. Monitor for paralytic ileus—auscultate bowel sounds.

f. Monitor dressing for intactness and signs of complications.

   i. Note bleeding along incision.

   ii. Monitor for signs of infection.

2. Promote proper body alignment.

a. Turn child or adolescent every 2 hours (log roll only).

b. Monitor for reddened areas and pressure.

c. Keep child or adolescent flat in bed until doctor orders activity (flat with log rolling only until body jacket arrives) (not always ordered with Harrington rod because child is out of bed by 2 to 4 days after surgery).

d. Institute passive range of motion exercises on second postoperative day.

3. Promote pulmonary ventilation.

a. Monitor vital signs as often as every 2 hours.

b. Have child or adolescent cough, turn, and deep breathe as often as every 2 hours.

c. Use incentive spirometer every 2 hours.

d. Monitor respiratory status every 2 hours until stable, and then every 4 hours.

4. Monitor fluid and electrolyte balance.

a. Monitor and record intake and output—intravenous fluids, urine, nasogastric drainage.

b. Monitor bowel sounds.

c. Advance diet as tolerated (clear liquid to regular diet).

d. Monitor for signs and symptoms of dehydration and fluid overload: dehydration—decreased urinary output, increased specific gravity, doughy skin, dry mucous membranes; fluid overload—increased apical pulse, increased respiratory rate, pulmonary congestion, dyspnea, edema initially of extremities.

5. Provide pain relief measures as necessary (may have epidural catheter and/or patient-controlled anesthesia) (see Appendix I).
   a. Medicate routinely every 2 to 4 hours for first 72 hours.
   b. Medicate before procedures.
   c. Provide diversional activities and relaxation techniques.

🏠 Discharge Planning and Home Care

Postoperative Care

1. Instruct child or adolescent and family about various aspects of care (which vary according to procedure).
   a. Physical restrictions and need for moderate physical exercise
   b. Use of body cast or jacket (thoracolumbar-sacral orthotics)
   c. Equipment (e.g., firm mattress), log-rolling technique
   d. Signs of infection (increased temperature, odor from cast)
   e. Incision site care
2. Encourage child or adolescent and family to express fears and body image concerns.
3. Refer to community resources (public health nurse, home health nurses) (see Appendix G).
4. Encourage adherence to follow-up care regimen (clinic visits for 6 to 12 months postoperatively).

Nonsurgical Interventions

1. Instruct child or adolescent and parents in use of Milwaukee brace or Orthoplast jacket, Charleston brace, or Boston Brace.
   a. Application and removal of brace or jacket
   b. Cleaning of brace or jacket
   c. Skin inspection for pressure sores or skin breakdown
   d. Bathing before application
   e. Use of undergarments
2. Instruct child or adolescent and parents in use of exercises, and reinforce instruction.

3. Instruct child or adolescent and parents about participation in sports and recreational activities.
4. Encourage child or adolescent to express feelings of concern and inadequacy concerning brace.
   a. Distortion of body image
   b. Feelings of rejection by peers
5. Emphasize that compliance with brace regimen leads to better results than noncompliance.
6. Initiate community referrals (see Appendix G).
   a. School nurse to facilitate school adaptation
   b. Financial assistance resources to cover costs incurred in treatment of condition
7. Instruct child or adolescent and family about cast care.
   a. Skin care (use alcohol only)
   b. Assessment for sensation and movement
   c. Exercise for unaffected extremities
   d. Assessment for signs of infection (musty odor, drainage on cast)
   e. Petal cast edges

CLIENT OUTCOMES

1. Child will maintain proper body alignment.
2. Child will have minimal pain during first 72 hours postoperatively.
3. Child and family will adhere to various aspects of postoperative home care.
4. Child will experience sense of mastery about the hospitalization and surgical experience.
5. Child will integrate positive body image of him- or herself following the recovery period.
6. Child will resume usual daily activities with minimal amount of disruption.

REFERENCES

Asher Marc et al: Safety and efficacy of isola instrumentation and arthrodesis for adolescent idiopathic scoliosis: Two to 12 year follow-up, *Spine* 29(18): 2013, 2004.

Lamontagne LL et al: Adolescent scoliosis: Effects of corrective surgery, cognitive-behavioral interventions, and age on activity outcomes, *Appl Nurs Res* 17(3): 168, 2005.

Lamontagne LL et al: Adolescents' coping with surgery for scoliosis: Effects on recovery outcomes over time, *Res Nurs Health* 27(4):237, 2004.

Lamontagne LL et al: Anxiety and postoperative pain in children who undergo major orthopedic surgery, *Appl Nurs Res* 14(3):119, 2001.

Lenssinck ML et al: Effect of bracing and other conservative interventions in the treatment of idiopathic scoliosis in adolescents: A systematic review of clinical trials, *Phys Ther* 85(12):1329, 2005.

Rahman T et al: The association between brace compliance and outcome for patients with idiopathic scoliosis, *J Pediatr Orthop* 25(4):420, 2005.

Sapontzi-Krepia DS et al: Perceptions of body image, happiness and satisfaction in adolescents wearing a Boston brace for scoliosis treatment, *J Adv Nurs* 35(5):683, 2001.

Schufflebarger HL et al: The posterior approach for lumbar and thoracolumbar adolescent idiopathic scoliosis: Posterior shortening and pedicle screws, *Spine* 29(3):269, 2004.

Zhang JG et al: The role of preoperative pulmonary function tests in the surgical treatment of scoliosis, *Spine* 30(2):218, 2005.

69

Seizure Disorders

PATHOPHYSIOLOGY

A seizure is a sudden, transient alteration in brain function as a result of abnormal neuronal activity and excessive cerebral electrical discharge. This activity can be partial or focal, originating in a specific area of the cerebral cortex—or generalized, involving both hemispheres of the brain. It is indicative of underlying brain pathology. Clinical manifestations vary, depending on the area(s) of brain involvement. The types of seizure affecting children and adolescents are listed in Box 69-1, which is the international classification of epileptic seizures created in 1981 by the International League Against Epilepsy. This classification is currently being revised.

If an area of the brain is affected, a *focal seizure* occurs, and if the whole brain is affected, a *generalized seizure* occurs. Any type of seizure can secondarily generalize. Before a focal seizure, a person may have a preictal (preseizure) phase consisting of varied symptoms, which may include a feeling, a subjective sensation, or a physical symptom signifying that a seizure will occur. In younger children the preictal phase may consist of a mood change or clingy type behavior that the parent will say occurs before the seizure.

A seizure is referred to as the ictal phase. Most seizures last less than 5 minutes, the majority less than 2 minutes. Seizure symptoms can include vocal, motor, cognitive, respiratory, and autonomic components, change in consciousness, and/or loss of consciousness. The postictal phase may occur after the seizure, and symptoms may include headache, fatigue, confusion, transient focal weakness (Todd's paresis or paralysis),

BOX 69-1

The International Classification of Epileptic Seizures

I. Partial (focal, local) seizures
   A. Simple partial seizures (consciousness not impaired)
      1. Motor abnormal movement of an arm, leg, or both (Jacksonian march)
      2. Somatosensory or special sensory (gustatory, olfactory, auditory)
      3. Autonomic (tachycardia, respiration, flushing)
      4. Psychic (déjà vu, fearful feeling)
   B. Complex partial seizures (with impairment of consciousness)
      1. Beginning as simple partial seizure and progressing to impairment of consciousness
         a. No other symptoms
         b. Motor, somatosensory, special sensory, autonomic, or psychic symptoms
         c. Automatisms
      2. With impairment of consciousness at onset
         a. No other symptoms
         b. Motor, somatosensory, special sensory, autonomic psychic symptoms
         c. Automatisms
   C. Partial seizures evolving to secondarily generalized seizures
      1. Simple partial seizure leads to generalized seizures
      2. Complex partial seizure leads to generalized seizures
      3. Simple partial seizure leads to complex partial seizure, which leads to generalized seizures
II. Generalized seizures (convulsive or nonconvulsive, all associated with loss of consciousness)
   A. Absence
      1. Onset in childhood; approximately 50% ending in adolescence and 50% supplanted by tonic-clonic seizures
      2. Symptoms include altered awareness or attention and blank stare; may include eye blinking lasting 5 to 30 seconds
      3. Can be mistaken as learning disabilities or behavior problems if unrecognized
   B. Myoclonic
      1. Characterized by short, abrupt muscular contractions of arms, legs, and/or torso

Continued

BOX 69-1

The International Classification of Epileptic Seizures—cont'd

  2. Symptoms include jerks that are symmetrical or asymmetrical, syncronus or asynchronous, and single or multiple; possible brief loss of consciousness
C. Clonic
  1. Symptoms include muscle contraction and relaxation, usually lasting several minutes
  2. Distinct phases may not be easily observable
D. Tonic
  1. Symptoms include an abrupt increase in muscle tone (contraction), loss of consciousness, and autonomic signs, lasting from 30 seconds to several minutes
E. Tonic-clonic
  1. Tonic phase—may begin with shrill cry caused by secondary expulsion of air due to abrupt closure of the epiglottis; rigidity, opisthotonos, extension of arms and legs; jaw may snap shut; temporary (up to 1 minute) cessation of respiration; nonreactive dilated pupils; decreased heart rate
  2. Clonic phase—begins suddenly and ends gradually, characterized by quick, bilateral, severe jerking movements; stertorous respirations; autonomic symptoms; lasts 2 to 5 minutes
  3. Postictal phase—muscle flaccidity; gradual return of consciousness; amnesia related to the seizure; patient may need 30 to 60 minutes of sleep following seizure activity
F. Atonic
  1. Characterized by abrupt loss of muscle tone followed by postictal confusion; injury likely
III. Unclassified epileptic seizures—cannot be classified because of inadequate or incomplete data; includes some neonatal seizures (e.g., rhythmic eye movements, chewing, and swimming movements)

Adapted from Commission on Classification and Terminology of the International League Against Epilepsy. Proposal for revised clinical and electroencephalographic classification of epileptic seizures. *Epilepsia* 22:489–501, 1981 currently under revision (p. 20, Dreifuss, 1996).

speech difficulty, amnesia, muscle aches, sleepiness, and so forth. Seizures can be further classified as *idopathic* if there is not identifiable cause, *symptomatic* if a cause is identified, or *cryptogenic* if an unidentified brain disorder is suspected.

The causes of seizure include perinatal factors, anoxia, congenital malformations of the brain, genetic factors, infectious disease (encephalitis, meningitis), febrile illness, metabolic disorders, trauma, neoplasms, toxins, circulatory disturbances, and degenerative diseases of the nervous system. Seizure triggers can include sleep deprivation, poor nutrition and hydration, photic stimulation, nonadherence to aspects of the treatment plan, stress, illness, certain medications, hormonal issues, and alcohol or drug use or withdrawal.

Epilepsy is a disorder characterized by recurrent, spontaneous, unprovoked seizures that are primarily of cerebral origin; it indicates the presence of underlying brain dysfunction. Epilepsy is not a disease in itself but a disorder, which can include possible effects on functional status, social status, emotional status, cognition, perception of health status, and quality of life. When a person is diagnosed with epilepsy, the seizure is classified according to type. Once the seizure type is known, the age of onset and the medical history, including development, physical examination, and electroencephalogram (EEG) pattern, are used to determine if the epilepsy fits into an epilepsy syndrome. Epilepsy syndromes common in children include juvenile absence epilepsy, benign centrotemporal epilepsy, and juvenile myoclonic epilepsy. Other disorders have clinical symptoms that can look like seizures. It is important to distinguish seizures from breath-holding spells, behavior disorders, cardiac arrrhythmias, anxiety attacks, migraine disorder, movement disorders, nonepileptic seizures, sleep disorders, and syncope.

INCIDENCE

1. Epilepsy and seizures affect 2.5 million Americans of all ages.
2. Of the general population, 10% will experience a seizure at some time in their life.

3. Of the American population, 3% will develop epilepsy by 75 years of age.
4. Epilepsy incidence is highest in those under 2 years and over 65 years of age.
5. Each year 45,000 children under age 15 years develop epilepsy.
6. Infections and metabolic disorders are the most common causes of seizure in children.
7. Etiology of epilepsy is unknown in two thirds of affected individuals.
8. Of all children between 6 months and 5 years of age, 2% to 5% will experience a febrile seizure.
9. Of children with febrile seizures, 2% to 5% will develop epilepsy.

CLINICAL MANIFESTATIONS

See Box 69-1 for clinical manifestations of seizure activity. Seizure disorders may also affect cognitive and functional abilities and emotional status during nonseizure periods.

COMPLICATIONS

Of Acute Seizure

1. Respiratory: aspiration pneumonia, respiratory arrest with possible cardiac arrest
2. Physical injuries such as lacerations, burns, drownings or near drownings

Of Epilepsy

1. Cognition: learning disabilities
2. Neurodevelopmental: attention deficit or attention deficit/hyperactivity disorders (ADD/ADHD); speech, gross motor, and fine motor disorders
3. Neurologic: headache, migraines, sudden unexplained death in epilepsy [SUDEP]
4. Psychiatric: behavioral, anxiety-depressive disorders
5. Social challenges: stigma, school or job performance, driving restrictions (different in each state)

LABORATORY AND DIAGNOSTIC TESTS

Tests are ordered based upon the child's history, examination findings, and seizure description. Refer to Appendix D for normal values and/or ranges of laboratory and diagnostic tests.

1. Complete blood cell count (CBC)—to rule out infection or possible side effects to medication or ketogenic diet–like anemias or bleeding issues
2. Electrolyte panel—to look for possible metabolic or electrolyte causes
3. Urine and serum toxicology screens—to rule out ingestion as possible cause
4. Lumbar puncture—to rule out infection if febrile or concerned about possible meningitis or encephalitis
5. Antiepileptic drug levels—trough level is done to evaluate adherence to plan of care, to determine whether level medication is effective, or to ascertain peak level to determine reasons for side effects or toxicity
6. Urine organic acids and/or serum quantitative amino acids—to detect inborn errors of metabolism as possible cause
7. Routine electroencephalogram (EEG)—standard test for nonfebrile seizure to determine seizure type, epilepsy syndrome, and risk for recurrence; it assists in treatment management decisions. A normal EEG does not rule out epilepsy, and an abnormal EEG does not confirm it. An EEG is a guide for diagnosis and treatment decisions. The EEG is usually done at least 48 hours after the seizure so as not to confuse the findings with postictal slowing. An EEG is usually performed in partially sleep-deprived children to assist in detecting any abnormalities. If possible, the EEG should be done without sedation.
8. Video-EEG: provides video recording of the patient simultaneous with an EEG—to assist in comparing the clinical symptoms with electrographic changes on EEG during the clinical event. It further aids in determining the seizure type and possible epilepsy syndrome. This test is typically used when evaluating treatment failure and/or evaluating a possible candidate for epilepsy surgery.

9. Computed tomography (CT) of the brain—may be done as an emergent scan for quick determination of signs like bleeding, trauma, or tumor when the patient has postictal focal deficits or has not returned to baseline after the seizure.

10. Magnetic resonance imaging (MRI) of the brain—preferred neuroimaging study conducted as more sensitive study of brain at the cellular level. An MRI is done to discover abnormalities that may affect treatment and management planning and as a component of the evaluation for possible epilepsy surgery.

11. Positron emission tomography (PET) or single photon emission computed tomography (SPECT) scans of the brain: nuclear imaging studies that use intravenously administered radioisotopes to evaluate any possible abnormalities of brain metabolic functioning—can help locate the onset of a focal epilepsy; also used as part of the evaluation for possible epilepsy surgery.

12. Speech evaluation—to ascertain the effect of epilepsy on speech reception, expression, and comprehension; also used as part of the evaluation for epilepsy surgery.

13. Neuropsychologic or psychologic evaluation—to ascertain the effect of epilepsy on cognitive skills, gross and fine motor skills, and emotional issues. These evaluations are used as part of the epilepsy surgery evaluation.

14. Physical therapy evaluation—as needed to ascertain gross motor functioning secondary to epilepsy.

15. Occupational therapy evaluation—as needed to determine fine motor problems secondary to epilepsy.

MEDICAL MANAGEMENT
Antiepileptic Drug Therapy

Antiepileptic drug (AED) therapy is the mainstay of medical management. Monotherapy is preferred to polytherapy to decrease potential side effects. The goal is no seizures and no side effects, although this is not always possible. The drug of choice is based on seizure type, epilepsy syndrome, and client variables. Polytherapy may be tried to achieve seizure control in intractable cases. Complete control is achieved in about two thirds of persons with epilepsy who remain on antiepileptic medication for an extended period. Febrile seizure disorder is not treated with antiepileptic drug therapy, since febrile seizures are not epilepsy; instead, fever and illness prophylaxis are taught to parents for management.

A child with a first unprovoked seizure may not be treated immediately with medication. The risk of a second seizure is about 33%. The risks of taking antiepileptic medications must be weighed with the child's history, neurologic examination findings, seizure type, and EEG findings. The drug of choice is also based upon these findings.

The mechanisms of action of antiepileptic drugs are complex and not completely understood. The possible mechanisms of action include altering intrinsic membrane properties and the synaptic function. These actions reduce neuronal firing, facilitate the increase of inhibitory and the decrease of excitatory neurotransmitters, or reduce the firing of the thalamic neurons. There are antiepileptic medications that are used for prophylaxis and rescue. If the child with epilepsy is seizure free for 1 to 2 years and is without reason to have further seizures, the child may be weaned from the antiepileptic medication(s). The following prophylactic antiepileptic medications are classified according to the seizure type and the known therapeutic drug levels.

Focal Seizures

Carbamazepine	4–12 mg/L
Lamotrigine	4–20 mg/L
Levetiracetam	5–40 mg/L
Oxcarbazepine	12–30 mg/L
Pregabalin	Not established
Topiramate	2–25 mcg/ml
Valproate, valproic acid	50–125 mg/L
Zonisamide	10–40 mcg/ml

Generalized Seizures

Lamotrigine	4–20 mg/L
Levetiracetam	5–40 mg/L
Topiramate	2–25 mcg/ml
Valproate, valproic acid	50–125 mg/L
Zonisamide	10–40 mg/ml

Broad-Spectrum (for More Than One Seizure Type)

Lamotrigine	4–20 mg/L
Levetiracetam	5–40 mg/L
Topiramate	2–25 mcg/ml
Valproate, valproic acid	50–125 mg/L
Zonisamide	10–40 mcg/ml

Prophylactic medications not included on the list are felbamate, phenobarbital, phenytoin, primidone, and tiagabine. Phenobarbital has a clinically established safety profile, is used for neonatal seizures, and is an excellent rescue medication, but it tends to cause hyperactivity and cognitive effects in children over 1 year of age. Phenytoin is an excellent rescue medication especially when its prodrug form, fosphenytoin, is used; but phenytoin can cause undesirable side effects like coarsening and broadening of the facies, hirsutism, and cerebellar atrophy. Intravenous fluids must be chosen carefully with phenytoin but not fosphenytoin.

Felbamate is a powerful broad-spectrum medication. Initially it was approved by the FDA, and then it was restricted, since it caused serious adverse effects of aplastic anemia and hepatotoxicity in a number of patients. Felbamate can also cause side effects of insomnia and appetite depression. It must be used with caution, and families must be counseled about potential adverse effects.

Neither gabapentin nor tiagabine have demonstrated efficacy as monotherapeutic agents, but they can be used as adjunct medications for focal seizures. Methsuximide and ethosuximide are older antiepileptic medications that are no longer used. Ethosuximide has been used for absence epilepsy but does not treat the tonic-clonic seizures that occur in 50% of patients with absence epilepsy. Adrenocorticoptropin hormone (ACTH; Acthar Gel) is used on a limited basis as the treatment of choice for infantile spasms, a potentially devastating epilepsy syndrome. Pyridoxine-dependent epilepsy is rarely diagnosed, and the treatment of choice is pyridoxine daily for life. Seizures sometimes break through the week before the menstrual cycle, and acetazolamide may be used during that week to decrease breakthrough seizures.

Recent research has noted the potential for osteopenia and osteoporosis to occur in patients on long-term antiepileptic medications. The addition of vitamin D and calcium supplements has been suggested to prevent these complications.

Rescue medications for prolonged seizures or status epilepticus can be administered via intravenous, intranasal, and rectal routes. Medications administered via the intravenous routes are Depacon, diazepam, fosphenytoin, lorazepam, phenobarbital, and phenytoin. Diastat can be administered rectally. Midazolam is administered intranasally.

Adverse effects that may occur with antiepileptic drugs affect multiple systems. Central nervous system effects can include somnolence, confusion, gait problems, dizziness, and slurred speech. Gastrointestinal effects can include nausea and vomiting, changes in appetite, stomach pain, and hepatotoxicity. Adverse metabolic effects can include electrolyte changes such as sodium alterations, osteopenia, and osteoporosis. Adverse dermatologic effects can include skin rash, jaundice, and photosensitivity symptoms. Genitourinary adverse effects can consist of kidney stones and urinary output changes. Hematologic effects that have been observed are repeated infections, anemias, and bruising.

Ketogenic Diet

It has been noted as far back as Biblical times that starvation stopped seizures. The ketogenic diet is a high-fat, low-carbohydrate and low-protein diet that is calorie restricted for the brain to use ketones instead of glucose as an energy source. The exact mechanism of action is not known, but ketosis appears to produce an anticonvulsant effect in the brain. The diet requires strict adherence and can also be given in liquid form via gastrostomy tube for those patients without oral intake abilities. The diet is not especially palatable; it may be easier for children to ingest who have cognitive and mobility limitations. The ketogenic diet is attractive to parents, because if seizure control is improved with the diet, then antiepileptic medications can be weaned away over time. The ketogenic diet is not difficult to learn but requires commitment from the family, the school, and the community.

Adherence to the ketogenic diet necessitates a team approach. A dietitian trained in how to calculate, teach, and manage the ketogenic diet is essential. Team members must include nurses and physicians who are aware of how to manage the ketogenic diet and antiepileptic treatments. It may be started in the hospital or at home.

Possible adverse effects of the ketogenic diet include elevated cholesterol and triglycerides, lethargy, hypoglycemia, acidosis, nausea, vomiting, and constipation. Other adverse effects can include abdominal pain, dehydration, anorexia, electrolyte disturbances (e.g., hypocalcemia, hypomagnesemia, acidosis), platelet disturbances (aggregation disorders), and vitamin deficiencies.

Supplements are given to prevent vitamin and mineral (electrolyte) deficiencies. Supplements can include sugar-free vitamins with mineral, calcium, magnesium, potassium, salt, selenium, carnitine, and so forth.

It is important to know that children may feel hungry on this diet. If this occurs, the calories and make-up of the diet should be reviewed and compared with the child's seizure status and height and weight. All involved in the child's care must be aware the ketogenic diet is being used.

The child cannot receive anything with glucose in it, including toothpaste. All foods must be reviewed with the dietitian since even "sugar-free" foods can have hidden carbohydrates that can affect the ketogenic diet. Medications are monitored for carbohydrate amount and calculated into the diet. When sugar-free medications are available, they are used.

Documentation of the child's current seizure treatment plan, including information about the ketogenic diet, should accompany the child if the child is transported to the emergency room or admitted to the hospital for an emergent condition, procedure, or prolonged seizure. In emergencies, the treatment of the patient overrides the ketogenic diet treatment. The diet can be restarted after the child's condition is stabilized. The medical team should remain alert for breakthrough seizures or status epilepticus in the event the diet is changed.

Family home care involves monitoring of the ketogenic diet with daily urine ketone checks. The family also monitors the child's growth in weight and height, since the rate of growth is slower than normal.

Laboratory monitoring is done periodically, in the fasting state. It typically includes complete blood cell count, and a comprehensive metabolic panel to include magnesium, lipid panel, and antiepileptic drug trough levels. A new laboratory value used in the ketogenic diet is the beta-hydroxybutyrate level, revealing serum ketosis. This laboratory evaluation is used to monitor the ketogenic diet and supplements.

Vagus Nerve Stimulation (VNS)

Since FDA approval in 1996, the VNS has been used as an adjunct treatment for intractable partial epilepsy. The VNS consists of a generator implanted subcutaneously in the left chest with an attached lead that is tunneled to the left vagus nerve. The left vagus nerve is used since it has more to do with innervation of the brain, whereas the right vagus nerve has more to do with the heart and intestines. The generator is programmed to deliver electrical stimulation to the lead, and impulses of predetermined duration are sent to widespread areas of the brain for a certain amount of time, such as 30 seconds of stimulation every 5 minutes. The mechanism of action is not understood, but there is metabolic activation of brain structures such as the thalamus, the brainstem, and limbic areas. There are also changes in neurotransmitter levels in the brain and the locus coeruleus, such as norepinephrine.

The degree of seizure reduction for the VNS is comparable to antiepileptic drugs. For those whose seizure control improves, AEDs may be decreased. A follow-up surgery to replace the battery or generator is needed every 8 to 10 years. Side effects that can occur during stimulation include hoarse voice, coughing, and minor throat discomfort. There are no cognitive side effects. There are no adherence issues, since the generator is programmed at the clinic office visit. There is a magnet that has a twofold purpose. It may be used during a seizure as a rescue method to stop or shorten the seizure, or to decrease postictal symptoms. The magnet is placed over the generator (it can be done over clothes) for a slow count of 3.

The generator then sets off an extra stimulation that is typically set higher and longer than the programmed stimulation to try to stop the seizure. Patients and families are taught to use the magnet as seizure rescue every 60 to 90 seconds for at least five attempts before going on to the next step in their seizure rescue treatment plan. The magnet can also be taped over the generator or placed in a shirt pocket over the generator to stop stimulation so a person's voice is not affected by the VNS stimulation. This may be helpful to those who want to sing or give a professional presentation without a noticeable effect on their voice. The magnet must be in place for at least 5 minutes to stop the cycle. When the magnet is removed, the VNS cycle will restart about 5 minutes later. The VNS stimulation builds up over time, so there is no risk in stopping stimulation for short periods.

Patients with a VNS cannot have an MRI of the body, owing to potential tissue damage from overheating and vagus nerve damage. A MRI of the brain with a head coil is possible if the VNS generator turned off before the procedure. The VNS is then turned back on after the brain MRI is completed. Other x-ray studies and CT scans can be done without a problem.

Epilepsy Surgery

Epilepsy surgery can be palliative or curative. A corpus callosotomy is done for children with intractable atonic seizures that cause daily multiple falls and potential injuries. A corpus callosotomy stops the atonic seizures, but the epilepsy is not cured; the seizure discharge is no longer generalized but merely confined to one hemisphere. Following the resection of the corpus callosum, the seizures are expressed differently. Typically a two-thirds resection of the corpus callosum to decrease seizure potential may result in adverse side effects such as personality changes and difficulty remembering how to do things like eating. A child must remain on antiepileptic medications after a corpus callosotomy.

A focal cortical resection or functional hemispherectomy can potentially end seizure activity. These types of epilepsy surgeries require an extensive evaluation to ensure that the patient will not lose eloquent brain function. The evaluation requires a multidisciplinary team including an epileptologist, neurosurgeon, epilepsy nurse specialist, psychologist, psychiatrist, social worker, physical therapist, occupational therapist, speech therapist, and neuroradiologist.

A hemispherectomy is performed for certain epilepsy disorders such as Sturge-Weber syndrome, hemimegalencephaly, and Rasmussen's encephalitis. The patient and the family must be made aware that following a hemispherectomy, there may be a hemiparesis that may or may not improve. Typically a patient with one of those disorders has a preexisting hemiparesis. The hemispherectomy carries a risk of hemorrhage, so the procedure tends to be done as a functional hemispherectomy, meaning the brain structures are disconnected but left in place to avoid potential hemorrhage.

A focal cortical resection is done in the area of the brain where the onset of seizure occurs. A temporal lobectomy has an 80% to 90% cure rate, and extratemporal resections result in a 40% to 70% cure rate. If a person is seizure free for 1 to 2 years after a focal cortical resection or hemispherectomy, antiepileptic medication may be eventually discontinued.

NURSING ASSESSMENT

1. See the Neurologic Assessment section in Appendix A.
2. Refer to Box 69-1 for specific types of seizure disorders.

NURSING DIAGNOSES

- Injury, Risk for
- Development, Risk for delayed
- Falls, Risk for
- Coping, Ineffective
- Self-esteem, Chronic low
- Spiritual distress, Risk for
- Knowledge, Deficient
- Memory, Impaired
- Social isolation
- Adjustment, Impaired
- Body image, Disturbed
- Parenting, Risk for impaired
- Coping, family, Compromised

NURSING INTERVENTIONS

Seizures

1. Protect child from injury.
   a. Do not attempt to restrain child or give food, liquids, or medications by mouth.
   b. If child is standing or sitting and there is threat of falling, ease child down to prevent fall.
   c. Do not place anything in child's mouth.
   d. Loosen restrictive clothing.
   e. Prevent child from hitting anything sharp by padding any objects that might be contacted and removing any sharp objects from area. Pad bed rails.
   f. Turn child on side to facilitate clearing airway of secretions.
2. Maintain detailed observation and recording of seizure (ictal) activity to assist in diagnosis or assessment of medication response.
   a. Time of onset and any precipitating events
   b. Preictal symptoms (warning that seizure is coming)
   c. Type of seizure or description of pupillary reaction, head and/or eye deviation to the left or right, skin color changes, symmetric or asymmetric motor movements, tone, presence or absence of incontinence, and cognitive level and/or level of consciousness
   d. Length of seizure
   e. Interventions during seizure (medication or safety measures)
   f. Postictal phase length and activities
   g. Vital signs
3. Provide for sleep or rest after seizure. Reassure patient as consciousness returns.
4. Monitor child's reaction to medication, VNS, ketogenic diet, and/or epilepsy surgery therapies.
5. Monitor drug levels and other laboratory evaluations as needed.

Status Epilepticus

1. Stabilize patent airway; suction as needed.
2. Provide supplemental 100% oxygen by face mask.

3. Monitor pulse oximetry and vital signs.
4. Place on electrocardiogram (ECG) monitoring.
5. Establish intravenous (IV) access for antiepileptic drug levels, other laboratory tests, and/or administration of rescue medication such as lorazepam, diazepam, fosphenytoin, phenytoin, or phenobarbital. Be prepared for further airway management if needed secondary to drug effects and prolonged seizure activity (more common if more than one medication is used or if multiple doses are given).
6. Know the facility's treatment protocol to promote best practice and outcome.

Comorbidities of Epilepsy

1. Assess for comorbidities of epilepsy, including depression, anxiety, behavioral issues, ADD/ADHD, learning disorders, language disorders, fine and gross motor disorders, headaches and migraines, and social challenges.
2. If a comorbidity exists, consider further evaluation appropriate to the concern, such as health care provider evaluation, neuropsychologic assessment, psychiatric or psychologic assessment, speech and language evaluation, physical therapy evaluation, and/or occupational evaluation.

🏠 Discharge Planning and Home Care

1. Provide information about seizures, antiepileptic medications, and any other seizure therapies including VNS, ketogenic diet, and/or epilepsy surgery. Address any knowledge deficits family may have.
2. Stress importance of taking medication regularly and complying with scheduled follow-up appointments to monitor seizure disorder and growth and development, and to evaluate for any subtle side effects of medications or other therapies.
3. List what steps family should take to manage seizures as they occur and when to seek emergency medical care. Encourage family to practice seizure drills so each person knows what to do and expect when a seizure occurs.

4. Provide anticipatory guidance regarding safety.
   a. Family to obtain medical alert bracelet
   b. If swimming, must have 1:1 observation by someone who is able to swim in case of seizure activity and potential drowning
   c. Avoidance of unprotected heights, cycling with helmet when off-road and on soft ground if there is potential breakthrough seizure activity
   d. Possible restrictions on operating machinery and electrical appliances
   e. Helmet for patients with atonic seizures, depending on seizure activity; some may need other protective gear like elbow and/or knee pads
   f. If child is old enough to warm up food, use microwave instead of stove or oven
   g. Keep water temperature below 120° F to prevent burns
   h. Use showers instead of baths, with bathroom door unlocked; may place sign on door so others know it is occupied
   i. Stay hydrated; use sunscreen; take frequent breaks in warm, sunny weather
   j. Avoid known seizure triggers
   k. Know state driving laws regarding persons with epilepsy
   l. Family may desire monitoring system when child is sleeping; may use nursery monitoring system or may consider TV monitoring system
5. Assist parent or caregiver in understanding process by which healthy self-concept is developed in presence of chronic condition. Reinforce need for consistent parenting and discipline.
6. Refer to Epilepsy Foundation of America for further information and support (www.efa.org).
7. Review potential issues that might arise for patient and family during adjustment to diagnosis, and need for support and intervention if adjustment problems occur. Educate family about the issue of stigma in epilepsy. Refer child and family for counseling as needed.
8. Refer to parenting and peer support groups.

CLIENT OUTCOMES

1. Child will have safety interventions in place to prevent injury from seizure activity.
2. Seizure activity will be prevented or controlled with antiepileptic medications and/or other seizure therapies like VNS, ketogenic diet, and/or epilepsy surgery.
3. Child will have positive self-esteem and self-image that will enhance wellness secondary to education received regarding epilepsy disorder.
4. Child will obtain optimal development and independence secondary to seizure assessment and treatment.
5. The family of a child with epilepsy will obtain optimal development and quality of life secondary to epilepsy education and support resources given.

REFERENCES

American Association of Neuroscience Nurses: *A guide to the care of the patient with seizures*, Glenville, Il, 2004, The Association.

Bergqvist AG et al: Fasting versus gradual initiation of the ketogenic diet: A prospective, randomized clinical trial of efficacy, *Epilepsia* 46(11):1810, 2005.

Dreifuss FE: Classification of the epilepsies: influence on management. In: Santilli N, editor: *Managing seizure disorders: A handbook for health care professionals*, Philadelphia, PA, 1996, Lippincott-Raven.

Epilepsy Foundation of America: *Epilepsy and mood disorders: Information for health care providers*. Maryland, 2005, The Foundation.

French JA et al: Efficacy and tolerability of the new antiepileptic drugs, I: Treatment of new-onset epilepsy: Report of the Therapeutics and Technology Assessment and Quality Standards Subcommittees of the American Academy of Neurology and the American Epilepsy Society, *Epilepsia* 45(8):401, 2004.

French JA et al: Efficacy and tolerability of the new antiepileptic drugs, II: Treatment of refractory epilepsy: Report of the Therapeutics and Technology Assessment and Quality Standards Subcommittees of the American Academy of Neurology and the American Epilepsy Society, *Epilepsia* 45(8):410, 2004.

Heck C, Helmers SL, DeGiorgio CM: Vagus nerve stimulation therapy, epilepsy, and device parameters: Scientific basis and recommendations for use, *Neurology* 59(suppl 4):S31, 2002.

Hirtz D et al: Practice parameter: evaluating a first nonfebrile seizure in children: Report of the Quality Standards Subcommittee of the American

Academy of Neurology, the Child Neurology Society, and the American Epilepsy Society 55(5):616, 2000.

Hirtz D et al: Practice parameter: Treatment of the child with a first unprovoked seizure: Report of the Quality Standards Subcommittee of the American Academy of Neurology and the Practice Committee of the Child Neurology Society, *Neurology* 60(2):166, 2003.

70

❖

Short Bowel Syndrome

PATHOPHYSIOLOGY

Short bowel syndrome (SBS) is the syndrome of malabsorption and malnutrition that occurs because of a congenitally malfunctioning bowel or after resection of small bowel necessitated by congenital or acquired conditions (Box 70-1). Symptoms of SBS include chronic diarrhea, impaired nutrient absorption, malnutrition, and poor growth and development. In addition, many affected children are chronically dependent on parenteral nutrition (PN), which can lead to liver dysfunction and disease.

SBS has three characteristic stages. Stage I begins in the immediate postoperative period and usually lasts for 7 to 10 days after the enterostomy is created. Characteristics of this stage include intractable diarrhea with massive water, fluid and electrolyte losses, dependence on parenteral nutrition and, possibly, bowel mucosa atrophy. Stage II begins 2 weeks later and can last up to 1 year after surgery. During stage II, gastric acid hypersecretion can lead to quick intestinal transit time and diarrhea, impaired pancreatic enzyme function, and gastric ulcers. At the end of stage II, stabilization of diarrhea and progression of enteral feedings occur. These changes signal an adaptive hyperplasia of the intestinal mucosa including elongation of both intestinal villi and crypts. Stage III is seen up to 2 years after the surgery. This stage represents control of diarrhea and increased tolerance of enteral nutrition (EN). Oftentimes stomas are reanastomosed at this time. Reaching this stage is dependent upon bowel adaptation, which is critical to the patient with SBS. Bowel adaptation is, in turn, dependent upon many factors, the first of which is intestinal length.

BOX 70-1
Etiology of Short Bowel Syndrome

- Congenital
- Multiple intestinal atresias
- Gastroschisis
- Omphalocele
- Cloacal extrophy
- Malrotation and volvulus
- Long segment Hirschsprung's disease
- Meconium ileus
- Intussusception
- Superior mesenteric artery deformities
- Acquired
- Necrotizing enterocolitis (NEC)
- Volvulus
- Inflammatory bowel disease
- Trauma
- Arterial or venous thrombosis
- Intussusception

Most surgeons agree the 25 cm of small bowel without an intact ileocecal valve (ICV), or 15 cm of small bowel with an intact ICV, is necessary for tolerance of enteral feedings. The second significant factor is the presence of the ICV. The ICV slows intestinal transit time, allowing increased nutrient and fluid absorption, and prevents contamination of the small bowel with colonic flora. Although important, the presence of the ICV is not absolutely necessary, depending on bowel length. The third factor important to bowel adaptation is the location of resection. The adaptive response is greater in the ileum than in the jejunum. Changes in the crypts and the villi allow the ileum to take over some of the functions of the jejunum, whereas the reverse is not true.

The fourth factor in bowel adaptation is the reintroduction of EN. Early and aggressive initiation and advancement of EN, especially human breast milk, protein hydrolysate formulas, or amino acid–containing formulas, appears to promote intestinal adaptation. The fifth factor is the age of the infant at resection. Because intestinal length doubles between the second trimester and full term, a preterm infant has a great capacity for adaptation. The final factor is individual response. Liver tolerance of chronic PN, the number and virulence of infections, and the development of bowel obstructions from strictures or adhesions all seem to play an important role in the overall outcome of patients with SBS.

INCIDENCE

1. Survival rate is reported to be 80% to 94%, with death occurring secondary to liver disease and sepsis.
2. Cost of treatment can range from $150,000 to $500,000 per patient per year.

CLINICAL MANIFESTATIONS

1. Diarrhea, ranging from acute to chronic
2. Poor tolerance of enteral nutrition
3. Poor and inconsistent growth—evidence of failure to thrive
4. Malnutrition (poor carbohydrate and fat absorption)
5. Jaundice
6. Anemia

COMPLICATIONS

1. Gastrointestinal: fluid and electrolyte imbalance, especially in the early postoperative period, diarrhea, gastric acid hypersecretion, gallbladder disease
2. Hematologic: sepsis, hepatomegaly indicative of PN-induced liver disease
3. Nutrition: difficulty advancing enteral feedings, poor growth, vitamin and mineral deficiency, osteopenia, poor healing
4. Integumentary: skin breakdown, especially in the buttocks and the perineum, and at the enterostomy site
5. Developmental: failure to meet developmental milestones; oral aversion
6. Other: need for multiple surgeries, particularly for bowel obstructions

LABORATORY AND DIAGNOSTIC TESTS

Refer to Appendix D for normal values and ranges of laboratory and diagnostic tests.

1. Complete blood count (CBC) with differential and platelet count—may see increased or decreased white blood cell count with sepsis, decreased platelets, and anemia secondary to liver dysfunction
2. Serum electrolytes, glucose, blood urea nitrogen, creatinine—to assess fluid and electrolyte imbalances, tolerance of PN
3. Liver function test—to assess liver tolerance of PN
4. Alkaline phosphatase levels—to assess liver function and monitor course of cholestasis
5. Dipstick or urinalysis for protein, glucose, blood, and ketones—to assess tolerance of PN
6. Gastric pH—to assess the presence of gastric acid hypersecretion
7. Stool hematest, reducing substances, stool ictotest—to assess tolerance of EN and check for the presence of bile in stool
8. Abdominal x-ray study—to check for dilated or obstructed loops of bowel
9. Ultrasound of liver and gallbladder—to check for cholestasis and gallstones
10. Liver scan—uses a radioactive isotope to help determine liver function
11. Liver biopsy—to diagnose liver disease

MEDICAL MANAGEMENT

The medical management of SBS focuses on the minimization of symptoms through medication and diet therapy. EN is initiated as soon as the postoperative ileus has resolved. Early initiation and aggressive advancement of EN will help promote intestinal adaptation and decrease complications of prolonged PN. Surgical interventions are offered as needed. A number of medications may be used for the complications, as shown in Box 70-2.

Nutritional interventions for patients in stage I SBS focus on postoperative fluid management and beginning the healing process. Initially, nutrition is provided entirely parenterally through a central venous catheter. PN must be monitored to assure sufficient calories, proteins, and amino acids for healing

BOX 70-2
Medications Used to Treat Complications

A. Diarrhea

1. Loperamide (Imodium)—an antidiarrheal opioid agent that slows transit time, thereby increasing absorption of water and nutrients
2. Cholestyramine—bile-salt binder to decrease secretory diarrhea
3. Octreotide acetate (Sandostatin)—decreases secretory diarrhea by inhibiting exocrine and endocrine, gastrointestinal, and pancreatic secretions (little is known about effects in infants; decreases insulin and growth hormone levels)
4. Fiber source (Benefiber or pectin)—decreases water content in stool

B. Gastric acid hypersecretion:

Ranitidine (Zantac)—H$_2$ blocker to increase gastric pH, slow transit time, and prevent ulcers and breakdown at anastomosis site (gastric acid hypersecretion should be temporary [up to 6 months]; these medications may promote bacterial overgrowth of the small intestine)

C. Liver dysfunction

1. Phenobarbital—increases liver enzyme induction
2. Ursodiol (Actigall)—increases bile excretion; absorbed in ileum
3. Cholecystokinin—initiates gallbladder contractions

D. Intestinal bacterial overgrowth

1. Trimethoprim (Bactrim)—use a half dose for antibiotic prophylaxis to "sterilize" the intestine and to prevent bacterial overgrowth, translocation, and sepsis.
2. Metronidazole (Flagyl)—same action as trimethoprim
3. Probiotics (CULTURELLE, Lactobacillus GG)—live, human-derived microorganisms that improve intestinal microbial balance

E. Vitamin and mineral deficiency

1. Multivitamin (ADEK pediatric drops)—fat-soluble vitamin supplementation
2. Cyanocabalamin (B$_{12}$)—injections usually needed after first few months as patient is weaned off PN

Continued

BOX 70-2

Medications Used to Treat Complications—cont'd

3. Mineral supplements—zinc aids in healing; selenium plays a role in antioxidant system.

F. Experimental Therapies

1. Human growth hormone—used to promote intestinal adaptation and reduce parenteral nutrition.

and sustained growth. In the immediate postoperative period, fluid and electrolyte losses are large, especially sodium. Sodium replacement must occur with a fluid other than PN. Once the postoperative gastrointestinal (GI) motility has returned, trophic low-volume feedings of human breast milk or dilute formula may be initiated. These feedings are advanced aggressively in both strength and volume, as tolerated, based on stool output. Rates as low as 1 ml/hr may prevent mucosal atrophy and decrease intestinal adaptation time.

Nutritional interventions in stages II and III SBS focus on intestinal adaptation and sustaining growth. Enteral feedings of human breast milk or an elemental formula such as Alimentum (Ross Laboratories) or Pregestimal (Mead Johnson) are continued. If the infant is premature, the enteral feedings should be changed gradually to premature formula once feedings are tolerated. Enteral feedings should be given through continuous infusion into the stomach through an orogastric or gastrostomy tube. Increased transit time will maximize absorption. Enteral feeding volumes are advanced based on stool volume output. Feedings are advanced until stool volume output increases by 50% or is greater than 40 to 50 ml/kg/day and/or significant malabsorption occurs. During this time, it is essential to provide an oral motor stimulation program to prevent oral aversion.

Parenteral nutrition should be customized to meet the patient's changing mineral needs. Supplements of zinc and selenium are often needed, and copper and manganese should be deleted if liver dysfunction develops. Later in stage II, cycling of parenteral nutrition may be attempted. Although this technique remains highly debated, it appears to decrease the incidence of cholestasis and allows for some time with greater freedom of movement for the patient.

Surgical interventions are designed to slow transit time, increase mucosal surface area, or increase intestinal length. Indications for surgical intervention include poor tolerance of EN; numerous complications of PN such as multiple catheter-related infections, which limit venous access; and liver dysfunction and disease. In order to improve nutrient absorption, some surgical interventions focus on slowing intestinal transit time. There are four possible procedures currently being used. The first procedure is the placement of an intestinal valve. Clinical experience is limited, but the intervention is designed to slow transit time in a process similar to the way the ileocecal valve functions. The second procedure is the placement of a reversed intestinal segment. A 3- to 6-cm segment of the child's own bowel is inserted in a position such that retrograde peristalsis occurs, thus increasing absorption time. It is most effective when placed in the distal bowel and is limited to patients who have longer small bowel length. In the third procedure, a colon interposition, a piece of the colon is placed between two segments of small bowel; this may slow transit time by virtue of the colon's inherently slow peristalsis. The fourth procedure is reversed electrical pacing; electrical signals are applied to the distal region of the small bowel to initiate retrograde peristalsis. This procedure is experimental with no successful clinical reports as yet, but further study is needed.

Surgical interventions that focus on increasing mucosal surface area are the tapering enteroplasty and the neomucosa. In the tapering enteroplasty, the caliber of the dilated small bowel is reduced to a more normal size. In theory, this should increase peristalsis within this segment and decrease bacterial overgrowth. Clinical experience with this procedure is limited. The neomucosa is the transplantation of a patch of intestine with new mucosa. This mucosa has been grown in the laboratory from a cut edge of the normal bowel. To date, this procedure has only been done in animal trials.

The final group of surgical interventions focuses on increasing intestinal length. This procedure includes the Bianchi and Iowa procedures. In the Bianchi procedure the dilated short bowel is divided lengthwise into two separate segments, which are joined together by creating an end-to-end anastomosis; the result is a doubling of length. This procedure has been performed many times with varying clinical results. The Iowa procedure is a two-step surgery. The first step involves securing a segment of bowel under the surface of the liver or the posterior abdominal wall musculature to help the bowel develop neovascularization. The second step of surgery involves longitudinal division of the newly vascularized bowel to increase the length. There is limited clinical experience with this procedure; however, early results are promising.

Bowel and multiple organ transplantation remain as a last option for those patients in end-stage liver disease or with complete intestinal failure. Success has been limited; however, survival rates have improved with more effective immunosuppressive therapy.

NURSING ASSESSMENT

1. See the section on Gastrointestinal Assessment in Appendix A.
2. Assess for fluid and electrolyte imbalances.
3. Assess hydration status.
4. Assess child's tolerance of PN.
5. Assess child's readiness for and tolerance of EN.
6. Assess child for presence of pain (see Appendix I).
7. Assess for signs and symptoms of infection.
8. Assess for signs of skin breakdown.
9. Assess child's height and weight, head circumference, and pattern of growth (see Appendix E).
10. Assess child's response to medications.
11. Assess family's response to hospitalization and child's condition (refer to Appendix F).
12. Assess family's readiness for discharge and ability to manage home treatment regimen.

NURSING DIAGNOSES

- Fluid volume, Deficient
- Nutrition: less than body requirements, Imbalanced
- Pain, Acute
- Infection, Risk for

- Growth and development, Delayed
- Family processes, Interrupted
- Therapeutic regimen management, Ineffective
- Skin integrity, Risk for impaired

NURSING INTERVENTIONS

1. Assess for fluid and electrolyte imbalances, hydration status, and tolerance of PN.
   a. Monitor vital signs, perfusion, and mucous membranes.
   b. Monitor urine output and dipstick results.
   c. Monitor serum and urine electrolytes and serum glucose.
   d. Monitor serum nutritional lab test results.
2. Monitor readiness for and tolerance of enteral nutrition.
   a. Record and monitor intake, stool and enterostomy output, and emesis.
   b. Measure abdominal girth.
   c. Perform stool hematest.
   d. Test stool for reducing substances.
3. Monitor for verbal and nonverbal pain behaviors; administer nonpharmacologic and pharmacologic pain measures (see Appendix I).
4. Assess for any signs or symptoms of infection.
   a. Monitor serum CBC, differential, and platelets as ordered.
   b. In newborn infants, monitor for temperature and glucose instability, lethargy, and poor perfusion.
   c. In older children, monitor for poor feeding, increased temperature, and irritability.
5. Monitor for growth deficiencies.
   a. Record daily weights.
   b. Record weekly length and head circumference (see Appendix E).
   c. Plot growth parameters on growth chart (see Appendix E).
   d. Monitor serum lab results, assessing nutritional status.
   e. Monitor for therapeutic and adverse effects of medications that may negatively affect growth.

6. Monitor for appropriate growth and development (see Appendix B).
   a. Initiate developmental evaluation and treatment plan.
   b. Initiate oral stimulation program.
   c. Encourage age-appropriate use of toys and activities.
   d. Encourage contact with peers (for older children).
7. Support the family.
   a. Involve parents and family in patient's care.
   b. Encourage therapeutic communication to discuss the range of emotions associated with raising a child with a chronic condition and long-term intensive home treatment regimen.
   c. Consider referral to social worker for evaluation and support.
   d. Assist family in identifying and using community resources and support systems (refer to Appendix G).
   e. Educate family on patient care and discharge planning.

🏠 Discharge Planning and Home Care

1. Instruct family about home administration of nutrition.
   a. PN—how to obtain and administer
   b. EN—how to obtain, mix, and administer
2. Instruct family about medications—administration and monitoring for desired and undesired effects.
3. Instruct family about care of the central venous catheter and other catheter care.
4. Instruct family about enterostomy care (if applicable).
5. Arrange for and instruct family about follow-up appointments with specialists and primary care physician.
6. Arrange any developmental and/or oral stimulation program follow-up (see Appendix G).
7. Employ family support strategies.
   a. Assist family in identifying support systems (parent support groups, family members, church members).
   b. Encourage open communication among family members and with providers.
   c. Encourage family to participate in child's care.
   d. Reinforce information, answer questions, and address concerns about child's long-term care needs.

CLIENT OUTCOMES

1. Patient will be able to be weaned from PN to EN.
2. Patient will be free of infections.
3. Family will be able to adhere to treatment regimen.
4. Child will achieve developmental milestones.

REFERENCES

Andorsky DJ et al: Nutritional and other postoperative management of neonates with short bowel syndrome correlates with clinical outcomes, *J Pediatr* 139(1):27, 2001.

Hwang ST, Shulman RJ: Update on management and treatment of short gut, *Clin Perinatol* 29(1):181, 2002.

Kim HB et al: Serial transverse enteroplasty for short bowel syndrome: A case report, *J Pediatr Surg* 38(6):881, 2003.

Wales PW et al: Neonatal short bowel syndrome: Population-based estimates of incidence and mortality rates, *J Pediatr Surg* 39(5):690, 2004.

Warner BW et al: What's new in the management of short gut syndrome in children, *Am J Coll Surg* 190(6):725, 2000.

71

❖

Sickle Cell Disease

PATHOPHYSIOLOGY

Sickle cell disease is a general term that is used to describe a group of related disorders that affect the red blood cells. The basic defect is a mutant autosomal gene that effects a substitution of valine for glutamic acid on the beta chain of hemoglobin. The result is a person with either a heterozygous or homozygous hemoglobinopathy. A person diagnosed with sickle cell trait (heterozygous form Hb AS) has inherited the sickle gene from only one parent and will not have any signs and symptoms of sickle cell disease. Sickle cell trait cannot change into sickle cell disease; however, there is a 50% chance that affected persons will pass the trait to their offspring. Sickle cell anemia, or homozygous sickle cell disease (Hb SS), is an inherited autosomal recessive disorder, which means that a person has inherited the sickle gene from both parents and will have signs and symptoms of disease. There are other variants of sickle cell anemia as well; Hb SC, Hb SB thalassemia, Hb SD, and Hb SE are the most common. Sickled red blood cells are crescent-shaped, have decreased oxygen-carrying capacity, and undergo destruction at a greater rate than normal red blood cells. The life span of sickled cells is diminished to 10 to 30 days (normal is 120 days). Sickled cells are extremely rigid because of the gelled hemoglobin, cellular dehydration, and an inflexible membrane. The rigid cells become trapped in the circulatory system, which leads to a vicious cycle of infarction and progressive sickling.

Splenic hypofunction and, later, splenic atrophy result in reticuloendothelial failure and an incidence of infection that

BOX 71-1
Early Detection: Newborn Screening Programs

- Morbidity and mortality can be significantly reduced with newborn screening and early intervention.
- Screening should include prenatal, maternal, and neonatal screening.
- Public education is critical for effective neonatal screening. Target groups include day care centers, schools, and the media.

Adapted from Commission on Classification and Terminology of the International League Against Epilepsy: Proposal for revised clinical and electroencephalographic classification of epileptic seizures, *Epilepsia* 22(4): 489, 1981, currently under revision. In: Dreifuss FE: Classification of the epilepsies: Influence on management. In: Santilli N, editor: *Managing seizure disorders: A handbook for health care professionals*, Philadelphia, 1998, Lippincott-Raven.

is 600 times higher in children with sickle cell disease than in the normal population. Children are born with fetal hemoglobin, which consists of a gamma chain; therefore, until approximately 6 months of age, when the hemoglobin begins to change to the adult type, symptoms of the disease do not usually occur (Box 71-1).

Sickle cell crises result from physiologic changes that decrease the oxygen available to the hemoglobin; they are typically precipitated by dehydration, infection, and hypoxia. Sickling of cells results in clumping of red blood cells in the vessels, decreased oxygen transport, and increased destruction of red blood cells. Ischemia, infarct, and tissue necrosis result from the obstruction of vessels and decreased blood flow. Three types of crisis occur: (1) vasoocclusive (painful), (2) splenic sequestration, and (3) aplastic. Sickle cell crises occur less frequently with age. Mortality in the first years of life is usually caused by infection and sequestration crisis.

INCIDENCE

1. Incidence of sickle cell trait among African Americans is estimated at 1 in 12, and incidence of sickle cell disease is estimated at 1 in 375. The disease has also been reported occasionally in those from certain areas of the Mediterranean basin (Turkey, Greece, Italy), the Caribbean, and South and

Central America, as well as in some with Arabian, Asiatic Indian, Native American, or East Indian ancestry.

2. Approximately 2000 infants are born with sickle cell disease each year in the United States.

3. Death occurs most frequently in children from 1 to 3 years of age from organ failure or thrombosis of major organs, most commonly the lungs and the brain.

4. With new treatments, 85% of affected individuals survive to the age of 20 years; 50% survive beyond 50 years.

CLINICAL MANIFESTATIONS

1. Vasoocclusive crisis (painful crisis) results from ischemia in tissue distal to occlusion. Crises can occur when the child has an illness that causes dehydration or a respiratory infection that lowers oxygen exchange. Other precipitating events can be exposure to cold, anesthesia, or high altitudes, or extremely strenuous exercise. Fifty percent of children will have a vasoocclusive crisis by 1 year of age, and close to 100% will suffer from one by the age of 6 years. Vasoocclusive crisis is characterized by the following symptoms:
   a. Irritability
   b. Vomiting
   c. Fever
   d. Anorexia
   e. Pain in extremities, back, or chest
   f. Dactylitis (hand-and-foot syndrome)—decreased range of motion and inflamed extremities (common in young infants)
   g. Abdominal crisis
   h. Cerebrovascular accidents (CVAs)
   i. Ocular hemorrhages

2. Sequestration crisis (usually seen in children from 5 to 36 months of age, with 76% of cases occurring before age 2 years) is due to the sequestration of sickled blood within the spleen over a period of hours, which rapidly decreases the hemoglobin level (blood pooled in the spleen is not available to the general circulation). Children are subject to

fatal splenic rupture and/or splenic atrophy. Signs and symptoms of sequestration crisis are as follows:
  a. Rapid and massive enlargement of spleen (splenomegaly)
  b. Rapid fall in hemoglobin level, anemia
  c. Tachycardia, dyspnea, pallor, syncope, and weakness (common)
  d. Nausea, vomiting
  e. Sudden, severe abdominal pain
  f. Enlargement of liver
  g. Circulatory collapse and shock
3. Aplastic crisis results from a transient suppression of red cell production while hemolysis continues at the same rate. It often occurs in association with an infection, when the strong compensatory mechanism is depressed (e.g., parvovirus B19, *Salmonella, Streptococcus, Mycoplasma,* Epstein-Barr virus infections). Aplastic crisis typically occurs in children younger than 10 years. Signs and symptoms of aplastic crisis are as follows:
  a. Weakness, fatigue, dizziness
  b. Pallor
  c. Fever
  d. Dyspnea
  e. Anorexia
  f. Arthralgia
  g. Tachycardia
  h. Decreased hemoglobin level, hematocrit, and reticulocyte count
  i. Shock

COMPLICATIONS

1. Increased risk of bacterial infection, primarily due to hypofunctional spleen: overwhelming sepsis, meningitis (children with sickle cell anemia have 36 times greater incidence of pneumococcal meningitis), pneumococcal pneumonia, *Salmonella* osteomyelitis
2. Reproductive and sexuality: delayed onset of puberty, impaired fertility, priapism
3. Gastrointestinal: gallstones

4. Respiratory: "acute chest syndrome"—respiratory distress with cough and tachypnea, high fever, chest pain, and infiltrate on chest radiographic studies
5. Cardiovascular: chronic heart, liver, and kidney disease, CVAs (10%, especially between ages of 3 and 10 years), avascular necrosis, leg ulcers, proliferative retinopathy
6. Genitourinary: enuresis
7. Psychiatric and psychosocial: depression, isolation, low self-esteem, risk for drug addiction (actual prevalence in this population is low, according to recent literature), strained parent-child relationships
8. Avascular necrosis

LABORATORY AND DIAGNOSTIC TESTS

Refer to Appendix D for normal values and ranges of laboratory and diagnostic tests.

1. Hemoglobin electrophoresis, preferably at birth for all infants as part of newborn screening—to quantify percentage of hemoglobin S present. If disorder is not identified at birth, diagnosis is rarely made before 6 to 12 months of age.
2. Tests of fetal blood or fetal cells—to make prenatal diagnosis possible between 9 and 11 weeks' gestation.

MEDICAL MANAGEMENT

Medical management focuses on pain control, oxygenation, hydration, and careful monitoring for complications of vasoocclusion. Administration of prophylactic penicillin to prevent septicemia should be initiated at 2 to 3 months of age and continued through 5 to 6 years of life. Immunizations are crucial to protect these children from infection. Specifically required are (1) pneumococcal conjugate vaccine (PCV7), four doses between 2 months and 2 years of age; (2) pneumococcal polysaccharide vaccine (PPV23) starting at 2 years of age; and (3) influenza vaccine every fall for children over 6 months of age. Meningococcal vaccine is sometimes recommended for asplenic children.

Transcranial Doppler ultrasonography is being used in some centers to identify children who are at high risk for developing a first stroke. Subsequent initiation of a long-term transfusion program for those with abnormal test results may decrease the incidence of stroke.

A program of hypertransfusion (transfusion every 3 to 4 weeks) is a current treatment (90% effective) for children who have had CVAs, progressive pulmonary disease, and possibly debilitating vasoocclusive crisis. The iron overload leads to hemosiderosis (iron deposits on organs), with the following complications occurring: cardiomyopathy, cirrhosis, insulin-dependent diabetes mellitus, hypothyroidism, hypoparathyroidism, delayed growth, and delayed sexual development. Deferoxamine (Desferal), administered either subcutaneously or by intravenous transfusion at regular intervals, will chelate the iron so that it can be excreted through the urine or bile to help reduce these complications.

Analgesics are used to control pain during a crisis period. Antibiotics may be used, because infection can trigger the crisis. Folic acid supplementation may be considered for children with significant hemolysis. Daily administration of oral hydroxyurea in adults 18 years and older is an effective pharmacologic intervention, although use in children has not been well studied. Treatment with hydroxyurea, which increases levels of fetal hemoglobin, has been shown to reduce pain events, hospital admissions, and the need for blood transfusions.

The only cure is thought to be a bone marrow transplant, which also involves risks. This may be a promising treatment modality in the near future.

NURSING ASSESSMENT

See the Cardiovascular Assessment and Respiratory Assessment sections in Appendix A and the Pain Assessment section in Appendix I.

NURSING DIAGNOSES

- Tissue perfusion, Ineffective
- Comfort, Impaired
- Infection, Risk for
- Injury, Risk for
- Pain, Acute

- Growth and development, Delayed
- Nutrition: less than body requirements, Imbalanced
- Coping, Compromised family
- Coping, Ineffective
- Therapeutic regimen management, Ineffective

NURSING INTERVENTIONS

1. Prevent or minimize effects of sickle cell crisis.
   a. Encourage avoidance of temperature extremes and high altitudes.
   b. Be aware that early assessment and action are keys to prevention of and intervention in crisis episode.
   c. Avoid cold and vasoconstriction during pain episode; cold promotes sickling.
   d. Provide for and promote hydration (1.5 to 2 times maintenance levels).
      i. Maintain strict intake and output measurements.
      ii. Assess for signs of dehydration.
   e. Promote oxygenation of tissues; monitor for signs of hypoxia—cyanosis and hyperventilation; increased apical pulse, respiratory rate, and blood pressure; and mental confusion.
2. Provide frequent rest periods to decrease oxygen expenditure.
3. Monitor use of oxygen equipment.
4. Administer and monitor use of blood products and chelation therapy; assess for signs of transfusion reaction—fever, restlessness, cardiac arrhythmias, chills and shaking, nausea and vomiting, chest pain, red or black urine, headache, flank pain, and signs of shock or renal failure.
5. Monitor for signs of circulatory overload—dyspnea, increased respiratory rate, cyanosis, chest pain, and dry cough.
6. Relieve or minimize pain (see Appendix I).
   a. Moist heat for first 24 hours
   b. Whirlpool or walking tank, especially if swelling has occurred
   c. Therapeutic exercises

    d. Administration of analgesics as ordered based on pain assessment. Acetaminophen with codeine may be adequate for mild to moderate pain. More severe crisis may be treated with intermittent or continuous intravenous morphine. Patient-controlled analgesia systems have been used effectively in children as young as 5 years of age.

    e. Use of nonpharmacologic methods such as guided imagery (see Appendix I).

7. Prevent infection.

    a. Assess for signs of infection—fever, malaise or irritability, and inflamed and swollen soft tissue and lymph nodes.

    b. Be aware that children are particularly susceptible to pneumococcal sepsis and pneumonia (children younger than 3 to 4 years of age) and *Salmonella* osteomyelitis.

8. Monitor for signs of complications.

    a. Infection

    b. Splenomegaly

    c. Heart, liver, kidney, joint disease

    d. Leg ulcers

    e. Stroke

    f. Decreased vision

    g. Chest pain or dyspnea

    h. Delay in growth and development

    i. Vascular collapse and shock

9. Provide age-appropriate explanation to child about hospitalization and procedures (see Appendix B).

10. Ensure good nutrition. Metabolic rate of children with sickle cell disease has been demonstrated to be higher than that of children without the disease.

11. Provide emotional support to child and family (see the Supportive Care section in Appendix F).

    a. Encourage performance of normal activities. School absences may put child behind expected grade level (see Appendixes B and G).

    b. Encourage networking with other children and families who have sickle cell anemia.

    c. Delayed puberty occurs frequently. Adolescent often needs additional support.

12. Encourage parents to screen their family members.
    a. Newborn screening for hemoglobinopathies
    b. Screening of siblings for disease and trait
13. Identification at birth makes possible early prophylaxis against infections. Use of prophylactic penicillin is recommended beginning in newborn period (2 to 3 months of age).

🏠 Discharge Planning and Home Care

1. Provide genetic counseling.
2. Counsel child on appropriate play, leisure activities, and sports participation (to prevent hypoxia resulting from strenuous physical exertion and excessive life stress).
3. Provide parent teaching and anticipatory guidance about prevention of infection to ensure that child is seen by physician at first signs of illness; teach parents procedure for taking temperature and methods to decrease temperature.
4. Counsel parents on the importance of encouraging the child's self-reliance as appropriate for age.
5. Provide parents with information about routine immunizations. Child should have annual vision screening.

CLIENT OUTCOMES

1. Child's respiratory rate, oxygen saturation, and arterial blood gas levels will be within normal limits, cyanosis will be absent, and urine output will be higher than 1 ml/kg/hr.
2. Child will indicate relief from pain.
3. Child and family will understand importance of medical follow-up and know when to seek medical attention.
4. Child will have minimal vasoocclusive, sequestration, and aplastic crises.
5. Child will demonstrate regular observable growth and achieve age-appropriate developmental milestones (see Appendix B).
6. Family will seek genetic counseling for other children.
7. Parents will be able to accurately describe disease process and identify special precautions necessary to prevent sickle cell crisis (Box 71-2).

BOX 71-2
Resources

- The Sickle Cell Information Center: www.SCInfo.org (404-616-3572)
- The Sickle Cell Disease Association of America: www.sicklecelldisease.org (800-421-8453)
- The Sickle Cell Disease Scientific Research Group: NHLBI Health Information Center: www.nhlbi.nih.gov (301-592-8573 or 240-629-3255 TTY)

REFERENCES

American Academy of Pediatrics: Health supervision for children with sickle cell disease, policy statement, *American Academy of Pediatrics Web Site* (serial online): http://aappolicy.aappublications.org/cgi/reprint/pediatrics;109/3/526.pdf. Accessed May 6, 2006.

Learn about sickle cell disease and sickle cell trait, 2004 edition (08–04-A), Channing Bete Company, pamphlet number PS21828.

The Sickle Cell Information Center: Sickle Cell information—Clinician summary, *The Sickle Cell Information Center* (serial online): www.scinfo.org/prod05.htm. Accessed May 6, 2006.

72

❖

Spina Bifida

PATHOPHYSIOLOGY

Spina bifida means cleft spine, which is the incomplete closure of the spinal column. Two distinct types of failure of fusion of the vertebral laminae of the spinal column occur during fetal development: spina bifida occulta and spina bifida cystica.

Spina bifida occulta is a defect in closure in which the meninges are not exposed on the surface of the skin. The vertebral defect is small, usually involving the lumbosacral region. External abnormalities (present in 50% of cases) may include a hair tuft, nevus, or hemangioma. A pilonidal sinus may require surgical closure if it becomes infected.

Spina bifida cystica is a defect in closure that results in protrusion of the spinal cord and/or its coverings. The two types of spina bifida cystica are meningocele and myelomeningocele.

Meningocele is a protrusion that includes the meninges and a sac containing cerebrospinal fluid (CSF); it is covered by normal skin. No neurologic abnormalities are present, and the spinal cord is not involved. Hydrocephalus occurs in 20% of cases. A meningocele usually is in the lumbosacral or the sacral area. Surgical correction is usually performed within days of birth.

Myelomeningocele is a protrusion of the meninges and a portion of the spinal cord, as well as a sac containing CSF. The site is most often the lumbar or the lumbosacral area. The lumbosacral area is affected in 42% of cases, the thoracolumbar area in 27%, the sacral area in 21%, and the thoracic or cervical in 10%. Infants with a myelomeningocele are prone to injury during the birth process. Hydrocephalus occurs in most affected children (85% to 90%); about 60% to 70% have a normal intelligence quotient, but impairments of conceptual reasoning abilities are common. Children with both myelomeningocele and hydrocephalus have other central nervous system malformations, of which Arnold-Chiari deformity is the most common. Surgical intervention usually is performed at birth, with neurosurgery for shunt placement to prevent hydrocephalus if indicated. More recently, experimental fetal surgical procedures (done about 7 weeks before birth) have demonstrated the potential to reduce the symptoms of spina bifida.

The specific cause of spina bifida is unknown. Multiple factors such as heredity and environment are thought to interact to produce these defects. The neural tube is normally complete 4 weeks after conception. The following have been identified as causative factors: low levels of maternal vitamins, including folic acid; the taking of clomiphene and valproic acid; and hyperthermia during pregnancy. It is estimated that nearly 75% of neural tube defects could be prevented if women took vitamins, including folic acid, before conception. Widespread public health efforts are now directed to encouraging women to take daily folic acid supplements (400 mcg daily) for 1 to 3 months before becoming pregnant.

Advances in interdisciplinary care have improved the long-term outcome for affected children. Treatment improvement, with the use of medications and neurosurgery, has contributed to extending their life spans.

Diminished self-esteem is common in children and adolescents with this condition. Adolescents express concerns about sexual adequacy, social mastery, peer relationships, and physical maturity and attractiveness. The perceived severity of disability is more directly related to self-perception of the disability than to the actual disability of the adolescent.

INCIDENCE

1. Annually, approximately 4000 infants are born with spina bifida in the United States.
2. In the United States, the incidence is 1 in 1000 live births.
3. The risk of the disorder increases by 5% with the second child.
4. Girls are more often affected than boys.

5. Nearly 72% of children with spina bifida have latex or natural rubber allergies.
6. Between 80% and 90% of individuals with myelomeningocele have shunts.

CLINICAL MANIFESTATIONS

A varying degree of dysfunction affecting the skeleton, the skin, and the genitourinary tract results from spina bifida, depending on the portion of the spinal cord involved:

1. Motor, sensory, reflex, and sphincter abnormalities—may occur in varying degrees
2. Flaccid paralysis of legs; lack or diminished sensation and reflexes
3. Hydrocephalus
4. Scoliosis
5. Bladder and bowel functions varying from normal to ineffective

COMPLICATIONS

Birth-related complications of spina bifida include the following:

1. Neuromuscular: cerebral palsy
2. Cognitive: mental retardation
3. Sensory: optic atrophy
4. Neurologic: epilepsy
5. Orthopedic: fractures
6. Other: painless ulcerations, injuries

Other long-term complications include the following:

1. Infectious and inflammatory: shunt infections, ventriculitis, meningitis, tendonitis, decubitus ulcer
2. Neurologic and neurosensory: increased intracranial pressure due to blocked shunt, blocked shunt (may be asymptomatic), tethered cord syndrome, benign intracranial hypertension, slit ventricle syndrome, visual deficits
3. Immune: latex sensitization and allergy
4. Gastrointestinal: bowel problems (incontinence), gastrointestinal disorders
5. Endocrine: obesity, impaired sexual and reproductive functioning

6. Integumentary: decubitus ulcer, traumatic injury to insensate areas
7. Orthopedic problems: foot deformities, bowed legs, dislocated hips, spinal curvature, osteoporosis, mobility limitations
8. Cognitive: learning disabilities
9. Psychologic: depression, anxiety disorders, low self-esteem, altered body image

LABORATORY AND DIAGNOSTIC TESTS

1. Antenatal period testing: serum alpha fetoprotein level between 16 and 18 weeks of gestation, ultrasonography of fetus, amniocentesis if other tests are inconclusive
2. Diagnostic examinations: chest radiographic study, ultrasonography, computed tomography, magnetic resonance imaging, amniocentesis
3. Routine preoperative testing: complete blood count, urinalysis, culture and sensitivity (C and S) testing, chest radiographic study

MEDICAL AND SURGICAL MANAGEMENT

Surgical repair of myelomeningocele is performed in the neonatal period to prevent rupture. Surgical repair of the spinal lesion and shunting of CSF in infants with hydrocephalus is performed at birth. Skin grafting is necessary if the lesion is large. Children with spina bifida are at risk for latex sensitization and allergy because they are exposed to surgeries and procedures in which latex gloves come into direct contact with blood vessels and mucosa. Risk factors associated with the development of latex sensitization and allergy are atopic diathesis and number of surgeries. Children who have latex allergy have clinical symptoms, whereas those with latex sensitization have immunoglobulin E antibodies with no clinical symptoms. Whether the child has latex allergy or sensitization, avoidance of contact with latex is recommended.

Prophylactic antibiotics are administered to prevent infection. Nursing interventions will depend on the presence and extent of dysfunction of various body systems. In addition, children with myelomeningocele will undergo a number of surgeries depending on their clinical problems, such as tethered spinal cord, orthopedic problems, decubitus ulcers, and a shunt that requires revision.

The following medications may be used depending on the child's clinical needs:

1. Antibiotics and/or antiseptics—used prophylactically to prevent urinary tract infections
2. Anticholinergics—to increase bladder tone
3. Alpha agonists—to tighten sphincter
4. Stool softeners and laxatives—used for bowel training and evacuation of stool
5. Medications—to control or treat other medical and mental health problems such as epilepsy, depression

NURSING ASSESSMENT

1. See the Musculoskeletal Assessment and Neurologic Assessment sections in Appendix A.
2. Assess parents' interactions with their infant and ability to cope with their child's condition.
3. Assess extent of motor and sensory involvement, and presence of reflexes.
4. Assess for signs and symptoms of dehydration or fluid overload.
5. Assess parents' need for preoperative and postoperative information and support (see Appendix F).
6. Assess for wound drainage and signs of infection.
7. Assess for increased intracranial pressure.
8. Assess parents' and child's ability to manage home treatment regimen.
9. Assess parents' and child's needs for community services (see Appendix G).

NURSING DIAGNOSES

- Grieving, Risk for dysfunctional
- Family processes, Interrupted
- Caregiver role strain, Risk for
- Mobility, Impaired physical
- Nutrition: more than body requirements, Imbalanced
- Infection, Risk for

- Injury, Risk for
- Urinary elimination, Impaired
- Bowel incontinence
- Skin integrity, Impaired
- Knowledge, Deficient
- Body image, Disturbed
- Sexuality pattern, Ineffective
- Growth and development, Delayed
- Therapeutic regimen management, Ineffective
- Self-care deficit, Bathing/hygiene
- Self-care deficit, Dressing/grooming
- Self-care deficit, Feeding
- Self-care deficit, Toileting

NURSING INTERVENTIONS
Preoperative Care
1. Encourage parental expression of grief over loss of "perfect" child.
   a. Feelings related to guilt, self-blame
   b. Feelings of anger about child's condition
   c. Feelings of inadequacy for procreating infant
   d. Feelings of being overwhelmed with the situation and the unknown
2. Provide emotional support to parents (see the Supportive Care section in Appendix F).
3. Monitor infant's vital signs and neurologic status.
   a. Evaluation of temperature, apical pulse, respiratory rate, and blood pressure as often as every 2 hours
   b. Neurologic assessment (see the Neurologic Assessment section in Appendix A)
4. Promote optimal preoperative hydration and nutritional status.
   a. Monitor for dehydration or fluid overload.
   b. Monitor administration of maintenance fluids (by mouth or intravenous [IV] route).
   c. Monitor and record intake and output.
   d. Record weight daily.
5. Maintain integrity of defect; prevent further injury.

    a. Monitor for signs and symptoms of infection—fever, drainage, odor, swelling, and redness.

    b. Maintain child in prone position.

    c. Maintain sterility of dressing.

6. Prepare parents and infant for surgery (refer to institutional manual for specific guidelines) (see Appendix F).

Postoperative Care

1. Maintain nutritional and fluid intake.
   a. Assess for signs of dehydration or fluid overload.
   b. Monitor for bowel sounds.
   c. Monitor administration of IV fluids.
   d. Monitor and record intake and output.
   e. Monitor and record weight daily.
2. Monitor for signs and symptoms of infections.
   a. Fever (obtain blood C and S when infant is febrile)
   b. Drainage from surgical site
   c. Redness and inflammation
   d. Increased irritability or lethargy
3. Promote healing of surgical site; use sterile technique when changing and reinforcing dressing.
   a. Avoid use of latex gloves and other latex-containing medical products.
4. Monitor vital signs and neurologic status.
   a. Monitor temperature, pulse, respirations, and blood pressure.
   b. Perform neurologic assessment (see the Neurologic Assessment section in Appendix A).
   c. Monitor head circumference.
5. Provide emotional support to parents (see the Supportive Care section in Appendix F).

🏠 Discharge Planning and Home Care

1. Instruct parents about long-term management of bowel and bladder training.
   a. Bladder training
      i. Prevention of bladder infections
      ii. Modification of fluid consumption for bladder control

iii. Clean intermittent catheterization
iv. Provide preparation and information about surgical procedures: augmentation, enterocystoplasty, artificial urinary sphincter, urethral sling, abdominal stoma, and urinary diversion
v. Provide preparation and information on methods for assessing renal functioning: urine cultures, measurement of serum electrolyte levels, renal scans, intravenous pyelograms, ultrasonography, and urodynamic testing

b. Bowel training—to implement regular evacuation program
   i. High-fiber diet with bulking agents
   ii. Use of stool softeners
   iii. Use of digital stimulation (i.e., glycerin suppositories)
   iv. Use of laxatives (casanthranol [Peri-Colace])
   v. Use of low-volume bowel irrigation or enemas
   vi. Importance of good bowel habits to promote good health (reduction of urinary problems, shunt problems)

2. Provide information to parent and child about techniques to facilitate mobility and independence.
   a. Use of casting, corrective appliances (to provide mobility and independence, prevent osteoporosis and contractures)
   b. Use of wheelchairs and assistive devices
      i. Prevention of complications such as decubitus ulcers
      ii. Problem solving with respect to malfunctions and equipment problems
      iii. Access to service providers for equipment repairs and maintenance
   c. Physical therapy regimen
      i. Reinforce importance of adherence to exercises and daily activities
      ii. Coordinate services with physical therapist such as scheduling of appointments and integrated approach to providing services

    d. Provide preparation and information on surgical procedures to treat medical needs and long-term complications (see Appendix F).

3. Instruct parents on importance of child's avoiding contact with latex or natural rubber.

    a. Notify health care professionals in all settings, such as dentists, school nurses.

    b. Review sources of latex in home and community.

       i. Clothing

       ii. Art supplies

       iii. Diapers

       iv. Toys (water toys, dolls)

4. Provide information about skin care and injury prevention.

    a. Loss of sensation of the skin below level of lesion.

    b. Some drugs used to assist in urinary continence may cause decreased sweating (may result in dry skin and overheating).

    c. Check skin daily for scratches, bruises, cuts, red marks.

    d. Always wear protective footwear (insensate feet can acquire serious injury).

    e. Use prescribed seat cushion in wheelchair.

    f. Relieve pressure from sitting surface frequently, shift weight every 15 minutes if wheelchair-bound.

    g. Prevent burns.

       i. Check bathwater temperature before bathing.

       ii. Avoid contact with hot surfaces (in hot weather: wheelchair footrest, seatbelt buckles).

       iii. Apply sunscreen lotion (at least PF15) to all exposed skin when outdoors.

5. Provide education to parents about normal growth and development and deviations from norm (see Appendix B).

    a. Call attention to special problems and needs of child with disability.

    b. Encourage positive expectations and hope for achieving of developmental milestones, with goal of living as independently and productively as possible.

    c. Act as liaison with parents, teachers, and school to establish developmentally and intellectually appropriate expectations (see Appendix G).

i. If special education student, work with family and individualized education plan (IEP) team to ensure that health-related needs that interfere with learning are considered in developing IEP objectives (see Appendix G)

d. Instruct adolescents and provide information about areas of concern such as recreational programs, procurement of driver's license, postsecondary programs, and peer relationships.

e. Provide sexual and reproductive counseling (based on evaluation of genital responsiveness).
    i. Birth control concerns
    ii. Increased risk for sexual abuse or exploitation
    iii. Latex barrier contraceptives should be avoided

f. Provide career and vocational counseling.
    i. Refer youth and family to secondary and postsecondary educational resources and job training youth programs in community

g. Provide counseling about independent living in inclusive community settings.

h. Provide counseling on weight-control measures as needed.
    i. Promote acquisition of self-advocacy and self-determination skills

CLIENT OUTCOMES

1. Child will function at developmentally appropriate level.
2. Child will experience minimal complications associated with spina bifida.
3. Child will be well hydrated and will maintain weight within normal parameters.
4. Child will be free of infection.
5. Child and parents will demonstrate ability to maintain long-term home care and keep child free of complications, with child eventually assuming responsibility for self-care.
6. Parents will demonstrate ability to access services and supports as needed for their child's long-term management needs.
7. Child will demonstrate ability to function as independently as is developmentally possible.

BOX 72-1

Resources

Organizations

- Spina Bifida Association of America
  4590 MacArthur Blvd, N.W., Suite 250
  Washington, DC 20007–4226
  800–621–3141
  sbaa@sbaa.org
- March of Dimes Birth Defects Foundation
  1275 Mamaroneck Ave.
  White Plains, NY 10605
  888–663–4637
  www.marchofdimes.com
- Easter Seals—National Office
  230 West Monroe Street, Suite 1800
  Chicago, IL 60606
  800–221–6827
  www.easterseals.org
- National Rehabilitation Information Center (NARIC)
  4200 Forbes Blvd, Suite 202
  Lanham, MD 20706
  800–346–2742
  301–459–5984 (TTY)
  www.naric.com
- National Dissemination Center for Children with Disabilities
  (NICHCY)
  P.O. Box 1492
  Washington, DC 20013
  800–695–0285
  www.nichcy.org

Publications

- Lutkenoff M, editor: *Children with spina bifida: A parents' guide,* Bethesda, MD, 1999, Woodbine House. Contact publisher at 800–843–7323 or www.woodbinehouse.com.
- Lutkenoff M, Oppenheimer S: *SPINabilities: A young person's guide to spina bifida,* Bethesda, MD, 1997, Woodbine House. Contact publisher at 800–843–7323 or www.woodbinehouse.com.
- Spina Bifida Association of America: Health guide for adults with spina bifida (website): www.sbaa.sbaa.org.

REFERENCES

Behrman R et al editors : *Nelson textbook of pediatrics*, ed 17, Philadelphia, 2004, WB Saunders.

Gleeson RM, Malone A: *Skin care steps to take when caring for children with spina bifida*, Wilmington, DE, 2004, Alfred I duPont Institute.

Grosse SD et al: Reevaluating the benefits of folic acid fortification in the United States: Economic analysis, regulation, and public health, *Am J Pub Health* 95(11):1917, 2005.

Jones KL: *Smith's recognizable patterns of human malformation*, ed 5, Philadelphia, 1997, WB Saunders.

Rendeli C et al: Latex sensitisation and allergy with myelomeningocele, *Child Nerv Syst,* 22(1):28, 2005.

73

❖

Substance-Related Disorders

PATHOPHYSIOLOGY

Substance-related disorders are a major public health problem affecting young people in the United States. They are the leading cause of preventable death in 15- to 24-year-olds. Substances used can be any of a number of drugs taken for toxic or side effects. Such substances include alcohol, amphetamines, cannabis, cocaine, hallucinogens, inhalants, nicotine, opioids, anxiolytics, and phencyclidine (PCP). The effects of substance intoxication vary widely depending on the individual and the substance used. Generally, intoxication causes physiologic, cognitive, and psychosocial effects. A diagnosis of substance abuse is made when drug use causes adverse consequences such as physically hazardous behaviors, legal problems, and interference with school functioning.

A more serious problem is substance dependence. Prolonged, heavy use of a substance results in dependence. Over time, increasing amounts of the substance are needed to achieve intoxication; this is referred to as tolerance. When blood concentrations of the substance diminish, unpleasant withdrawal symptoms are experienced. Once dependence develops, the individual uses the substance primarily to relieve withdrawal symptoms. Withdrawal from certain drugs such as alcohol and benzodiazepines (e.g., Valium) is potentially life threatening. Hospitalization to manage detoxification may be indicated.

Alcohol, tobacco, and marijuana are the substances most frequently abused by children and adults. Inhalant use, which is often perceived as harmless by adolescents, accounts for a large number of deaths of teenagers. Both inhalant and heroin use are on the rise in the United States. Steroids are also one of the drugs being used with increased frequency by adolescents. Steroids became popular in athletics to improve performance by increasing muscularity. Because steroids do not increase endurance, they are mostly used by athletes who participate in football, wrestling, weight lifting, powerlifting, and bodybuilding.

The use of steroids by adolescents may or may not be for sports performance. Some abusers of steroids have muscle dysmorphia or "bigorexia," which is when an individual is obsessed with being unreasonably muscular and with low body fat. Some see muscle dysmorphia as an antithesis to anorexia nervosa. The connection is strengthened by the fact that many male and female steroid abusers have been victims of sexual and physical abuse.

Most steroid abusers are considered to be psychologically normal when they start using steroids. Gym dosing is typically 10 to 100 times the dosage for medical use. As with other illicit drugs, the problem with steroids is cessation. One of the major consequences of cessation of administration is depression. Use has decreased, possibly because of the press given to negative consequences suffered by professional athletes. Programs that have failed to reduce steroid use are drug testing–only programs, physical training or nutrition education, and education-only programs that do not focus on changing the perception of risk.

A number of psychosocial, developmental, cultural, attitudinal, and personality factors put a youth at risk for drug experimentation. The most significant predictor for substance use is drug use by peers. Other risk factors include poor self-image, problems with school performance, difficult temperament, hyperactivity, and genetic predisposition. Risk factors include problems associated with family dysfunction, including abuse and neglect, overly rigid or permissive parents, parental rejection, and divorce. The following are factors associated with resistance to illicit substance use: nurturing parents, positive school experience, negative attitudes toward drugs, committed religious attitudes, positive self-esteem, and social competence.

Generally, the younger the age of initial drug use, the higher the risk for serious long-term health consequences and adult abuse. Cigarette, alcohol, and marijuana use has been associated with ready access to these substances in the child's home.

Gateway phenomenon is a term denoting the pattern of using an increasing variety of substances, ultimately leading to polysubstance abuse. Evidence for this phenomenon is that youth who smoke tobacco and drink alcohol are more likely to use marijuana, and those who use marijuana are more likely to use cocaine. An adolescent may initially begin using to achieve a false sense of maturity, but eventually he or she is likely to develop drug dependence. Substance abuse is associated with depression, low self-esteem, risk for school underachievement, teenage pregnancy, and delinquency. Illicit drug use creates a greater risk of contracting human immunodeficiency virus (HIV) infection and hepatitis C.

Box 73-1 presents the criteria from the American Psychiatric Association's *Diagnostic and statistical manual of mental disorders* (DSM IV-TR) for substance abuse, substance dependence, substance intoxication, and substance withdrawal.

BOX 73-1

Substance Abuse

The DSM-IV-TR defines substance abuse as a maladaptive pattern of substance use manifested by recurrent and significant adverse consequences related to repeated use of the substance. Criteria include the following:

1. Recurrent substance use resulting in a failure to fulfill major role obligations at work, school, or home
2. Recurrent substance use in situations in which it is physically hazardous
3. Recurrent substance-related legal problems
4. Continued substance use despite having persistent or recurrent social or interpersonal problems caused or exacerbated by the effects of the substance

Substance Dependence

The DSM-IV-TR defines substance dependence by the following criteria:

BOX 73-1

Substance Abuse—cont'd

1. Evidence of tolerance, as identified by either of the following:
   a. A need for increased amounts of the substance to achieve intoxication or the desired effect
   b. Markedly diminished effect with continued use of the same amount of the substance
2. Evidence of withdrawal symptoms, as manifested by either of the following:
   a. The characteristic withdrawal syndrome for the substance
   b. The same (or closely related) substance is taken to relieve or avoid withdrawal symptoms
3. The substance is often taken in larger amounts or over a longer period than was intended.
4. There is a persistent desire or unsuccessful effort to decrease or control substance use.
5. A great deal of time is spent in activities necessary to obtain or use the substance or to recover from the effects of the substance.
6. Important social, occupational, or recreational activities are given up or reduced because of substance use.
7. The substance use is continued despite knowledge of having a persistent or recurrent physical or psychologic problem that is likely to have been caused or exacerbated by the substance.

Substance Intoxication

The DSM-IV-TR defines substance intoxication by the following criteria:

1. The development of a reversible substance-specific syndrome caused by recent ingestion of or exposure to a substance.
2. Clinically significant maladaptive behavior or psychologic changes that are caused by the effect of the substance on the central nervous system (CNS) and that develop during or shortly after use of the substance.
3. The symptoms are not caused by a general medical condition and are not better accounted for by another mental disorder.

Substance Withdrawal

The DSM-IV-TR defines substance withdrawal by the following criteria:

1. The development of a substance-specific syndrome caused by the cessation of or reduction in heavy and prolonged substance use.

Continued

BOX 73-1
Substance Abuse—cont'd

2. The substance-specific syndrome causes clinically significant distress or impairment in social, occupational, or other important areas of functioning.
3. The symptoms are not caused by a general medical condition and are not better accounted for by another mental disorder.

From American Psychiatric Association: Diagnostic and statistical manual of mental disorders, ed 4, text revision (DSM-IV-TR), Washington, DC, 2000, The Association.

INCIDENCE

1. Half the children in America (36 million) live in a home where a parent or other adult drinks heavily, uses illicit drugs, or smokes tobacco.
2. Children whose parents are alcoholics or drink heavily are 4 times more likely to use alcohol or develop alcohol-related problems compared to peers whose parents are not alcoholics.
3. The prevalence rate depends on the substance; substance use among adolescents has declined, but the use of steroids, opiates, LSD, and inhalants have shown periodic increases.
4. Of high school seniors, 64% have experimented with illicit drugs.
5. Nearly 50% of teenage suicides and accidental deaths have been associated with illegal substance use.
6. Of high school seniors, 6% report using illicit drugs on a regular basis.
7. Nearly 90% of adolescents ages 18 years and younger report having used alcohol.
8. During the past decade, the use of inhalant drugs (glue, aerosols) has increased threefold in the 12- to 17-year-old age group.
9. During the past decade, marijuana and inhalants have become the two most commonly used illicit drugs by the 12- to 17-year-old age group.
10. The age at which experimentation begins has been declining, especially for inhalants.

11. Depression is a comorbidity in 33% to 50% of those with opioid dependence or abuse, and in 40% of those with alcohol dependence.
12. Drug use disorders are strongly associated with anxiety, mood, and personality disorders.
13. Substance abusers are 20 times more likely to commit suicide than the general population; substance abuse is a major precipitating factor for suicide.
14. Substance abuse is generally higher in males than in females.
15. The earlier the onset of drug use and the faster the progression to stronger drugs, the higher the risk of substance abuse disorder.

CLINICAL MANIFESTATIONS

1. Most adolescents experiment with cigarettes and alcohol, some will advance to marijuana, and a smaller portion will advance to other drugs.
2. Craving for the substance
3. Reddened eyes
4. Changes in cognition: impaired concentration, disturbance of thinking, and changes in attention span and perception.
5. Signs of trauma that result from needle use, violent behaviors, injuries due to intoxication, and high-risk behavior.
6. Behavioral changes that include lethargy, agitation, disinhibition, hyperactivity, hypervigilance, and somnolence.
7. Impairment in psychosocial and academic functioning is the hallmark of substance abuse disorder.
8. Isolation of self from family members and friends.
9. All of the substances used are illegal for adolescents; some of the negative consequences are from the illegal nature of the substance rather than from use of the substance.
10. The course varies, but abuse is often discontinued in early adulthood, whereas dependence is more likely to continue.

COMPLICATIONS
Alcohol

1. General: bodily injury
2. Integumentary: diaphoresis, alopecia, spider nevi, telangiectases, angioma, palmar erythema, rosacea, superficial infection

3. Head, eyes, ears, nose, and throat (HEENT): rhinorrhea, sneezing, lacrimation
4. Cardiopulmonary: myocardial infarction, tachycardia, respiratory depression, cardiomyopathy, arrhythmias, hypertension, subacute bacterial endocarditis, chronic upper respiratory infection (URI), aspiration pneumonia
5. Gastrointestinal (GI): inadequate or poor nutritional status, abdominal tenderness, splenomegaly, hepatomegaly, GI bleeding, weight loss, diarrhea, esophagitis, gastritis, gastric ulcers, pancreatitis, pancreatic cancer
6. Musculoskeletal: muscle aches or cramps
7. Endocrine: testicular atrophy, gynecomastia, sexual dysfunction, amenorrhea
8. Neuropsychiatric: cerebrovascular accident, depression, anxiety, nystagmus, emotional lability, irritability, peripheral neuropathy, hallucinations (especially tactile), insomnia, headache, seizure, coma, convulsions, delirium, unsteady gait, difficulty standing, impaired judgment, Wernicke-Korsakoff syndrome (alcoholic encephalopathy)
9. Hematologic: anemia, leukopenia, thrombocytopenia

Complications Related to Stimulant or Opioid Abuse

1. Integumentary: diaphoresis
2. HEENT: Erosion of nasal septum (from cocaine use), dilated pupils, mydriasis
3. Cardiopulmonary: cardiac arrhythmias, myocardial infarction, tachycardia, chest pain, respiratory depression, hypertension, cardiac arrest (from overdose), subacute bacterial endocarditis, bradycardia, hypotension
4. Gastrointestinal: inadequate or poor nutritional status, abdominal tenderness, splenomegaly, hepatomegaly, GI bleeding, weight loss, nausea, vomiting
5. Genitourinary: impotence
6. Musculoskeletal: psychomotor retardation, muscle cramps, fatigue
7. Endocrine/immunologic: hypothermia, human immunodeficiency virus (HIV), hepatitis from intravenous use

8. Neuropsychiatric: cerebrovascular accident, depression, anxiety, emotional lability, irritability, hallucinations, insomnia, panic episodes, restlessness, agitation, elated mood, grandiosity, mood swings, headache, seizure, dystonia, dyskinesia, nightmares

Complications Related to Depressant Agents

Neuropsychiatric: dysphoria, anxiety, mood swings, ataxia, disinhibition, paranoia, drowsiness, slurred speech, hallucinations, lack of impulse control, impaired attention, impaired memory, impaired judgment

Complications Related to Hallucinogens*

1. General: deterioration of health status; sudden death
2. Integumentary: diaphoresis, alopecia, spider nevi, telangiectases, angioma, palmar erythema, rosacea, superficial infection
3. HEENT: dilated pupils, blurred vision
4. Cardiopulmonary: tachycardia, palpitations
5. Neuropsychiatric: tremors, ataxia, nystagmus, mood swings, panic episodes, flashbacks, aggression, hallucination, paranoia, impaired concentration, impaired memory, inability to make decisions, incoordination

Complications Related to Cannabis†

1. Mouth and throat: dry mouth
2. Cardiovascular: tachycardia
3. GI: increased hunger
4. Neuropsychiatric: paranoia, confusion, time distortion, hallucinations, anxiety, depersonalization, derealization, euphoria, disinhibition, impaired attention, reaction time, and judgment

Complications Related to Inhalants

1. General: accident or injury while intoxicated

---

*Hallucination intoxication usually lacks a withdrawal symptoms.
†Cannabis usually lacks withdrawal symptoms. After long-term heavy use, individual may have a postural tremor, sweating, irritability, anxiety, and muscle aches.

2. Integumentary: residue of inhalant on skin, face, hands, and clothes; diaphoresis
3. HEENT: irritation of the eyes and nose, rash around nose and mouth, unusual breath odor
4. Mouth and throat: irritation of throat and lungs
5. Cardiopulmonary: cardiac arrhythmias, respiratory depression, tachycardia, hypertension, asphyxiation, cardiac arrest
6. GI: nausea and vomiting, anorexia, weight loss, hepatic damage
7. Genitourinary: kidney damage
8. Musculoskeletal: permanent muscle damage associated with rhabdomyolysis
9. Neuropsychiatric: ataxia, anxiety, agitation, confusion, stupor, delusions, hallucinations, irritability, psychosis, delirium, dementia, brain atrophy, decreased intelligence quotient (IQ), temporal lobe epilepsy, nystagmus

Complications Related to Steroids

1. Integumentary: severe acne
2. HEENT: alopecia
3. Cardiopulmonary: tachycardia, cerebrovascular disease, hypertension
4. Genitourinary: kidney tumor, gynecomastia, sexual dysfunction, testicular atrophy, prostate cancer, reduced sperm count or infertility (females), amenorrhea, alopecia, facial hair, enlarged clitoris, deepened voice
5. Endocrine: liver cancer, jaundice, HIV infection, hepatitis, tetanus (from use of contaminated needle), increased low-density lipoprotein (LDL), decreased high-density lipoprotein (HDL), stunted growth or premature skeletal maturation
6. Neuropsychiatric: tremor, depression, aggression, delusions, paranoia, manic symptoms, irritability, jealousy, mood swings, impaired judgment

LABORATORY AND DIAGNOSTIC TESTS

Refer to Appendix D for normal values and ranges of laboratory and diagnostic tests.
1. Toxicologic analysis—used for identification of substance, differential diagnosis

2. Urine drug screen (UDS)—indicates type of substance used and time of use (limitations include civil liberties issues, short "window" of detection of metabolites, and intermittent pattern of abuse; also, tests vary in sensitivity, expense, and time)
3. Blood alcohol level—to detect level of alcohol in the blood
4. Complete blood count—low white blood cell (WBC) count, increased prothrombin time (PT), anemia
5. Liver enzymes—increased in alcohol dependence
6. Breathalyzer—measures the level of blood alcohol concentration (BAC) using a breath sample
7. Psychologic evaluations—screening tests for assessment of substance abuse
   a. CAGE questionnaire:
      i. Have you ever felt you should **cut** down on your drinking?
      ii. Have people **annoyed** you by criticizing your drinking?
      iii. Have you ever felt bad or **guilty** about your drinking?
      iv. Have you ever had a drink first thing in the morning to steady your nerves or get rid of a hangover (**eye opener**)?
   b. Self-administered alcohol screening test (SAAST)—to screen for alcoholism: there are two formats, one for individuals who may have an alcohol problem and another for a person (e.g., friend, classmate) who knows the individual
   c. Brief drug abuse screening test (B-DAST), self-administered 20-item test—to identify individuals abusing psychoactive drugs
   d. Addiction severity index (ASI)—to assess the severity of the substance abuse

MEDICAL MANAGEMENT

Treatment for substance abuse is typically done on an outpatient basis. Inpatient hospitalization is indicated if the client is suicidal or requires detoxification. Controlling drug use should never be the end target of treatment. Harm reduction is effective in reducing the use and the adverse effects of substances, increasing level of functioning, and reducing frequency and severity of relapse, while client learns skills to deal with substance abuse. Improved self-confidence may increase the chances of abstinence.

Comprehensive treatment programs include individual and group psychotherapy, family therapy, recreational therapy, and social skills training. Intensive initial treatment, whether provided on an inpatient or outpatient basis, is associated with positive outcomes. Concurrent attention to interpersonal deficits, coexisting psychiatric symptomatology, family functioning, and educational or vocational functioning improves treatment outcomes. It is important that the youth be connected to community resources that can support achievement of long-term outcomes. Linkages to education, training, rehabilitation, and job development programs can be of assistance.

Treating comorbid conditions is a major part of substance abuse disorder. Care must be given to using psychotropic medications with adolescents who have substance problems because of the increased potential for unintentional or intentional overdose, either with these medications or in combination with some substance of abuse. Cognitive behavioral therapy (CBT) is effective in treating conduct disorder, which is the most common comorbid disorder, and can be used to focus on substance abuse issues.

Prevention efforts that emphasize development or enhancement of protective factors (strengthening self-esteem, and problem solving, coping, and communication skills) are most effective. These programs emphasize resistance to peer pressure and highlight that most children and youth do not use drugs. Interactive learning models such as role playing and small-group learning sessions are more effective than educational programs. Prevention programs, referred to as universal, selective, or indicated, should be targeted to specific audiences. Universal programs address the needs of the general public, selective programs provide outreach to at-risk populations such as children of abusing parents, and indicated programs are directed to youths who use illicit substances.

NURSING ASSESSMENT

1. Obtain thorough history of illegal and illicit drugs of choice, time of last use, amount used, frequency and duration of use, and routes of administration (intravenous, oral, and inhalant forms provide more rapid effect).
2. Conduct physical assessment with emphasis on respiratory, cardiovascular, and neurologic systems (see Appendix A).
3. Note any signs of trauma or injury (e.g., needle puncture marks).
4. Assess for depression and suicide potential (refer to Chapter 75). Refer for further evaluation if the answer is yes to two or more of the following questions:
   a. Are you feeling suicidal?
   b. Do you have a plan (gun, knife, rope)?
   c. Do you have access to materials to carry out your plan?
   d. Are you able to contract not to harm yourself?
   e. Do you know anyone who has attempted or committed suicide?
5. Assess for youth and family drug- and alcohol-related problems.
6. Obtain information about school performance.
7. Assess level, type, and frequency of social activities, after-school activities, and peer relationships.
8. Assess level and quality of family and social support.

NURSING DIAGNOSES

- Injury, Risk for
- Denial, Ineffective
- Knowledge, Deficient
- Self-esteem, Chronic low
- Coping, Compromised family

NURSING INTERVENTIONS

1. Assess specific safety requirements by obtaining history of type of substance used and level of toxication (urine toxicology screen may be more accurate than client report), amount and time last consumed, amount consumed on

a daily basis, when client started using and frequency of use, signs and severity of withdrawal symptoms.
2. Institute necessary safety precautions.
   a. Orient client to reality and surroundings.
   b. Remove potentially harmful objects.
   c. Monitor vital signs as acute symptoms subside.
3. Use caring confrontation regarding rationalizing and fantasizing about drug lifestyle, and provide information to correct misperceptions about substance abuse.
4. Encourage sharing of feelings, anxieties, and fears while encouraging and reinforcing independent positive decision making.
5. Assess client's readiness to learn and preferred learning method to teach psychologic and physiologic effects of drug dependence, starting with simple and moving on to more complex concepts.
6. Teach assertiveness techniques and effective communication utilizing client's strengths and accomplishments.
7. Assess family communication, coping, and support; provide support and information about enabling; and involve family in discharge referral plans.
8. Encourage linkages to community-based resources and services.

🏠 Discharge Planning and Home Care

1. Provide realistic and credible information about risks and consequences associated with drug use.
2. Provide parental anticipatory guidance on need to create clearly delineated expectations for their youth's behavior and their responsibility to serve as appropriate role models.
3. Provide parental anticipatory guidance regarding use of home drug test kits—that they have limitations and can generate false-positive results, and that their use does not substitute for open communication or parental supervision.
4. Provide information to parents about relationship between their use of tobacco and alcohol, child and adolescent, and adolescent substance use and abuse.
5. Advise parents that treatment programs must include comprehensive interdisciplinary approach that involves juvenile

justice, social services, mental health services, and primary care

CLIENT OUTCOMES

1. Adolescent will stop or decrease illicit drug use.
2. Adolescent will verbally take responsibility for own behavior and acknowledge association between personal problems and substance use.
3. Adolescent will develop more positive coping skills.
4. Family members will learn to communicate and interact with each other more effectively.

REFERENCES

American Academy of Child and Adolescent Psychiatry: Practice parameter for the assessment and treatment of children and adolescents with substance use disorder, *J Am Acad Child Adolesc Psychiatr* 44(6):609, 2005.

American Psychiatric Association: *Diagnostic and statistical manual of mental disorders,* ed 4, text revision (DSM-IV-TR), Washington, DC, 2000, The Association.

Colliver J et al: Development in the epidemiology of drug use and drug use disorders, *Am J Psychiat* 162(8):1494, 2005.

Jonnson L et al: Teen drug use down but progress halts among youngest teens. University of Michigan News and Information Services: Ann Arbor, MI, *Monitor the Future* (serial online): http://monitorthefuture.org. Accessed April 26, 2007.

National Institute on Drug Abuse: *NIDA infofacts: Steroids (anabolic androgenic)* (website): www.drugabuse.gov/infofacts/steroids.html. Accessed February 28, 2006.

Simkin D: Adolescent substance abuse. In: Sadock B and Sadock V: *Kaplan & Sadock's comprehensive textbook of psychiatry,* ed 8, Philadelphia, 2005, Lippincott, Williams & Wilkins.

Townsend MC: Unit Two—Alterations in psychiatric adaptation. Chapter 4. Substance-related disorders. In: Townsend M, Ed.: *Nursing diagnosis in psychiatric nursing: Care plans and psychotropic medications,* ed 6, Philadelphia, 2004, FA Davis.

74

Sudden Infant Death Syndrome

PATHOPHYSIOLOGY

Sudden infant death syndrome (SIDS) is defined as "the sudden death of an infant under 1 year of age which remains unexplained after a thorough case investigation, including performance of a complete autopsy, examination of the death scene, and review of the clinical history" (Willinger, James, & Catz, 1991, p. 681). The autopsy report can include the following findings. External examination reveals a body that appears well developed and nourished. There is a small amount of mucous, or watery or bloody secretions present at the nares. Cyanosis of the lips and nail beds is almost always present. The internal examination findings indicate a subacute inflammation of the upper respiratory tract and petechiae on the pleura, the pericardium, and the thymus (this is found in 80% of cases). There is pulmonary edema and congestion. The autopsy reveals symptoms of chronic hypoxemia including brainstem changes; persistence of brown fat, especially around the adrenals; and hepatic erythropoiesis. Some of these autopsy findings are demonstrated in about 80% of SIDS cases, and their absence does not exclude the diagnosis. Risk factors associated with the incidence of SIDS are listed in Box 74-1.

The pathophysiology of SIDS remains unclear, but current research is focused in the following six areas:

1. Abnormalities of the central nervous system (CNS): There are two areas of focus within this category. The first is delayed myelination or gliosis (or scarring) in the respiratory control

BOX 74-1
Risk Factors

Infant Risk Factors

- Prematurity, particularly with birth weight <2500 g
- Low birth weight for gestational age
- African American and Native American heritage
- Male sex (risk increased by 50%)
- Multiple births
- Low Apgar scores
- Central nervous system disturbances
- Respiratory disorders such as bronchopulmonary dysplasia
- Neonatal intensive care history

Familial Risk Factors

- Low socioeconomic status
- Low educational level
- Young maternal age
- Young married mother <20 years old
- History of smoking during pregnancy
- History of drug abuse (including marijuana, methadone, cocaine, heroin, or psychedelics)
- High parity
- Low interpregnancy interval
- Anemia

areas of the brainstem. The second is altered neuronal pathways within the brainstem, which prevent an infant from responding to life-threatening hypercapnea, hypoxemia, hyperthermia, or cardiovascular episodes during sleep.

2. Primary cardiac arrhythmias, particularly those causing bradycardia secondary to a decrease in vagal nerve tone and occurring simultaneously with central apnea and prolonged QT interval.

3. Carbon dioxide rebreathing and airway obstruction associated with the prone sleeping position and soft bedding: This position can cause an increased frequency of oxygen desaturation in the blood, exposing the infant to periods of hypoxemia and hypercapnea as well as pharyngeal collapse that causes a functional obstruction of the infant's airway.

4. Impaired temperature regulation and its effects on the respiratory pattern, chemoreceptor sensitivity, and cardiac control

5. Infant sleep state: Infants sleeping in the prone position may have more time in quiet sleep and less time in active sleep. In quiet sleep, an infant experiences fewer awakenings and an increased arousal threshold.

6. Infectious agents, particularly viral septicemia

INCIDENCE

1. Sudden infant death syndrome is the most common cause of death before 1 year of age.

2. Since the introduction of the "Back to Sleep" campaign in 1992, which resulted in a steady decrease in the prone sleeping rate, the SIDS rate has decreased from 1.2 deaths per 1000 live births to 0.56 death per 1000 live births in 2001. This represents a 53% decrease.

3. Age range of peak incidence is 2 to 3 months; it is uncommon before 2 weeks of age or after 6 months of age.

4. It has seasonal occurrence in the winter months, particularly during January; however, there has been a decrease in seasonality over the past 5 years.

5. Occurrence of death is most frequently between midnight and 9 am.

6. SIDS death rates are 2 to 3 times the national average in African American and American Indian and Alaska Native children.

7. SIDS accounts for an estimated 7000 to 10,000 infant deaths per year worldwide.

NURSING ASSESSMENT

1. Assess the infant, familial, and maternal risk factors (see Box 74-1) associated with SIDS.

2. Assess family's ability to manage in-home apnea monitoring, as appropriate for selected groups of infants.

3. Assess family's need for support and resources during the acute grieving period (refer to Appendixes G and H).

NURSING DIAGNOSES

- Therapeutic regimen management, Ineffective
- Family processes, Interrupted
- Grieving, Risk for dysfunctional

NURSING INTERVENTIONS

Prevention

1. Complete a thorough history and physical examination to determine the presence of risk factors.
2. Perform newborn teaching with parents before discharge, stressing the need for follow-up care with a pediatrician and the use of the American Academy of Pediatrics 2005 updated guidelines discouraging the use of the prone sleeping position (refer to Box 74-2).
3. Promote American Academy of Pediatrics (AAP) and the "Back to Sleep" recommendations that include the following:
   a. Supine sleeping position, wholly on the back, for every sleep
   b. No sleeping on soft surfaces—a firm crib mattress covered by a sheet is recommended
   c. Limit soft materials or objects such as stuffed animals and toys in the crib.
   d. Separate but proximate sleeping environment
   e. Do not smoke during pregnancy. Protect infant from secondhand smoking by parents or caretaker.

BOX 74-2
Modifiable Risk Factors

- Prone sleeping
- Soft sleep surfaces and loose bedding
- Overheating
- Maternal smoking during pregnancy
- Cosleeping
- Preterm birth and low birth weight
- Protective factors include breast-feeding and use of pacifiers
- Apnea monitors may be appropriate for infants with underlying disease such as bronchopulmonary dysplasia

f. Offer a pacifier at nap and bedtime.

g. Avoid overheating with excessive clothing, warm room temperature, and excessive blankets.

h. Avoid devices marketed to reduce the risk of SIDS.

i. Do not use home monitors as a strategy to reduce the risk of SIDS.

j. Avoid development of positional plagiocephaly (a persistent flattened spot on the back or one side of the head) by encouraging "tummy time" when awake and avoiding excessive time in car or bouncer seats.

k. Outreach efforts are directed to parents, health care professionals, and especially child care providers. The Back to Sleep program was initiated jointly by the U.S. Public Health Service, the AAP, the SIDS Alliance, and the Association of SIDS and Infant Mortality Programs.

4. Refer mothers who use tobacco to smoking cessation programs.

5. Monitor ability of family members to participate in in-home apnea monitoring and use of cardiopulmonary resuscitation when applicable.

Care after SIDS

1. Support the family during the acute grieving period.

2. Counsel parents and reassure them that they are not responsible for the infant's death.

3. Encourage parents to express their feelings of guilt and remorse.

4. Employ therapeutic listening skills to assist parents in the grieving process.

5. Allow sufficient privacy for parents to be alone with infant as needed.

6. Refer family to appropriate community-based support group (i.e., Compassionate Friends, Candlelighters; refer to Appendix G).

🏠 Discharge Planning and Home Care

1. During bereavement period, refer family to appropriate resources to deal with issues such as chronic grief (Box 74-3, Appendix G).
2. Follow up with phone call and sympathy card from staff.

CLIENT OUTCOMES

1. Family will be knowledgeable about community resources.
2. Family will demonstrate appropriate grieving behaviors.

BOX 74-3

Resources

- National SIDS and Infant Death Resource Center
  8280 Greensboro Dr., Suite 300
  McClean, VA 22102
  703–821–8955
  866–866–7437
  www.sidscenter.org
- Back to Sleep
  31 Center Dr., Rm 2A32
  Bethesda, MD 20892–2425
  800–505-CRIB
  www.nichd.nih.gov/SIDS
- American Sudden Infant Death Syndrome Institute
  509 Augusta Dr.
  Marietta, GA 30067
  800–232-SIDS
  www.sids.org
- SIDS Alliance/First Candle
  1314 Bedford Ave. Suite 210
  Baltimore, MD 21208
  800–221–7437
  410–653–8226
  www.sidsalliance.org

REFERENCES

American Academy of Pediatrics Task Force on Sudden Infant Death Syndrome: The changing concepts of sudden infant death syndrome: Diagnostic coding shifts, controversies regarding the sleeping environment, and new variables to consider in reducing risk, *Pediatrics* 116(5):1245, 2005.

Anonymous: Assessment of infant sleeping positions—selected states, *MMWR Morb Mortal Wkly Rep* 47(41):873, 1998.

Hymel K and the Committee on Child Abuse and Neglect, American Academy of Pediatrics Clinical Report: Distinguishing sudden infant death syndrome from child abuse fatalities, *Pediatrics* 118(1):421, 2006.

Malloy M, MacDorman M: Changes in the classification of sudden unexpected infant deaths: United States, 1992–2001, *Pediatrics* 115(5):1247, 2005.

Mathews TJ, Menacker F, MacDorman F: Infant morality statistics from the 2002 period linked birth/infant death data set, *Natl Vital Stat Rep* 53 (10):1, 2004.

Paris J, Remler R, Daling J: Risk factors for sudden infant death syndrome: Changes associated with sleep position recommendations, *J Pediatrics* 139 (6):771, 2001.

Patel A et al: Occurrence and mechanisms of sudden oxygen desaturation in infants who sleep face down, *Pediatrics* 111(4):e328, 2004.

Raydo L, Reu-Donlon C: Putting babies "back to sleep": Can we do better? *Neonat Network* 24(6):9, 2005.

Spitzer A: Current controversies in the pathophysiology and prevention of sudden infant death syndrome, *Curr Opin Pediatr* 17(2):181, 2005.

Willinger M, James L, Catz C: Defining the sudden infant death syndrome (SIDS): Deliberations of an expert panel convened by the National Institute of Child Health and Human Development, *Pediatr Pathol* 11(5):677, 1991.

75

❖

Suicide

PATHOPHYSIOLOGY

Suicide is the third leading cause of death among youth in the United States. Risk of suicide is the most frequent reason for inpatient psychiatric hospitalizations of adolescents. Suicidal behaviors represent a continuum ranging from the completed act to suicide attempts and self-inflicted injury. Suicidal ideations are recurrent thoughts of death and of killing oneself. Suicidal ideations do not necessarily include a plan or intention to kill oneself but may be a precursor to suicidal behavior. A carefully formulated suicide plan is an indicator that the youth has serious intentions of carrying out his or her plan.

Contributing factors to youth suicide are complex and fall within the following areas: psychiatric illnesses, family problems, major life changes, and demographics. Mood disorders, especially untreated depression and substance abuse, place the youth in considerable jeopardy. Family history of emotional problems, multiple family moves, problematic parent-child relationships, sexual abuse, emotional neglect, parental divorce, and family violence are risk factors for suicide. Significant recent life changes such as loss of a parent, end of a romantic relationship, and a recent move are also associated with suicidal behaviors. Demographic risk factors include being a member of a single-parent family or in a noncustodial living arrangement, being male, and being in one's late teens. Ready access to firearms in the home is positively associated with suicide attempts.

Suicide clusters have been identified among adolescents who imitate their peers in committing suicide. Three or more suicides or attempts occurring within 3 months within a specific geographic area constitute a *suicide cluster*. During adolescence the sense that death is final may not be entirely grasped. The youth may fantasize about being at his or her own funeral and observing other's reactions to his or her death. Suicide methods used by adolescents include poisoning, hanging, jumping from a high place, jumping out of a car, inhaling carbon monoxide fumes, drowning, and overdosing from medications. Use of a firearm is the most common method used to commit suicide in the United States, by adults as well as youth. Females use less violent methods of suicide than males. Males are 4 times more likely to die from suicide attempts than females.

INCIDENCE

1. Depression with functional impairment occurs in 2% to 10% of children and adolescents who complete suicide.
2. Mood disorders account for most suicide attempts.
3. Suicide is the third leading cause of death in 15- to 19-year-olds and the fourth leading cause in 10- to 14-year-olds.
4. American Indians and Alaska Natives have the highest suicide rate in the 15- to 24-year age-group.
5. For every suicide among high school students, there are approximately 350 unsuccessful suicide attempts.
6. Suicide rates in the United States are highest in the spring and lowest in the winter.
7. Adolescent suicide risk increases sevenfold with maternal suicide attempts and fivefold with marital discord.
8. Use of firearms is the method most often employed in completed suicides among those 10 to 14 years old, followed by hanging and drug overdose.
9. Use of firearms, hanging, and drug overdose are the methods used most often by 15- to 24-year-olds who complete suicide.

CLINICAL MANIFESTATIONS

1. Prolonged unhappiness, sadness, tearfulness, and moodiness
2. Social withdrawal from friends, family, and usual social activities

3. Acting out and aggressive behaviors, fighting with peers and/or siblings
4. Sense of hopelessness and despair
5. Delinquent behaviors: stealing, lying, property destruction (e.g., graffiti)
6. Sleep disorders and disturbances such as nightmares, excessive sleeping, and insomnia
7. Eating disorders; changes in weight and appetite
8. Changes in school performance
9. Somatic complaints such as abdominal pain and headaches
10. Feelings of shame and guilt
11. Low self-esteem as evidenced by self-deprecating remarks, sense of worthlessness, and behavior

MEDICAL MANAGEMENT

The suicide risk must be assessed by a professional. Assessment must include inquiry into suicidal ideation, plan, intention, and available means to carry out a suicide plan. If the child or youth reports suicidal ideations with a plan, and has the means and the intention to carry out the plan, the individual should be continually supervised or monitored until he or she is evaluated by a mental health professional. Children and youths who attempt suicide should receive emergency treatment.

If the suicide risk is acute, hospitalization is necessary for stabilization, intensive monitoring, and comprehensive diagnostic evaluation. Follow-up in outpatient treatment is imperative and may include individual and family psychotherapy as well as medication. Depression underlies most suicidality and is best treated with a combination of psychotherapy (i.e., cognitive behavioral or psychodynamic approaches) and medications. When mood disorder symptoms interfere with the child's functioning, antidepressants are typically indicated.

Youths taking antidepressants are at risk during the early stage of medication treatment for behavioral activiation, or a switch to mania and suicidal thoughts. For this reason the U.S. Food and Drug Administration recently issued warnings on the use of antidepressants in children. During the first 4 weeks of antidepressant treatment, children and adolescents should be followed once a week by a mental health provider such as a psychiatric nurse practitioner or psychiatrist, then every other week for the next 4 weeks and finally, when dosage and symptoms are stabilized, every 4 months. If the youth has a problem with drug and/or alcohol abuse, chemical dependency treatment should be rendered concurrently with the psychiatric interventions.

NURSING ASSESSMENT

1. Do not be afraid to ask child or youth about suicidal thoughts and whether he or she has a plan and/or intentions to carry out plan. Does he or she have history of past suicides attempts, access to drugs or medications, or weapons?
2. Assess for alcohol and drug use (when under influence of alcohol and other drugs that cause disinhibition, child or youth may act impulsively on suicidal thoughts).
3. Assess for significant changes in behavior (refer to Clinical Manifestations section in this chapter).
4. Assess level of social and family support.

NURSING DIAGNOSES

- Injury, Risk for
- Violence, Risk for self-directed
- Coping, Ineffective
- Coping, Compromised family
- Thought processes, Disturbed
- Therapeutic regimen management, Ineffective

NURSING INTERVENTIONS

1. Recognize warning signs of mood disorders and suicidal behaviors.
2. Identify children and youths at risk for suicide and refer for comprehensive interdisciplinary treatment services (e.g., crisis intervention team).
3. Refer child or youth to psychotherapist, school psychologist, or counselor for ongoing treatment.
4. Encourage sharing of feelings and family's active listening to child's or youth's concerns.

5. Promote use of positive coping strategies; focus on emphasizing child's or youth's strengths.
6. Provide support for problem solving and positive use of alternative strategies.
7. Restrict access to firearms and lethal weapons.
8. Provide access number for crisis hotline.
9. Elicit contract from child or youth not to harm self.
   a. Ask child or youth, "Are you able to verbally contract not to harm yourself, and can you inform (name of specific adult) if you have thought of harming yourself?"

🏠 Discharge Planning and Home Care

1. Provide information to parents about association between ready access to guns in home and increased risk of adolescent suicide. Encourage parents to limit access to firearms or remove them from home.
2. Advocate positive parent-child relationships and positive communications; refer to family-centered therapy services, parenting skills programs, psychotherapy, and psychoeducational programs.
3. Facilitate referrals for children and youths to peer support programs.
4. Coordinate prevention efforts with educational and community-based colleagues focused on self-awareness for mood disorders and suicide, and methods to enhance self-esteem.

CLIENT OUTCOMES

1. Child or youth suicide plan or attempt will be prevented.
2. Child or youth will develop new, more positive, coping strategies.
3. Child or youth will identify sources of support (e.g., friends, family members).

REFERENCES

Dopheide JA: Recognizing and treating depression in children and adolescents, *Am J Health Syst Pharm* 1:63(3):233, 2006.

Kochanck KD et al: Deaths: Final data for 2002. *Natl Vital Stats Rep,* 53(5):1, 2004.

Murphy K: What can you do to prevent teen suicide? *Nursing* 35(12):43, 2005.

National Institute of Mental Health: *Suicide facts and statistics* (website): www.nimh.nih.gov/suicideprevention/suifact.cfm. Accessed March 10, 2006.

76

❖

Systemic Bacterial Infection

PATHOPHYSIOLOGY

Infants and toddlers with a systemic bacterial infection often present with few, nonspecific signs of illness. The younger the child, the more difficult it is to recognize a bacterial infection by history. If a systemic bacterial infection is suspected, urgent investigation is performed, which is called a septic workup, and immediate intravenous antibiotic therapy is administered to prevent the illness from becoming life-threatening.

The risk of a systemic bacterial illness is generally believed to be higher in febrile infants under 3 months of age than in older febrile infants. The types of systemic bacterial infections are *septicemia, occult bacteremia,* and *meningitis. Septicemia* is the presence of microorganisms in the blood, with a localized or systemic diseaase in an ill-appearing child. *Occult bacteremia* is a bacteremia with a benign appearance and no other apparent source of serious infection. Factors increasing the risk of bacteremia are young age, premature birth, previous serious illness, chronic illness, ill appearance, fever, elevated white blood cell (WBC) count, and elevated absolute neutrophil count. *Meningitis* is an acute inflammation of the meninges and cerebrospinal fluid from a bacterial pathogen.

The most common serious bacterial infections in children older than 3 months of age are meningitis, bacteremia, urinary tract infection, pneumonia, soft-tissue infections, and enteric infections. The occurrence of a child having an acute episode of fever with a systemic illness is greater in children older than 3 months of age. Conversely, owing to an infant's immature immune system, infants younger than 1 month of age rarely become febrile, and more often hypothermia is seen with systemic bacterial infections. However, most febrile young children have self-limited viral infections.

INCIDENCE

1. In febrile infants under 3 months of age with a rectal temperature of 100.4° F (38.0° C) or higher, the prevalence of serious bacterial illness is approximately 8% to 10%.
2. The risk of occult bacteremia in children 3 to 36 months of age with fever but without localizing signs is approximately 2% to 10%.
3. Group B *Streptococcus* (GBS) now accounts for most bacterial infections in infants younger than 3 months of age.
4. *Streptococcus pneumoniae* is the most prevalent bacterial infection in healthy children older than 3 months of age.
5. Fever in children from 3 to 36 months of age is seen more often between November and March.
6. Approximately 10% of children with bacteremia will develop a systemic bacterial infection.
7. Hearing impairment is the most common sequela from meningitis.

CLINICAL MANIFESTATIONS

1. "Not doing well"; vague symptoms reported by caregiver
2. Fever, hypothermia
3. Apnea, tachypnea, grunting, retractions
4. Duskiness, mottling, cyanosis
5. Tachycardia
6. Poor feeding, weight loss
7. Vomiting, diarrhea
8. Fussiness, irritability, lethargy, altered sleep patterns
9. Hypotonicity
10. Rash, petechiae, purpura, vesicles
11. Bulging fontanelle, seizure activity, high-pitched cry

COMPLICATIONS

1. Infectious: meningitis, urosepsis, septic shock
2. End-organ failure

3. Neurologic: hearing impairment, neurologic devastation
4. Death

LABORATORY AND DIAGNOSTIC TESTS

Refer to Appendix D for normal values and ranges of laboratory and diagnostic tests.

1. Complete blood count with differential—to evaluate any evidence of infection
2. Erythrocyte sedimentation rate, C-reactive protein level—to assess for an inflammatory process
3. Blood culture—to detect and identify bacterial pathogens
4. Urinalysis and urine culture of specimen obtained by catheterization or suprapubic tap; 20% of children with urinary tract infection (UTI) have normal urinalysis but can have subsequent positive culture results
5. Lumbar puncture, cerebrospinal fluid detects bacterial and viral pathogens
6. Stool smear for WBCs and culture if gastroenteritis is suspected—to detect enteral pathogens
7. Chest radiographic studies—to detect lung abnormalities such as pneumonia

MEDICAL MANAGEMENT

The goals of therapy are to treat the underlying process causing the infection and reduce the incidence of negative sequelae. Bacterial infections should be treated with appropriate antimicrobial therapy. Febrile infants younger than 1 month of age who appear toxic should receive intravenous (IV) antimicrobials in the hospital with 48 to 72 hours of observation. Infants from 30 to 60 days of age who appear ill and/or have abnormal laboratory studies should be admitted to a hospital for IV antimicrobials and observed for 48 to 72 hours. There continues to be debate on treatment approaches for infants older than 3 months of age. Well-appearing infants older than 3 months of age without abnormal laboratory values may be followed at home or hospitalized for 48 to 72 hours of observation. If infants are followed at home, careful observation by the caregivers and assurance of follow-up with the health care provider is required.

NURSING ASSESSMENT

1. Monitor vital signs closely.
   a. Apical heart rate, respiratory rate at rest, rectal temperature, pulse oximetry
2. See the Cardiovascular, Respiratory and Neurologic Assessment sections in Appendix A.
3. Assess for signs of dehydration.
   a. Urine output, skin turgor, sunken fontanelle, capillary refill
4. Assess child's response to medications.
   a. Allergic reactions
   b. Decrease in febrile state

NURSING DIAGNOSES

- Infection, Risk for
- Tissue perfusion, Ineffective
- Hypothermia
- Hyperthermia
- Nutrition: less than body requirements, Imbalanced
- Anxiety
- Knowledge, Deficient
- Coping, Ineffective
- Coping, Compromised family

NURSING INTERVENTIONS

1. Monitor child's vital signs and neurologic status (including palpation of anterior fontanelle) as often as condition warrants.
2. Observe for rashes, petechiae, purpura, and/or vesicles.
3. Administer intravenous antibiotics; monitor for side effects.
4. Institute isolation procedures; simple isolation may be acceptable if cerebrospinal fluid (CSF) gram stain is without organisms (check hospital policy).
5. Monitor child's hydration status (IV and oral intake, urine output, skin turgor, edema, daily weights).
6. Monitor for cardiovascular compromise (skin color, skin temperature, capillary refill, level of consciousness).
7. Sponge with tepid water and unbundle child to reduce fever.
8. Administer antipyretics.
9. Continue the infant or child on a regular diet, if tolerated.

10. Monitor for fluid overload from additional IV fluid volume while administering IV antimicrobials.
11. Provide emotional support to child during lumbar puncture and other tests; restrain child to prevent injury (refer to Appendix F).
12. Provide emotional support to family; provide and reinforce information about condition and hospitalization (refer to Appendix F).

🏠 Discharge Planning and Home Care

1. Instruct parents verbally and with written reinforcement about administration of medications and monitoring for side effects.
2. Instruct parents to follow up with health care provider, as instructed.
3. Provide with home health referral if child is going home with IV antimicrobials.
4. Instruct parents on good handwashing practices for children with viral infections and/or enteropathies.
5. Instruct parents to maintain adequate fluid and nutritional intake and observe for signs of dehydration.
6. Repeat hearing screen for those infants and children with meningitis.

CLIENT OUTCOMES

1. Child will be free from complications of infection.
2. Child will remain normothermic.
3. Child will have consistent weight gain.
4. Child will remain hemodynamically stable.
5. Family will use effective coping mechanisms in managing anxiety.
6. Family will understand home care and follow-up care.
7. Child will adapt positively and resume age-appropriate activities.

REFERENCES

Byington CL et al: Serious bacterial infections in febrile infants 1 to 90 days old with and without viral infection, *Pediatrics* 113(6):1662, 2004.

Hannah FS, Macias CG: *Evaluation and management of fever in the neonate and young infant (less than three months of age)* (website): www.utdol.com/utd/content/topic.do?topicKey=ped_emer/2114&view=print. Accessed February 23, 2006.

Jaskiewicz JA: Febrile infants at low risk for serious bacterial infection: An appraisal of the Rochester criteria and implications for management, *Pediatrics* 94(3):390, 1994.

Lee GM, Harper MB: Risk of bacteremia for febrile young children in the post-haemophilus influenzae type b era, *Arch Adolesc Med* 152(7):624, 1998.

McCarthy PL: Fever, *Pediatr Rev* 19(12):401, 1998.

Pantell RH et al: Management and outcomes of care of fever in early infancy, *JAMA* 291(10):1203, 2004.

77

❖

Tetralogy of Fallot

PATHOPHYSIOLOGY

Tetralogy of Fallot (TOF) is a cyanotic congenital heart defect composed of four structural components: (1) ventricular septal defect (VSD); (2) pulmonic stenosis, which can occur at any level (infundibular, valvular, supravalvular) and causes obstruction of blood flow into the pulmonary arteries; (3) right ventricular hypertrophy; and (4) overriding of the aorta. In children with TOF, the diameter of the aorta is larger than normal, whereas the pulmonary artery is smaller than normal.

The pulmonic stenosis causes portions of the deoxygenated blood from the right ventricle to shunt across the VSD into the aorta (right to left shunt) and results in cyanosis. The degree of cyanosis is related to the severity of the pulmonic stenosis, with more severe cyanosis associated with more severe obstruction. The degree of cyanosis ranges from none (pink TOF) in children with minimal right to left shunting to profound in children with more significant right to left shunting (blue TOF).

INCIDENCE

1. TOF affects boys and girls equally.
2. Incidence is higher with older maternal age.
3. Few affected individuals survive beyond 20 years without surgery.
4. TOF accounts for 8% to 10% of congenital defects and is the most common cyanotic defect beyond the first week of life.
5. For patients with uncomplicated repair, the mortality rate is 2% to 3% during the first 2 years.

CLINICAL MANIFESTATIONS

1. Cyanosis—appears after neonatal period, although children with mild degree of right ventricular outflow obstruction may be acyanotic
2. Hypercyanotic spells during infancy, also known as "tet spells"
   a. Increased rate and depth of respiration
   b. Increased cyanosis
   c. Increased irritablity and prolonged crying that may lead to an alteration in consciousness and, if untreated, may ultimately result in seizures, cerebrovascular accident, and death
   d. Decreased intensity of cardiac murmur
3. Clubbing—late sign seen in unrepaired older children
4. Initially normal blood pressure—can increase after several years of marked cyanosis and polycythemia in unrepaired older children
5. Preference for classic squatting position—decreases venous return from lower extremities and increases pulmonary blood flow and systemic arterial oxygenation during spells or after exercise; rarely seen now owing to earlier repair of the defect
6. Anemia (if severe hypoxia and polycythemia are present)—contributes to worsening of symptoms
7. Decreased exercise tolerance
8. Murmur (systolic ejection murmur at upper left sternal border)
9. May have a palpable thrill

COMPLICATIONS

1. Severe hypoxia
2. Arrhythmias
3. Hypercyanotic spells
4. Bacterial endocarditis
5. Residual pulmonic stenosis
6. Pulmonic insufficiency

Postoperative complications

1. Bleeding—especially prominent in children with polycythemia
2. Arrhythmias
3. Low cardiac output or heart failure

4. Pleural effusion (surgical complication related to multiple cardiac procedures)
5. Phrenic nerve damage (surgical complication related to multiple cardiac procedures)
6. Cerebral embolism or thrombosis—risk greater with polycythemia, anemia, or sepsis
7. Complications specific to Blalock-Taussig shunts: congestive heart failure (CHF) if the shunt is too large, persistent cyanosis if the shunt is too small; shunt occlusion

LABORATORY AND DIAGNOSTIC TESTS

1. Chest radiograph—indicates increase or decrease in pulmonary flow, size of heart, and borders
2. Electrocardiogram (ECG)—to monitor right ventricular hypertrophy due to the pressure overload of the right ventricle; may also find left ventricular hypertrophy in patients with increased pulmonary blood flow due to collaterals or large shunts
3. Oxygen saturation by pulse oximetry—to monitor cyanosis as a clinical indication of the degree of pulmonic stenosis
4. Hematocrit or hemoglobin level—to monitor oxygen-carrying capacity and viscosity of blood, and for the development of iron deficiency anemia
5. Echocardiogram—to evaluate anatomy, pressure gradient across the obstruction
6. Cardiac catheterization; most patients with TOF do not require cardiac catheterization unless there is concern regarding the pulmonary artery anatomy

Preoperative

Refer to Appendix D for normal values and ranges of laboratory and diagnostic tests.

a. Complete blood count: sodium, potassium, chloride, carbon dioxide—to establish a baseline hemoglobin, hematocrit, white blood cell count, and platelet count and to rule out infectious illness
b. Baseline electrolytes and renal function panel: urinalysis, blood urea nitrogen level—to evaluate renal function and metabolic status

c. Liver function test—to evaluate baseline liver function
d. Blood coagulation studies: prothrombin time, partial thromboplastin time, platelet count—to establish baseline as well as rule out any previously unknown coagulopathies
e. Type and cross-match—to have blood products available perioperatively
f. Chest radiograph and ECG—to provide baseline data, assess for cardiac enlargement and/or chamber hypertrophy, and assess lung fields
g. Serum glucose level—to determine base data

MEDICAL AND SURGICAL MANAGEMENT

Several medications may be used to medically manage TOF. The specific medication or combination of medications used depends on the child's phsyiology. Propranolol (Inderal) is a beta-blocker that may be used to prevent or treat hypercyanotic spells and to treat arrhythmias. Diuretics, such as furosemide, may be used to promote diuresis. Though most children with TOF do not develop CHF because the pulmonic stenosis limits pulmonary blood flow, diuretics may be particularly useful in children with large ventricular septal defects and minimal pulmonic stenosis. In these same children, digitalis may be prescribed to improve cardiac performance by improving contractility and decreasing venous pressures. Further, digitalis slows conduction through the atrioventricular node and can therefore be used to treat selected cardiac arrhythmias (rarely given before correction unless shunt is too large).

Hypercyanotic spells are a medical emergency. A child experiencing a hypercyanotic spell should be placed in a knee-chest position and be given 100% oxygen by face mask. The knee-chest position improves venous return to the heart and therefore improves pulmonary blood flow. Oxygen is a potent pulmonary vasodilator and will also improve pulmonary blood flow. There are several medications that may also be helpful. Morphine is a sedative that decreases irritability, suppresses the respiratory center, and abolishes hyperpnea. Children with hypercyanotic spells quickly become acidotic. Therefore sodium bicarbonate, a potent systemic alkalizer, may be used to treat acidosis.

Definitive Surgical Repair

Historically, complete repair of TOF was postponed until the preschool years. Advances in surgical technique and medical management now allow for earlier repair. Single-stage repair is performed in most centers before the age of 6 months while the pulmonary artery dimensions are favorable. There are numerous benefits to earlier repair, including normal growth and development of organs, elimination of cyanosis at an earlier age, decreased incidence of late arrhythmias, and better late ventricular function. Repair requires cardiopulmonary bypass and is accomplished through a median sternotomy incision. Deep hypothermia may be used for some infants. If a previous shunt is in place, it is removed. Ideally, the surgeon will repair the defect through a right atrial incision. A right ventriculotomy is avoided when possible because of the potential for impaired ventricular function. The right ventricular outflow obstruction is resected and widened, using Dacron with pericardial backing. Care is taken to avoid pulmonary insufficiency. In cases of severe right ventricular outflow tract obstruction, a conduit may be inserted. The ventricular septal defect is closed with a Dacron patch to complete the operation.

Palliative Surgical Procedures

Owing to the preference for earlier complete repair, the need for palliative procedures is diminishing. Historically, a Blalock-Taussig (BT) shunt was placed to increase the pulmonary blood flow until complete repair could be performed. A classic BT shunt is created when the subclavian artery opposite the side of the aortic arch is ligated, divided, and anastomosed to the contralateral pulmonary artery. The advantages of this shunt procedure are the ability to construct very small shunts that grow with the child and the ease of shunt removal during definitive repair. Collateral circulation will develop to ensure adequate arterial flow to the arm, although a blood pressure reading will not be obtainable in that arm.

More commonly used is the modified Blalock-Taussig shunt, which is essentially the same but uses a prosthetic material to connect the pulmonary artery to the subclavian artery. With the modified BT shunt, the size can be better controlled, which is critical in preventing CHF while providing adequate pulmonary blood flow. The modified BT shunt allows for placement despite aortic arch anomalies; however, a right-sided shunt is most often performed to ensure ease of removal at the time of complete repair. The removal of either the classic or the modified BT shunt is generally uncomplicated.

Both the classic and the modified BT shunts increase pulmonary blood flow by providing a means for systemic blood to enter the pulmonary circulation through the subclavian artery. This increases pulmonary blood flow under low pressure and avoids pulmonary congestion. This stabilizes pulmonary blood flow and improves cardiac and respiratory status until conditions are more favorable for complete repair.

NURSING ASSESSMENT

1. See the Cardiovascular Assessment section in Appendix A.
2. Assess child's level of activity and achieving of developmental milestones (preoperatively) (see Appendix B).
3. Assess for changes in cardiopulmonary status (specific attention to the development of hypercyanotic spells).
4. Important additional postoperative assessments include assessment for complications in addition to those previously mentioned: bleeding, CHF, arrhythmias, pulmonary insufficiency, low cardiac output, pulmonary hypertension, pleural effusion, electrolyte imbalances, fluid overload, hepatomegaly, and neurologic complications.
5. Assess for postoperative pain (see Appendix I).

NURSING DIAGNOSES

- Cardiac output, Decreased
- Tissue perfusion, Ineffective
- Pain, Acute
- Fluid volume, Excess
- Fluid volume, Risk for deficient
- Infection, Risk for

- Injury, Risk for
- Fear
- Anxiety
- Family processes, Interrupted
- Coping, Ineffective
- Nutrition: less than body requirements, Imbalanced
- Activity intolerance
- Growth and development, Risk for delayed
- Therapeutic regimen management, Ineffective

NURSING INTERVENTIONS
Maintenance Care

1. Monitor for changes in cardiopulmonary status as described in the Nursing Assessment section in this chapter.
2. Monitor and maintain hydration status.
   a. Daily weight, intake and output, urine specific gravity
   b. Signs of dehydration (pallor, sunken fontanelles, decreased urine output, dry mucous membranes)
3. Monitor child's response to medications (see the Medical Management section in this chapter).
   a. Antibiotics—administered before, during, and after surgery as prophylaxis against subacute bacterial endocarditis and other perioperative infections
   b. Diuretics (furosemide)—monitor for signs of excessive diuresis, such as urine output greater than expected for weight or more than eight wet diapers daily in an infant
   c. Digitalis—monitor heart rate for signs of toxicity— (anorexia, nausea, vomiting, diarrhea, restlessness, fatigue, prolonged PR interval, profound sinus bradycardia, and serum digoxin level >2 ng/mL)
4. Provide foods high in iron (to prevent iron deficiency anemia) and protein (to promote healing).
   a. Iron-fortified formula and/or cereal for infants, cereals, egg yolk, and meat for older children
   b. Administer supplemental iron with orange juice if possible to increase absorption
5. Protect child from potentially infectious contacts and promote preventive practices (to prevent subacute bacterial endocarditis).

    a. Screen visitors for infections.
    b. Instruct child and family about good dental care.
       i. Brushing and flossing of teeth
      ii. Frequent dental checkups for detection of caries and gingival infections
     iii. Importance of antibiotic prophylaxis for dental work
    c. Provide close surveillance for and timely reporting of fever.
    d. Administer antibiotic prophylaxis for some invasive medical procedures such as dental extractions or fillings, as ordered.
6. Monitor for signs of complications and child's response to treatment regimen.
    a. Hypercyanotic spells
    b. Arrhythymias
    c. Anemia or polycythemia
7. Monitor growth and development to ensure timely achievement of developmental milestones.

Preoperative Care

1. Prepare child for surgery by obtaining assessment data. See Laboratory and Diagnostic Tests in this chapter for details of what tests are needed and why.
2. Use age-appropriate explanations for preparation of child and family (see the Preparation for Procedures or Surgery section in Appendix F).
3. Do not take blood pressure readings or make arterial punctures in potential shunt arm.

Postoperative Care

TOF corrective surgery—monitor child's clinical status for postoperative complications.

1. Monitor child's cardiac function frequently per institutional policy.
    a. Vital signs, including rectal temperature
    b. Color
    c. Peripheral pulses and capillary refill time
    d. Arterial blood pressure and central venous pressure
    e. Hepatomegaly

    f. Periorbital edema
    g. Pleural effusion
    h. Pulsus paradoxus
    i. Heart sounds
    j. Ascites (rare)
2. Arrhythmias
    a. Right bundle branch block caused by right ventriculotomy or ventricular septal defect repair
    b. Complete heart block
    c. Supraventricular arrhythmia
    d. Ventricular tachycardia
3. CHF or ventricular dysfunction (more likely if ventricular incision is required)
4. Hemorrhage
    a. Assess child's chest tube output frequently per institutional policy.
    b. Assess for bleeding from other sites.
    c. Maintain strict intake and output.
    d. Assess for ecchymotic lesions and petechiae.
5. Low cardiac output as evidenced by irritability, fatigue, poor feeding, change in neurologic responsiveness, tachycardia, auscultation of a gallop, diaphoresis, oliguria, pallor, peripheral cyanosis, and decreased capillary refill
6. Neurologic complications (refer to section in this chapter on Complications)
7. Pulmonary insufficiency as evidenced by rales, wheezing, increased respiratory effort, use of accessory muscles for respiratory effort, and cyanosis
8. Residual ventricular septal defect as evidenced by ongoing failure and echographic findings
9. Monitor child's response to medications.
    a. Inotropic support may be required such as dopamine, or milrinone.
    b. Digitalis and diuretics may be needed for several weeks to months after surgery to control CHF.
10. Monitor and maintain child's fluid and electrolyte balance.
    a. Infuse intravenous fluids per institutional policy.
    b. Assess for signs and symptoms of dehydration (decreased skin turgor, dry mucous membranes, soft or sunken

fontanelle, irritability, reduction or absence of tears, decreased urine output, and increased capillary refill).
11. Monitor and maintain child's respiratory status.
    a. Perform chest physiotherapy
    b. Place child in semi-Fowler position
    c. Humidify air
12. Monitor for chylothorax as evidenced by persistent pleural effusions.
13. Provide for child's and family's emotional needs (see the Supportive Care section in Appendix F).
14. Monitor and alleviate child's pain (see Appendix I).
15. Provide developmentally appropriate stimulation and/or activities (see Appendix B).

Surgical Palliation
1. Assess child's clinical status.
    a. Immediately after surgery, expect arm with involved subclavian artery to be cool and without blood pressure (BT anastomosis).
2. Note pulse pressure since a wide pulse pressure may indicate a large shunt.
    a. Note quality of pulses, since bounding pulses may indicate a large shunt.
    b. Note cyanosis, hypoxemia, or signs of acidosis, since they may indicate early occlusion of shunt.
3. Monitor child for any postoperative complications.
    a. Bleeding as evidenced by decreased or unstable blood pressure, tachycardia, increased chest tube output, decreased O_2 saturation, and decreased hematocrit
    b. CHF if shunt is too large or pulmonary hypertension is present
    c. Increased pulmonary blood flow and pulmonary hypertension
4. Monitor child's response to administered medications—digitalis and diuretics are administered if needed.
5. Monitor and maintain fluid and electrolyte balance.
    a. Monitor intake and output and daily weights.
    b. Administer fluids per institutional policy.

6. Promote and maintain optimal respiratory status.
   a. Perform percussion and postural drainage every 2 to 4 hours.
   b. Use suction as needed.
   c. Use spirometer, if developmentally appropriate, every 1 to 2 hours for 24 hours, then every 4 hours.
   d. Monitor chest tube output frequently.
7. Monitor and alleviate child's pain (see Appendix I).

🏠 Discharge Planning and Home Care

1. Instruct parents or caregivers on home care treatment regimen.
   a. Administer appropriate wound care.
   b. Observe for signs and symptoms of infection.
   c. Give instructions regarding exercise limitations for first 6 weeks following surgery to allow time for sternum to completely heal.
   d. Avoid stress to the sternum by supporting the child's head and shoulders with one arm and the lower body with the other.
   e. Give information regarding administration of medications and monitoring child's response to them.
   f. Instruct parents in cardiopulmonary resuscitation (CPR).
   g. Instruct parents on the importance of well-child care and routine immunizations.
   h. Instruct parents on monitoring developmental status and providing age-appropriate opportunities for social and recreational activities.
   i. Advise parents that antibiotic prophylaxis is required for dental work and surgery.
   j. Instruct parents on child-rearing practices for child recovering from surgery for TOF.
      i. Need to maintain usual expectations for behavior and misbehavior
      ii. Continuance of disciplinary measures
      iii. Methods and strategies to assist child in living normally and dealing with concerns

CLIENT OUTCOMES

1. Child's vital signs will be within normal limits for age.
2. Child will participate in physical activities appropriate for age.
3. Child will be free of postoperative complications.

REFERENCES

Allen H et al: *Moss & Adams' heart disease in infant's, children, and adolescents,* Philadelphia, 2001, Lippincott, Williams & Wilkins.

Callow L, Suddaby E: Cardiovascular system. In: Slota M, editor: *Core curriculum for pediatric critical care nursing,* St. Louis, 2006, Saunders.

Jonas R: *Comprehensive surgical management of congenital heart disease,* New York, 2004, Oxford University Press.

Koenig P, Hijazi ZM, Zimmerman F: *Essential pediatric cardiology,* New York, 2004, McGraw-Hill.

Mavroudis C, Backer C: *Pediatric cardiac surgery,* St. Louis, 2003, Mosby.

Park M: *The pediatric cardiology handbook,* St. Louis, 1997, Mosby.

Park M: *Pediatric cardiology for practitioners,* St. Louis, 2002, Mosby.

Pye S, Green A: Caring for your baby after heart surgery, *Adv Neonat Care* 3(3):157, 2003.

Pye S, Green A: Parent education after newborn congenital heart surgery, *Adv Neonat Care* 3(3):147, 2003.

Spilman L, Furdon S: Recognition, understanding, and current management of cardiac lesions with decreased pulmonary blood flow, *Neonat Network* 17(4):7, 1998.

78

❖

Transplantation:
Hematopoietic Stem Cell

PATHOPHYSIOLOGY

Hematopoietic stem cell transplantation (HSCT), formerly known as bone marrow transplantation, is performed for the treatment of malignancies (leukemia, lymphoma, and solid tumors), bone marrow dysfunction and failure, immunodeficiencies, and congenital metabolic disorders (Box 78-1). The bone marrow, where all blood cells originate, is involved in a number of functions: (1) transportation of oxygen throughout the body by the erythrocytes; (2) infection protection by granulocytes, lymphocytes, and monocytes; and (3) control and prevention of bleeding by platelets. The goal of HSCT is to restore bone marrow and its hematologic, and immune functions, and to reverse immune dysfunction or failure. HSCT also is used to treat and prevent further progression of genetic diseases by replacing the enzyme-deficient cells with genetically normal bone marrow and subsequently normal blood cells.

In HSCT, donor stem cells are removed, which is termed harvesting, and then transplanted into the recipient. Once the stem cells are infused into the recipient on the day of transplant, they migrate to the marrow's spaces and eventually begin to produce new cells. Additional information on the process of transplantation is provided in the Medical Management section of this chapter.

Stem cells harvested from and transplanted back into the recipient are termed autologous; those collected from someone other than the recipient are termed allogeneic and may be

BOX 78-1

Conditions Treated with Hematopoietic Stem Cell Transplantation

Malignancies: Leukemias, Lymphomas, and Solid Tumors

- Acute lymphocytic leukemia (ALL)
- Acute myelogenous leukemia (AML)
- Brain tumors
- Burkitt's lymphoma
- Chronic myelogenous leukemia
- Ewing's sarcoma
- Germ cell tumor
- Histiocytosis
- Hodgkin's disease
- Juvenile chronic myelogenous leukemia
- Myelodysplastic syndrome
- Neuroblastoma
- Non-Hodgkin's lymphoma
- Primitive neuroectodermal tumor
- Retinoblastoma
- Rhabdomyosarcoma
- Wilms' tumor

Bone Marrow Dysfunction or Failure

- Blackfan-Diamond anemia
- Chronic granulomatous disease
- Congenital neutropenia
- Fanconi's anemia
- Immune dysfunction
- Infantile agranulocytosis
- Leukocyte adhesion defects
- Osteopetrosis
- Severe aplastic anemia
- Severe combined immunodeficiency syndrome
- Sickle cell disease
- Thalassemia

Immunodeficiencies

- Chédiak-Higashi syndrome
- Glanzmann's thrombasthenia
- Wiskott-Aldrich syndrome
- Chronic mucocutaneous candidiasis
- Kostmann's agranulocytosis

BOX 78-1

Conditions Treated with Hematopoietic Stem Cell Transplantation—cont'd

Congenital Metabolic Disorders
- Adrenoleukodystrophy
- Hunter's syndrome
- Hurler's syndrome
- Lesch-Nyhan syndrome
- Maroteaux-Lamy syndrome
- Metachromatic leukodystrophy
- Mucopolysaccharoidosis

matched related (from a sibling), syngeneic (from a twin sibling), matched unrelated (from a donor pool), or mismatched. Stem cells can be collected from bone marrow, peripheral blood, or the placenta and umbilical cord blood obtained after birth. Cord blood stem cells show neonatal naiveté and have less risk of viral transmission and graft versus host disease (GVHD) when compared to other sources of stem cells. Rate of engraftment following transplantation for all types of stem cells is dependent on a number of factors such as cell dose, the conditioning regimen, the recipient's disease, and post-transplant infection. Peripheral blood stem cells engraft faster and are associated with a decreased risk of tumor contamination when compared to autologous bone marrow.

INCIDENCE

1. Survival rates following transplantation are 60% to 90%.
2. Of children under the age of 10 years, 10% develop GVHD between the second and tenth week after HSCT.
3. Among older children, 30% to 60% develop GVHD.
4. More than 70% of children lack a human lymphocyte antigen (HLA)–matched sibling.
5. Children transplanted early in their disease for chronic myelogenous leukemia have disease-free survival rates between 70% and 86%.

6. Survival rates for individuals with acute leukemia following transplantation are 30% to 60%.
7. HSCT remains the most successful treatment for children with acute myelogenous leukemia (AML) in second remission; disease-free survival is 40% in allogeneic HSCT, and 35% for autologous.
8. Patients with AML or acute lymphocytic leukemia (ALL) who receive HSCT while in remission have relapse rates of 5% to 30%. Those who receive an HSCT during a more advanced stage of disease have relapse rates of 40% to 80%.

CLINICAL MANIFESTATIONS

Clinical manifestations experienced by children during the transplant process are commonly related to the toxicities of the preparative regimen (chemotherapy with or without radiation), infection, and the occurrence of GVHD in the posttransplant period:

1. Impaired skin integrity
   a. Maculopapular rash beginning on soles, palms, and ears, and spreading throughout body; blister formation and desquamation in severe cases of acute GVHD; dryness, pigmentation changes, and hardening of the skin, as seen in autoimmune diseases such as scleroderma, are associated with chronic GVHD.
   b. Pruritus
   c. Stomatitis and esophagitis
   d. Perianal redness, abscesses, fissures
   e. Hair loss
2. Respiratory infections, pulmonary edema
   a. Tachypnea
   b. Rales, rhonchi, wheezing
   c. Retractions
3. Hepatomegaly, venoocclusive disease, ascites
   a. Right upper quadrant pain
   b. Jaundice
   c. Weight gain
   d. Bleeding

4. Encephalopathy
   a. Changes in vital signs
   b. Alteration in level of consciousness
5. Renal insufficiency (increased or decreased fluid volume)
   a. Signs of fluid overload: input greater than output, weight gain, hypertension, edema, rales, and rhonchi
   b. Signs of dehydration and electrolyte imbalance: output greater than input, poor skin turgor, lethargy, leg cramps, twitching
6. Gastrointestinal effects
   a. Nausea, vomiting, anorexia
   b. Abdominal cramping, diarrhea
   c. Symptoms of dehydration
   d. Weight loss
7. Musculoskeletal changes
   a. Muscle weakness and/or atrophy
   b. Contractures
   c. Limping, inability to bear weight
8. Thrombocytopenia
   a. Bleeding from gums, mouth, nose
   b. Hematuria
   c. Bruising, petechiae
9. Anemia
   a. Pallor (especially of mucous membranes, conjunctiva, or palmar creases)
   b. Tachycardia
   c. Dizziness, syncope
   d. Headaches
   e. Dyspnea
10. Pain

COMPLICATIONS

1. Bone marrow suppression: Approximately 7 to 10 days following the preparative regimen, all cell lines will be eradicated, causing profound neutopenia, anemia, and thrombocytopenia. During this very vulnerable period, children are at risk for (a) infection (due to immunosuppression and low or absent bacteria fighting ability); (b) adverse effects of anemia such as lethargy, dizziness,

headaches, and pallor; and (c) bleeding due to low platelet count and reduced clotting ability. Supportive care to minimize the risks of these complications until engraftment includes (a) the administration of colony-stimulating factors (G-CSF, GM-CSF) starting immediately after transplant to stimulate recovery of neutrophil count and engraftment; (b) administration of packed red blood cells and platelets to correct anemia; and (c) thrombocytopenia and/or bleeding.

2. Infection: Infection is a leading cause of morbidity and mortality among children undergoing HSCT. They are at increased risk for bacterial, viral, and fungal infections owing to their immunocompromised state. In the first 30 days posttransplant, the most common infections are gram-negative bacteremia and herpes simplex infections; from 30 to 100 days, children are at most risk for fungal infections such as *Aspergillus* and *Candida*, cytomegalovirus, and *Pneumocystis jiroveci;* following the 100-day phase and up to 1 year after HSCT, the most prevalent infections are viral infections including varicella zoster (shingles) and herpes infections. Prophylactic antiviral therapy to prevent reactivation of viruses is an essential part of the supportive care plan. Aggressive and appropriate antibiotic therapy is instituted with the onset of fevers, and early addition of antifungal therapy for unresolved fever in a posttransplant patient receiving antibiotic therapy is recommended to decrease the mortality rate due to sepsis. Common indicators of infection include fever, change in vital signs from baseline, diaphoresis, irritability, pain and/or erythema at affected site, behavioral changes, pain on urination, cough, and new onset of drainage from any site.

3. GVHD: This is one of the most serious complications of allogeneic HSCT. GVHD occurs when transplanted T lymphocytes from the donor's bone marrow react against the immunocompromised host tissues. GVHD is classified as acute if it develops in the first 100 days following a stem cell transplant. Chronic GVHD may occur following the acute phase and up to 1 year after the transplantation. Severity of manifestations vary once vital organs are involved, and death can occur. Signs and symptoms of acute

GVHD appear in the following order from the mildest (stage 1) to the most severe (stage 4) (Table 78-1):

a. A maculopapular rash on the palms of the hands and soles of the feet, which may spread over the entire body. The rash may progress to the formation of blisters, bullae, or desquamation and skin sloughing.

b. Chronic skin GVHD includes dryness, pigmentation changes, and hardening of the skin, as seen in autoimmune diseases such as scleroderma.

c. Gastrointestinal symptoms range from mild indigestion, nausea, anorexia, abdominal pain, and watery diarrhea containing gut tissue with life-threatening complications of intestinal ileus, bleeding, and perforation.

TABLE 78-1
GVHD Staging

Stage	Skin	Liver	Gut
1	Rash on <25% of skin	Bilirubin 2.0–3.0 mg/dl	Diarrhea <500 ml/day (280 ml/m^2 in children) or persistent nausea
2	Rash on 25% to 50% of skin	Bilirubin 3.1–6.0 mg/dl	Diarrhea >1000 ml/day (>555 ml/m^2 in children)
3	Rash on >50% of skin	Bilirubin 6.1 > 15.0 mg/dl	Diarrhea >1500 ml/day (>833 ml/m^2 in children)
4	Generalized erythroderma with bullous formation	Bilirubin >15.0 mg/dl	Severe abdominal pain with/without ileus

GVHD, Graft versus host disease.

   d. Hepatic GVHD causing liver dysfunction can occur, resulting in right upper quadrant pain, ascites, and jaundice. Liver enzymes become elevated including serum bilirubin, alkaline phosphatase, serum transaminases, and gamma glutamyl transferase (GGT).

   Acute GVHD is staged by the degree of organ involvement (skin, gut, and liver), and these stages are summed into an overall grade (Table 78-2). This system is used by health care providers as a universal measurement of GVHD for diagnosis, management, and evaluation of treatment for this disease.

4. Gastrointestinal: Stomatitis and esophagitis secondary to chemotherapy and radiation appears with oral lesions and mucosal breakdown, dysphagia, and sloughing of the mucosal lining of the gut. This occurs immediately after transplant following chemotherapy and usually resolves with engraftment, with a recovering white blood cell count at 2 to 3 weeks after transplant. Changes in taste or sensation and dry mouth (hyposalivation) are all side effects of the preparative regimen. Antibacterial mouthwashes, topical analgesia, and systemic pain medications are essential to support the patient with these symptoms. Anorexia, nausea, and vomiting are common during the high-dose emetogenic chemotherapy. Antinausea medications are often given continuously or at scheduled intervals. Patients require enteral feeding

TABLE 78-2
GVHD Grading System

Grade	Skin	Liver	Gut
0	None	None	None
I	Stages 1 to 2, and	None, and	None
II	Stage 3, and/or	Stage 1, and/or	Stage 1
III	None—stage 3 with	Stages 2 to 3, or	Stages 2 to 4
IV	Stage 4, or	Stage 4	

GVHD, Graft versus host disease.

or total parenteral feeding to provide nutrition during this period of mucositis to promote healing and maintain caloric intake. Diarrhea can occur also as a result of chemotherapy but also may be due to GVHD or infection.

5. Dental: Dental caries, enamel changes, and poor root development are common in patients after HSCT, especially if they received total body irradiation (TBI) or radiation to the mandible or head. Dental follow-up and care is an essential part of posttransplant care. Also, all patients must have a complete dental evaluation before HSCT to rule out any caries or infection, since this can be a source of abscess or infection, in the transplant phase.

6. Pulmonary: Pulmonary edema due to capillary leak syndrome may be experienced in the first 2 weeks after transplant. Cytomegalovirus (CMV) pneumonitis occurs because of reactivation of CMV approximately 2 to 4 months after HSCT. These patients experience low-grade fever, tachypnea, cough, and increased oxygen requirements owing to interstitial lung disease.

7. Renal insufficiency: Acute renal failure may develop as a result of damage to the epithelial cells of the lining of the renal tubules. This can be due to chemotherapy used in preparative regimen, antimicrobial use, and immunosuppressive medications. Blood chemistries including blood urea nitrogen (BUN) and creatinine are monitored carefully, and medications are renal-dosed to reduce the risk of further renal damage.

8. Genitourinary: Hemorrhagic cystitis sometimes develops in the posttransplant period. This may occur if cyclophosphamide or ifosfamide are used as preparative chemotherapy because, when excreted, these drugs irritate the bladder wall and cause bleeding. Viruses such as BK virus and adenovirus also can cause a similar picture. These patients require vigorous hydration to flush the bladder wall. Mesna may be given in cases of chemotherapy-related cystitis. Analgesia and antispasmodic medications are given to relieve the symptoms. If hematuria is severe, bladder irrigation may be needed. These symptoms can occur within 24 hours

after transplant and continue for up to 2 months. Platelet transfusions are administered more frequently when there is evidence of bleeding.

9. Relapse: Relapse of the primary malignancy after HSCT is associated with poor prognosis, and limited treatment options remain available. Relapse is more common in patients with aggressive disease.

10. Endocrine dysfunction: Thyroid dysfunction can occur in patients who have received TBI. Patients show an increase in thyroid-stimulating hormone (TSH) and a decrease in thyroid hormone (T_4), requiring thyroid replacement therapy. Growth and development delays are common in the growing child who receives TBI or steroid therapy, or who suffers from GVHD. Careful monitoring of growth patterns with each visit is essential, and early intervention with growth hormone replacement is essential to promote optimal development and prevent early closure of growth plates. Impaired fertility is a risk related to specific chemotherapy agents received in HSCT. Prepubertal patients are affected less than those treated during or after puberty, and girls are usually less affected than boys.

11. Secondary malignancies: Risk factors for the development of secondary tumors include preoperative combination chemotherapy, TBI, viral infections, chronic GVHD, and genetic cancer predisposition. The most common secondary malignancies are leukemia and lymphoma.

12. Posttransplant lymphoproliferative disease (PTLD) occurs in approximately 1% of posttransplant patients owing to Epstein-Barr virus (EBV) causing a lymphoma in an immunocompromised host. Children or adolescents with normal immune systems may have EBV but have immunity to keep it under control. Prognosis to date for PTLD has been very poor; however, emerging therapies such as alpha interferon and rituximab (monoclonal antibodies) and modifications to immunosuppression are making an impact on this disease.

LABORATORY AND DIAGNOSTIC TESTS

Refer to Appendix D for normal values and ranges of laboratory and diagnostic tests.

1. HLA typing—to identify compatibility of potential donors
2. Mixed lymphocyte culture analyses—to determine histoincompatibility between HLAs of potential donor and recipient
3. Microlymphocytotoxicity test—to identify HLAs
4. Type and cross-match—to determine if the donor is ABO-compatible with the recipient
5. Complete blood count, differential, and platelet count—to assess for adequate blood cell counts before harvesting
6. Chemistry panel, levels of electrolytes, creatinine, magnesium—to monitor renal function and to assess for any electrolyte imbalances
7. Liver function tests, hepatitis screen (A, B, C and E)—to assess liver function
8. Coagulation tests—to determine clotting ability and risk for bleeding
9. Immunoglobulins: IgG, IgA, IgM, and IgE—to assess immune functioning
10. Viral testing: cytomegalovirus, herpes simplex virus, varicella-zoster virus, Epstein-Barr virus, human immunodeficiency virus, toxoplasmosis—to determine presence of viral infection
11. Urinalysis and culture—to determine presence of infection or bleeding
12. Endocrine function testing—to assess for post-HSCT endocrine dysfunction
13. Pregnancy test for all adolescent females before preconditioning therapy
14. CT chest, abdomen, pelvis, and sinuses, chest x-ray—to rule out infection
15. Cardiac evaluation: electrocardiogram, echocardiogram, multiple-gated acquisition—to assess cardiac function before HSCT and to provide baseline to monitor for post-HSCT complications
16. Pulmonary function tests—to assess for post-HSCT pulmonary complications
17. Glomerular filtration rate, renogram—to determine the presence of renal insufficiency before and after HSCT

18. Disease staging: X-ray, computed tomography (CT), magnetic resonance imaging (MRI), bone scan, surgical biopsy, lumbar puncture, or bone marrow evaluation dependent on disease—to determine the extent of the disease

19. Neuropsychologic or developmental evaluation—to determine HSCT effects upon neuropsychologic and developmental functioning

20. Interdisciplinary evaluations—to assess and determine the need for ancillary services such as audiology, dentistry, nutrition, ophthalmology, occupational therapy, physical therapy, child life services, social work, and pastoral care

21. Counseling regarding sperm banking and egg donation should be included in all pretransplant evaluations.

MEDICAL MANAGEMENT

There are three types of hematopoietic stem cell transplants: autologous, allogeneic, and syngeneic. Autologous transplantation (auto-HSCT) uses the child's own bone marrow and is performed for treatment of malignant diseases. Auto-HSCT is used as a form of consolidation therapy when an initial remission is achieved, when there is progressive disease, or when a patient's relapse is showing poor response to conventional therapy. In these patients, transplantation is used as "rescue therapy" so that higher bone marrow–ablative doses of chemotherapy may be administered in an effort to cure the disease. Allogeneic transplantation (allo-HSCT), the most frequent type of HSCT, uses bone marrow from someone other than the child. The donor of choice is first a sibling, followed by a matched unrelated donor (obtained through a national registry). Alternative donor matching options include mismatched related donors (including haplotype parent donors), and matched or mismatched unrelated donors. Syngeneic HSCT is used when stem cells are used from an identical twin. The chances of a sibling match are about 35%; parents and relatives have only a remote chance of being matches, so increasing numbers of children with no matched siblings are transplanted from a closely matched unrelated donor located through the national bone marrow and cord blood stem cell transplantation registries.

Critical to ensuring appropriate matching between donor and recipient is HLA typing. HLA matching is important to minimize the complication of GVHD. Rejection risk increases as the incompatibility between the donor and recipient increases. A majority of transplants are allogeneic, but methods to decrease graft rejection and GVHD have improved. HLAs are protein antigens on the surface of cells that are used for immune recognition. The HLA system is responsible for recognizing foreign tissues and activating an immune response. There are approximately 100 HLA antigens. The most important HLAs for matching tissue for HSCT are HLA-A, HLA-B, HLA-DR, and HLA-DQ antigens. The three most important genes to match for compatibility as a predictor of GVHD are HLA-A, HLA-B, and HLA-DR. HLAs may be typed by a blood test or buccal swabs.

Before the transplantation, a conditioning (ablative) regimen is followed. Conditioning destroys cancer cells to prevent relapse, suppresses the immune system to prevent rejection of the marrow, and enables engraftment of the infused stem cells to occur in the child's marrow. In autologous transplants, the stem cells may be treated with tumor antibodies to eradicate any residual disease before the stem cells are infused. The conditioning regimen involves high-dose cytotoxic drugs with or without TBI. Common chemotherapeutic agents used in conditioning regimens include cyclophosphamide, busulfan, cytosine arabinoside, melphalan, thiotepa, carmustine, carboplatin, cisplatin, and etoposide. Once the conditioning is completed, the harvested marrow is infused into the child via a central venous access catheter. With auto-HSCT, stem cells are either harvested from the bone marrow of the donor's iliac crest under general anesthesia or collected peripherally via a pheresis process, and frozen several weeks before the HSCT. With allo-HSCT, stem cells are harvested, processed, sometimes manipulated to remove red cells and/or T cells, and infused directly into the recipient within a 48- to 72-hour period. Between 12 and 56 days after the transplantation, engraftment occurs. This is dependent on stem cell dose and source, and the patient's diagnosis, condition, and prior history of therapy. Engraftment is demonstrated by an absolute neutrophil count (ANC) greater than 500 for 3 consecutive days following discontinuation of colony-stimulating factors and a platelet count greater than 20,000/mm^3 for 3 consecutive days without the transfusion of platelets.

The most serious complication of allogeneic HSCT is GVHD (see the Complications section of this chapter). Acute GVHD usually occurs within 30 days of the transplantation (the most critical posttransplantation period). Immunosuppressive agents such as cyclosporine, methotrexate, antithymocyte globulin, steroids, tacrolimus, sirolimus, daclizumab, mycophenolate mofetil (MMF), or azathioprine (Imuran) are used to prevent or treat GVHD and prevent graft rejection. Those who undergo HSCT for leukemia and experience the complications of GVHD (acute or chronic form) have less risk of experiencing relapse of their leukemia. This immune effect is called the graft versus leukemia effect, providing immunity from donor cells against their disease.

NURSING ASSESSMENT

1. Assess psychologic status before and after HSCT.
2. Assess for signs and symptoms of sepsis.
3. Assess for gastrointestinal complications of GVHD.
4. Assess for hepatic complications of GVHD (venoocclusive disease).
5. Assess for renal complications of GVHD.
6. Assess skin and mucous membranes for breakdown, infection, or GVHD.
7. Focus of assessments identified in items 2 through 5 is on monitoring for life-threatening effects.

NURSING DIAGNOSES

- Anxiety
- Skin integrity, Impaired
- Tissue integrity, Impaired
- Infection, Risk for
- Fluid volume, Risk for imbalanced
- Oral mucous membrane, Impaired
- Nausea

- Diarrhea
- Pain
- Fatigue
- Nutrition: less than body requirements, Imbalanced
- Mobility, Impaired physical
- Growth and development, Delayed
- Therapeutic regimen management, Ineffective
- Body image, Disturbed
- Family processes, Interrupted
- Coping, Compromised family
- Social isolation

NURSING INTERVENTIONS

1. Answer parent's questions and reinforce information about research on HSCT, alternative treatments, and transplant centers.
2. Answer child's questions and reinforce information using age-appropriate terminology and explanations (see Appendixes B and F).
3. Provide orientation and reinforce information about HSCT routines, restrictions of personal items, isolation procedures and policies, and average length of hospital stay (see Appendix F).
4. Provide meticulous oral and dental care.
5. Provide meticulous skin care.
6. Monitor for signs and symptoms of infection (refer to Complications section).
7. Monitor hydration status, intake, and output.
8. Monitor side effects and complications of conditioning drug therapies (refer to Complications section).
9. Monitor for signs and symptoms of GVHD (refer to Complications section).
10. Monitor bone marrow infusion and assess for reactions (nausea, vomiting, fever, rigors, hypertension, tachycardia, tachypnea).
11. Assess pain status, and administer pharmacologic and nonpharmacologic therapies (see Appendix I).
12. Ensure adequate nutritional support.

13. Serve as service coordinator and communication liaison regarding treatment and care concerns.
14. Provide psychosocial support to child and family as indicated by psychologic assessment and ongoing needs (see Appendix F).
15. Refer to child and/or family mental health professional as needed for counseling to deal with the challenges of living in social isolation during HSCT process (see Appendix F).
16. Encourage child or youth's expression of feelings using age-appropriate methods (see Appendix F).
17. Ensure continuity with child or youth's lifestyle activities as condition permits (academics, peers, hobbies).
18. Use behavioral techniques (i.e., hypnosis, muscle relaxation, visual imagery) for chemotherapy-related symptoms of anxiety, nausea, and vomiting.

🏠 Discharge Planning and Home Care

At selected HSCT centers, early discharge with intensive clinic follow-up and home care is being implemented. Discharge criteria under these circumstances are the following: child must be afebrile and have an ANC of 500 polymorphonuclear cells/mm^3 for up to 72 hours before discharge.

1. Instruct family and child about disease, long-term treatment, medication administration, symptom recognition, and complications.
2. Coordinate with school personnel. Children with autologous transplants return to school in 3 to 6 months; those with allogeneic transplants, in 9 to 12 months (see Appendix G).
3. Instruct about long-term effects.
   a. Impaired growth and development
   b. Impaired fertility and endocrine dysfunction
   c. Restrictive lung disease and infections
   d. Cataracts
   e. Skin changes (similar to scleroderma)
   f. Musculoskeletal dysfunction
4. Refer child and family to community resources based on individualized needs (mental health services, community support groups) (refer to Appendix G).

CLIENT OUTCOMES

1. Child will experience minimal complications.
2. Child will achieve maximum potential for growth and development.
3. Parents will be competent in care of child.
4. Parents will recognize signs and symptoms of infection, GVHD and toxicities related to the therapy.
5. Child will remain disease-free.

REFERENCES

Alcoser P, Rodgers C: Treatment strategies in childhood cancer, *J Pediatr Nurs* 18(2):103, 2003.

Benjamin DK et al: Infections diagnosed in the first year after pediatric stem cell transplantation, *Pediatr Infect Dis J* 21(3):227, 2002.

Gonzales L et al: Hematopoietic stem cell transplantation, In: Baggot et al, editors: *Nursing care of children and adolescents with cancer,* ed 3, Philadelphia, 2002, WB Saunders.

Guinan, EC, Krance, RA, Lehman LE: Stem cell transplantation in pediatric oncology, In: Pizzo PA, Popock DG, editors. *Principles and practice of pediatric oncology,* ed 5, Philadelphia, 2005, Lippincott, Williams & Wilkins.

Lennard AL, Jackson GH: Stem cell transplantation, *West J Med* 175(1):42, 2001.

Norville R, Monroe R, Forte K: Hematopoietic stem cell transplantation, In: Kline NE, editor: *Essentials of pediatric oncology nursing: A core curriculum,* ed 2, Glenview, IL, 2004, Association of Pediatric Oncology Nurses.

Ringden O et al: Allogeneic hematapoietic stem cell transplantation for inherited disorders: Experience in a single center, *Transplantation* 81(5):718, 2006.

Senior K: Umbilical cord blood transplants as good as bone marrow? *Lancet* 357 (9273):2031, 2001.

79

Transplantation: Organ

PATHOPHYSIOLOGY

Tremendous strides have been made in pediatric transplantation in the last decade. Organ transplantation is an acceptable form of treatment for end-stage organ failure. Advances in immunosuppression, improvements in surgical techniques, and experience in postoperative management have contributed to the improved results. Kidney, liver, and heart transplantations have become routine, and lung and small bowel transplantations are increasing in numbers. Primary diseases that can lead to the need for renal transplantation include acquired diseases such as chronic glomerulonephritis, lupus erythematosus, pyelonephritis, hemolytic-uremic syndrome, and bilateral Wilms' tumor. It is also the treatment for congenital conditions such as polycystic disease, obstructive uropathy, cystinosis, and Alport syndrome. The major indications for liver transplantation include biliary atresia, alpha$_1$-antitrypsin deficiency, tyrosinemia, and posthepatic cirrhosis. Indications for cardiac transplantation include cardiomyopathy, hypoplastic left heart syndrome, and other lethal, complex, congenital heart anomalies.

The major problem associated with transplantation is rejection. Rejection can result from any of a variety of causes: cellular and/or humoral immune response, infection, and noncompliance with treatment regimen. Other causes of graft failure include technical failure, infection, and medication toxicity.

The survival rates have improved significantly in recent years and range from 85% to 95% at 1 year after transplantation. Factors restricting transplantation currently are the limited availability of organs and the need for lifelong immunosuppression. Growth may be delayed, but pubertal development proceeds normally after successful transplantation.

INCIDENCE

1. Occurrence of organ transplantation is 15 to 20 per 1 million population.
2. One-year graft survival rate for kidney transplants is 90% to 95%.
3. One-year graft survival rate for heart transplants is 90%.
4. One-year graft survival rate for liver transplants is 85% to 90%.
5. Survival rates are decreased with subsequent grafts.

CLINICAL MANIFESTATIONS

Refer to chapters dealing with disorders of specific organ.

COMPLICATIONS (POSTTRANSPLANTATION)

1. Hyperacute, acute, or chronic rejection
2. Poor organ function
3. Hypertension
4. Bleeding at transplant site
5. Infection (*Candida,* cytomegalovirus, polyomavirus, other viruses)
6. Medication toxicity
7. Surgical complications
8. Increased risk of cancer

LABORATORY AND DIAGNOSTIC TESTS
Preoperative Evaluation

1. Extensive serologic studies including chemistry panel, complete blood count (CBC) with differential, platelet count, viral screening, blood cultures
2. Meticulous search for infection, including dental examinations, sinus radiography
3. Electrocardiogram, chest radiographic study, echocardiogram, possible cardiac biopsy
4. Urinalysis, urine culture, and sensitivity testing
5. Histocompatibility testing
   a. ABO blood type

b. Antibody screening
c. Human leukocyte antigen (HLA) typing (A, B, C, D, DR)

Postoperative Evaluation

1. Metabolic panel, liver panel, CBC
2. Cyclosporine or tacrolimus levels
3. Biopsy of the transplanted organ (diagnostic for rejection)

MEDICAL MANAGEMENT

Immunosuppression regimens vary by center, but most include a combination of cyclosporine, azathioprine, tacrolimus, mycophenolate mofetil, sirolimus, and corticosteroids to prevent rejection. Rejection is treated with high-dose steroids or polyclonal or monoclonal antibodies. Other medications include nystatin as a prophylactic for *Candida* infection, antihypertensives and diuretics for hypertension and edema, antibiotics, and antacids. The average length of hospital stay following transplantation is 2 weeks. Medications must be taken for life, and close medical follow-up is required.

NURSING ASSESSMENT

1. See the Renal Assessment and Cardiovascular Assessment sections in Appendix A.
2. Assess hydration status.
3. Assess for signs and symptoms of infection.
4. Assess for signs and symptoms of rejection.

NURSING DIAGNOSES

- Infection, Risk for
- Fluid volume, Excess
- Body image, Disturbed
- Fear
- Coping, Ineffective

NURSING INTERVENTIONS
Preoperative Care

Prepare recipient and family for transplantation.
1. Provide information about presurgical routine.

2. Reinforce information given about surgery.
3. Provide age-appropriate preprocedural or preoperative preparation.

Postoperative Care

1. Monitor for and report signs of rejection.
2. Monitor vital signs and report significant changes, because they may be indicators of rejection, bleeding, infection, or hypovolemic shock. Check vital signs every hour for 24 hours; if stable, then check vital signs every 4 hours.
3. Monitor urinary output; report any significant changes.
4. Observe for drainage on dressing.
   a. Circle extent of drainage.
   b. Notify physician if drainage increases significantly.
5. Observe for child's therapeutic response to and untoward effects of medications.
6. Observe for and report signs and symptoms of possible complications.

🏠 Discharge Planning and Home Care

1. Instruct child and family about therapeutic responses and untoward reactions to medications.
2. Reinforce necessity of complying with medical regimen.
3. Reinforce information provided about nutritional needs.
4. Instruct about proper dental care (brushing and flossing).
5. Refer to appropriate community resources, clinics, agencies, or personnel for psychosocial needs.

CLIENT OUTCOMES

1. Child will have normal graft function.
2. Child will remain free of infection.
3. Child and family will understand and remain compliant with medication and follow-up regimens.

REFERENCES

Flavio V: A decade of progress in kidney transplantation, *Transplantation* 77(9): S52, 2004.

Harmon W et al: Trends in immunosuppressive strategies in pediatric transplantation, *Am J Transplant* 3(5):285, 2003.

Harmon W et al: Pediatric transplantation, *Am J Transplant* 5(4 Part 2):887, 2005.

Magee J et al: Pediatric transplantation, *Am J Transplant* 4(Supplement 9):54, 2004.

Saunders R et al: Rapamycin in transplantation: A review of the evidence, *Kidney Int* 59(1):3, 2001.

80

Traumatic Brain Injury

PATHOPHYSIOLOGY

Traumatic brain injury (TBI) is a common injury in children and the most common cause of traumatic death. TBI is often caused by a primary injury, and is followed by a secondary injury. The primary injury is the actual trauma itself, because it occurs at the time of impact on the central nervous system and may cause damage and/or death to the brain cells. A hypoxic insult may also cause a primary injury. The secondary injury is caused by the brain's response to the trauma and evolves over a period of hours to days after the injury. The secondary injury can result in the loss of cerebral autoregulation, development of cerebral edema, and breakdown of the blood-brain barrier. The secondary injury is exacerbated by systemic hypotension or hypertension, ischemia, hypoxia, or hypercapnia.

There are several types of brain injury:

1. Open head injuries are caused by bullets or other penetrating objects, which include but are not restricted to depressed skull fracture(s) with scalp laceration.
2. Closed head injuries are the more common of the two and usually are caused by a rapid movement of the head, during which the brain is forced back and forth within the skullcap. Such injuries are commonly found in motor vehicle crashes, falls, and recreational sports related activities (i.e., football, bicycling).

Brain injuries are also commonly classified in terms of severity (i.e., mild, moderate, severe).

1. Mild brain injury (Glasgow Coma Scale: 13–15) is commonly referred to as a concussion, which may involve a brief

loss of consciousness, loss of memory of events immediately preceding and/or following the injury, alteration in mental status at the time of the injury, and/or neurologic deficits that may or may not be transient. Characteristics most common of mild brain injury include physical, cognitive, and/or behavioral, and are listed below.

2. Moderate brain injury (Glasgow Coma Scale: 8–12) results in a loss of consciousness lasting from minutes to hours, followed by days and/or weeks of confusion. This is usually associated with physical, cognitive, and/or behavioral impairments, which may be transient or permanent.

3. Severe brain injury (Glasgow Coma Scale: <8 for at least 6 hours after injury) always results in prolonged loss of consciousness or coma lasting from days to sometimes months, depending on the severity and location of the injury. Diffuse axonal injury (DAI) is a common finding in severe brain injuries on radiographic investigation. DAI is defined as impaired function and gradual loss of some axons, which are the long extensions of a nerve cell that enable such cells to communicate with each other and integrate global function. Such injuries may leave patients with severe and permanent disabilities involving physical, cognitive, and/or behavioral impairments.

INCIDENCE

1. Males are twice as likes as females to suffer head injuries.
2. Concussions are the most frequent type of TBI.
3. Among children ages 0–14 years, 475,000 TBIs occurred each year between 1995 and 2001 in the United States. Of those, 435,000 children were treated for TBI in the emergency department (ED) each year, 37,000 were hospitalized, and 2685 died.
4. TBI is the leading cause of acquired disability in childhood.
5. Causes of TBI vary with age: very young children ages 0 to 4 years had the highest rate of TBI-related ED visits (1035.0 per 100,000 population).
   a. Infants to 2 years—frequently results from child abuse
   b. Ages 2 to 5 years—frequently results from falls and motor vehicle collisions in which the child was an unrestrained passenger

   c. Ages 5 to 12 years—frequently results from pedestrian
      injuries and falls from bikes, roller blades, all-terrain
      vehicles, skateboards
   d. Ages 15 to 19 years—frequently results from motor vehi-
      cle collision and violent assaults
6. Posttraumatic seizures develop in 7% to 12% of children
   with cerebral contusions.
7. Exposure to guns and access to a loaded firearm increase the
   risk of unintentional brain injury and death in a child. The
   unintentional death rate among children 14 years of age and
   younger is 9 times higher in the United States than in 25
   other industrialized countries combined.

CLINICAL MANIFESTATIONS

1. Bump or bruise on head
2. Headache, dizziness, light-headedness, or loss of balance
3. Bleeding or clear drainage from laceration, nose, or ears
4. Seizures
5. Nausea, vomiting
6. Irritability and agitation, sleep problems, fatigue, anxiety,
   depression, emotional lability
7. Loss of consciousness or cognitive impairment, decreased
   attention span, concentration or mental speed; short-term
   memory loss
8. Focal deficit including impaired motor function of limbs
   such as hemiparesis or hemiplegia
9. Decorticate or decerebrate posturing
10. Battle sign—bruising behind ear
11. Raccoon sign—bruising around eyes
12. Increased sensitivity to lights, sounds, or distractions
13. Loss of sense of smell or taste
14. Ringing in the ears
15. Slowness in thinking, speaking, acting, or reading

COMPLICATIONS

Depending on the type, severity, and location of the head injury,
deficits may be multiple and include motor, communicative,
cognitive, sensory, behavioral, and emotional problems or delay
in reaching developmental milestones not yet achieved. A variety of complications involving the nervous system and other

organ systems may be seen. These complications can occur from either the primary or secondary injury to the brain.

Primary Brain Injury

Traumatic brain injury (TBI) is defined as a physiologic disruption of brain function resulting from both external (an object striking the head or the head striking an object) and/or internal trauma (the rapid acceleration/deceleration of the brain within the skullcap).

Primary injuries include the following:

1. Concussion results from shearing and stretching forces in the brain that produce no structural damage. This is the least serious type of injury that requires close monitoring for complications. With a concussion, the child usually has a momentary loss of consciousness. Recovery generally takes place within 24 hours, with a return to the preinjury level of activity and orientation.

2. Cerebral contusion is localized brain injury that consists of bruising, tearing, bleeding, and swelling of the brain, with temporary or permanent structural damage. This may occur directly under the area of impact or on the opposite side of the brain as it hits the skull. A contusion causes a disruption of cerebral tissue to varying degrees with possible surrounding edema. Signs and symptoms reflect the extent of injury and blood loss and may include loss of consciousness, mild motor and sensory deficits, changes in visual awareness, seizures, or coma.

3. Skull fractures may take the form of a linear skull fracture in which the dura mater is not penetrated and usually does not require surgery for repair; a depressed skull fracture, in which bone fragments are indented and can affect underlying brain tissue and produce a hematoma or contusion; or a compound skull fracture, in which a laceration and depressed fracture are present. The skull fragment may lacerate the dura as it is displaced into the brain tissue.
   A basilar skull fracture is a break in the base of the skull that often results in a dural laceration, which may involve drainage of cerebrospinal fluid through the ear or nose.

4. Hematoma is the accumulation of blood under the skull. An epidural hematoma occurs when there is a blood clot that collects between the skull and the dura mater. This is most common in older children and commonly results from a tear of the middle meningeal artery. Clinically, a loss of consciousness may occur, and thus a hematoma should be excluded by radiographic investigation, if there is a basal or temporal skull fracture. Children with this type of hematoma should be assessed for decreased level of consciousness, development of headache, dilation of the pupil on the affected side, and focal deficit such as hemiparesis or plegia. Surgical evacuation of an epidural hematoma is a common treatment if the child is symptomatic, or if the clot is large enough that there is compression of underlying neural tissue. Recovery from an epidural hematoma is excellent if recognized and treated in an appropriate time frame. Symptoms of a subdural hematoma may be delayed for hours or days since the source of bleeding is venous. A subdural hematoma occurs when blood collects between the dura mater and the brain and is often associated with a contusion. This type of hematoma can become life threatening if it compresses vital centers of the brain or causes cerebral edema. Children with this type of hematoma should be assessed for loss of consciousness, unilateral pupil dilation, focal seizures, and/or hemiparesis. Treatment for symptomatic hematomas, no matter where they are located, is surgical evacuation of the hematoma by a craniotomy procedure. The prognosis for the child with a subdural hematoma is less favorable than that for a child with an epidural hematoma, even after surgical evacuation, owing to the associated damage to the underlying brain tissue.

5. Subarachnoid hemorrhage results from a tear of the subarachnoid arterial vessels resulting from large shearing forces encountered during a severe TBI. It appears as diffuse blood spread thinly over the surface of the brain. This type of hemorrhage is frequently seen in the abused child, as well as resulting from motor vehicle crashes and falls. Children should be assessed for nuchal rigidity,

headache, decreasing levels of consciousness, and retinal hemorrhages.

6. Diffuse axonal injury is frequently seen in children with severe head trauma, such as those with shaken baby syndrome and those who have been involved in a motor vehicle crash. This may result in a generalized global decline of the neurologic exam, affecting mental status, motor function, and brain stem function. This type of injury may result in widespread cerebral edema, neuronal dysfunction, and prolonged coma. The prognosis for this type of injury ranges from moderate disability to death.

Secondary Brain Injury

Secondary brain injury results from the severity of the primary brain injury and may be made worse by hypotension, hypertension, deoxygenation, and ischemia. Consequences of secondary injury include the following:

1. Cerebral edema either is caused by the primary injury or is a result of hypoxia, hypercapnia, or cerebral ischemia. Edema usually peaks in 24 to 72 hours after injury, and often results in a deterioration of neurologic status. Cerebral edema may result in increased intracranial pressure (ICP) and decreased cerebral perfusion pressure (CPP); if adequate intervention is not taken, this may result in irreversible brain dysfunction, herniation, and death, if not treated.

2. Meningitis may result from an infection of the cerebrospinal fluid (CSF). Clinically, the child will develop fever, decreased level of consciousness, nuchal rigidity, and irritability; sampling of the CSF will reveal a pleocytosis of the white blood cells.

LABORATORY AND DIAGNOSTIC TESTS

1. Radiographic study of skull—to identify fractures
2. Computed tomography (CT) scan of brain—to identify hematomas, edema, increased ICP, DAI
3. Magnetic resonance imaging (MRI) of brain—to identify hematomas, edema, increased ICP, DAI
4. Test for presence of glucose in drainage from ears or nose—identification of CSF leak

MEDICAL MANAGEMENT

Management goals are to avoid, prevent, and minimize secondary injury to the brain. As with any severe injury, the first step of treatment is management of the airway, breathing, and circulation. Treatment is then based on the neurologic assessment, which includes use of the pediatric Glasgow Coma Scale (GCS). The GCS rates the child's performance in three major areas: eye opening, motor response, and verbal response. The highest score that can be achieved is 15 (least injured); the lowest is 3 (poorest outcome). Scores of 8 or lower indicate a severe brain injury; scores of 9 to 12 indicate a moderate injury; and scores of 13 to 15 indicate a minor injury.

1. Minor injury (GCS score of 13 through 15) with normal radiologic studies and vital signs. It is recognized that a small percentage of children with normal exams and absence of other findings may still have positive radiographic findings, such as contusion or small epidural or subdural hematoma. It is therefore recommended to perform a head CT scan to exclude this possibility. In the absence of such findings, a child may be discharged to a reliable, knowledgeable parent. Appropriate discharge instructions include the following:
   a. Wake the child every 2 hours to look for changes in mental status.
   b. Return to the emergency department if any of the following occur:
      i. Vomiting
      ii. Sleepiness or weakness
      iii. Headaches
      iv. Confusion
      v. Restlessness
      vi. Personality changes
      vii. Inconsolable irritability
      viii. Seizures
      ix. Clear drainage (rhinorrhea) or blood from nose or ears
2. Moderate injury (GCS score of 9 through 12): child should be admitted for observation even if radiologic studies are normal. Frequent neurologic checks should be performed

and an additional surveillance CT scan obtained if symptoms develop.

3. Severe injury (GCS score of 3 through 8): child should be admitted or transferred to a pediatric intensive care unit. May require surgical evacuation of subdural or epidural hematoma or craniectomy to allow for brain swelling, along with supportive management. ICP monitoring and CSF drainage is generally indicated to monitor and manage cerebral edema. Fluid management, sedation, chemical paralysis, and hyperosmolar therapy are all current modes of head injury management.

In all cases of TBI, the goal of therapy is a return of function. In some cases, function is lost or limited, which results in disability. Factors most predictive of disability(s) in a severe injury include the GCS motor score 3 days after injury, level of oxygenation in the ED, presence of intracranial hematoma, duration of ICP elevation and decreased CPP, and presence and severity of extracranial injuries. Children with a severe injury will require an intensive rehabilitation program designed to promote a return to an optimal level of function. This is best managed in a pediatric inpatient rehabilitation unit, followed by outpatient therapy. In addition to rehabilitation of lost physical function such as impaired motor skills of the upper and lower extremities and language and swallowing abilities, cognitive rehabilitation is also critical to minimize the severity of disability. If a child's development is in progress before the head injury, cognitive impairment as a consequence of head injury may further limit or impair completion of developmental milestones. For children, a return to school is a major goal. For those with a severe TBI, a special individualized education plan (IEP) will have to be developed to continue with the cognitive rehabilitation. Children may also be provided with school-based physical, occupational, and speech-language therapies; services for the hearing and visually impaired; behavior management; and counseling.

NURSING ASSESSMENT

1. Assess airway, breathing, and circulation.
2. See the Neurologic Assessment section in Appendix A.

3. Assess level of consciousness.
4. Assess for signs of increased ICP such as new onset of irritability, nausea, vomiting, or focal deficits.
5. Assess for skin bruising or swelling, rhinorrhea, or ear drainage.
6. Assess cause of injury and identify potential child abuse.
7. Assess for signs of pain and discomfort.

NURSING DIAGNOSES

- Gas exchange, Impaired (if severe)
- Tissue perfusion, Ineffective (brain) (if severe)
- Injury, Risk for
- Pain, Risk for
- Knowledge, Deficient
- Family processes, Impaired
- Caregiver role strain, Risk for

NURSING INTERVENTIONS

1. Ensure that patent airway, breathing, and circulation are present. Maintain adequate oxygenation using pulse oximeter or other oxygen-saturation monitoring device, and suction at bedside.
2. Monitor for, prevent, and intervene in case of increased ICP.
   a. Elevate head of bed 30 degrees to promote venous return and optimize cerebral blood flow.
   b. Monitor for signs of increased ICP.
      i. Increased respiratory rate, decreased heart rate, elevated blood pressure
      ii. Decreased level of consciousness
      iii. Seizure activity
      iv. Vomiting
      v. Alteration in pupil size and reactivity
3. Ensure safe environment, using safety restraints as necessary or chemical sedation.
4. Maximize pain control by identifying agents that will minimize patient's pain source and limit effect on neurologic assessment.
5. Assess for signs and symptoms of disability.
6. Apply ice to areas of soft tissue swelling, lacerations, or other areas of bruising.

7. Administer skin care under cervical collar, if used.
8. Promote team participation within child's care to include physical, occupational, and speech therapy assessments and interventions as necessary.
9. Educate child and parents about causes and prevention of TBI.

🏠 Discharge Planning and Home Care
Preventive Care

Instruct children and family about importance of prevention. Examples include use of helmets in sports in which injury to head is possible following a fall, prevention of pedestrian–motor vehicle or bicycle–motor vehicle accidents, and avoidance of high-risk behaviors in older children. Offer both oral and written instructions, because families can be overwhelmed at discharge.

Long-Term Care

1. Educate patient and family regarding the need for and administration of medications, particularly antiepileptic (AED) medications.
2. Identify need for outpatient physical and occupational therapy, cognitive retraining, expressive and receptive language retraining, oral motor retraining (speech therapy), behavior management, and counseling.
3. Support child and family with the school reentry process.
   a. Development of IEP
   b. Neuropsychologic testing for baseline cognitive performance
   c. Appropriate stimulation; too many competing external stimuli can increase agitation
   d. Gradual reentry back into school with full school faculty involvement in the education process

CLIENT OUTCOMES

1. Child will return to optimal level of neurologic functioning.
2. Child will maintain adequate CPP, and vital signs will be within normal parameters.
3. Family will demonstrate positive coping strategies in situations where disability results from TBI.

REFERENCES

Adelson PD, Bratton SL, Carney NA: Guidelines for the acute medical management of severe traumatic brain injury in infants, children, and adolescents, *Pediatr Crit Care Med* 4(3 Suppl):S72, 2003. Lippincott, Williams & Wilkins.

American Association of Neurological Surgeons: Traumatic brain injury, *What is neurosurgery?* (serial online): www.neurosurgerytoday.org/what/patient_e/head.asp.

Brain Injury Association of America: *Brain injury: The ABC years; Understanding and preventing pediatric brain injury* (website): www.biausa.org. Accessed June 14, 2006.

Centers for Disease Control, National Center for Injury Prevention and Control: *Traumatic brain injury in the United States: Emergency department visits, hospitalizations, and deaths* (website): www.cdcgove/nicpc/pub-res/TBI_in_US_04/TBI_ED.htm). Accessed June 14, 2006.

Centers for Disease Control, National Center for Injury Prevention and Control: *What is traumatic brain injury?* (website): www.cdc.gove/ncipc/tbi/TBI.htm).

Centers for Disease Control, National Center for Injury Prevention and Control: *Overview* (website): www.cdc.gov/ncipc/tbi/Overview.htm. Accessed June 14, 2006.

81

Turner Syndrome

PATHOPHYSIOLOGY

Turner syndrome is a genetic condition that occurs only in females, in which there is an X chromosome missing or abnormally structured. This results in short stature, ovarian dysgenesis, and infertility. It was first observed by Henry Turner in 1938, when he treated seven female patients for dwarfism and lack of sexual development. Through the years, the knowledge base about Turner syndrome has increased dramatically. Early treatments with pituitary extracts were ineffective; however, current treatments with growth hormone injections and other hormone therapies are creating much more positive outcomes for these girls.

The chromosomal abnormality occurs on chromosome 45. It can be a complete absence of X, a structural abnormality with partial deletion of X, or mosaicism, which is a mixture of the two. In mosaicism, some cells will have the typical 46 chromosomes and some will have 45. The gene has been identified at the *SHOX* or short stature homeobox–containing gene. Two copies of the *SHOX* gene are required for normal growth.

Girls with Turner syndrome may or may not be diagnosed in infancy. There may be a slight intrauterine growth restriction, and growth may be slow during infancy in early childhood.

There will be no pubertal growth spurt. Many body systems are affected by Turner syndrome, although not all girls with the syndrome will have all manifestations.

INCIDENCE

1. Occurs in 1 to 2000 to 2500 live births.
2. Occurs only in females.

3. Approximately 1% to 2% of all fetuses have 45,X chromosome pattern; 99% spontaneously abort.
4. Some pregnancies that progress to second trimester have complications that are associated with fetal death.

CLINICAL MANIFESTATIONS
Very Common: >50% of girls
1. Short stature
2. Gonadal dysgenesis or failure and infertility
3. Deep-set, hyperconvex nails
4. Unusual shape or rotation of ears, tendency toward ear infections
5. Narrow maxilla and dental crowding
6. Spatial-visual difficulties
7. Tendency toward overweight or obesity

Frequent: <50% of girls
1. Hearing loss
2. Thyroid problems
3. Webbed neck
4. Short metacarpals
5. Cubitus valgus
6. Osteoporosis
7. Hypertension
8. High arched palate
9. Low posterior hairline
10. Lymphedema of hands and feet
11. Kidney anomalies
12. Congenital cardiac anomalies
13. Pigmented nevi

Rare: <5% of girls
1. Gonadoblastoma, neuroblastoma, colon cancer
2. Scoliosis, kyphosis, or lordosis
3. Inflammatory bowel disease
4. Difficulty with carbohydrate metabolism
5. Liver disease

COMPLICATIONS

1. Cardiovascular: occurs in one of three girls, left-sided anomalies such as coarctation of the aorta and abnormalities of the aortic valve are the most common.

2. Neurologic: often have normal intelligence but may have difficulty with memory, attention, visual processing, and math. Psychosocial issues result from short stature and typical facial features that may cause teasing in school. Behavioral disorders may result from issues regarding self-esteem.

3. Renal: may have horseshoe kidney or malrotated kidney; does not affect renal function but may predispose the girl to urinary tract infections.

4. Musculoskeletal: short neck occurs in about 40%, owing to hypoplasia of cervical vertebra. Scoliosis, kyphosis, or lordosis may occur less commonly.

5. Endocrine: lack of secretion of growth hormone; no estrogen or other female hormones as a result of ovarian dysgenesis. Puberty is delayed or absent, infertility is common, premature menopause may occur. Hypothyroid conditions may also occur.

6. Lymph: lymphedema and cellular migration cause many features of Turner syndrome. The lymphedema occurs in 1 of every 3 infants affected; improves with age; may recur at puberty.

7. Nail dysplasia occurs in 50%, with small, narrow, hyperconvex nails, inserted at an acute angle; webbed neck occurs in about 25% and develops prenatally; low posterior hairline, bushy eyebrows, and low-set, posterior, rotated ears are common. Shield-shaped chest and widely spaced nipples are result of stretching of rib cage from fetal edema.

8. Sensory: strabismus or ptosis may be noted; recurrent otitis media occurs in 75% of cases and is related to anatomic differences.

9. Dermatology: nevi are common.

10. Orthopedic: hallmark of Turner syndrome is short stature; there is delay in skeletal maturation, and bone size is smaller. Bone mineral density is decreased. There may be

a shortening of the fourth metacarpal; knee abnormalities are seen in 60% of patients, scoliosis in 12%, and increased carrying angle of arms (cubitus valgus) in 45%. High arched palate and small chin are characteristic features.

11. Growth: short stature occurs in almost 100% of girls.

LABORATORY AND DIAGNOSTIC TESTS

1. Diagnosis is made by karyotype of chromosomal patterns—results will show a single X chromosome and absence of all or part of the second sex chromosome. Absence of X accounts for about 60% of Turner syndrome cases, and is known as 45,X.

2. A karyotype gene was recently identified as being responsible for part of the short stature in girls with Turner syndrome. It is known as the short stature homeobox (*SHOX*)–containing gene. This gene accounts for some of the short stature and the skeletal abnormalities.

MEDICAL MANAGEMENT

Nurses caring for children with Turner syndrome are most likely to see them in the hospital or the outpatient setting for other procedures or care. Medical management of a girl with Turner syndrome is very complex. It requires first a suspicion of the syndrome to lead to diagnosis. Diagnosis is based upon karyotype of chromosomes, which can be done prenatally with chorionic villus sampling or amniocentesis, and postnatally with a blood test. Most often, Turner syndrome is not diagnosed in infancy, and is suspected later in childhood because of growth failure. At that time, a very thorough work-up should be done.

Depending on the degree of involvement of different clinical manifestations, the long term management may require several specialists. At the least, a pediatric endocrinologist should be involved in management of growth hormone and other hormone replacement therapy.

Since most girls with Turner syndrome have short stature, growth hormone therapy has become the standard of care. This therapy is usually started after the child falls below the 5th percentile for age. Some will reach this marker at 2 years, and many girls start growth hormone at this time. It is generally thought that a minimum of 6 years of growth hormone therapy is required for a girl to reach maximal height.

Cardiovascular abnormalities are treated based upon etiology. Usually, the left side of the heart is involved. Common defects such as bicuspid aortic valve and coarctation of the aorta are repaired surgically as needed. Most girls with Turner syndrome and accompanying cardiovascular anomalies require prophylactic administration of antibiotics for dental or surgical procedure. Some girls with Turner syndrome will also develop hypertension. Careful monitoring of cardiovascular status is important as part of well-child exams.

Other sensory issues should be assessed and monitored routinely. There may be vision and/or hearing difficulties. Referral to an ophthalmologist for initial evaluation at time of diagnosis (if not made prenatally or after birth) should be considered for all affected girls. Regular hearing assessments should be part of all well-child exams.

Since there are a variety of other problems occurring with Turner syndrome, such as craniofacial abnormalities, thyroid dysfunction, obesity, orthopedic problems, and carbohydrate metabolism difficulties, it is crucial that the health care provider monitoring the child with this syndrome be aware of these and manage or refer as appropriate. This child should have annual well-child exams to screen for other issues that may arise throughout childhood. Support groups for girls with Turner syndrome can be invaluable in dealing with self-esteem and other psychosocial issues. Working with the educational team and school nurse at the child's school can facilitate school success for the girl with Turner syndrome.

NURSING ASSESSMENT

1. Cardiovascular: auscultate for murmurs indicative of coarctation of the aorta or other left sided cardiac anomalies.
2. Neurologic: assess for possible difficulties in learning at school.
3. Renal: monitor for increased incidence of urinary tract infections.
4. Musculoskeletal: look for typical facial features as described above, along with typical hand features, cubitus valgus, and short stature.

5. Endocrine: monitor for delayed puberty and lack of growth spurt.

NURSING DIAGNOSES

- Self-esteem, Risk for situational low
- Body image, Disturbed
- Knowledge, Deficient
- Growth, Risk for disproportionate
- Cardiac output, Decreased (if girl has associated cardiovascular defects)
- Infection, Risk for (if the girl has immune or renal involvement)
- Sensory perception, Disturbed (if there is visual or auditory involvement)

NURSING INTERVENTIONS

1. Demonstrate acceptance of the child and family during admission or outpatient care.
2. Educate child (if developmentally appropriate) and parents about Turner syndrome multisystem involvement and potential problems to watch for; provide information regarding support groups and websites with accurate and complete information.
3. Teach child (if developmentally appropriate) and parent about administration of growth hormone injections and other hormonal supplements.
4. Encourage parents to work with school system regarding best possible educational situation for child.
5. Provide education and appropriate nursing care for other affected systems; will need to be individualized based upon organ and/or system involvement for each patient; that is, postoperative care after cardiac surgery, information regarding orthopedic issues such as scoliosis treatment, education regarding thyroid medications and hormone replacement therapy, and so on.

🏠 Discharge Planning and Home Care

1. Ensure that parents and child have adequate supplies for administration of growth hormone and other medications,

and that they have demonstrated proficiency in administering these.

2. Ensure that parents and child are adequately educated regarding the multisystem involvement with Turner syndrome.
3. Ensure that parents are connected with appropriate referral and support systems (e.g., pediatric endocrinologist, Turner syndrome support group).

CLIENT OUTCOMES

1. Child will experience adequate growth and development based upon treatment with growth hormone injections and other hormonal support.
2. Child will maintain good state of health (adequate cardiac output, minimal urinary tract infections, good self-esteem) based upon clinical manifestations present.

REFERENCES

Barclay L: Growth hormone supplementation may be helpful in Turner syndrome, *Medscape* (serial online): www.medscape.com/viewarticle/501983. Accessed December 29, 2005.

Frias JL, Davenport ML: Health supervision for children with Turner syndrome, *Pediatrics* 111(3):692, 2003.

National Institutes of Health: *Table 1. Incidence of phenotypes* (website): http://turners.nichd.nih.gov/ClinFrTables.html. Accessed January 14, 2006.

Ross JL, St. Dennis-Feezle LK, Weber C: Turner syndrome: Toward early recognition and improved outcomes, *Medscape* (serial online): www.medscape.com/viewprogram/2115_pnt. Accessed December 29, 2005.

Rudy C: When will I start my periods? *J Pediatr Health Care* 18(1):39, 2004.

Turner Syndrome Society: *Turner Syndrome Society* (website): www.turner-syndrome-us.org. Accessed January 14, 2006.

82

❖

Urinary Tract Infections

PATHOPHYSIOLOGY

Urinary tract infection (UTI) is the colonization of bacteria any-where along the urinary tract. Infections can be of the lower urinary tract (urethra or bladder, also known as cystitis) or the upper urinary tract (ureters or the kidney, also known as pyelo-nephritis). The infectious agent is generally enteric in nature, most commonly *Escherichia coli*, followed by *Klebsiella, Proteus, Enterococcus* and coagulase-negative staphylococci. The presence of urine and stool around the urinary meatus allows the bacteria to proliferate and ascend upward to the urethra. Voiding is the first line of defense in preventing the causative agent from invading the urethra and bladder walls. Females have a shorter urethra, and bacteria enter at the end of micturition; males have a longer urethra and antibacterial properties that help to contribute to lower incidence of infection. UTI is second in frequency of occurrence of infections to upper respiratory tract infections.

There is an increased incidence in infants and young children learning to toilet-train. Children at risk are those with disorders that do not allow for full bladder emptying such as underlying defects of the urinary system, chronic disease, and neurologic disorders. Immunocompromised children are also at risk.

INCIDENCE

1. Neonatal-infancy period—boys increased incidence over girls
2. Beyond 1 year of life—girls have an increased incidence over boys (10:1)
3. Peak incidence not caused by structural abnormalities is 2 to 6 years

4. *E. coli* causes 80% of infections.
5. Most recurrence occurs after 3 to 6 months, with 60% to 80% of girls having a recurrence within 18 months.
6. Incidence of symptomatic UTI is lower than that of asymptomatic UTI.
7. UTI rarely leads to permanent damage, end-stage renal disease, or chronic pyelonephritis.
8. Uncircumcised boys typically experience two or three UTIs in childhood.

CLINICAL MANIFESTATIONS
Infants (Initially Seen with Vague Symptoms)
1. Colic
2. Jaundice
3. Poor eating, failure to thrive
4. Vomiting
5. Diarrhea
6. Fever
7. Lethargy
8. Irritability
9. Squirming
10. Increased number of wet diapers
11. Foul-smelling urine
12. Diaper rash

Preschool Children
1. Fever (most common)
2. Weak urinary stream or dribbling
3. Foul-smelling urine
4. Hematuria
5. Enuresis
6. Abdominal pain
7. Frequency
8. Urgency
9. Dysuria

School-Aged Children
1. Diarrhea
2. Strong urine

3. Hematuria
4. Dysuria
5. Frequency
6. Urgency
7. Personality changes

Children of All Ages

1. Abdominal distention
2. Dehydration
3. Flank pain
4. Costovertebral angle tenderness
5. Chills and fever
6. Constipation

COMPLICATIONS

1. Reinfection
2. Chronic pyelonephritis
3. Renal insufficiency
4. Urosepsis

LABORATORY AND DIAGNOSTIC TESTS

1. Urine culture (definitive diagnosis)—to determine presence and amount of microorganisms (obtain sample from midstream urine or urethral catheterization)
2. Suprapubic aspiration—to obtain sterile urine
3. Intravenous pyelogram—to visualize kidney and bladder
4. Voiding cystourethrogram—to establish presence of vesicoureteral reflux and abnormalities
5. Cystoscopy—to visualize interior of bladder and urethra (not routinely performed)
6. Retrograde pyelography—to visualize contour and size of ureters and kidneys
7. Cystometry—to assess filling capacity of bladder and effectiveness of detrusor reflux

MEDICAL MANAGEMENT

Before treatment is initiated, a diagnosis must be made based on the child's symptoms and results of the culture and sensitivity testing identifying the organism. Most of the commonly acquired UTIs can be effectively treated with 7 to 14 days of antibiotic therapy. The most commonly used antibiotics are trimethoprim-sulfamethoxazole, nitrofurantoin, amoxicillin, sulfisoxazole, ceftriaxone, ampicillin, and gentamicin. Preferred treatment is the oral route; however, infants younger than 3 months of age or children with suspected pyelonephritis may require intravenous (IV) antibiotic therapy.

NURSING ASSESSMENT

1. See Renal Assessment section of Appendix A.
2. Assess urine output for frequency, urgency, presence of odor, and dysuria.
3. Assess for elevated temperature.
4. Assess for pain (see Appendix I).
5. Assess for behavioral changes.

NURSING DIAGNOSES

- Urinary elimination, Impaired
- Hyperthermia
- Pain, Acute
- Therapeutic regimen management, Ineffective
- Injury, Risk for
- Knowledge, Deficient

NURSING INTERVENTIONS

1. Monitor child's therapeutic response to and untoward effects of medication.
   a. Obtain urinalysis including culture and sensitivity test (using right test for age of patient) before administration of drugs.
   b. Repeat urinalysis 48 to 72 hours after antibiotics are initiated and 1 week after therapy has ended.
2. Encourage intake of fluids according to normal guidelines.
   a. First 10 kg—100 ml/kg/24 hr
   b. Second 10 kg—150 ml/kg/24 hr
   c. Above 20 kg—170 ml/kg/24 hr
3. Administer antibiotics as ordered.
4. Monitor patient's clinical status (if patient is admitted to hospital).

a. Vital signs
b. Intake and output
c. Signs of urosepsis (signs and symptoms of shock)

🏠 Discharge Planning and Home Care

Primary concern is to prevent reinfection.

1. Instruct family and child about importance of completing 7- to 14-day course of antibiotic treatment.
2. Instruct child to void frequently (retention of urine serves to maintain infection).
3. Instruct about proper perineal cleaning (e.g., anterior-to-posterior wiping).
4. Instruct about avoidance of bubble baths.

CLIENT OUTCOMES

1. Child will be free of signs and symptoms of UTI.
2. Child will not experience recurrent UTIs.
3. Child and family will adhere to treatment regimen.
4. Child will remain free of complications.

REFERENCES

Alper BS, Curry SH: Urinary tract infection in children, *Am Fam Physician* 72(12):2483, 2005.

Behrman RE, Kiegman R, Jenson HB: *Nelson textbook of pediatrics*, ed 17, Philadelphia, 2004, WB Saunders.

Bonny AE, Brouhard BH: Urinary tract infections among adolescents, *Adolesc Med Clin* 16(1):149, 2005.

Hockenberry MJ et al: *Wong's nursing care of infants and children*, ed 7, St. Louis, 2004, Mosby.

Ma JF, Shortliffe LM: Urinary tract infection in children: Etiology and epidemiology, *Urol Clin North Am* 31(3):517, 2004.

Malhotra SM, Kennedy WA: Urinary tract infections in children: Treatment, *Urol Clin North Am* 31(3):527, 2004.

83

Ventricular Septal Defect and Repair

PATHOPHYSIOLOGY

A ventricular septal defect (VSD) is a communication or abnormal opening between the right and left ventricles of the heart. VSDs are classified according to location in the ventricular septum as either membranous or muscular. The size of the communication varies widely. Many small, muscular VSDs close spontaneously. The defect is frequently associated with other cardiac defects such as transposition of the great arteries, pulmonary stenosis, atrial septal defect, and coarctation of the aorta. The altered physiology can be described as follows:

1. Pressure is higher in the left ventricle, and thus oxygenated blood shunts from the left ventricle to the right ventricle.
2. Increased blood volume is pumped into the lungs, which eventually may become congested with blood. Over time, this may lead to increased pulmonary vascular resistance.
3. If the pulmonary resistance is high, right ventricular pressure may increase, causing a reversal of the shunt. The unoxygenated blood then flows from the right ventricle to the left, which produces cyanosis (Eisenmenger's syndrome).

INCIDENCE

1. VSD is the most common congenital heart defect, occurring at a rate of 2 per 1000 live births and accounting for 20% of all congenital heart defects.

2. VSD is also the most common congenital heart defect in children with chromosomal abnormalities such as Down syndrome.
3. Male/female ratio is 1:1.
4. Congenital heart defects are more common in the offspring of those who had a VSD.

CLINICAL MANIFESTATIONS

1. Loud systolic murmur generally heard best at left lower sternal border; the size of the defect does not correlate with intensity of the murmur, since louder murmurs may be associated with smaller defects.
2. Thrill may be palpable at left lower sternal border.
3. Signs and symptoms vary with size of the defect and pressure differences between the right and left ventricle.
   a. Children with small VSDs are asymptomatic.
   b. Children with moderate to large VSDs become symptomatic by 2 to 3 months of age and may demonstrate poor growth, poor feeding, repeated pulmonary infections, and congestive heart failure (CHF).

COMPLICATIONS

1. Cardiac: CHF, development of aortic insufficiency or pulmonary stenosis, progressive pulmonary vascular disease, damage to ventricular conduction system
2. Infectious disease: infective endocarditis
3. Growth and development: failure to thrive

Postoperative Complications

1. Cardiac: aortic insufficiency, tricuspid insufficiency, electrocardiogram (ECG) changes such as right bundle branch block, arrhythmias including heart block, ventricular dysfunction with potential for low cardiac output (especially if pulmonary hypertension and/or ventriculotomy), residual VSD
2. Hematologic: hemorrhage
3. Growth and development: neurodevelopmental sequelae of cardiopulmonary bypass

LABORATORY AND DIAGNOSTIC TESTS

Refer to Appendix D for normal values and ranges of laboratory and diagnostic tests.

1. Chest radiograph—varying degrees of cardiomegaly, with increased pulmonary vascular markings
2. ECG—normal with a small VSD; may have left ventricular hypertrophy (LVH) with larger defects
3. Echocardiogram—to identify size and location of defect, identify associated defects, and estimate the magnitude of the left to right shunt
4. Cardiac catheterization—may not be required unless there are other associated defects or concerns regarding elevated pulmonary vascular resistance
5. Preoperative laboratory data
   a. Complete blood count—used to screen hematologic status preoperatively including evaluation of baseline white blood cell count, hemoglobin, and hematocrit
   b. Baseline electrolyte levels and renal function panels—sodium, potassium, chloride, carbon dioxide, blood urea nitrogen, and creatinine to assess renal function and metabolic status preoperatively
   c. Blood coagulation studies—prothrombin time, partial thromboplastin time, platelet count
   d. Type and cross-match—blood products may be required to prime the cardiopulmonary bypass pump and may be required intraoperatively or postoperatively

MEDICAL AND SURGICAL MANAGEMENT

Management strategies vary according to the child's symptoms. Digoxin, diuretics, and afterload-reducing agents are prescribed for children with CHF. For children with associated growth delay, calorically dense formula (greater than 20 kcal/ounce) may be prescribed to maximize growth, and oral feedings may be supplemented with nasogastric tube feedings. No exercise restriction is necessary unless the child has Eisenmenger's syndrome.

1. Cardiac glycosides—improve myocardial contractility, modulate the autonomic nervous system, and decrease elevated ventricular filling pressures (e.g., digoxin)

2. Diuretics—decrease circulatory congestion (e.g., furosemide)
3. Angiotensin-converting enzyme (ACE) inhibitors—reduce afterload (e.g., captopril)

Ventricular Septal Defect Repair

Early surgical repair (in the first 3 months of life) is preferable if the defect is large, particularly if there is CHF and growth failure that does not improve with maximal medical management. Because many VSDs resolve spontaneously or decrease in size, asymptomatic infants and infants whose symptoms can be adequately managed medically are followed clinically. The size of the defect and magnitude of the left-to-right shunt are evaluated at around 6 to 12 months of age. Significant left-to-right shunts are repaired in that time frame. Those with small, insignificant left-to-right shunts may not require repair. Pulmonary artery banding is rarely performed in lieu of complete repair unless there are additional lesions or complications that make complete repair difficult.

Repair is accomplished through a median sternotomy, and cardiopulmonary bypass is required. Hypothermia is used for some infants. For many defects, a right atrial incision allows the surgeon to repair the defect by working through the tricuspid valve. Otherwise, a right or left ventriculotomy is necessary. Generally, a Dacron or pericardial patch is placed over the lesion, although direct suturing may be used if the defect is minimal. Surgery should produce a hemodynamically normal heart, although any damage caused by pulmonary hypertension is irreversible.

NURSING ASSESSMENT

1. See the Cardiovascular Assessment section in Appendix A.
2. Assess for complications.
3. Assess growth and development.

NURSING DIAGNOSES

- Cardiac output, Decreased
- Tissue perfusion, Ineffective
- Breathing pattern, Ineffective

- Fluid volume, Deficient bleeding
- Fluid Volume, Risk for imbalanced
- Pain, Acute
- Anxiety
- Infection, Risk for
- Injury, Risk for
- Family processes, Interrupted
- Knowledge, Deficient
- Growth and development, Delayed
- Therapeutic regimen management, Ineffective
- Coping, Ineffective

NURSING INTERVENTIONS
Preoperative Care

1. Monitor child's baseline status.
   a. Vital signs
   b. Color of mucous membranes
   c. Quality of peripheral pulses
   d. Capillary refill time
   e. Temperature of extremities
2. Assist and support child during preoperative laboratory and diagnostic tests.
3. Prepare child and family with age-appropriate explanations before surgery (see the Preparation for Procedures or Surgery section in Appendix F).

Postoperative Care

1. Monitor child's postoperative status per institutional policy.
   a. Vital signs
   b. Color
   c. Quality and intensity of peripheral pulses
   d. Capillary refill time and core and skin temperatures
   e. Edema
   f. Arterial and intracardiac pressures
   g. Cardiac rhythm
2. Monitor and maintain child's respiratory status.
   a. Have child turn, cough, and deep breathe.
   b. Carefully monitor chest tube patency and output.

    c. Perform chest physiotherapy.

    d. Humidify air.

    e. Monitor for chylothorax.

3. Monitor for hemorrhage.

    a. Measure chest tube drainage per institutional policy.

    b. Assess for clot formation in chest tube.

    c. Assess for ecchymotic lesions and petechiae.

    d. Assess for bleeding from other sites.

    e. Record blood output for diagnostic studies.

    f. Monitor strict intake and output.

    g. Administer fluids as ordered.

    h. Administer blood products as indicated.

4. Monitor child's hydration status.

    a. Skin turgor

    b. Moistness of mucous membranes

    c. Urine specific gravity

    d. Daily weights

    e. Urine output

5. Maintain skin temperature at 36.0° to 36.5° C (96.8° to 97.7° F) and rectal temperature at 37° C (98.6° F).

6. Provide pain medications as needed (see Appendix I).

7. Provide opportunities for child to express feelings through age-appropriate means (see the relevant section in Appendix F).

8. Encourage parental presence and appropriate involvement with care.

9. Perform wound care according to institutional policy.

10. Monitor for signs and symptoms of infection.

11. Provide education and emotional support to parents (see the Supportive Care section in Appendix F).

12. Monitor for complications (see the Complications section in this chapter).

🏠 Discharge Planning and Home Care

1. Instruct parents on home care management.

    a. Appropriate wound care according to institutional policy

    b. Observe for signs and symptoms of infection.

    c. Activity limitations as instructed by the health care team

    d. Appropriate lifting techniques for infants and toddlers: avoid grabbing the child under the arms; support the child's head and shoulders with one arm, and the lower body with the other

    e. Pain management (refer to Appendix I)

    f. Administration of medications and monitoring child's response

    g. Importance of follow-up with medical appointments

    h. Good dental hygiene and antibiotic prophylaxis before and after invasive procedures to prevent bacterial endocarditis

    i. Importance of routine well-child care and immunizations

    j. Importance of developmentally appropriate social and recreational activities (refer to Appendix B)

    k. Importance of maintaining expectations for behavior and discipline and of supporting the child's complete recovery

CLIENT OUTCOMES

1. Child's vital signs will be within normal limits for age.
2. Child will participate in physical activities appropriate for age.
3. Child will be free of postoperative complications.
4. Child's pain will be adequately managed.

REFERENCES

Craig J, Smith JB, Fineman LD: Tissue perfusion. In: Curley MAQ, Moloney-Harmon PA, editors: *Critical care nursing of infants and children*, ed 2, Philadelphia, 2001, WB Saunders.

Craig J et al: Cardiovascular critical care problems. In: Curley MAQ, Moloney-Harmon PA, editors: *Critical care nursing of infants and children*, ed 2, Philadelphia, 2001, WB Saunders.

Koenig P, Hijazi ZM, Zimmerman F: *Essential pediatric cardiology*, New York, 2004, McGraw-Hill.

Mavroudis C, Backer CL: *Pediatric cardiac surgery*, ed 3, St. Louis, 2003, Mosby.

Park M: *Pediatric cardiology for practitioners*, ed 4, St. Louis, 2002, Mosby.

Pye S, Green A: Caring for your baby after heart surgery, *Adv Neonat Care* 3(3):157, 2003.

Pye S, Green A: Parent education after newborn congenital heart surgery, *Adv Neonat Care* 3(3):147, 2003.

84

❖

Wilms' Tumor

PATHOPHYSIOLOGY

Wilms' is typically a large, encapsulated, single tumor arising from the renoblast cells located in the renal parenchyma. A membranous capsule usually encloses the tumor. Wilms' tumors may be multifocal, extend to surrounding structures, involve both kidneys, cause obstruction of the inferior vena cava, invade local retroperitoneal lymph nodes, and/or obstruct the intestines. Metastasis most often occurs in the lungs, followed by the liver and the contralateral kidney, and in rare cases spreads to the bone. Ten percent of Wilms' patients have associated congenital anomalies such as WAGR syndrome (*W*ilms', *a*niridia—absence of pupils, *g*enitourinary [GU] abnormalities, and mental *r*etardation) hypospadias, cryptorchidism, Denys-Drash syndrome (pseudohermaphroditism, GU ambiguity), cardiac malformations, and aniridia. Another 10% have phenotypic or overgrowth syndromes (syndromes characterized by overgrowth of organs or features) such as hemihypertrophy, and Simpson-Golabi-Behmel and Beckwith-Wiedemann. Children with overgrowth syndromes should be screened for Wilms' using renal ultrasound every 3 months until they are 10 years of age.

Wilms' tumor grows rapidly, and typically it is very large when detected. Tissue type varies from "favorable" to "unfavorable" and is the most significant prognostic characteristic. Children with favorable histologic characteristics have 95% survival. Within this favorable category is a cystic, partially differentiated nephroblastoma variant that has 100% survival with surgery alone. Unfavorable histologic characteristics include various degrees of anaplasia (e.g., enlarged nucleus; hyperploidy, which increases the potential for metastasis) that account for more aggressive disease and are more common in children over 2 years of age. The more areas of anaplasia seen, the more aggressive the tumor. Clear-cell sarcoma and rhabdoid tumors are aggressive renal tumors and are not classified as Wilms' tumor. Congenital mesoblastic nephromas are benign renal tumors that are also not considered in the Wilms' family of tumors. Nephroblastomatosis is a focus of cells that, if found, indicate a precursor lesion with a higher risk of development of tumor in the contralateral kidney. These are resting cells, also known as "nephrogenic rests," with a propensity to become Wilms'.

A small percentage of Wilms' tumors are hereditary. Hereditary forms account for the majority of bilateral Wilms'. Chromosomal abnormalities linked to specific genes such as *WT1* and *WT2* are now known to be associated with the predisposition to Wilms' tumor. *WT1* gene has been found on short arm of chromosome 11p13. *WT2* has been mapped to 11p15 location and is associated with Beckwith-Weidemann syndrome. These genetic mutations can occur sporadically or be inherited.

INCIDENCE

1. Wilms' tumor accounts for 6% of childhood cancers and 8% of all solid tumors in children. It is the most common renal malignancy in children. There are 500 children diagnosed annually in the United States.
2. Age range of peak incidence is 2 to 3 years; it is rarely seen after age 6.
3. Of Wilms' tumors, 5% are bilateral, affecting both kidneys, and 1% to 2% are familial.
4. Prognosis varies according to the stage of the disease at the time of diagnosis and histologic characteristics of the tumor cells.
5. Overall survival rate of children with Wilms' tumors is 90%.
6. Girls are affected slightly more often than boys.

CLINICAL MANIFESTATIONS

The first three of the following symptoms are the predominant clinical manifestations.

1. Flank mass
2. Pain
3. Hematuria
4. Hypertension
5. Fever
6. Malaise
7. Weight loss and anorexia
8. Shortness of breath
9. Constipation or diarrhea
10. Anemia

COMPLICATIONS

1. Metastasis to lungs, liver, contralateral kidney, bone marrow
2. Hepatic: local tumor extension resulting in lymphatic blockage and causing ascites
3. Cardiovascular: local tumor extension causing vena cava clots
4. Gastrointestinal: bowel obstruction from tumor, ileus, adhesions
5. Renal: renal dysfunction or failure; hypertension
6. Short- and long-term adverse reactions to chemotherapy and/or radiation therapy

LABORATORY AND DIAGNOSTIC TESTS

1. Computed tomography (CT), ultrasonography, and/or magnetic resonance imaging of the kidneys—to detect mass, tumor thrombus in renal veins, enlarged lymph nodes, and tumor relationship to adjoining structures
2. Liver function tests (alanine transaminase [ALT], aspartate transaminase [AST], total and direct bilirubin)—to detect liver involvement
3. Complete blood count (CBC)—to assess anemia and possible bone marrow involvement
4. Urinalysis—to assess for hematuria
5. Urinary catecholamine levels—tumor markers used to rule out neuroblastoma
6. Blood urea nitrogen, creatinine, and electrolyte levels—to assess renal function
7. Chest CT scan or chest x-ray study—to assess for metastasis

8. Additional testing of liver, bone, and brain only if additional symptoms indicate involvement

MEDICAL AND SURGICAL MANAGEMENT

Skillful surgery is essential for successful treatment of Wilms' tumor. A nephrectomy, or removal of the affected kidney, is performed to remove the tumor and to provide tissue for diagnosis, histologic examination, and staging. It also provides an opportunity to explore and biopsy lymph nodes and abdominal organs for involvement. Surgery allows staging, which is the exact determination of the extent of the disease at the time of diagnosis. The National Wilms' Tumor Study (NWTS) group staging system consists of five stages that reflect the extent of disease. Exact staging is essential to determine the appropriate further treatment, which will include chemotherapy with or without radiation therapy. See Table 84-1 for the NWTS-5 summary of staging and recommended treatment. Bilateral tumors require separate staging, and since resection of both kidneys is not feasible, a second surgery after chemotherapy is required to examine the potential for resection of remaining disease.

Wilms' tumor is radiosensitive. The decision to use radiation therapy is based on the histologic features and stage of the tumor and the success of surgery. Radiation doses delivered to the flank of the affected kidney are now given evenly over the vertebrae to eliminate the risk of scoliosis. The chemotherapy drugs and dosage chosen are highly individualized and are also based on extent of disease, histologic features, and the degree of surgical success. The following drugs may be given: vincristine, actinomycin D, doxorubicin, cyclophosphamide, etoposide, and ifosfamide. Use of single-, intensive-dose and shortened-interval chemotherapy rather than longer-duration chemotherapy has been found to improve cure rates and decrease toxicity. Dosing of doxorubicin and dactinomycin are decreased during radiation to limit side effects.

NURSING ASSESSMENT

1. See Renal Assessment section in Appendix A (acites, urine output assessment).

TABLE 84-1
Wilms' Tumor Staging and Treatment

Stage	Staging Characteristics	Histology	Treatment	
			Radiation	Chemotherapy
I	Tumor completely in the kidney, completely resected with capsule intact	Favorable or Unfavorable	None	Vincristine and actinomycin for 18 weeks
II	Local extension to fatty tissue or blood vessel next to kidney with complete resection	Favorable	None	Vincristine and actinomycin for 18 weeks
		Unfavorable focal anaplasia	None	Vincristine, actinomycin, and doxorubicin for 24 weeks
		Diffuse		Vincristine, doxorubicin, etoposide, and cytoxan for 24 weeks

Continued

TABLE 84-1
Wilms' Tumor Staging and Treatment—cont'd

Stage	Staging Characteristics	Histology	Treatment	
			Radiation	Chemotherapy
III	Residual local spread: abdominal or pelvic nodes, peritoneal penetration or seeding, unclear margins postoperatively, tumor spillage, tumor biopsy without removal, or tumor removal in more than one piece	Favorable, focal anaplasia	Flank or whole abdomen	Vincristine, actinomycin, and doxorubicin for 24 weeks
		Diffuse anaplasia	Whole abdomen and whole lung if metastases seen on chest x-ray study	Vincristine, cytoxan, doxorubicin, and etoposide for 24 weeks

IV	Hematogenous metastasis to liver, lungs, bone, or brain or distant lymphatic spread	Favorable, focal anaplasia	Whole abdomen if renal tumor is stage III; none if stage I or II and distant sites	Vincristine, actinomycin and doxorubicin for 24 weeks
		Unfavorable, diffuse	As above	Vincristine, cytoxan, doxorubicin and etoposide for 24 weeks
V	Bilateral kidney involvement	Each kidney is separately staged	Whole abdomen and distant site according to staging and metastases	Presurgery and postsurgery chemotherapy based on staging of each tumor and resection later

2. Assess preoperatively for enlarged abdomen in flank areas (do not palpate tumor).
3. Assess for bowel sounds and abdominal distention postoperatively.
4. Assess for preoperative and postoperative pain (see Appendix I).
5. Assess wound for drainage and signs of infection.
6. Assess for complications of all aspects of treatment including surgery, chemotherapy, and radiation therapy.
7. Assess child's and family's responses to illness and surgery.
8. Assess child's developmental level (see Appendix B).
9. Assess knowledge and learning needs of family and caregivers.

NURSING DIAGNOSES

- Tissue integrity, Impaired
- Injury, Risk for
- Gas exchange, Impaired
- Fluid volume, Risk for imbalanced
- Nutrition: less than body requirements, Imbalanced
- Infection, Risk for
- Anxiety
- Pain, Acute
- Fatigue
- Coping, Ineffective
- Family processes, Interrupted
- Therapeutic regimen management, Ineffective
- Growth and development, Delayed

NURSING INTERVENTIONS
Preoperative Phase

1. Avoid palpation of abdomen to prevent seeding of tumor.
2. Monitor child's clinical status; observe for signs and symptoms of complications (refer to Complications section in this chapter).
   a. Vital signs
   b. Signs and symptoms of vena caval obstruction (facial plethora and venous engorgement)
   c. Signs and symptoms of renal failure (refer to Chapter 64)

    d. Bone pain

    e. Anemia and bleeding tendencies

    f. Hypertension (refer to Chapter 39)

3. Provide age-appropriate preprocedural and presurgical explanations to child to alleviate anxiety (see Preparation for Procedures or Surgery section in Appendix F).

4. Encourage child and parents to express concerns, questions, and fears about diagnosis (see the Supportive Care section in Appendix F).

Postoperative Care

1. Monitor child's clinical status.

    a. Vital signs (monitor as often as every 2 hours after surgery)

    b. Intake, output (especially urine output at least 1 ml/kg/hr) and weight

    c. Hypertension based on norms for age (caused by removal of kidney)

2. Monitor child's abdominal functioning.

    a. Patency of nasogastric (NG) tube

    b. Bowel sounds and stool output

    c. Signs and symptoms of obstruction—vomiting, distended and painful abdomen, decreased or absent stool, abnormal bowel sounds (either absent or hyperactive)

    d. Postoperative adhesion formation long-term

3. Promote fluid and electrolyte balance.

    a. Monitor infusion of intravenous solutions.

    b. Monitor for electrolyte imbalances.

    c. Monitor for metabolic alkalosis—high pH and bicarbonate elevation (results from NG drainage, which is acidic).

    d. Monitor for third spacing—ascites, dependent or peripheral edema, decreased urine output (most marked on second postoperative day).

4. Maintain and support respiratory status.

    a. Perform pulmonary toilet.

        i. Have child turn, cough, and deep breathe. Use incentive spirometry every hour.

        ii. Assess respiratory effort, O_2 saturation, and lung sounds. Use suction as needed.

   iii. Change child's position every 2 hours.
   iv. Have child ambulate as soon as feasible.
   b. Provide adequate pain control so the foregoing interventions are possible (refer to Appendix I).
5. Monitor incisional site for appropriate healing.
   a. Observe and record drainage for amount and color; change dressings when needed.
   b. Monitor for incision for appropriate closure.
   c. Monitor for signs and symptoms of infection (i.e., redness, warmth, inflammation, fever).

Chemotherapy and Radiation Phase

1. Provide for child's hygienic needs.
   a. Oral and rectal care (especially important because child is immunosuppressed)
   b. Assess skin, including line sites, and provide skin care—dry between folds of skin and lubricate
2. Protect child from infection resulting from immunosuppression. Educate family about symptoms to report.
   a. When in hospital, maintain reverse isolation. Practice good handwashing and use antibacterial foam when child is neutropenic (refer to institutional policy); wash fresh fruits and vegetables well.
   b. Limit ill contacts.
   c. Educate families to immediately report fever, chills, lethargy, skin breakdown, fainting, or any signs of infection.
   d. Educate about the importance of pneumocystis prophylaxis using trimethoprim-sulfa until off treatment for 3 months.
   e. Educate about the importance of ongoing immunizations except live vaccines during therapy.
3. Monitor side effects of radiotherapy; tumor is remarkably sensitive to radiation.
   a. Nausea, vomiting, and diarrhea
   b. Fatigue
   c. Burn skin at site and/or radiation recall, which is a reburn at a site of previous radiation therapy.

4. Monitor and minimize side effects of chemotherapy. Provide anticipatory guidance for family regarding treatment-related side effects and preventive and management measures. The following are a few side effects that necessitate specific teaching or specific interventions. The list is not inclusive. All can contribute to anorexia and weight loss (refer to Table 49-1 in Leukemia chapter for additional information).
   a. Actinomycin D—pancytopenia, nausea and vomiting, and radiation recall
   b. Vincristine—constipation and neuropathy
   c. Doxorubicin—pancytopenia, nausea and vomiting, alopecia, red urine, radiation recall, and cardiomyopathy
   d. Cyclophosphamide—pancytopenia, hemorrhagic cystitis, nausea and vomiting, alopecia
   e. Carboplatin—nausea and vomiting, alopecia, and delayed pancytopenia
   f. Etoposide—nausea and vomiting, alopecia, pancytopenia, and low blood pressure during infusion
   g. Ifosfamide—hemorrhagic cystitis, alopecia, pancytopenia, nausea and vomiting
5. Maintain aseptic care of intravenous access device (IVAD).
   a. Educate about the role of dental prophylaxis with amoxicillin 1 hour before any dental manipulation, including cleaning.
6. Maintain adequate nutritional status.
   a. Assess weight at least weekly during aggressive phases of therapy.
   b. Supplement oral diet with enteral or supplements if weight gain is not adequate.
   c. Offer frequent, high-calorie meals.
7. Monitor and alleviate child's pain (see Appendix I).
8. Provide education about symptoms of anemia and thrombocytopenia and the risks and benefits of transfusions when needed.
9. Forewarn parents and youth that fatigue from therapy can worsen neuropathy from vincristine secondary to disuse.

10. Provide developmentally appropriate stimulation and/or activities for child (see Appendix B).
    a. Refer to child life specialist for procedural preparation.
    b. Assist with the use of positive coping strategies to deal with stresses associated with hospitalization, painful treatments, and uncertainty of disease course.
    c. Promote normal developmental activities for patient and his/her siblings.

🏠 Discharge Planning and Home Care

1. Instruct parents about various aspects of medical management.
    a. Assessment and care of the wound and symptoms to report
    b. Activity considerations after surgery
    c. Therapeutic response to medications and correct dosing
    d. Untoward reactions to medications
    e. Attendance at scheduled clinic visits
    f. Monitoring of axillary and oral temperature (no rectal temperatures)
    g. When and how to call physician or nurse if any signs or symptoms of infection or other complications are noted
    h. Importance of physical activity to support recovery
    i. Review constipation management
2. Provide information to parents about available resources.
    a. Community (i.e., school) resources (see Appendix G)
    b. Financial resources
    c. Genetic counseling for inherited types
    d. CureSearch website (www.curesearch.org) for tumor-specific information in lay terms
3. Provide emotional support and referral to support groups for parents, siblings, and affected child (refer to Appendix F).
4. Encourage normal parenting and discipline. Facilitate ongoing school performance.
5. Instruct parents to monitor and be aware of long-term effects.

   a. Linear growth can be affected by radiation and nutritional deficiencies.

   b. Second malignancies and infertility can result from radiation and/or chemotherapy.

   c. Adhesions from abdominal surgeries and radiation can contribute to bowel obstruction.

   d. Cardiomyopathy from doxorubicin is compounded if whole lung is irradiated.

CLIENT OUTCOMES

1. Child will be free of complications and learn to recognize possible side effects and how to prevent and deal with them appropriately.
2. Child's level of anxiety before procedures and surgery will be minimized.
3. Child and family will adhere to long-term treatment regimen.
4. Child's development will be physically, socially, and emotionally typical for age.
5. The family will remain intact and adapt the diagnosis and its management into their routines.

REFERENCES

Dome JS et al: Wilms' tumor. In: Pizzo PA, Poplack DG, editors. *Principles and practice of pediatric oncology*, ed 5, Philadelphia, 2006, Lippincott, Williams & Wilkins.

Drigan R, Androkites AL: Wilms' tumor. In: Baggott CR et al, editors: *Nursing care of children and adolescents with cancer*, ed 3, Philadelphia, 2002, WB Saunders.

Duffy-Lind E: Tumors of the kidney. In: Kline NE, editor: *Essentials of pediatric oncology nursing: A core curriculum*, ed 2, Glenview, IL, 2004, Association of Pediatric Oncology Nurses.

National Childhood Cancer Foundation Children's/Oncology Group: Wilms' Tumor, *CureSearch* (serial online): www.curesearch.org/for_parents_and_families/newlydiagnosed/article.aspx?ArticleId=3226&StageID=1&TopicId=1&Level=1. Accessed March 9, 2006.

U.S. National Institutes of Health: Wilms' tumor and other childhood kidney tumors (PDQ): Treatment, *National Cancer Institute* (serial online): www.cancer.gov/cancertopics/pdq/treatment/wilms/healthprofessional/. Accessed March 9, 2006.

II

❖

Pediatric Diagnostic Tests and Procedures

❖

General Nursing Action

These nursing actions are applicable to all the procedures discussed in this section.

NURSING ASSESSMENT
Assess the following:
1. Developmental level of cognitive capacity as it relates to ability to understand procedure
2. Previous experience with procedure
3. Acuity level
4. Coping abilities
5. Available parental support
6. Parental understanding of procedure
7. Allergies
8. Reaction to medications taken previously
9. Health literacy

NURSING INTERVENTIONS
Preprocedural Care
1. Explain procedure in age-appropriate language, including anticipation of sensations; younger child may want to practice selected aspects of procedure (e.g., lying on abdomen).
2. Prepare child for preparatory procedural assessment (e.g., complete blood count or urinalysis).
3. Obtain information about usual reaction and sensitivity.
4. Reinforce information given to parents about child's or infant's condition; explain purpose and anticipated outcome of procedure.

Postprocedural Care
1. Provide opportunities for child to discuss procedure and for clarification of misconceptions.

2. Monitor child's clinical status.
   a. Vital signs
   b. Level of consciousness
3. Provide foods and fluids when tolerated.
   a. Discontinue intravenous fluids when child is awake.
   b. Initially offer small amounts of clear fluids; assess tolerance before progressing to full liquids and solids.

85

❖

Cardiac Catheterization

Cardiac catheterization is an invasive procedure used to measure the intracardiac pressure of the heart chambers and the great vessels, as well as oxygen saturation. In addition, angiography is performed when contrast or dye is injected to outline the anatomic details of any cardiac malformation. A radiopaque catheter is inserted percutaneously through a large-bore needle into a large artery, such as the femoral artery. Measurements of chamber pressures, oxygen saturation, cardiac output, and shunt flow, as well as pulmonary vascular resistance, are obtained and recorded (Box 85-1). In children, cardiac catheterization is used primarily to accurately diagnose complex cardiac defects.

Cardiac catheterization is also performed in an interventional manner, using balloon catheters or coiled stents for such purposes as dilating stenotic valves or vessels, and using coils or umbrella catheters for closing septal defects. Interventional cardiac catheterization can delay or negate the need for surgery. Cardiac catheterization is also performed for electrophysiologic studies to diagnose arrhythmias and treat those that are refractory to medication.

NURSING ASSESSMENT

1. Assess cardiopulmonary status.
   a. Respiratory rate and quality of lung sounds
   b. Color
   c. Heart rate and cardiac sounds
   d. Pulses distal to insertion site
   e. Skin temperature and color
   f. Complete blood count (to obtain values necessary for hemodynamic calculations in the catheterization laboratory), blood coagulation studies, and type and cross-match

BOX 85-1

Normal Heart Chamber and Great Vessel Pressures and Oxygen Saturations

Heart Chamber and Great Vessel Pressures

The pressures in the systemic circuit, or on the left side of the heart, are normally higher than those in the pulmonary circuit, or on the right side of the heart.

- Superior vena cava mean pressure: 3 to 5 mm Hg
- Right atrium mean pressure: 3 to 5 mm Hg
- Right ventricle systolic/diastolic pressure: 25/3 mm Hg
- Pulmonary artery systolic/diastolic pressure: 25/10 mm Hg
- Left atrium mean pressure: 8 mm Hg
- Left ventricle systolic/diastolic pressure: 100/6 mm Hg
- Aorta systolic/diastolic pressure: 100/60 mm Hg

Oxygen Saturation Levels

It is normal for oxygen in the blood to be extracted by the tissues so that blood returns to the right side of the heart with an oxygen level about 30% lower than the level when it entered the left atrium from the lungs. Blood entering the left atrium is less than 97% to 100% saturated because there is mixing with blood passing through pulmonary arteriovenous and other small shunts.

- Right atrium saturation: 65% to 75%
- Right ventricle saturation: 65% to 75%
- Left atrium saturation: 95%
- Left ventricle saturation: 95%

2. Assess whether nothing-by-mouth orders were carried out.
3. Assess child's and parents' knowledge of procedure and level of anxiety.

NURSING INTERVENTIONS

Preprocedural Care

1. Prepare child and parents for procedure and describe cardiac catheterization room.
2. Administer sedative and monitor child's response according to institutional guidelines. Allow parents to remain with child until asleep.
3. Mark pulses distal to insertion site.
4. Record baseline oxygen saturation.

5. Ensure safe transport to catheterization laboratory.
    a. Monitor heart rate, respiratory activity, and oxygen saturation.
    b. Provide equipment for airway management, including oxygen, suction, and ventilation bag and mask, as well as additional airway equipment for intubation should the need arise.

Postprocedural Care

1. Assess physiologic status.
    a. Monitor vital signs per institutional policy.
    b. Assess pulses below catheterization site for quality and symmetry.
    c. Assess color and temperature of affected extremity.
2. Assess insertion site.
    a. Intactness of dressing
    b. Signs of bleeding
    c. Formation of hematoma
3. Maintain bed rest for 6 to 12 hours after catheterization if arterial catheterization was performed, and for 4 to 6 hours if venous catheterization was performed (or per order of physician).
4. Begin administration of clear liquids and advance diet as tolerated.
5. Assess for other complications or adverse effects such as pain, hemorrhage, cold stress (infants), arrrhythmias, dye reactions, or nausea and vomiting.
6. Provide opportunities for distraction, relaxation, and play.

REFERENCES

Lock JE: *Diagnostic and interventional catheterization in congenital heart disease,* Boston, 1987, Martinus Nijhoff.

Tremko LA: Understanding diagnostic cardiac catheterization, *Am J Nurs* 97(2): 16K, 1997.

Uzark K: Therapeutic cardiac catheterization for congenital heart disease—A new era in pediatric care, *J Pediatr Nurs* 16(5):300, 2001.

86

Computed Tomography

Computed tomography is an invasive (when carried out with use of contrast dye) or noninvasive radiographic procedure that is performed to detect differences in tissue radiodensity. It is used for the entire body; for example, it provides a 360-degree view of the brain in 1-degree increments, giving an image of the intracranial structures and showing precise location of abnormalities. It is a diagnostic tool used in the assessment of various pathologic conditions. Serial evaluations can be performed because the amount of radiation is minimal.

NURSING ASSESSMENT

1. Assess infant's or child's ability to remain still for 5 to 45 minutes.
2. Assess for allergies if contrast dye is to be administered.
3. Assess child's previous experience with and reaction to similar procedures and need for sedation.

NURSING INTERVENTIONS

1. Provide age-appropriate explanation of procedure as it is performed (include anticipation of sensations).
2. Monitor infant's or child's reaction to sedation.
   a. Record pulse, respiration, and pulse oximetry readings (and blood pressure, if special equipment is available) every 5 minutes.
   b. Monitor untoward allergic reactions.
   c. Secure infant or child safely on scanning table.
3. Monitor infant's or child's pretest reaction to contrast medium; report any signs or symptoms of allergic reaction.

4. If procedure is performed on outpatient basis, instruct parents about monitoring sedated child after procedure.
   a. Child should rest or sleep until sedation has worn off.
   b. Ensure that parents understand importance of maintaining open airway when child is sleeping from sedation (especially in car seat).

REFERENCES

Behrman RE, Kiegman R, Jenson HB: *Nelson textbook of pediatrics*, ed 17, Philadelphia, 2004, WB Saunders.

Hockenberry MJ et al: *Wong's nursing care of infants and children*, ed 7, St. Louis, 2004, Mosby.

87

Electrocardiography

Electrocardiography is a noninvasive procedure that measures the electrical activity of the heart and records it on graph paper. Electrocardiograms (ECGs or EKGs) can be used diagnostically to demonstrate hypertrophy or enlargement of the heart chambers, electrolyte imbalances, myocardial infarction, and myocardial ischemia, as well as the effects of various drugs. The ECG is used to detect cardiac arrhythmias and conduction defects, as well as cardiac rhythms that are diagnostic of a specific cardiac disorder or congenital heart defect.

NURSING ASSESSMENT

1. Assess child's previous experience with procedures.
2. Assess child's developmental and cognitive levels.
3. Assess child's and parents' understanding of procedure.

NURSING INTERVENTIONS

1. Explain procedure to child before it is performed.
2. Encourage child to ask questions.
3. Reassure child and encourage him or her to lie quietly during procedure.
4. Assist in gently holding infant or child (to limit motion during procedure).
5. Remove conduction gel after procedure is completed.

REFERENCE

Park M: *Pediatric cardiology for practitioners*, St. Louis, 2002, Mosby.

88

❖

Endoscopy

Fiberoptic endoscopy of the upper and lower intestines is used for the diagnosis and treatment of a variety of intestinal diseases. Endoscopy provides visualization of the mucosa of the gastrointestinal (GI) tract, allows tissue samples to be obtained (biopsy), and permits performance of therapeutic procedures. Upper intestinal tract endoscopy allows direct visualization of the esophagus, the stomach, and the duodenum. Indications for an upper intestinal tract endoscopy include prolapsed gastropathy, "a more accurate description of an old and possibly common cause of upper gastrointestinal bleeding in children" (Gilger, 2001), vomiting, failure to thrive, recurrent abdominal pain, ingestion of foreign body or caustic substance, and stricture. Lower intestinal tract endoscopy allows the physician direct visualization of the mucosa of the colon. Indications for colonoscopy include bleeding, chronic inflammatory bowel disease, and chronic diarrhea. There are few contraindications to endoscopy, and it is most often performed in an outpatient setting. Conscious sedation is used not only to sedate but also to minimize discomfort during the procedure. Complaints of sore throat and neck pain are usually mild and of no consequence. Some children may feel some soreness in their abdomen the day after the procedure. Adverse effects of endoscopy include but not limited to the following: infection, allergic and/or adverse reaction to anesthesia, aspiration, bleeding, and perforation of the GI tract.

There is an increased trend in the therapeutic use of endoscopy in children. These include pediatric endoscopic retrograde cholangiopancreatography to diagnose infant cholestasis, endoscopic treatment of pancreatitis, and antireflux operations (endoscopic fundoplication). Computer-assisted virtual endoscopy and the wireless videoendoscope are also now available for the pediatric population.

Computer-assisted virtual endoscopy and the wireless videoendoscope may soon replace conventional endoscopy as a diagnostic tool. Advances in medical technology contribute to enhanced performance of newer capsule endoscopy for children; for example, providing improved visualization of the small bowel mucosa and higher diagnostic yield. Administration of sedation or use of contrast media or anesthesia is not necessary.

NURSING ASSESSMENT

1. Assess child's compliance with preprocedural preparation such as ingestion of nothing by mouth and bowel preparation as ordered.
2. Assess child's and parents' understanding of procedure.

NURSING INTERVENTIONS

1. Explain procedure to child and caregivers before it is performed.
2. Monitor vital signs, including oxygen saturation, during and after procedure.
3. Ensure proper positioning of child.
4. Assist with airway maintenance.
5. Observe for evidence of bleeding or excessive abdominal pain and/or distention.

REFERENCES

American Academy of Pediatrics, Pickering LK, editor: *2003 Red book: Report of the Committee on Infectious Diseases*, ed 26, Elk Grove Village, Ill, 2000, The Academy.

Gilger M: Gastroenterologic endoscopy in children: Past, present and future, *Curr Opin Pediatr* 13(5):429, 2001.

Hay WW et al: *Current pediatric diagnosis and treatment*, ed 17, New York, 2005, McGraw-Hill.

Perlstein PH et al: Implementing an evidence-based acute gastroenteritis guideline at a children's hospital, *Jt Comm J Qual Improv* 28(1):20, 2002.

Wong DL et al: *Maternal child nursing care*, ed 3, St. Louis, 2006, Mosby.

89

Hernia (Inguinal) and Hernia Repair

PATHOPHYSIOLOGY

An inguinal hernia is generally the result of a patent processus vaginalis caused by congenital weakness or failure of the processus vaginalis to close. Normally the layers of the proximal portion of the processus vaginalis atrophy around the eighth month of gestation, and the peritoneal cavity is then closed off from the inguinal canal. Failure of the processus vaginalis to close allows abdominal fluid or contents (such as intestine) from the abdominal cavity to enter the inguinal ring and possibly the scrotum.

A communicating hydrocele is present if only fluid from the peritoneal cavity enters the scrotal sac. Although present at birth, the hernia may not be detected for several weeks, until enough abdominal pressure is built up and opens the sac. The child is initially seen with an intermittent lump or bulge in the groin, the scrotum, or the labia. It becomes prominent with intraabdominal pressure such as that resulting from crying or straining. Contents of the hernia sac usually can be reduced with gentle pressure. Surgical repair (herniorrhaphy) is usually performed on an outpatient basis. Early repair eliminates the risk of incarceration.

INCIDENCE

1. Of full-term newborns, 3.5% to 5% will have an inguinal hernia. Incidence of bilateral hernias approaches 50% in premature and low birth weight infants. The majority of

infantile inguinal hernias are diagnosed in the first month of life.

2. If premature infants, incidence ranges from 9% to 11% and as high as 30% in very low birth weight infants.
3. Incidence is highest during infancy (more than 50%), with the remaining cases generally occurring before 5 years of age.
4. Boys are affected more frequently than girls at a ration of 5:1 or 6:1.
5. Sixty percent of hernias occur on the right side, 30% on the left side, and 10% bilaterally.

CLINICAL MANIFESTATIONS

1. Asymptomatic bulge in the groin
   a. More prominent with crying, straining, laughing, or coughing
   b. Smooth, firm, sausage-shaped, mildly tender mass
   c. May spontaneously reduce when child relaxes
2. Scrotal or labia swelling

If Hernia is Incarcerated

1. Bulge or swelling to groin or scrotum (intermittent)
2. Pain
3. Continuous crying
4. Vomiting
5. Abdominal distention
6. Bloody stools
7. Scrotal color changes (redness)

COMPLICATIONS

1. Incarceration (nonreducible) of hernia
2. Strangulation leading to gangrene of the bowel
3. Gonadal or bowel infarction
4. Recurrence of hernia
5. Atrophy of gonad

LABORATORY AND DIAGNOSTIC TESTS

1. None indicated; diagnosis is by physical exam

2. Scrotal ultrasound—to differentiate inguinal hernia from hydrocele.

SURGICAL MANAGEMENT

Children with reducible hernias are scheduled for elective surgery on an outpatient basis. A 1- to 2-cm transverse incision is made in the area overlying the inguinal canal. Children with suspected incarcerated hernias are admitted to the hospital, with immediate surgical repair performed to avoid bowel necrosis and, in boys, testicular infarction. Postoperatively these children are observed for at least 24 hours to be assessed for adequate return of gastrointestinal function and to receive prophylactic intravenous antibiotics. Analgesic medications are used for pain management, oral feedings are begun when adequate peristalsis is established, and the wound is often covered with a protective sealant after surgery.

NURSING ASSESSMENT

1. See the Gastrointestinal Assessment section in Appendix A.
2. Assess for presence of lump in area of groin, scrotum, or labia.
3. Assess for scrotal swelling or redness.
4. Assess for pain.

NURSING DIAGNOSES

- Tissue integrity, Impaired
- Fluid volume, Deficient
- Pain, Acute
- Knowledge, Deficient

NURSING INTERVENTIONS
Preoperative Care

1. Assess child's clinical status before surgery.
   a. Monitor vital signs
   b. Signs of infection
   c. Hemoglobin level higher than 10 g/dl
2. Explain anticipated preoperative and postoperative events using age-appropriate means.

Postoperative Care

1. Monitor child's clinical status.
   a. Measure vital signs as often as every 2 hours for first 24 hours, then every 4 hours (depending on hospital protocol).
   b. Assess for signs and symptoms of infection.
   c. Check temperature and observe for drainage from site, redness, inflammation.
   d. Change diaper frequently (to reduce irritation or infection of incision).
2. Monitor for signs and symptoms of complications.
   a. Recurrence of hernia
   b. Development of wound infection
3. Promote nutritional and fluid intake.
   a. Record intake and output.
   b. Monitor for signs of dehydration.
   c. Advance diet as tolerated.
4. Promote and maintain respiratory function.
   a. Have child turn, cough, and deep breathe.
   b. Perform postural drainage and percussion.
   c. Change child's position every 2 hours.
   d. Keep head of bed in semi-Fowler position.
5. Alleviate child's pain as needed.
   a. Maintain position of comfort.
   b. Use recreational and diversional activities and toys.
   c. Administer analgesics as ordered.
6. Provide and reinforce information given to parents about child's condition.

🏠 Discharge Planning and Home Care

1. Instruct parents about care of dressing (if present).
   a. Keep incision covered with plastic-coated dressing.
   b. Give sponge bath or bathe child with incision covered by dressing.
   c. Do frequent diaper changes at home (protect incision from fecal and urinary contamination and irritation).
2. Instruct parents about short- and long-term management.
   a. Allow no major physical activity for 1 to 3 weeks after surgery.

b. Administer acetaminophen (Tylenol) or ibuprofen (Motrin, Advil) for pain as needed.
c. Monitor for complications.
d. Scrotal swelling and bruising are very common after surgery and may last 1 to 3 weeks.

CLIENT OUTCOMES

1. Child's gastrointestinal function will return to normal.
2. Child's pain will be eliminated.
3. Child will remain free of infection.
4. Child will not develop complications.
5. Child and family will understand home care and follow-up needs.

REFERENCES

Behrman RE, Kiegman R, Jenson HB: *Nelson textbook of pediatrics,* ed 17, Philadelphia, 2004, WB Saunders.

Hockenberry MJ et al: *Wong's nursing care of infants and children,* ed 7, St. Louis, 2004, Mosby.

McCollough M, Sharieff GQ: Abdominal pain in children, *Pediatr Clin North Am* 53(1):107, 2006.

McCollough M, Sharieff GQ: Abdominal surgical emergencies in infants and young children, *Emerg Med Clin North Am* 21(4):909, 2003.

Intravenous Pyelogram (Excretory Urography)

The intravenous pyelogram (IVP) is also called an excretory urography. This test assists with visualization of the following:

- Presence, size, configuration, and function of the kidneys, the renal pelvis, the ureters, and the bladder
- Renal function (assessed by timing the clearance of the contrast medium through the kidneys)
- Urinary or kidney abnormalities (e.g., tumors, polycystic kidney disease, renovascular hypertension, hydronephrosis, renal calculi, vesicoureteral reflux, or abscess)
- Distortions, strictures, scarring, and distention from obstruction
- Displacement of the kidneys, the ureters, or the bladder may indicate the presence of a mass or other abnormality.
- Renal and/or urinary system trauma

Intravenous (IV) radiopaque contrast material is injected and assessed as it passes through the kidney, the ureters, and the bladder. The dye is filtered by the kidney and passes through renal tubules. Traditionally, visualization is achieved through a sequence of x-ray films taken at set intervals over the 30 to 45 minutes. Computed tomography (CT) and magnetic resonance imaging (MRI) are newer techniques being used for urography imaging.

Congenital abnormalities such as absent or displaced kidneys, horseshoe kidneys, and abnormalities of the ureter are detected by assessing size and position of the structures compared to normal. Retroperitoneal tumors are detected by assessing kidney displacement and/or compression of renal structures. Extrinsic or intrinsic tumors, cysts, stones, or scar tissue can be detected by assessing the flow of dye through the renal pelvis, the ureter, and the bladder. IVP after trauma to the urinary system may reveal urinary leakage outside the urinary system. Renal hematomas are detected by assessing kidney contours. If renal arterial blood flow is interrupted (e.g., renal artery blood clots, artery laceration), the contrast media may not be visualized or the clearance time may be significantly increased. If glomerular disease is present (e.g., glomerulonephritis), a delay in clearance time reflects the decreased glomerular filtration rate.

NURSING ASSESSMENT

1. Obtain a careful history, assessing for contraindications for IVP and conditions that are related to increased risk of complications including:
   a. Allergies: allergy or sensitivity to iodine (shellfish allergy) or current treatment for asthma or other severe allergies
   b. Organ failure: combined renal and hepatic disease, cardiac failure, oliguria (severe renal failure), severely elevated blood urea nitrogen (BUN)
   c. Increased risk of negative effects from nephrotoxic dye: multiple myeloma, sickle cell disease, pheochromocytoma, or other inability to tolerate procedures that can result in dehydration
2. Assess the child's developmental level and previous experience with medical procedures. Plan and implement preparation as appropriate for the individual child.

NURSING INTERVENTIONS
Preprocedural Care

1. Inform radiology staff and health care provider if allergies, sensitivity to iodine or shellfish, and/or other significant medical problems are present. Premedicate with steroids and diphenhydramine (Benedryl), if ordered, for prophylaxis in cases of suspected sensitivity to the contrast material.

2. Ensure the availability of antihistamines, epinephrine, vasopressors, steroids, oxygen, normal saline, IV fluids, and resuscitation equipment in case they are needed for treating an anaphylactic response to the dye.

3. Administer cathartic, laxative, and/or enema the evening before and the morning of the procedure, as ordered. Infants and young children are generally excluded. Fecal material, barium, and gas in the bowel can impair visualization of renal structures.

4. Maintain food and fluid restrictions. Frequently, solid foods are restricted 8 to 12 hours before the procedure. Clear fluids may or may not be permitted according to institutional policies. High IV infusion rates may have to be decreased before the IVP. Although slight dehydration assists with concentrating the dye, adequate hydration before and after the procedure is needed to prevent complications related to the contrast medium.

5. Assess fluid, electrolyte, and renal status (serum BUN and creatinine levels). Report any lab results that indicate renal failure and/or dehydration, since the dye may worsen renal function.

Postprocedural Care

1. Observe for reactions to the dye. Many patients experience transient warmth, facial flushing, or salty or metallic taste. Mild reactions may include nausea, vomiting, and occasional wheals. Serious reactions are related to anaphylactic allergic reaction to the dye. Promptly notify the physician if any reaction occurs. Be prepared to administer antihistamines if symptoms persist. If anaphylaxis occurs (rare), be prepared to resuscitate using oxygen, positive pressure ventilation, diphenhydramine, steroids, epinephrine, fluid bolus, and vasopressors as indicated.

2. Ensure adequate oral or IV hydration to replenish fluids and to avoid dehydration. Assess for adequacy of urine output. Instruct parents to report any decrease in normal urine output following the procedure, since it may indicate renal impairment.

3. Observe for signs of extravasation at the IV insertion site (elevate extremity, apply warm soaks, and implement other interventions as needed).
4. Instruct family to assess for and report delayed response to the dye and other abnormalities to their health care provider.

REFERENCES

Kawashima A, Glockner JF: CT urography and MR urography, *Radiol Clin North Am* 41(5):945, 2003.

Kee JL: *Handbook of laboratory and diagnostic tests*, ed 5, Upper Saddle River, NJ, 2005, Prentice-Hall.

Kee JL: *Laboratory and diagnostic tests with nursing implications*, ed 7, Upper Saddle River, NJ, 2005, Prentice-Hall.

U.S. National Library of Medicine, National Institutes of Health Intravenous Pyelogram, *MedlinePlus* (serial online): www.nlm.nih.gov/medlineplus/ency/imagepages/9481.htm. Accessed March 10, 2006.

WebMD: Intravenous Pyelogram, *WebMD* (serial online): www.webmd.com/hw/health_ guide_atoz/hw231427.asp. Accessed March 10, 2006.

91

Magnetic Resonance Imaging

Magnetic resonance imaging (MRI) is an imaging method that provides a clear anatomic display of the body. This display provides excellent tissue discrimination, and the study may be done in any plane without the use of radiation. The MRI scan is found to be superior to the computed tomographic (CT) scan because MRI uses no radiation, and it depicts subtle contrasts between body tissues. Magnetic resonance images are created by sending radio waves to the child, who is lying in an external magnetic field. The image is created from interaction of the body tissue with the radio waves in the magnetic field. To prevent artifacts caused by movement, children are frequently sedated with either chloral hydrate or pentobarbital (Nembutal).

Client and environmental safety issues are paramount in the MRI room because the magnet is always on. The resulting magnetic field will attract any ferrous object (e.g., beepers, watches, infusion pumps, and oxygen tanks) into the scanner. Individuals are screened before entry for internal and external objects that may retain heat from the radio waves and cause burns.

NURSING ASSESSMENT

1. Screen child for pregnancy or implanted metal devices before scanning (metal devices may include, but are not limited to, metal pins or screws in bones, joints, or soft tissues; Harrington rod; pacemaker; and artificial heart valve).
2. Assess for adequate oxygenation during procedure if sedated.
3. Assess child's and parents' understanding of procedure.

NURSING INTERVENTIONS

1. Do not allow anyone to enter scan room with prohibited items.
   a. Hearing aid
   b. Cochlear or lens implant
   c. Jewelry, watch, tie pin, or tie tac
   d. Cardiac pacemaker
   e. Coins, magnetic-strip credit cards, or money clips
   f. Keys, safety pins, bobby pins or hairpins, or barrettes
   g. Beeper or metal stethoscope
2. Explain procedure to parents and child before entering scan room.
3. Monitor child's reaction to sedation.
   a. Record pulse oximetry value every 5 minutes until child is awake.
   b. Monitor untoward allergic reactions.

REFERENCE

Hockenberry M et al: *Wong's nursing care of infants and children*, ed 7, St. Louis, 2004, Mosby.

92

Myringotomy with/without PE Tubes

PATHOPHYSIOLOGY

A myringotomy is a surgical procedure that involves making a small hole in the ear drum to insert pressure-equalizing tubes in the tympanic membrane. This allows for ventilation of the middle ear space, relieves the negative pressure the child often feels in the ears, and allows for drainage of fluid congestion that builds up in the middle ear space. This fluid congestion occurs as a result of frequent and/or unresolved otitis media infections (see Chapter 59). The procedure can relieve symptoms of chronic otitis media with effusion, and allow a sample of middle ear fluid to be taken for culture. This procedure is performed on children with chronic ear infections that have not resolved with antibiotic therapy, and those who have a persistent middle ear effusion.

During the myringotomy procedure, an opening is made in the ear drum to relieve the effusion and/or to insert tympanostomy tubes. This is almost always done on both ears during the same procedure. The ear drum will heal around the tubes and secure them in place. The tubes may be shaped like a bobbin; these fall out in 9 to 12 months. There are also T-shaped tubes; these stay in longer and may need surgical intervention for removal. Tubes are either plastic or metal. Myringotomy with tube insertion is usually done by an ear, nose, throat specialist. It is usually done in an ambulatory or outpatient surgical setting.

INCIDENCE

1. About 1 million children have tubes placed annually.
2. Most are placed in 1- to 3-year-old children.
3. About 30% of children having tubes placed will need an additional set within 5 years.
4. By the time a child is about 5 years old, the eustachian tube becomes wider and longer, making it less likely that a child will get ear infections.

CLINICAL MANIFESTATIONS/INDICATIONS FOR PROCEDURE

1. Persistent ear infections that do not respond to antibiotic use
2. Fluid in the ears for more than 3 months following resolution of otitis media
3. Hearing loss associated with chronic otitis media
4. Changes in the actual structure of the eardrum from chronic otitis media

COMPLICATIONS

1. Anesthesia complications may occur.
2. Complications related to procedure include accidental cutting of outer ear, scarring of ear, and permanent perforation of ear drum.
3. Complications if procedure is not done include long-term hearing loss and, possibly, language acquisition delays.

LABORATORY AND DIAGNOSTIC TESTS

1. Tympanogram may be flat, indicating chronic middle ear effusion.
2. Acoustic impedance tests may show fluid behind tympanic membrane.
3. Child may fail hearing screenings.

MEDICAL MANAGEMENT

Children with recurrent otitis media are treated based upon the current guidelines from the American Academy of Pediatrics. After recurrent otitis media and persistent effusion, a myringotomy and tube placement is often performed. After surgery, the child will require administration antibiotic ear drops for a short period of time.

NURSING ASSESSMENT

1. Assess for pain in ears.
2. Assess for hearing loss.

NURSING DIAGNOSES

- Anxiety (preoperative)
- Pain, Acute (preoperative and/or postoperative)
- Sensory perception, Disturbed (from hearing loss)

NURSING INTERVENTIONS

Preoperative Interventions

1. Perform admission of the child to the preoperative area.
2. Take medical history from parent.
3. Assess vital signs preoperatively.
4. Complete preoperative teaching through play at age-appropriate level.

Postoperative Interventions

1. Assess airway, breathing, and circulation as child arrives in recovery.
2. Monitor vital signs.
3. Monitor neurologic status as child awakens.
4. Monitor for otorrhea and/or bleeding.
5. Monitor pain and provide pain medication as needed.
6. Bring parents into recovery area when appropriate.

🏠 Discharge Planning and Home Care

1. Instruct parents to keep ears dry by using ear plugs for shampooing hair and during swimming.
2. Instruct parents to use ear drops as prescribed upon return home.
3. Instruct parents to monitor for ear drainage and to expect some in the week after surgery.
4. Ensure that parents have follow-up visit date scheduled with surgeon.

5. Instruct parents regarding other possible complications that may occur from anesthesia.
6. Instruct parents to have child's hearing checked after follow-up appointment with surgeon.

CLIENT OUTCOMES

1. Child will be free of ear pain and have minimal middle ear effusion.
2. Child's hearing and language skills will improve to normal level.

REFERENCES

Barclay L: Prompt use of tympanostomy tubes may not improve developmental outcomes at age six years, *Medscape* (serial online): www.medscape.com/viewarticle/510438. Accessed on January 9, 2006.

Goldstein NA et al: Water precautions and tympanostomy tubes: a randomized controlled trial, *Laryngoscope* 115(2):324, 2005.

Nomura Y et al: Effect of myringotomy on prognosis in pediatric acute otitis media, *Int J Pediatr Otorhinolaryngol* 69(1):61, 2005.

Paradise JL et al: Developmental outcomes after early or delayed insertion of tympanostomy tubes, *N Engl J Med* 353(6):576, 2005.

U.S. National Library of Medicine and the National Institutes of Health: Ear tube insertion, *MedlinePlus* (serial online): www.nlm.nih.gov/medlineplus/ency/article/003015.htm. Accessed on January 14, 2006.

93

Peritoneal Dialysis

Peritoneal dialysis (PD) removes toxic substances, body wastes, and excess fluids using the peritoneum (a semipermeable membrane) as an exchange surface. Solutes move from the bloodstream into the peritoneum and then into the dialysate. This occurs through diffusion (movement from an area of higher concentration to one of lower concentration). The dialysate is a hypertonic dextrose solution with a concentration similar to plasma. A higher percentage of dextrose will lead to a greater osmotic effect and more fluid removal.

The PD catheter is placed through a small abdominal incision or through a trocar-induced puncture hole into the peritoneal cavity. This catheter is connected to a system of fluid bags and tubing. A PD exchange consists of three steps: (1) filling (fluid flows into the abdomen), (2) dwell or equilibrium time (fluid remains in the abdomen), and (3) drain (fluid flows out of the abdomen). The "fill" bag is raised above the patient. Opening the clamp allows fluid to flow into the abdomen (approximately 10 minutes). During the dwell time, equilibration between plasma and dialysis fluid leads to removal of solutes and excess fluid. Typically, this ranges from 15 to 60 minutes, but it can last several hours depending on the type of PD. After the prescribed dwell or equilibrium time, the "drain" bag is placed below the patient to enable gravity drainage of the PD fluid (approximately 10 minutes). Fill and drain times will be affected by patency of the catheter, height of the fluid bags, patient position, and other factors. The type of dialysate, equilibrium times, and number of exchanges per day will be prescribed. It is important to maintain an accurate record of the exact amount of fluid instilled and drained.

PD is an alternative to hemodialysis in the treatment of acute and chronic renal failure in children. PD may be contra-indicated for use or used with extreme caution with the following conditions:

- Abdominal defects that prevent effective PD or have an increased risk of infection (e.g., diaphragmatic hernia, omphalocele, gastroschisis, bladder extrophy, irreparable hernia)
- Extensive abdominal adhesions or loss of peritoneal functioning may lead to difficulty with catheter flow and effectiveness of PD.
- Body size limitation of either too small or too large. The abdominal cavity may be too small and/or unable to tolerate dialysate volume. Morbid obesity may also cause issues related to healing, effectiveness of treatment, and/or increased caloric absorption from dextrose in dialysate.
- Inflammatory or ischemic bowel disease (e.g., necrotizing enterocolitis, frequent episodes of diverticulitis) may lead to exacerbation of infection.
- Abdominal wall or skin infection may lead to contamination during catheter placement.
- Recent placement of an intraabdominal foreign body (e.g., ventricular-peritoneal shunt) may lead to leakage and/or peritonitis. Adequate healing time is needed.
- Severe malnutrition may be associated with problems with wound healing and/or peritoneal protein loss.
- Inability to tolerate PD volumes and/or inability to achieve desired clearance leads to the need for alternative methods of dialysis.
- Frequent peritonitis or other PD-related complications may warrant switching to hemodialysis.

NURSING ASSESSMENT

1. Assess the child's underlying condition including medical diagnosis and conditions that PD may be contraindicated, fluid and electrolyte status, hemodynamic stability, body weight, and other related factors.
2. Assess the child's ability to tolerate the procedure and therapy.

3. Assess the child's response to therapy and the resolving of symptoms or improvement in underlying condition.
4. Assess for complications related to peritoneal dialysis.

NURSING INTERVENTIONS

1. Prepare the child for catheter placement.
   a. Perform preprocedural teaching. Obtain informed consent (see Appendix F).
   b. Monitor the child's reaction to sedation and pain medication (see Appendix I).
   c. Maintain sterile technique when assisting with placement (e.g., use surgical mask and sterile gloves).
   d. Monitor the child's condition and intervene as needed. Assess for retroperitoneal bleeding from perforation (decreased hematocrit, abdominal discoloration, signs of hypovolemia).
2. Perform peritoneal dialysis as prescribed.
   a. Use sterile technique when priming and connecting dialysate solution, drainage bags, tubing, and catheters. Use "no touch" connection devices and other procedures to prevent contamination whenever possible. Clean connections thoroughly.
   b. Maintain patency of the dialysis catheter. Assess for leakage at the insertion site.
      i. Assess for catheter occlusion by monitoring ease of flow by gravity.
      ii. Reposition child as needed to improve flow (e.g., turn side to side, raise or lower head of bed).
      iii. Position catheter and tubing without kinks, with fluid bags at the appropriate level. Secure catheter and tubing with a sterile dressing and tape or tubing immobilization device.
      iv. Keep clamps in appropriate position.
      v. Report chronic and/or unresolved flow problems. Anticoagulants may have to be added to the dialysate.
3. Monitor response to therapy and PD-related complications
   a. Monitor for signs of respiratory distress from abdominal distention and/or fluid overload. Raise the head of the bed to assist with breathing as needed. Monitor for signs

of respiratory distress (i.e., tachypnea, accessory muscle use, retractions, agitation, decreased oxygen saturation, respiratory acidosis, carbon dioxide retention) from abdominal distention and/or fluid overload. Raise the head of the bed, reposition the airway, and administer oxygen or other supportive measures to assist with breathing as needed.

b. Monitor temperature, since infants and young children may become hypothermic if dialysate is not warmed before instillation.

c. Assess lab results of blood urea nitrogen, creatinine, and blood chemistry tests.

   i. Assess for signs of electrolyte imbalance, since electrolytes will be removed during PD.

   ii. Assess for hyperglycemia, particularly when using a dialysis solution with a high concentration of dextrose.

   iii. If the child is hypokalemic, potassium can be added to the dialysate.

d. Assess fluid status. Assess for signs of dehydration (i.e., tachycardia, hypotension, sunken eyeballs, decreased peripheral perfusion, change in level of consciousness). Hypotension may result if fluid is withdrawn too rapidly and circulatory volume is depleted.

e. Assess for bowel sounds and abdominal complications.

f. Monitor for infection at the catheter insertion site and/or peritoneal cavity.

   i. Maintain intact system while avoiding entering the line. Use sterile technique when entering the line or changing drainage bags.

   ii. Maintain a sterile dressing over the catheter insertion site. Clean site with nonirritating solution. Replace the dressing per routine and as needed when the dressing is wet or soiled.

   iii. Assess for signs of infection (i.e., fever, chills, increased abdominal tenderness, redness or swelling at the catheter insertion site, increased serum white blood cell count, cloudy dialysate drainage solution).

iv. Obtain and send dialysate fluid for microbiology cultures as ordered.

v. Administer antibiotics as ordered.

g. Assess nutritional status and monitor for protein loss. Promote adequate nutritional intake and protein replacement.

h. Assess comfort level and ability to resume activities of daily living. Assess for back pain, cramping, incision site pain, and other areas of discomfort. Use analgesic agents and nonpharmacologic techniques as indicated (see Appendix I).

i. Monitor for sleep pattern disturbance. Promote comfort and adequate rest periods.

4. Prepare child and family for home peritoneal dialysis (as appropriate) through teaching and arranging home care support, equipment, and follow-up. Families will need instruction regarding technique, complications, trouble shooting and emergencies, medications, fluid and nutritional needs, follow-up, supplies, activities, travel, and other topics related to PD therapy.

a. The most common PD methods used at home are continuous ambulatory peritoneal dialysis (CAPD) and continuous cycling PD (CCPD):

i. CAPD does not use a machine to fill the abdomen. Fluid is allowed to remain in the abdomen for several hours. An exchange at night is done with an overnight dwell time. During the day, the dwell time is generally 4 to 6 hours. This enables the child to go to school and/or participate in other activities. The child's abdomen will most likely be distended from the dialysate. This may lead to discomfort, clothing not fitting properly, and disturbed body image. Teaching and support should be provided.

ii. CCPD is a combination of the use of a machine (cycler) at night to perform automatic exchanges and one manual exchange with a dwell time that lasts the entire day. For some children, an additional manual exchange may be done in the middle of the day to achieve better clearance of fluid and solutes.

REFERENCES

ANNA Pediatric Nephrology Special Interest Group: Pediatric ESRD and peritoneal dialysis fact sheet, Pitman, NJ, 2005, American Nephrology Nursing Association.

Chada V, Warady BA: Adequacy of peritoneal dialysis in pediatric patients. In Nissenson AR, Fine RN, editors: *Dialysis therapy,* ed 3, Philadelphia, 2002, Harley & Belfus.

Holoway MS: Peritoneal dialysis orders in children. In: Nissenson AR, Fine RN, editors: *Dialysis therapy,* ed 3, Philadelphia, 2002, Harley & Belfus.

National Kidney Foundation: K/DOQI clinical practice guidelines for peritoneal dialysis adequacy, 2000, *Am J Kidney Dis* 37(suppl 1):S65, 2001.

National Kidney and Urologic Diseases Information Clearinghouse: *Treatment methods for kidney failure* (website): http://kidney.niddk.nih.gov/kudiseases/pubs/peritoneal. Accessed on March 31, 2006.

National Kidney and Urologic Diseases Information Clearinghouse: *Treatment methods for kidney failure in children* (website): http://kidney.niddk.nih.gov/kudiseases/pubs/childkidneydiseases/treatment_methods. Accessed on March 31, 2006.

Neu AM: Infant and neonatal peritoneal dialysis. In: Nissenson AR, Fine RN, editors: *Dialysis therapy,* ed 3, Philadelphia, 2002, Harley & Belfus.

Zabat E: When your patient needs peritoneal dialysis, *Nursing 2003* 33(8):52, 2003.

94

Ph Probe Monitoring

The presence of acid reflux in the distal esophagus is detected by pH probe monitoring. A thin, flexible probe is inserted transnasally and advanced to the distal esophagus 1 to 4 cm above the lower esophageal sphincter. It is attached to a portable recording device that permits monitoring of infants and children in a physiologic setting with normal dietary intake. Usually, the physician or practitioner will use a diary to record physical events that may suggest reflux activities such as coughing, gagging, hiccupping, burping, abdominal "soreness" or pain, "sour taste" in the mouth; and, for small infants, episodes or presence of arching and irritability, cyanosis, bradycardia, and apnea. This diary is used to compare the computer reading to the child's activities. The test runs for approximately 18 to 24 hours. Occasionally, older children are permitted to go home with the tube in place. Maneuvers that increase intraabdominal pressure such as bending over or exercise may increase episodes of reflux. There is an initial increase in bicarbonate-containing saliva following placement of a nasogastric tube, which can cause gastroesophageal reflux (GER) to be underestimated.

The physician or practitioner may consider repeating a negative pH probe in patients with symptoms of GER, especially if the duration of the study was less than 24 hours. A negative pH probe in a symptomatic child does not entirely eliminate the diagnosis of reflux. However, it has a very high specificity, so a positive result confirms the diagnosis of GER.

NURSING ASSESSMENT

1. Assess child's previous experience with procedures.
2. Assess child's and parents' understanding of procedure.

NURSING INTERVENTIONS

1. Explain procedure to child and parents before it is performed.
2. Probe should be securely taped to infant's or child's face to maintain placement. Reinforce as needed to prevent dislodgement or removal by infant or child.
3. Instruct parents to document starting and ending time of feedings, position changes, vomiting, apnea, and so on. Careful documentation is necessary to ensure accurate results.
4. Instruct family and/or parents to avoid placing tension on probe or electrode wire.
5. Normal pH is 5.5 to 7.0; pH readings on meter that are higher than 8 or that are negative number indicate machine malfunction.

REFERENCES

Hay WW et al: *Current pediatric diagnosis and treatment,* ed 17, New York, 2005, McGraw-Hill.

Perlstein PH et al: Implementing an evidence-based acute gastroenteritis guideline at a children's hospital, *Jt Comm J Qual Improv* 28(1):20, 2002.

Wong DL et al: *Maternal child nursing care,* ed 3, St. Louis, 2006, Mosby.

95

Polysomnogram Sleep Studies

Polysomnography refers to the continuous and simultaneous monitoring and recording of various physiologic parameters of sleep. In order to meet international standards, measured parameters must include one electroencephalography (EEG) channel, two electrooculogram (EOG) channels to measure eye movement, and one electromyography (EMG) channel to record rapid eye movement (REM) sleep.

Other parameters often monitored include additional EEG and EMG channels, airflow, electrocardiography, pulse oximetry, and respiratory effort; and sound recordings of snoring are often made. The data are reviewed and interpreted by a practitioner specially trained in sleep study and polysomnography interpretation.

A sleep study or polysomnography is indicated for children with sleep-related breathing disorders, neuromuscular disease, or sleep-related symptoms. Current evidence suggests that at least 2 nights of study may provide more accurate patient data.

NURSING ASSESSMENT

1. Assess child's previous experience with procedures.
2. Assess child's and parents' understanding of procedure.
3. Assess child's routine daily activities and sleep patterns.
4. Assess child's developmental and cognitive levels.

NURSING INTERVENTIONS

1. Explain procedure to child and parents before it is performed.

2. Instruct child and parents to maintain regular sleep-wake rhythm and to avoid strenuous activity on the day of the study.
3. Instruct parents to hold medications per physician direction, especially if they may stimulate or sedate child.
4. Provide supportive environment with favorite toy, pillow, or music to facilitate child's sleep.

REFERENCES

Armon C, Roy A, Nowack WJ: Polysomnography: Overview and clinical application, eMedicine (serial online): www.eMedicine.com/neuro/topic566.htm. Accessed March 14, 2006.

Montgomery-Downs HE, O'Brian LM, Gozal D: Polysomnographic characteristics in normal preschool and early school-aged children, *Pediatrics* (serial online): http://pediatrics.aappublications.org/cgi/reprint/117/3/741. Accessed March 14, 2006.

96

❖

Tonsillectomy with/without Adenoidectomy

PATHOPHYSIOLOGY

A tonsillectomy with and a tonsillectomy without an adenoidectomy are considered two of the most frequent major surgical procedures among children today in the United States, second only to myringotomy with tube insertion. In the past, adenotonsillectomy (T and A) was performed by general surgeons. Today, because of surgical specialization related to ear, nose, and throat (ENT) disorders, the T and A procedures are primarily performed by otolaryngologists.

In the twentieth century, the tonsillectomy was performed because of infectious etiologies. Today the tonsillectomy is primarily performed because of tonsillar hyperplasia causing sleep apnea related to airway obstruction, and cardiopulmonary complications such as failure to thrive, tonsillitis resulting in febrile seizures, developmental delays, learning and behavior disorders, and chronic infection syndromes. The adenoidectomy is performed because of chronic throat infections, otitis media, dental abnormalities, snoring, speech delays, and perceptions of low intelligence. Continued clinical trials and attitudes demonstrate through clinical experience and treatment modalities the efficacy of the T and A.

The tonsils and adenoids are a group of lymphoid tissue called Waldeyer's ring in the oral cavity and the nasopharynx; they begin growth in the third month of fetal development. The term *tonsil* typically refers to the palatine tonsil, which is located on both sides of the pharynx and bound anteriorly by the palatopharyngeus muscle (anterior tonsillar pillar) and posteriorly by the palatopharyngeus muscle (posterior tonsillar pillar). The palatine tonsils form the lateral aspects of Waldeyer's ring. The lingual tonsil is located at the base of the tongue and forms the inferior aspect of Waldeyer's ring.

The tonsils and adenoids are considered part of the immune system and primarily induce secretory immunity and regulate the production of secretory immunoglobulins. Their anatomic positioning provides a primary defense against foreign matter. The lymphoid defenses of Waldeyer's ring are most immunologically active between the ages of 4 to 10 years and decrease in efficiency after puberty. No major immunologic deficiency has been noted after either a tonsillectomy or an adenoidectomy.

Acute inflammation, intermittent or endemic, of the lymphatic tissue of the pharynx involves the palatine or facial tonsils. Inflammation is primarily due to infection by group A beta-hemolytic streptococci found in school-aged children and can cause sequelae such as rheumatic fever, carditis, or nephritis. Other responsible infectious organisms include Epstein-Barr virus, *Staphylococcus* species (in particular, *S. aureus*), *Streptococcus pyogenes, Haemophilus influenzae, Moraxella catarrhalis, and Streptococcus pneumoniae* and are identified by throat culture and/or serology testing. However, the etiology of the condition is largely irrelevant in determining whether a tonsillectomy is indicated.

INCIDENCE

1. Approximately 67% of children with sinus disease and failed medical therapy respond well to an adenoidectomy alone.
2. The prevalence of obstructive sleep apnea in pre–school-aged children is approximately 1% to 3% and is related to the increased size of the adenoids and the tonsils compared with the child's airway.
3. Adenotonsillectomy is the first-line treatment for obstructive sleep apnea, and the cure rate runs between 75% and 100%.
4. Adenotonsillectomy is considered a generally safe procedure; it has a reported mortality rate of up to 1 in 16,000.

CLINICAL MANIFESTATIONS
Preceding Tonsillectomy

Children who manifest abnormalities of the tonsils typically have problems related to obstruction, infection, or malignancy. The following are general manifestations.

General Malaise

1. Fever
2. Pharyngeal pain
3. Difficulty swallowing—dysphagia
4. Cervical lymphadenopathy
5. Changes in speech and hearing
6. Obstructive sleep apnea
7. Halitosis
8. Snoring
9. Enlarged and red tonsils with yellow or white exudates
10. Psychologic and behavioral problems—decreased ability to learn or concentrate, irritability, and fatigue

Preceding Adenoidectomy

The triad of hyponasality, mouth breathing, and snoring is indicative of obstructive adenoid hyperplasia.

1. Rhinorrhea
2. Postnasal drip
3. Chronic cough
4. Headache
5. Speech delays
6. Ear infections
7. Recurrent or persistent otitis media in children ages 3 to 4 years and older
8. Recurrent sinusitis

COMPLICATIONS

The most vulnerable group appears to be children under the age of 3 years associated with the following:

1. Cardiorespiratory: respiratory compromise related to a narrow oropharynx, potential for circulatory collapse, airway obstruction due to general edema or pulmonary edema, hematoma formation, or central apnea

2. Oral cavity: aspiration, severe pain causing reduced oral intake, difficulty swallowing, bleeding leading to increased hospital stays, nasal pharyngeal stenosis, velopharyngeal insufficiency (characterized by hypernasal speech and regurgitation of fluids through the nasal cavity)
3. Fluid and electrolyte balance: dehydration and facial edema
4. Muscular: refractory torticollis, Grissel's syndrome (a result of laxity, infection, or possible positioning of the transverse ligament of the axial vertebral body)
5. Hematologic: hemorrhage—complication that is most feared by physicians, patients, and parents; defined in two ways: primary—occurs in the first 24 hours, and secondary—which can occur 24 hours thereafter
6. Ophthalmic: otitis media
7. Psychologic: Emotional trauma
8. Eagle's syndrome—can occur when the elongated styloid process is in contact with the tonsillar fossa. Once the tonsils are removed postoperative edema and inflammation can cause scarring around the process, leading to chronic pain syndrome
9. Anesthesia risks: malignant hyperthermia, cardiac arrhythmias, vocal cord trauma, aspiration resulting in bronchopulmonary obstruction and/or infection; residual anesthesia causing potential hypothermia, hypoxemia, acid-base imbalance, hypocarbia, hypercarbia, and hypovolemia, and prolonged muscular paralysis
10. Velopharyngeal insufficiency—complication of adenoidectomy, characterized by hypernasal speech and regurgitation of fluids through the nasal cavity

LABORATORY AND DIAGNOSTIC TESTING

1. Throat culture—to identify causative agent(s)
2. Complete blood count (CBC)—to identify anemia or platelet abnormalities
3. Chemistry panel—performed as general baseline panel suggested by American Academy of Otolaryngology (AAO)
4. Coagulation studies—these tests include bleeding time, prothrombin time, and/or partial thrombin time—to

investigate suspected coagulation disorders (basic coagulation panel recommended by the AAO)
5. Urinalysis—to determine baseline kidney function
6. Pregnancy screening—performed for menstruating females
7. Full-night polysomnography (PSG)—to diagnose severe obstructive sleep apnea; this diagnostic test is expensive and use of it is limited owing to availability and access to sleep laboratory

MEDICAL AND SURGICAL MANAGEMENT

Preoperative screening and evaluation procedures are used to eliminate risks factors based on diagnosis, type of procedure required or available, preexistent medical problems, family history, and potential anesthesia risks, and to complete a physical examination.

According to the AAO—Head and Neck Surgery, "Children with three or more infections of the tonsils or adenoids per year despite adequate medical therapy are candidates for tonsillectomy." Tonsil infections are typically identified by the following criteria: dysphagia, fever >101° F, cervical adenopathy, positive group A beta-hemolytic streptococci culture, and tonsil exudates. Children considered candidates for tonsillectomy are those who have adenotonsillar hypertrophy related to obstructive sleep apnea, tonsil hyperplasia, and peritonsillar abscess unresponsive to medical management, symptomatic infectious mononucleosis, or tonsillitis resulting in febrile seizures. Tonsillectomy is indicated for children with inherited or immunodeficiency diseases such as acquired immunodeficiency syndrome (AIDS), X-linked lymphoproliferative disorder, posttransplant immunosuppression, and various lymphomas related to significant airway obstruction from adenotonsillar hyperplasia that occur in a large number of individuals infected with the Epstein-Barr virus.

Children are also considered candidates for adenoidectomy who have chronic or persistent otitis media (typically children 4 years old or younger); sinusitis, either recurrent or chronic; speech problems; or severe orofacial or dental abnormalities from adenoid hyperplasia, chronic otitis media, or suspected neoplasia.

There are a variety of effective and safe techniques available for the tonsillectomy and adenoidectomy procedures (Box 96-1). Surgical techniques are based on postoperative criteria such as pain and return to normal diet and activity, preoperative

BOX 96-1

Surgical Techniques for Tonsillectomy and Adenoidectomy

1. **Traditional cold-knife (steel) dissection**—Involves the removal of the tonsils by the use of a scalpel. The tonsils are completely removed with minimal postoperative bleeding.

2. **Electrocautery**—Electrocautery burns the tonsillar tissue and thus assists in the reduction of postoperative blood loss. Research has found the heat of the electrocautery ($400°$ C) can result in thermal injury to the adjacent tissues. This may result in increased postoperative pain. Currently this is the most popular technique to decrease intraoperative time and blood loss.

3. **CO_2 or potassium titanyl phosphate (KTP) laser-assisted surgical procedures**—Tonsils are removed using laser. Studies have demonstrated less postoperative pain, decreased healing time, less blood loss, and shorter intraoperative time using the CO_2 or KTP laser.

4. **Harmonic scalpel dissection**—The ultrasonic technology is used to cut and coagulate at lower temperatures than with electrocautery. Energy is created by vibratory rather than electrical current. Studies have found significant improvements in pain management.

5. **Tonsillar ablation and coblation**—This technique uses a combination of radio frequency energy and a electrolyte solution to create a plasma field to liquefy or excise the tonsils at low temperatures (between $40°$ to $70°$ C), thereby preserving the integrity of the healthy tissue adjacent to the tonsils.

6. **Intracapsular power-assisted partial tonsillectomy**—Studies have shown that if the tonsil capsule is left intact, the underlying pharyngeal musculature is undisturbed and isolated from secretions; however, tonsil regrowth is a potential side effect. Chronic tonsillitis is a contraindication for this technique. Less postoperative pain and speedier recovery is associated with the use of this procedure.

and postoperative hemorrhage, operating room time, and cost. Children who have tonsillectomies and adenoidectomies require intensive postanesthesia care associated with the potential for organ system dysfunction. Airway obstruction focus is on respiratory, circulatory, or neurologic compromise, and can result from surgical manipulation and/or bleeding.

Tonsillectomy or adenoidectomy is contraindicated in children who are at risk for anesthesia-related complications owing to uncontrolled medical illness. Other contraindications can include anemia, high fever, severe bleeding disorder, velopharyngeal insufficiency, and children with Down syndrome who have atlantoaxial laxity.

Postoperative pain and nausea are common following a tonsillectomy. Currently, some physicians are using local anesthetics to reduce postoperative pain and intraoperative and/or postoperative dexamethasone to reduce surgical site edema or respiratory compromise, and also as an antiemetic. Adjuvant antibiotic therapy has been shown to decrease inflammation of pharyngeal tissues following a tonsillectomy due to bacterial colonization. In addition, the benefits can include pain reduction, increased oral intake and, possibly, reduced postoperative bleeding.

NURSING ASSESSMENT

1. Obtain baseline health assessment including vital signs.
2. Obtain height and weight.
3. Obtain allergy history.
4. Ensure that necessary preoperative laboratory testing and imaging has been conducted.
5. Ensure child's nothing-by-mouth (NPO) status.
6. Assess child's and parents' understanding of the surgical procedure and sequence of recovery events.

NURSING DIAGNOSES

- Anxiety
- Knowledge, Deficient
- Airway clearance, Ineffective
- Fluid volume, Risk for deficient
- Pain, Acute

- Imbalanced nutrition: less than body requirements, Risk for
- Therapeutic regimen management, Ineffective

NURSING INTERVENTIONS
Preoperative Care

1. Encourage parents to communicate their concerns over surgical procedures, risks and benefits, and age-related anesthesia risks.
2. Carry out psychologic preparation for both the child and the family (refer to Appendix F). Preparation techniques include interactive books, Internet visits to associated facilities, and interventions by child-life specialists who facilitate preoperative visits to the hospital and offer interactive play focusing on the surgical procedure (see specific facility for availability of presurgical visits or online interactive modalities).
3. Inform parents of fasting requirements, based on the specific facility or anesthesia criteria. Typically most facilities require NPO status after midnight the night before surgery for children over the age of 2 years.
4. Inform parents of the registration process before the day of surgery to decrease anxiety and facilitate intake procedures (required insurance cards and driver's license or picture identification for all children must be available). In the case of adoption or temporary custody, court-approved papers must be available.
5. Inform parents of the preoperative, postoperative, and discharge course to reduce anxiety and instill confidence in associated health care providers.

Postoperative Recovery Care

1. Conduct initial patient assessment according to diagnosis, surgical procedure, intraoperative status, and patient history. Patient assessment, level of consciousness, and vital signs are taken every 15 minutes.
2. Manage airway.
   a. Administer supplemental oxygen (cooled humidified aerosol, or regular oxygen administration) following general anesthesia.

    b. Monitor for bleeding, respiratory failure, and/or airway obstruction (cardinal symptoms of bleeding: decreased blood pressure, tachycardia, pallor, changes in level of consciousness). Notify the anesthesiologist immediately.

    c. Be aware of extra airway swelling and/or injury, congenital anomalies, or drug-induced loss of functional residual capacity resulting in atelectasis.

    d. Have available bag valve mask, intubation tray, and anesthesia induction medications.

       i. Reversal agents should be kept available: flumazenil (0.1 mg/kg, by intravenous [IV] route) and naloxone (1–10 mcg/kg, titrated, by IV) in the event hypoventilation or changes in level of consciousness should occur; notify the anesthesiologist immediately.

3. Elevate head of bed 45 degrees or place child in tonsillar position (on side with face down).

4. Encourage child to expectorate secretions and to limit coughing, clearing the throat, blowing the nose, or talking excessively.

5. Monitor fluid and electrolyte balance.

    a. Monitor IV therapy—hourly rates are based on weight in kilograms.

    b. Monitor need for additional fluids related to nausea, vomiting, hypotension, dehydration, or changes in patient status.

    c. Assess child's tolerance to progress to soft diet (e.g., Jell-O, Popsicles, noodles, eggs).

6. Use pharmacologic and nonpharmacologic interventions (see Appendix I).

7. Apply ice collar (if tolerated, to decrease pain and swelling to surgical site).

8. Administer and monitor child's response to antiemetics for nausea and vomiting.

9. Transfer child to the pediatric unit or outpatient unit to be monitored and discharged according to surgeon and anesthesia discharge criteria.

🏠 **Discharge Planning and Home Care**

1. Inform parents both verbally and with postoperative, written instructions that follow-up care with the surgeon should be 5 to 10 days postoperatively unless otherwise indicated by physician.

2. Inform parents that 7 to 11 days postoperatively scabs begin to slough from surgical site, and parents may see minimal bleeding. If bleeding continues or if blood is bright red, they are to notify their physician immediately (in the case of tonsillectomy).

3. Inform parents that after a tonsillectomy, a white shaggy eschar forms in the tonsillar fossae (surgical site of tonsils) that may last from 3 to 4 weeks.

4. Children who have persistent pain, fever of 101° F or greater, bleeding, inability to take oral fluids, and signs of dehydration (i.e., pallor, lethargy, rapid pulse rate) should be evaluated by a physician.

5. Inform parents with children at risk for velopharyngeal insufficiency (see section in this chapter on Complications following a tonsillectomy and/or adenoidectomy) that they must use caution with feedings and be aware of the signs and symptoms: hypernasal speech and regurgitation of fluids through nasal cavity. This is rare following a tonsillectomy.

6. Teach about tonsillectomy diet—soft foods, puddings, eggs, noodles, ice cream, and so on, to minimize pain and risk of bleeding. Diet's duration varies from several days to 2 weeks or more.

7. Teach about adenoidectomy diet—soft to regular as tolerated.

8. Inform parents that oral fluid intake (hydration) is essential to prevent the vicious cycle of poor fluid intake, dehydration, and throat pain. Fluids include water, apple juice, Gatorade, Popsicles. Avoid citrus juices, since they may cause operative site pain; colas and other red liquids may be mistaken for blood.

9. Review pain management—oral acetaminophen with/without codeine, Vicodin, and/or physician preference, in keeping with any history of allergies and sensitivities.

10. Review nonpharmacologic pain management therapeutic modalities such as deep breathing and diversional activities such as TV, drawing, assisting with care, and puzzles.
11. Antibiotics are usually prescribed (amoxicillin for 7 to 10 days unless contraindicated related to allergies, history, or physician preference).
12. Teach about ear drops—as indicated per physician (adenoidectomy).
13. Recommended activity level is light; no active sports should be played for 2 weeks.
14. Inform parents that children after tonsillectomies have sore throats, halitosis, otalgia.
15. Provide parents with physician name and number for follow-up and/or emergencies.

CLIENT OUTCOMES

1. Child will have reduction in frequency or elimination of ear, nose, and throat infections.
2. Child's pain will be reduced and eventually alleviated.
3. Child will have fewer school absences and improved school performance.
4. Child will have fewer physician visits and sick days.
5. Child will experience good sleep at night.
6. Child will experience sense of mastery related to the surgical experience.
7. Child's daily activities will return to those typical for age.

REFERENCES

Behrman RE, Kiegman R, Jenson HB: *Nelson textbook of pediatrics*, ed 17, Philadelphia, 2004, WB Saunders.

Bluestone, CD et al: *Pediatric otolaryngology*, ed 3, Vol 2, Philadelphia, 2003, WB Saunders.

Drain CB: *Perianesthesia nursing: A critical care approach*, ed 4, Philadelphia, 2003, WB Saunders.

Drake A et al: Tonsillectomy, *eMedicine*, (serial online): www.emedicine.com/ent/topic315.htm. Accessed June 15, 2005.

Gigante J: Tonsillectomy and adenoidectomy, *Pediatr Rev* 26(6):199, 2005.

Hamunen K, Kontinen V: Systematic review on analgesics given for pain following tonsillectomy in children, *ScienceDirect* (serial online): www.sciencedirect.com/science?_ob=ArticleURL&_udi=B6T0K-4GWJ8MV-1&_user=964951

&_coverDate=09%2F30%2F2005&_alid=559147324&_rdoc=1&_fmt=full
&_orig=search&_cdi=4865&_sort=d&_docanchor=&view=c&_ct=1&_acct=
C000000593&_version=1&_urlVersion=0&_userid=964951&md5=e3043e577
39005d7bc90bd824077b6a8. Accessed March 22, 2007.

McClay J et al: Adenoidectomy, *eMedicine*, (serial online): www.emedicine.com/
ent/topic316.htm. Accessed August 14, 2006.

Rudolph CD et al: *Rudolph's pediatrics*, ed 21, New York, 2003, McGraw-Hill.

Simon L: Why we converted to coblation tonsillectomy, *Outpatient Surg Mag*
6(8):18, 2005.

Sterni LM, Tunkel DE: Obstructive sleep apnea in children: an update, *Pediatr
Clin North Am* 50(2):427, 2003.

Terris (ed): Sleep-disordered breathing, *Otolaryngol Clin North Am* 36(3):519,
2003.

Appendixes

A

Nursing Assessments

MEASUREMENTS

1. Temperature
2. Pulse
3. Respirations
4. Blood pressure
5. Height
6. Weight
7. Head circumference (under 2 years of age)

CARDIOVASCULAR ASSESSMENT

1. Pulses
   a. Apical pulse—rate, rhythm, and quality
   b. Peripheral pulses—presence or absence; if present, rate, rhythm, quality, and symmetry; major differences between extremities
   c. Blood pressure—all extremities
2. Chest examination and auscultation
   a. Chest circumference
   b. Presence of chest deformity
   c. Heart sounds—murmur
   d. Point of maximum impulse
3. General appearance
   a. Activity level
   b. Height, weight
   c. Behavior—apprehensive or agitated
   d. Clubbing of fingers and/or toes

4. Skin
   a. Pallor
   b. Cyanosis—mucous membranes, extremities, nail beds
   c. Diaphoresis
   d. Abnormal temperature
5. Edema
   a. Periorbital
   b. Extremities

RESPIRATORY ASSESSMENT

1. Breathing
   a. Respiratory rate, depth, and symmetry
   b. Pattern of breathing—apnea, tachypnea
   c. Retractions—suprasternal, intercostal, subcostal, and supraclavicular
   d. Nasal flaring
   e. Position of comfort
2. Chest auscultation
   a. Equal breath sounds
   b. Abnormal chest sounds—rales, rhonchi, wheezing
   c. Prolonged inspiratory and expiratory phases
   d. Hoarseness, cough, stridor
3. Chest examination
   a. Chest circumference
   b. Shape of chest
4. General appearance
   a. Color—pinkness, pallor, cyanosis, acrocyanosis
   b. Activity level
   c. Behavior—apathetic, inactive, restless, and/or apprehensive
   d. Height and weight

NEUROLOGIC ASSESSMENT

1. Vital signs
   a. Temperature
   b. Respirations
   c. Heart rate
   d. Blood pressure
   e. Pulse pressure

2. Head examination
   a. Fontanelles—bulging, flat, sunken
   b. Head circumference (under 2 years of age)
   c. General shape
3. Pupillary reaction
   a. Size
   b. Reaction to light
   c. Equality of responses
4. Level of consciousness (see Glasgow Coma Scale in Table A-1)
   a. Alertness—response to name and command
   b. Irritability
   c. Lethargy and drowsiness
   d. Orientation to self, others, and environment
5. Affect
   a. Mood
   b. Lability

TABLE A-1
Glasgow Coma Scale

Symptom	Score
Eyes Open	
Spontaneously	4
To speech	3
To pain	2
Not at all	1
Best Verbal Response	
Oriented to time, place, and person	5
Verbal response indicating confusion and disorientation	4
Inappropriate words making little sense	3
Incomprehensible sounds	2
None	1
Best Motor Response	
Compliance with command to move body part	5
Purposeful attempt to stop painful stimuli	4
Decorticate pain response (arm flexion)	3
Decerebrate pain response (arm extension and internal rotation)	2
None	1

6. Seizure activity
   a. Type
   b. Length
7. Sensory function
   a. Reaction to pain
   b. Reaction to temperature
8. Reflexes
   a. Superficial and deep tendon reflexes (see Table B-1 in Appendix B for infant reflexes)
   b. Presence of pathologic reflexes (see Table B-1 in Appendix B)
9. Intellectual abilities (according to developmental level)
   a. Ability to write or draw
   b. Ability to read

GASTROINTESTINAL ASSESSMENT

1. Hydration
   a. Skin turgor
   b. Mucous membranes
   c. Intake and output
2. Abdomen
   a. Pain
   b. Rigidity
   c. Bowel sounds
   d. Vomiting—amount, frequency, and characteristics
   e. Stooling—amount, frequency, and characteristics
   f. Cramping
   g. Tenesmus

RENAL ASSESSMENT

1. Vital signs
   a. Pulse
   b. Respirations
   c. Blood pressure
2. Kidney function
   a. Flank or suprapubic tenderness
   b. Dysuria
   c. Voiding pattern—steady or dribbling
   d. Frequency or incontinence

   e. Urgency
   f. Ascites
   g. Edema—scrotal, periorbital, of lower extremities
3. Character of urine and urination
   a. Appearance—clear or cloudy
   b. Color—amber, pink, red, reddish brown
   c. Odor—ammonia, acetone, maple syrup
   d. Specific gravity
   e. Crying upon urination
4. Hydration
5. Genitalia
   a. Irritation
   b. Discharge

MUSCULOSKELETAL ASSESSMENT

1. Gross motor function
   a. Muscle size—presence of atrophy or hypertrophy of muscles; symmetry in muscle mass
   b. Muscle tone—spasticity, flaccidity, limited range of motion
   c. Strength
   d. Abnormal movements—tremors, dystonia, athetosis
2. Fine motor function
   a. Manipulation of toys
   b. Drawing
3. Gait—arm and leg swing, heel-to-toe gait
4. Posture control
   a. Maintenance of upright position
   b. Ataxia
   c. Swaying
5. Joints
   a. Range of motion
   b. Contractures
   c. Redness, edema, pain
   d. Abnormal prominences
6. Spine
   a. Spinal curvature—scoliosis, kyphosis
   b. Pilonidal dimple

7. Hips
   a. Abduction
   b. Adduction

HEMATOLOGIC ASSESSMENT

1. Vital signs
   a. Pulse
   b. Respirations
2. General appearance
   a. Signs of congestive heart failure (refer to Chapter 16)
   b. Restlessness
3. Skin
   a. Abnormal color—pallor, jaundice
   b. Petechiae
   c. Bruises
   d. Bleeding from mucous membranes or from injection or venipuncture sites
   e. Hematomas
4. Abdomen
   a. Enlarged liver
   b. Enlarged spleen

ENDOCRINE ASSESSMENT

1. Vital signs
   a. Pulse
   b. Respirations—Kussmaul respirations
   c. Blood pressure
2. Hydration status
   a. Polyuria
   b. Polyphagia
   c. Dry skin
   d. Excessive thirst
3. General appearance
   a. Height and weight
   b. Mood
   c. Irritability
   d. Hunger
   e. Headache
   f. Shakiness

B

Growth and Development

INFANT (0 TO 1 YEAR)
Physical Characteristics
Age 0 to 6 Months
1. Weight
   a. Birth weight doubles by 6 months.
   b. Weight gain is approximately 1½ lb/mo.
2. Height
   a. Average height at 6 months is 26 inches.
   b. Height increases at rate of 1 in/mo.
3. Head circumference
   a. Head circumference reaches 17 inches at 6 months.
   b. Circumference increases by ½ in/mo.
4. Teeth
   a. Lower central incisor erupts between 6 and 10 months.

Age 6 to 12 Months
1. Weight
   a. Birth weight triples by end of 1 year.
   b. Approximate weight at 1 year is 22 lb.
   c. Weight gain is 1 lb/mo.
2. Height
   a. Most extensive growth occurs in trunk.
   b. Height increases ½ in/mo.
   c. Total height increases by 50% by 1 year.
3. Head circumference
   a. Head circumference increases by ¼ in/mo.
   b. Circumference at 1 year is 20 inches.

4. Teeth

Upper and lower central incisors and lateral incisors begin to erupt between 6 and 12 months of age.

Gross Motor Development
Age 1 to 4 Months
1. Raises head when prone
2. Can sit for short periods with firm support
3. Can sit with head erect
4. Bounces when held on lap in standing position
5. Attains complete head control
6. Lifts head while lying in supine position
7. Rolls from back to side
8. Arms and legs assume less flexed posture
9. Makes precrawling attempts

Age 4 to 8 Months
1. Holds head erect continuously
2. Bounces forward and backward
3. Rolls from back to abdomen
4. Can sit with support for short intervals

Age 8 to 12 Months
1. Sits from standing position without help
2. Can stand erect with support
3. Cruises
4. Momentarily stands erect alone
5. Pulls self to crawling position
6. Crawls
7. Walks with help

Fine Motor Development
Age 1 to 4 Months
1. Makes purposeful attempts to grab objects
2. Follows objects from side to side
3. Attempts to grasp objects but misses
4. Brings objects to mouth
5. Watches hands and feet

6. Grasps objects with both hands
7. Holds objects momentarily in hands

Age 4 to 8 Months

1. Uses thumb and fingers for grasping
2. Explores grasped objects
3. Uses shoulder and hand as single unit
4. Picks up objects with cupped hands
5. Is able to hold objects in both hands simultaneously
6. Transfers objects from hand to hand

Age 8 to 12 Months

1. Releases objects with uncurled fingers
2. Uses pincer grasp
3. Waves with wrist
4. Can locate hands for play
5. Can put objects in containers
6. Feeds crackers to self
7. Drinks from cup with help
8. Uses spoon with help
9. Eats with fingers
10. Holds crayons and makes marks on paper

Feeding Behaviors

1 to 4 Months

1. Feeding schedule is established at 2 months.
2. Bottle-fed infants are fed every 3 to 4 hours.
3. Breast-fed infants have more frequent feedings.
4. Night feedings diminish.

4 to 8 Months

1. Solid foods are introduced between 4 and 6 months.
2. Has 2 to 3 servings of solid foods per day at 6 months.
3. Early teething may begin at 4 months; teething usually begins at 6 months.
4. Increased drooling may occur because of saliva production and tongue thrust reflex.

8 to 12 Months

1. Begins to drink from cup
2. Uses fingers to feed self

Sensory Development
Age from Birth to 1 Month
1. Distinguishes sweet and sour taste
2. Withdraws from painful stimuli
3. Distinguishes odors—able to detect mother's scent
4. Turns head away from aversive odors
5. Discriminates sounds of different pitch, frequency, and duration
6. Responds to changes in brightness
7. Begins to track objects but easily loses location
8. Prefers human face to other objects in visual field
9. Has visual acuity of 20/400—able to focus on objects up to 8 inches away
10. Quiets at sound of voices

Age 1 to 4 Months
1. Discriminates mother's face and voice from those of female stranger
2. Evidences accurate visual tracking
3. Discriminates between visual patterns
4. Distinguishes familiar and unfamiliar faces

Age 4 to 8 Months
1. Responds to changes in color
2. Follows object from midline to side
3. Follows objects in any direction
4. Tries to locate sounds
5. Attempts hand-eye coordination
6. Has highly developed sense of smell
7. Reaches adult limits of visual acuity
8. Responds to unseen voice
9. Demonstrates taste preference

Age 8 to 12 Months
1. Has increased depth perception
2. Knows own name

Cognitive Development (Sensorimotor Stage—Birth to 2 Years)
Child learns through physical activities and sensory modalities (Table B-1).

TABLE B-1
Infant's Reflexes

Reflex	Description	Appearance	Disappearance
Babinski	Fanning of toes with upward extension when sole of foot is stroked	Birth	9 months
Galant	Arching of trunk toward stimulated side when infant is stroked along spine	Birth	Neonatal period
Moro (startle)	Sudden outward extension of arms with midline return when infant is startled by loud noise or rapid change in position	Birth	4 months
Palmar (grasp)	Grasping of object with fingers when palm is touched	Birth	4 months
Parachute	Extension forward of arms and legs in protective manner when infant is held in horizontal prone and downward-moving position	8 months	Indefinite
Placing	Attempt to raise and place foot on edge of surface when foot is touched on top	Birth	12 months
Plantar	Inward flexion of toes when balls of feet are stroked	Birth	12 months

Continued

TABLE B-1
Infant's Reflexes—cont'd

Reflex	Description	Appearance	Disappearance
Righting	Attempt to maintain head in upright position	Birth	24 months
Rooting	Turning of head toward stimulated side of cheek when touched	Birth	6 months
Sucking	Initiation of sucking when object is placed in mouth	Birth	Indefinite
Swimming	Mimicking of swimming movement when held horizontally in water	Birth	4 months
Walking	Initiation of stepping movements when held upright with feet touching a surface	First weeks; reappears at 4-5 months	12 months

Age from Birth to 1 Month
1. Involuntary behavior
2. Primarily reflexive
3. Autistic orientation
4. No concept of self or others

Age 1 to 4 Months
1. Reflexive behavior gradually replaced by voluntary movement
2. Activity centered around body
3. Makes initial attempts to repeat and duplicate actions
4. Engages in much trial-and-error behavior
5. Attempts to modify behavior in response to varied stimuli (e.g., sucking breast versus bottle)
6. Demonstrates symbiotic orientation
7. Is unable to differentiate self from others
8. Engages in activity because it is pleasurable

Age 4 to 8 Months
1. Demonstrates purposeful repetition of actions
2. Demonstrates emergence of goal-directed behavior
3. Discriminates differences in intensity (sounds and sights)
4. Imitates simple actions
5. Demonstrates beginnings of object permanence
6. Anticipates future events (e.g., feedings)
7. Demonstrates awareness that self is separate from others

Age 8 to 12 Months
1. Anticipates event as pleasant or unpleasant
2. Demonstrates emergence of intentional behavior
3. Demonstrates goal-directed behavior
4. Evidences object permanence
5. Looks for lost objects
6. Can imitate larger number of actions
7. Understands meaning of simple words and commands
8. Associates gestures and behaviors with symbols
9. Becomes more independent of mothering figure

Language Development
Age 1 Month
1. Coos
2. Makes vowel-like sounds
3. Makes whimpering sounds when upset

4. Makes gurgling sounds when content
5. Smiles in response to adult speech

Age 1 to 4 Months

1. Makes sounds and smiles
2. Can make vowel sounds
3. Vocalizes
4. Babbles

Age 4 to 8 Months

1. Uses increasing number of vocalizations
2. Uses two-syllable words ("boo-boo")

Age 8 to 12 Months

1. Speaks first word
2. Uses sounds to identify objects, persons, and activities
3. Imitates wide range of word sounds
4. Can say series of syllables
5. Understands meaning of prohibitions such as "no"
6. Responds to own name and those of immediate family members
7. Evidences discernible inflection of words
8. Uses three-word vocabulary
9. Uses one-word sentences

Psychosexual Development (Oral Stage—Infancy)

1. Body focus—mouth
2. Developmental task—gratification of basic needs (food, warmth, and comfort) as supplied by primary caretakers
3. Developmental crisis—weaning; is forced to give up pleasures derived from breast or bottle feedings
4. Common coping skills—sucking, crying, cooing, babbling, thrashing, and other forms of behavior in response to irritants
5. Play—derives physical pleasure from being held, cuddling, rocking, and sucking; pleasurable body sensations are generalized, although focused on oral needs
6. Role of parents—tactile stimulation and attachment behaviors of cuddling, rocking, and feeding provided by primary caretakers
7. Age-specific characteristics
   a. 1 to 4 months
      i. Initially (first month) behavior is reflexive; pleasurable sensations are centered around the mouth

ii. From 4 months to 8 months—pleasurable sensations associated with oral gratification from breast- or bottle-feeding and attachment behaviors of cuddling, rocking, and feeding by primary caretakers

iii. From 8 months to 12 months—pleasurable sensations focused on gratification of oral needs; bodily sensations derived from caretaker attachment behaviors of cuddling, stroking, rocking; frustration or tension ensues with the transition from being breast- or bottle-fed to introduction of solid foods and drinking from a cup

Psychosocial Development (Trust versus Mistrust)

1. Developmental task—development of sense of trust with primary caretaker
2. Developmental crisis—weaning from breast or bottle
3. Play—interactions with caretakers form the basis for development of relationships later in life
4. Role of parents—infant formulates basic attitudes toward life based on experiences with parents; parents can be perceived as reliable, consistent, available, and caring (sense of trust) or as the negative counterpart (sense of mistrust)
5. Plan—provide consistent, predictable support and love that foster child's attachment to primary caretakers and sense of trust about the environment

Socialization Behaviors

Age from Birth to 1 Month

Smiles indiscriminately

Age 1 to 4 Months

1. Smiles at human face
2. Is awake greater portion of day
3. Establishes sleep-awake cycle
4. Crying becomes differentiated
5. Distinguishes familiar and unfamiliar faces
6. Prefers gazing at familiar face
7. "Freezes" in presence of strangers

Age 4 to 8 Months
1. Is constrained in presence of strangers
2. Begins to play with toys
3. Fear of strangers emerges
4. Is easily frustrated
5. Flails arms and legs when upset

Age 8 to 12 Months
1. Plays simple games (peekaboo)
2. Cries when scolded
3. Makes simple requests with gestures
4. Demonstrates intense anxiety with separation from primary caregiver
5. Prefers caretaker figures to other adults
6. Recognizes family members

Moral Development
Moral development does not begin until the toddler years, when initial cognition is evident.

Faith Development (Undifferentiated Stage)
Feelings of trust and interactions with caretakers form the basis for subsequent faith development.

TODDLER (1 TO 2 YEARS)
Physical Characteristics
1. Weight
   a. Weight gain is approximately 5 lb/yr.
   b. Weight gain decelerates considerably.
2. Height
   a. Height increases by approximately 3 in/yr.
   b. Body proportions change; arms and legs grow at faster rate than head and trunk.
   c. Lumbar lordosis of spine is less evidenced.
   d. Less pudgy appearance is being achieved.
   e. Legs have "bowing" appearance (tibial torsion).
3. Head circumference
   a. Anterior fontanelle closes by 15 months.
   b. Head circumference increases by 1 in/yr.

4. Teeth
   a. Once teeth have begun to erupt, a new tooth erupts each month.
   b. Upper and lower first and second molars and canines erupt first.
   c. Most of the 20 primary teeth will have erupted by 2 years of age.

Gross Motor Development
Age 15 Months
1. Walks alone with wide-base gait
2. Creeps up stairs
3. Can throw objects
Age 18 Months
1. Begins to run; seldom falls
2. Climbs up and down stairs
3. Climbs onto furniture
4. Plays with pull toys
5. Can push light furniture around room
6. Seats self on chair
Age 24 Months
1. Walks with steady gait
2. Runs in more controlled manner
3. Walks up and down stairs using both feet on each step
4. Jumps crudely
5. Assists in undressing self
6. Kicks ball without losing balance
Age 30 Months
1. Can balance momentarily on one foot
2. Uses both feet for jumping
3. Jumps down from furniture
4. Pedals tricycle

Fine Motor Development
Age 15 Months
1. Builds tower of two blocks
2. Opens boxes
3. Pokes fingers in holes

4. Uses spoon but spills contents
5. Turns pages of book

Age 18 Months

1. Builds tower of three blocks
2. Scribbles in random fashion
3. Drinks from cup

Age 24 Months

1. Drinks from cup held in one hand
2. Uses spoon without spilling
3. Builds tower of four blocks
4. Empties contents of jar
5. Draws vertical line and circular shape

Age 30 Months

1. Holds crayons with fingers
2. Draws cross figure crudely
3. Builds tower of six blocks

Cognitive Development (Sensorimotor and Preoperational Stages—1 to 2 years)

Child learns through physical activities and sensory modalities.

1. Object permanence solidifies
2. Learns about objects through active manipulation of objects
3. Uses objects to represent something else
4. Has egocentric view of the world
5. Develops concept of time associated with daily activities such as meals, activities of daily living
6. Cognitive abilities associated with preoperational stage begin to emerge (refer to Cognitive Development in Preschooler section)

Language Development (1 to 2 years)

12 to 17 Months

1. Imitates simple words
2. Uses two- and three-word sentences, "no milk" "daddy car"
3. Vocabulary consists of about six words
4. Understands about 25 words
5. Uses same word sounds structures to objects, e.g., "wuwu," "lulu"

6. Indicates requests by pointing, grabbing at objects
7. Points at object says or babbles word derivative, e.g., "baw" for bottle

18 to 23 Months

1. Vocabulary of 5 to 20 words (18 months)
2. Vocabulary of 50 words (23 months)
3. Uses primarily nouns
4. Understands simple commands
5. Uses holophrastic expressions (uses one word to express several ideas such as 'sit' meaning 'Daddy sit here')
6. More than half of speech is understandable
7. Uses two-word questions, e.g., "where that?" "have some?"
8. Able to retrieve an object from another location when requested
9. Can play "patty-cake"
10. Starts to use pronouns such as "me"
11. Makes animal sounds such as "meow"
12. Can name familiar foods

AGE 30 MONTHS

Psychosexual Development (Anal Stage)

1. Body focus—anal area
2. Developmental task—learning to regulate elimination of bowel and bladder
3. Developmental crisis—toilet training
4. Common coping skills—temper tantrums, negativism, playing with stool and urine, regressive behaviors such as thumb sucking, curling hair into knot, crying, showing irritability, and pouting
5. Play—enjoys playing with excreta as evidenced by fecal smearing; sensations of pleasure are associated with excretory functions; actively explores body
6. Role of parents—foster achievement of continence without overly strict control or overpermissiveness
7. Age-specific characteristics
   2 years—learning self control of urine and stool; experiences level of frustration and, with new controls imposed on behavior, becomes irritable and fussy; can be inconsolable; has temper tantrums; demonstrates curiosity about body

Psychosocial Development (Autonomy versus Shame and Doubt)

1. Developmental task—learning to assert self in expression of needs, desires, and wants
2. Developmental crisis—toilet training; experiences, for the first time, social constraints on behavior by parents
3. Common coping skills—temper tantrums, crying, physical activity, negativism, breath holding, affection seeking, play, nightmares and sleep difficulties, and regression to infantile behaviors such as thumbsucking, bladder or bowel incontinence
4. Play—initiates and seeks play opportunities and activities; seeks attention from caretakers; explores body; enjoys sensations from gross and fine motor movements; plays actively with objects; learns to interact in socially approved ways
5. Role of parents—serve as socializing agents for basic rules of conduct; impose restrictions for first time on child's behavior; direct focus from primary and immediate gratification of child's needs
6. Plan—provide consistency in setting limits on child's behavior yet encourage child's exploration with environment and learning of new skills

Socialization Behaviors

1. Dinner is a family social event enabling one of the first learning activities: the rules of social conduct.
2. Learning of what is and what is not acceptable behavior (e.g., aggressive behaviors such as hitting, biting).
3. Rules of social interactions with playmates and adults are being learned.
4. Limited language competencies necessitate the use of physical actions for expression.
5. Limit-setting and parental discipline create frustration and aggressive responses from toddlers.

Moral Development (Preconventional Stage)

1. Concept of right and wrong is limited.
2. Parents have significant influence on conscious development.

Faith Development (Intuitive-Projective Stage)

1. Faith beliefs are learned from parents.
2. Family's religious practices and gestures are imitated.

PRESCHOOLER (3 TO 6 YEARS)
Physical Characteristics

1. Weight
   a. Weight gain is less than 5 lb/yr.
   b. Mean weight is 40 lb.
2. Height
   a. Preschooler grows 2 to 2½ in/yr.
   b. Mean height is 42 inches.
3. Posture
   Lordosis is no longer present.
4. Teeth
   a. Primary teeth (baby teeth) begin to be lost at 6 years of age.
   b. First primary tooth to be lost is typically the central incisor.
   c. First permanent tooth is usually the first molar.

Gross Motor Development
Age 3 Years
1. Dresses and undresses self
2. Walks backward
3. Walks up and down stairs, alternating feet
4. Balances momentarily on one foot
Age 4 Years
1. Hops on one foot
2. Climbs and jumps
3. Throws ball overhand with increased proficiency
Age 5 Years
1. Jumps rope
2. Runs with no difficulty
3. Skips well
4. Plays catch
Age 6 Years
1. Runs skillfully
2. Runs and plays games simultaneously

3. Begins to ride bicycle
4. Draws a person with body, arms, and legs
5. Includes features in drawing such as mouth, eyes, nose, and hair

Fine Motor Development
Age 3 Years
1. Strings large beads
2. Copies cross and circle
3. Unbuttons front and side buttons
4. Builds and balances 10-block tower
Age 4 Years
1. Uses scissors
2. Cuts out simple pictures
3. Copies square
Age 5 Years
1. Hits nail on head with hammer
2. Ties laces on shoes
3. Can copy some letters of alphabet
4. Can print name
Age 6 Years
1. Is able to use a fork
2. Begins to use a knife with suspension

Sensory Development
Age 36 Months
1. Comprehends temperature differences, "cold"
2. Learning object properties
3. Can identify some common colors
4. Learning to balance
Age 4 Years
1. Has very limited space perception
2. Can identify names of one or two colors
Age 5 Years
1. Can identify at least four colors
2. Can make distinctions between objects according to weight
3. Imitates parents and other adult role models

AGE 6 YEARS
Cognitive Development (Preoperational Stage— 2 to 7 Years)

Child progresses from sensorimotor behavior to the formation of symbolic thought.

1. Develops ability to form mental representations for objects and persons
2. Develops concept of time
3. Has egocentric perspective; supplies own meaning for reality
4. Has belief that objects have feelings, consciousness, and thoughts as humans do (animism)
5. Believes that a powerful agent (natural or supernatural) causes the occurrence of events (artificialism)
6. Able to focus on only one aspect of a situation (concentration)
7. Believes that events occur to meet the needs and desires of the child (participation)
8. Uses a specific explanation for an event as a way to explain situations that are different in nature from the original one (syncretism)
9. Employs a rudimentary form of association and reasoning; connects two events but does not imply causal relationship (juxtaposition)
10. Uses a rudimentary form of association and reasoning; associates nonsignificant facts in a causal relationship (transduction)
11. Is unable to reverse the process of thinking; inability to backtrack through the content of thoughts from conclusion to beginning (irreversibility)

Language Development
Age 3 Years
1. Constantly asks questions
2. Talks whether audience present or not
3. Uses telegraphic speech (without prepositions, adjectives, adverbs, and so on)
4. Enunciates the following consonants: *d, b, t, k,* and *y*

5. Omits *w* from speech
6. Has vocabulary of 900 words
7. Uses three-word sentences (subject-verb-object)
8. States own name
9. Makes specific sound errors (*s, sh, ch, z, th, r,* and *l*)
10. Pluralizes words
11. Repeats phrases and words aimlessly

Age 4 Years

1. Has vocabulary of 1500 words
2. Counts to three
3. Narrates lengthy story
4. Understands simple questions
5. Understands basic cause-effect relationships of feelings
6. Conversation is egocentric
7. Makes specific sound errors (*s, sh, ch, z, th, r,* and *l*)
8. Uses four-word sentences

Age 5 Years

1. Has 2100-word vocabulary
2. Uses five-word sentences
3. Uses prepositions and conjunctions
4. Uses complete sentences
5. Understands questions related to time and quantity (how much and when)
6. Continues specific sound errors
7. Learns to participate in social conversations
8. Can name days of week

Age 6 Years

1. Speech-sound errors disappear
2. Understands cause-effect relationships of physical events
3. Uses language as medium of verbal exchange
4. Speech resembles adult form in terms of structure
5. Expands vocabulary according to environmental stimulation

Psychosexual Development (Phallic Stage)

1. Body focus—genitals
2. Developmental task—increased awareness of sex organs and interest in sexuality
3. Developmental crisis—Oedipus or Electra complex; castration fears; fear of intrusion to body; development of

prerequisites for masculine or feminine identity; identification with parent of same sex (in families with only one parent, resolution of crisis during this stage may be more difficult)

4. Common coping skills—reaction formation; transition of feelings toward parent of opposite sex from negative to positive; masturbation during periods of stress and isolation; amount of jealousy and behaviors vary according to child's past experiences and family environment
5. Play—dramatic play in which parental roles and same-sex roles are enacted
6. Role of parents—encourage fantasy play, explain parental role behaviors when questions arise; demonstrate non-judgmental and supportive attitudes; provide reassurance and comfort in response to anxious and fearful behaviors; teach differences associated with private parts; answer questions in response to child's curiosity about body and facts on reproduction
7. Age-specific characteristics
   a. Age 3 years—demonstrates an awareness of gender differences related to physical differences; aware of differing societal expectations for behavior based on gender; can identify gender
   b. Age 4 years—sexual exploration evident as means of learning gender differences; modesty begins to emerge
   c. Age 5 years—decreased sex play; child is modest and evidences less exposure; interested in where babies come from; aware of adult sex organs
   d. Age 6 years—mild sex play, with increased exhibitionism; mutual investigation of sexes

Psychosocial Development (Initiative versus Guilt)

1. Developmental task—development of conscience; increased awareness of self and ability to function in the world
2. Developmental crisis—modeling appropriate sex roles; learning right and wrong
3. Common coping skills—beginning problem-solving skills, denial, reaction formation, somatization (usually in

gastrointestinal system), regression, displacement, projection, and fantasy; changes in eating behaviors, uncontrollable crying, nail biting, biting, angry and aggressive, sleep difficulties, nightmares, bedwetting, accident-prone

4. Play—has active fantasy life; evidences experimentation with new skills in play; increases play activities in which child has control and uses self

5. Role of parents—supervision and direction are accepted by 5-year-olds; 6-year-olds respond more slowly and negatively to parental requests and directions; parents are role models for the preschooler, and their attitudes have a great influence on the child's behavior and attitudes; child's confidence in developmental competence enhanced with parental encouragement

6. Plan—provide appropriate play activities and self-care opportunities

Socialization Behaviors

1. Sees parents as most important figures
2. Is possessive; wants things own way
3. Is able to share with peers and adults
4. Imitates parents and other adult role models

Moral Development (Preconventional Stage)

1. Parental rules are viewed as rigid and inflexible.
2. Negative consequences are viewed as punishment for misdeeds.
3. Parents are seen as the ultimate authorities for determining right and wrong.
4. Internalization of the sense of right and wrong begins.

Faith Development (Intuitive-Projective Stage)

1. Religious practices, trinkets, and symbols begin to have practical meaning for the preschooler.
2. God is viewed in human terms.
3. God is understood as being part of nature, such as in the trees, flowers, and rivers.
4. Evil can be imagined in frightening terms such as monsters or the devil.

SCHOOL-AGED CHILD (7 TO 12 YEARS)
Physical Characteristics
1. Weight
   a. Weight gain is between 4 and 7 lb/yr.
2. Height
   a. Growth spurt begins.
   b. Great variation in growth may be normal, since developmental charts are for reference only.
   c. At 8 years of age, arms grow longer in proportion to body; height increases at age 9.
3. Teeth
   a. Baby teeth continue to be lost.
   b. Last primary tooth is lost by 12 years of age, typically the cuspid or molar.
   c. By age 8, child has 10 to 11 permanent teeth.
   d. By age 12, child has approximately 26 permanent teeth.
4. Puberty
   a. Girls may begin to develop secondary sex characteristics.
   b. Girls begin menstruation.
   c. Age of onset has decreased in the past decade.

Gross Motor Development
Age 7 to 10 Years
1. Gross motor skills under conscious, cognitive control
2. Gradual increase in rhythm, smoothness, and gracefulness of muscular movements
3. Increased interest in perfection of physical skills
4. Strength and endurance increase
Age 10 to 12 Years
1. High energy level
2. Increased directing of and control over physical abilities

Fine Motor Development
1. Shows increased improvement in fine motor skills because of increased myelinization of central nervous system
2. Demonstrates improved balance and eye-hand coordination
3. Is able to write rather than print words by age 8

4. Demonstrates increased ability to express individuality and special interests such as sewing, building models, and playing musical instruments
5. Exhibits fine motor skills equal to those of adults by 10 to 12 years of age

Cognitive Development (Concrete Operational Stage—Age 7 to 11 Years)

Child's thinking becomes increasingly abstract and symbolic in character; ability to form mental representations is aided by reliance on perceptual senses.

1. Weighs a variety of alternatives in finding best solutions
2. Can reverse operations; can trace the sequence of events backward to beginning
3. Understands concepts of past, present, and future
4. Can tell time
5. Can classify objects according to classes and subclasses
6. Understands concepts of height, weight, and volume
7. Is able to focus on more than one aspect of a situation

Language Development

1. Uses language as medium for verbal exchange
2. Words may be recognized before their meaning is understood
3. Is less egocentric in orientation; able to consider another perspective
4. Understands most abstract vocabulary
5. Uses all parts of speech, including adjectives, adverbs, conjunctions, and prepositions
6. Incorporates use of compound and complex sentences
7. Vocabulary reaches 50,000 words at end of this period

Psychosexual Development (Latency Stage)

1. Body focus—sexual concerns become less conscious; more recent thinking suggest this is not a latent or neutral period of sexual development
2. Developmental task—gradual integration of previous sexual experiences and reactions

3. Developmental crisis—increased reference to preadolescent sexual concerns, beginning at approximately 10 years of age
4. Common coping skills—nail biting, dependence, increased problem-solving skills, denial, humor, fantasy, and identification
5. Play—begins to engage in activities with the opposite sex; sexually curious about the body
6. Role of parents—major role in educating child about rules and norms governing sexual behavior and sexuality and in influencing gender-specific behavior
7. Age-specific characteristics
   a. Age 7 years—decreased interest in sex and less exploration; increased interest in opposite sex, with beginning of girl-boy "love" feelings
   b. Age 8 years—high sexual interest; increase in activities such as peeping, telling dirty jokes, and wanting more sexual information about birth and sexual lovemaking; girls have increased interest in menstruation
   c. Age 9 years—increased discussion with peers about sexual topics; division of sexes in play activities; relating of self to process of reproduction; self-consciousness about sexual exposure; interest in dating and relationships with opposite sex in some children
   d. Age 10 years—increasing interest in own body and appearance; many begin to "date" and relate to opposite sex in group and couple activities
   e. Age 11 to 12 years—concerns about appearance; social pressures to look thin and attractive are source of stress; many have misconceptions about intercourse and pregnancy

Psychosocial Development (Industry versus Inferiority)

1. Developmental task—learns to develop a sense of adequacy about abilities and competencies as opportunities for social interactions and learning increase; strives to achieve in school

2. Developmental crisis—danger of developing a sense of inferiority if child does not feel competent in the achievement of tasks
3. Common coping skills—becomes withdrawn, school refusal, has difficulty with schoolwork and/or homework, has difficulty concentrating on tasks on hand, talks back to parents or adult authority figures, somatic complaints such as stomach aches and headaches, fearful, has nightmares, trouble sleeping, loss of appetite, urinary frequency, nail biting
4. Play—enjoys engaging in loosely structured activities with peers (e.g., baseball or foursquare); play tends to be sex-segregated; rough-and-tumble play is characteristic of outdoor unstructured play; personal interests, activities, and hobbies develop at this age
5. Role of parents—parents are becoming less significant figures as agents for socialization; association with peers tends to diminish the predominant effect parents have had previously; parents are still perceived and responded to as the primary adult authorities; expectations of teachers, coaches, and religious figures have significant impact on child's behavior
6. Plan—promote involvement in age-appropriate school-related activities (e.g., clubs and sports), after-school groups (e.g., 4-H and Boy and Girl Scouts), and social and community groups (e.g., volunteering) to develop a sense of accomplishment and pride

Socialization Behaviors

1. Social network expands beyond the family network.
2. Learns to become and function as a member of a social group for common purpose (e.g., sports team, Boy Scouts, Girl Scouts, 4-H Club).
3. Adult role models are sought out for mentorship purposes, especially in family-disadvantaged circumstances.
4. Social sense of responsibility begins to emerge.

Moral Development (Conventional Stage)

1. Sense of morality is determined by external rules and regulations.

2. Social relationships and contacts with authority figures influence his or her sense of right and wrong.
3. Sense of right and wrong is strict and rigid.

Faith Development (Mythical-Literal Stage)
1. Beliefs are heavily influenced by authority figures.
2. Differentiation commences between what is natural versus what is supernatural.
3. Personal sense of God begins to develop.

ADOLESCENT (13 TO 19 YEARS)
Physical Characteristics
1. Weight
   a. Many adolescents are overly concerned with weight.
   b. Fluctuations in weight gains and loss are evident.
   c. Eating disorder diagnoses such as anorexia nervosa and bulimia are associated with adolescent girls.
   d. Obesity is a growing epidemic amongst adolescents.
2. Height
   a. Higher averages occur in boys because of greater velocity of growth spurt and 2-year delay in puberty.
   b. Lordosis and scoliosis may be diagnosed and treated.
3. Teeth
   a. Dentition is completed during late adolescence.
   b. Eighty percent of adolescents need to have one or more wisdom teeth removed.
   c. Malocclusion of the teeth may be evident.
4. Puberty
   a. Girls mature an average of 2 years earlier than boys because of rapid maturation of central nervous system.
   b. Average age of onset is 12½ years in females and 15½ years in males (Table B-2).
   c. Nocturnal emissions are commonly reported at 14½ years (age range is 11½ to 17½ years).
   d. Menarche is the identification criterion for pubertal status in girls; average age is 12½ to 13 years.
   e. Emotions are heightened because of hormonal changes.

TABLE B-2
Changes During Puberty

Male	Female	Both Sexes
Thickening and strengthening of pelvic bone structure	Increase in diameter of internal pelvis	Increased broadening of body frame
Increase in size of scrotum and testicles	Enlargement of breasts, ovaries, and uterus	Darkening and coarsening of pubic hair
Increase in sensitivity of genital area	Increase in growth of labia	Increase in axillary hair
Increase in size of penis	Increase in size of vagina	Changes in vocal pitch

Gross Motor Development

1. Initial awkwardness in gross motor activity
2. Increases in control of gross motor skills are due to neurologic development and increased skill practice

Fine Motor Development

1. Improvement in fine motor control is evident
2. Skill acquisition due to neurologic changes and skills practice

Cognitive Development (Formal Operational Stage—11 Years and Up)

The ability to think approaches a level comparable with adult competencies.

1. Acquires the capacity to reason symbolically about more global and altruistic issues
2. Uses a more systematic approach to problem solving
3. Takes another perspective into account when processing information
4. Thinking is not limited by actual circumstances; can apply theoretic concepts to hypothesized or imagined situations

5. Develops an altruistic orientation (fairness and justice)
6. Develops own value system
7. Can form deductive and inductive conclusions

Language Development

1. Uses language as medium to convey ideas, opinions, and values
2. Incorporates complex structural and grammatical forms
3. Makes evident use of slang and peer-accepted terminology

Psychosexual Development (Genital Stage)

1. Body focus—genital region
2. Developmental task—integration of developmental tasks learned in previous stages; extent to which developmental tasks have been previously achieved and resolved will influence the extent to which the individual functions at this stage; stage is characterized by a renewed sexual interest and sexual attraction to others (of the same or opposite sex)
3. Developmental crisis—resolving and integrating the conflicts of previous stages to function and perform as an integrated adult; adult behavior is evidenced by the ability to engage in pleasurable intimate sexual relationships with a partner, become a responsible and caring parent, work productively, and be a contributing community member
4. Common coping skills—increased problem-solving skills, healthy lifestyle (exercise, proper eating, and sufficient sleep), prosocial behaviors, humor, fantasy, anger, denial, use of illicit substances, aggressive and criminal behaviors, "acting out" depression, and eating disorders
5. Play—preoccupied with physical appearance as evidenced by dress style, use of cosmetics, dieting, and fitness activities; sexually active
6. Role of parents—primary role of parents is to educate youth about appropriate sexual behavior and sexuality and rules of conduct in all social situations such as intimate relationships, social relationships, and work and community settings; parents and/or adult authority figures provide reproductive counseling and discuss prevention of sexually transmitted disease

7. Age-specific characteristics
    a. Age 14 to 16 years—concerns about appearances; social pressures to look thin and attractive are source of stress; pressure to conform to norms of peer group; social comparisons to social concepts of "popularity" influence social interactions; social relationships directed to include opposite sex; pairing of youths within larger social group activities becomes apparent; "steady" or monogamous dating patterns emerge; sexual activity is evident within this age group; teenage pregnancy is a risk
    b. Age 17 to 19 years—concerns about appearances continue; social pressures to look thin and attractive continue to be a source of stress; pressure to conform to norms of peer group continues; social comparisons to social concepts of "popularity" continue to influence social interactions; social relationships remain directed to include opposite sex; pairing of youths within larger social group activities continues to be apparent; "steady" or monogamous dating patterns continue to emerge; risks include teenage marriage, pregnancies, and sexually transmitted diseases

Psychosocial Development (Identity versus Role Confusion)

1. Developmental task—development of a sure sense of one's own unique individuality based on needs, desires, preferences, values, and belief system
2. Developmental crisis—feels a sense of role confusion; cannot identify accurately what factors are necessary for optimal self-growth; is heavily influenced by opinions and judgments of peers
3. Play—strenuous and structured physical activities (e.g., football and soccer) tend to be sex-segregated; heterosexual relationships evolve, laying the foundation for intimate long-term relationships; strong, intimate friendships develop; cliques appear, providing strong social and emotional support; begins to engage in adult activities (e.g., voting, drinking, and working); uses fantasy to imagine sexual encounters and relationships; enhances sexuality by focusing

on male and female stereotypic activities such as driving fast cars, wearing "sexy" clothing, and lifting weights; romance novels become popular, and activities such as shopping and spending time in clothing and department stores increase with adolescent girls

4. Common coping skills—problem solving; use of defenses (e.g., reaction formation, displacement, identification, suppression, rationalization, intellectualization, denial, conversion reaction); use of humor, increased socialization, engaging in high-risk behaviors such as consumption of alcohol or illicit substances, reckless driving, decreased or increased appetite or intake of food, nail biting, sleep disturbances, acts in rebellious manner, acts irresponsibly, withdrawn, isolates self from family and friends

5. Role of parents—conflicts with parents may arise, primarily out of adolescent's need to be independent; parents are influential, subconsciously and unconsciously, in the adaptation and use of values and beliefs in making decisions

6. Plan—facilitate and support social development

Socialization Behaviors

1. Peers acquire increasing importance as source of psychosocial and emotional support.
2. Influence of parents shifts to less than primary importance as peer influence increases.
3. Conflicts may emerge as adolescent attempts to resolve conflicts in values and beliefs between peers and family.
4. Sense of belonging to peer group can result in behavioral conformity as it relates to attitudes, activities, speech, dress, and lifestyle.
5. Membership in groups and clubs based on areas of mutual interest (e.g., sports, hobbies, recreational interests, cultural, volunteer).
6. Strong relationships exist with small group of friends.

Moral Development (Postconventional Stage)

1. Postconventional stage is not universally attained by adolescents.
2. May apply ideals to moral predicaments (justice, charity).

Faith Development (Individuating-Reflexive Stage)

1. Rejection of religious beliefs or becoming very religious may occur.
2. Regression to earlier stages may occur to obtain comfort.
3. Acceptance and rejection of beliefs may be influenced by peer group.

REFERENCES

American Dental Association: Tooth Eruption Charts, *American Dental Association,* (serial online): www.ada.org/public/topics/tooth_eruption.asp. Accessed April 11, 2007.

American Speech-Language-Hearing Association: How does your child hear and talk? *American Speech-Language-Hearing Association* (serial online): www.asha.org/public/speech/development/child_hear_talk.htm. Accessed January 17, 2006.

Atherton JS: Piaget's developmental theory, *Learning and Teaching* (serial online): www.learningandteaching.info/learning/piaget.htm. Accessed January 14, 2006.

Betz C, Hunsberger M, Wright S: *Family-centered nursing care of children,* ed 2, Philadelphia, 1994, WB Saunders.

Bowlby J: *Attachment and loss,* vol. 5, New York, 1980, Basic Books.

Child Development Institute: Language development in children, *Child Development & Parenting Information* (serial online): www.childdevelopmentinfo.com/development/language_development.shtml. Accessed January 17, 2006.

DeBord K: *Helping children coping with stress,* Raleigh, NC: North Carolina State University, College of Agriculture and Life Sciences, North Carolina Extension Service (website): www.ces.ncsu.edu/depts/fcs/human/pubs/copestress.html. Accessed January 14, 2006.

Elkind D: Egocentrism in adolescence. *Child Development,* 38(4):1025, 1967.

Erikson E: *Childhood and society,* New York, 1950, Norton.

Erikson E: *Identity and the life cycle: Selected papers, psychological issues* (Monograph Vol. 1, No. 1). New York, 1959, International Press.

Green, M et al, editors: *Bright futures: Guidelines for health supervision of infants, children, and adolescents, Pocket Guide—2001 Update,* ed 2, Washington, DC, 2001, National Center for Education in Maternal and Child Health(website): www.brightfutures.org/pocket/pdf/i_xvii.pdf. Accessed January 17, 2006.

Huitt W: Socioemotional development, *Educational Psychology Interactive,* Valdosta, GA, 1997, Valdosta State University (website): http://chiron.valdosta.edu/whuitt/col/affsys/erikson.html. Accessed January 4, 2006.

Huitt W, Hummel J: Piaget's theory of cognitive development, *Educational Psychology Interactive,* Valdosta, GA, 2003, Valdosta State University (website): http://chiron.valdosta.edu/whuitt/col/cogsys/piaget.html. Accessed January 4, 2006.

Kohlberg L: Stages in the development of moral thought and action, New York, 1969, Holt, Reinhart, & Winston.

Learning Disabilities Association of America: Speech and language milestone chart, *LD OnLine* (website): www.ldonline.org/ld_indepth/speech-language/lda_milestones.html. Accessed January 17, 2006.

Lucile Packhard Children's Hospital at Stanford: Dental and oral health: Anatomy and development of the mouth and teeth, *Lucile Packhard Children's Hospital at Stanford* (serial online) www.lpch.org/DiseaseHealthInfo/HealthLibrary/dental/teethanat.html. Accessed January 14, 2006.

Oesterreich L: Ages & stages—three-year-olds, In: L. Oesterreich, B. Holt, and S. Karas, *Iowa family child care handbook,* Ames, IA, 1995, Iowa State University Extension. National Network for Child Care (website): www.nncc.org/Child.Dev/ages.stages.3y.html. Accessed January 19, 2006.

Piaget J: *The psychology of the child,* New York, 1972, Basic Books.

Piaget J: *The psychology of intelligence,* Towota, NJ, 1976, Littlefied, Adams.

Piaget J: *The child's conception of the world,* New York, 1990, Littlefield, Adams.

Piaget J, Inhelder B: The growth of logical thinking from children to adolescence, New York, 1958, Basic Books.

Powell J, Smith CA: The 1st year. In: *Developmental milestones: A guide for parents,* Manhattan, KS, 1994, Kansas State Universiy Cooperative Extension Seervice (website): www.nncc.org/Child.Dev/mile1.html. Accessed January 17, 2006.

Zero to Three: *Helping Your Child Learn to Talk* (website): www.zerotothree.org/site/PageServer?pagename=ter_reg_language_tipstalking&AddInterest=1145. Accessed June 5, 2007.

C

❖

Immunizations

Two major roles played by the nurse caring for infants and children are educating parents about immunizations and reviewing the immunization status of each child. The following are some risk factors for failure of children to be immunized: low educational level and/or low socioeconomic status of the parent(s), nonwhite race, young parental age, large family size, single parent, lack of prenatal care, lack of parental knowledge regarding immunizations, misconceptions regarding immunizations, and late start with immunizations. Nurses should be aware of these risk factors and target those populations for education. Ongoing active immunization efforts are necessary to ensure that infectious disease continues to be a rare occurrence in the United States. All 50 states have immunization requirements that must be met for a child to enroll in school. This has resulted in immunization rates of close to 100% for school-aged children in the United States.

Some terms must be understood. *Immunity* is the resistance to or protection against a specific disease or infectious agent. There are basically three types of immunity: active, artificial, and passive. *Active immunity* is a long-lasting immunity that results when the body is stimulated to produce its own antibodies. *Artificial immunity* is a type of active immunity in which antibody production is caused by the introduction of antigens in the form of toxoids and vaccines rather than by a specific disease entity. A toxoid is a bacterial toxin that has been chemically treated or heat-treated to reduce its virulence without destroying its ability to stimulate the production of antibodies (e.g., the diphtheria and tetanus toxoids). A suspension of the actual microorganisms in weakened or killed form is a vaccine.

Typhoid, pertussis, measles, mumps, and rubella are examples of diseases for which there are vaccines. Finally, *passive immunity* is a form of immediate but transient protection against infectious disease. This type of immunity can be obtained through the administration of preparations of convalescent serum or adult blood products that contain antibodies previously formed against an infectious agent. Passive immunity provides only limited protection against infectious disease.

Box C-1 gives a recommended schedule for the immunization of normal or well children. Because there are frequent changes to the immunization schedule, the reader should double-check information with the American Academy of Pediatrics (AAP) Committee on Infectious Diseases.

VARIOUS VACCINES AND TOXOIDS
Diphtheria, Tetanus, and Pertussis

The diphtheria, tetanus, and acellular pertussis (DTaP) vaccine is made up of a mixture of three antigens (diphtheria and tetanus toxoids and acellular pertussis vaccine) and a mineral substance that prolongs and enhances the antigenic properties by delaying absorption. Although the diphtheria toxoid does not produce absolute immunity, when it is given on the recommended schedule, protective levels of antitoxin continue for 10 years or more. There are three forms of the tetanus immunizing agent: tetanus toxoid, tetanus immune globulin (human), and tetanus antitoxin (usually horse serum). A new tetanus toxoid (Tdap, adolescent preparation) is recommended for adolescents, aged 11 to 12 years who have received previous (DTaP/DTP) vaccinations and have not received the (Td) booster dose. The recommended dose and route are 0.5 ml intramuscularly (IM). A booster of tetanus and diphtheria (Td) vaccine should be given (0.5 ml IM) every 10 years.

Poliomyelitis

Inactivated poliovirus vaccine (IPV) is used in providing immunity to all three types of poliovirus that cause paralytic poliomyelitis. The recommended dose and route are 0.5 ml subcutaneously (subQ) or IM.

BOX C-1

ACIP, AAP, and AAFP Immunization Recommendations

HBV
- Birth to 2 months
- 1 to 4 months
- 6 to 18 months

DTP
- 2 months
- 4 months
- 6 months
- 12 to 18 months
- 4 to 6 years

HapA
- 12 to 23 months
- 2 years
- 2 years + 6–18 months

HIB
- 2 months
- 4 months
- 6 months
- 12 to 15 months

PCV7
- 2 months
- 4 months
- 6 months
- 12–15 months

Polio (Inactivated Poliovirus)
- 2 months
- 4 months
- 6 to 18 months
- 4 to 6 years

MMR
- 12–15 months
- 4–6 years

BOX C-1
ACIP, AAP, and AAFP Immunization Recommendations—cont'd

Tdap
- 11–12 years

MCV4
- 11–12 years

Varicella
- 12 to 18 months

Recommended Ages for Immunizations and Screenings
- Birth: HBV
- 2 months: DTP, IPV, HBC, HBV
- 4 months: DTP, IPV, HBC, HBV*
- 6 months: DTP, HBC, HBV
- 12 months: tuberculin test (depending on the risk of exposure, it may be administered yearly or every other year after this age), varicella vaccine (12 to 18 months)
- 15 months: MMR, HBC
- 12 to 18 months: DTP, IPV, HBC
- 15 to 18 months: DTaP, HBC
- 4 to 6 years: DTP, IPV
- 10 to 14 years: MMR
- 11 to 12 years: Tdap, MCV4

AAFP, American Academy of Family Physicians; AAP, American Academy of Pediatrics; ACIP, Advisory Committee on Immunization Practices; DTaP, diphtheria and tetanus toxoids and acellular pertussis vaccine; DTP, diphtheria and tetanus toxoids with pertussis vaccine; HAV, hepatitis A vaccine; HBC, *Haemophilus* influenzae type B conjugate vaccine; HBV, hepatitis B vaccine; Hib, *Haemophilus* influenzae type B3 conjugate vaccine; MMR, live measles, mumps, and rubella viruses combined in a vaccine; PCV7, 7-valent, pneumococcal polysaccharide-protein conjugate vaccine; Td, tetanus and diphtheria vaccine.
*not needed if monovalent HepB vaccine used.

Measles, Mumps, and Rubella
Live viruses for measles, mumps, and rubella (MMR) are usually combined into one vaccine. This one vaccine may provide lifelong immunity to each disease. The rubella portion is extremely important in controlling congenital rubella syndrome. The recommended dose and route are 0.5 ml subQ.

Haemophilus Influenzae Type B

The *Haemophilus influenzae* type B vaccine is a polysaccharide inactive vaccine. Three types of this vaccine are currently available, all of which appear to be equally effective: HBOC, PRP-OMP, and PRP-D (refer to AAP guidelines for recommendations for vaccine regimen). This vaccine provides protection against the *H. influenzae* bacteria, which can cause meningitis, epiglottitis, septic arthritis, sepsis, and bacterial pneumonia. The recommended dose and route are 0.5 ml IM.

Hepatitis B

Hepatitis B is a potentially fatal viral infection that can cause cirrhosis or liver cancer. The hepatitis B virus (HBV) vaccine can be administered at different sites simultaneously with the diphtheria-tetanus-pertussis (DTP), MMR, and *H. influenzae* B conjugate (HBC) vaccines. Pain and soreness at the injection site are the most common side effects. Infants should receive the vaccine before discharge from the hospital. Hepatitis B can be given in 4 doses when it is given in combination with other vaccines following birth dose, 4 month dose not needed if monovalent HepB vaccine administered. Hepatitis B vaccine is considered appropriate for all children, for adolescents who are sexually active with multiple partners, for persons with developmental disabilities, and for health care professionals. Protection is estimated to last a lifetime. The recommended dose and route are 0.5 ml IM.

Varicella

Children targeted for vaccination against varicella are infants between 12 and 18 months of age and older school-aged children who have not had varicella and who have not been previously immunized. Adolescents over the age of 13 should receive two doses of the vaccine, at least 4 weeks apart. This vaccine can be given with diphtheria, tetanus, DTP, polio, hepatitis B, and *H. influenzae* type B vaccines. Duration of immunity is not known. The recommended dose and route are 0.5 ml subQ.

Pneumococcal Infection

Infection with *Streptococcus pneumoniae* may cause meningitis and pneumonia. Pneumococcal infection is the leading cause of bacterial meningitis in the United States. The recommended dose and route are 0.5 ml IM.

Meningococcal Disease

On January 14, 2005, the Federal Drug Administration recommended that all children ages 11 to 12 years and unvaccinated teens ages 15 years entering high school should receive the meningococcal vaccine (MCV4). It is also recommended that entering college students (freshmen) who will be living in college dorms receive the MCV4 vaccine or the meningococcal vaccine (MPSV4).

Hepatitis A

Hepatitis A is transmitted via the oral-fecal route. Poor handwashing is a known contributor to its transmission. HapA vaccine series is now recommended for all children 1 year of age. The two doses of HapA are administered 6 months apart. The recommended dose and route for the vaccine are 0.5 ml IM.

POSSIBLE REACTIONS

Slight reactions to the DTP vaccine are not unusual. Local reactions (redness and edema) at the injection site are common. Mild to moderate temperature elevations and irritability may occur, but they usually resolve within a few hours. Seizures or neurologic damage occur on rare occasions after the administration of the DTP vaccine. If severe reactions occur (such as hypotonia or seizure), the pertussis portion of the vaccine may be eliminated in future vaccinations. Very rarely, vaccine-induced disease results; however, this event usually occurs only in immunosuppressed children. Fever and rash have occurred after the administration of the MMR vaccine. Side effects of the varicella vaccine include a maculopapular rash with up to five lesions at the injection site or elsewhere, and pain or redness at the injection site. Possible pneumococcal vaccine side effects are soreness, redness, or swelling at the injection site or low-grade fever. Most children who receive hepatitis type A vaccine are asymptomatic; however, some may have nonspecific symptoms such as fever and nausea.

CONTRAINDICATIONS

Any time an acute febrile illness is present, immunizations should be postponed. Administration of live-virus vaccines is contraindicated in individuals with leukemia, lymphoma, malignancies, or immunodeficiency diseases; children with marked sensitivity to eggs, chicken, or neomycin; children on immunosuppressive therapy; children who have recently received immune serum globulin plasma or blood products; and pregnant females. A physician's consent must be obtained before administering other immunizations to such individuals. The pertussis vaccine is contraindicated in those children with a history of previous reaction to the DTP vaccine. Anaphylactic reaction to any vaccine contraindicates future administration of that vaccine.

BOX C-2
Resources

- American Academy of Pediatrics: www.aap.org
- Children's Vaccine Program: www.childrensvaccine.org
- ImmunoFacts: www.immunofacts.com
- National Immunization Program of the Centers for Disease Control and Prevention: www.cdc.gov/nip

REFERENCES

Advisory Committee on Immunization Practices, American Academy of Pediatrics, and American Academy of Family Physicians: *Recommended childhood immunization schedule—United States, 2006* (website): www.cdc.gov/preview/mmwrhtml/mm545/-Immunizational.htm. Accessed June 5, 2007.

Center for Disease Control: 2007 Childhood & Adolescent Immunization Schedule, 2005 (website): www.cdc.gov/nip/recs/child-schedule-color-print.pdf. Accessed June 5, 2007.

Evers DB: Teaching mothers about childhood immunizations, *MCN* 26(5):253, 2001.

Paulson PR, Hammer AL: Pediatric immunization update 2002, *Pediatr Nurs* 28(2):173, 2002.

D

Laboratory Values

The following are normal laboratory values unless otherwise stated.

1. Acetone, ketone bodies (serum)
   a. Newborn to age 1 week: slightly higher than values for ages over 1 week
   b. Ages over 1 week
      i. Acetone: 0.3 to 2.0 mg/dl (51.6 to 344 μmol/L) (International System [SI] units)
      ii. Ketones: 2 to 4 mg/dl
2. Alanine transaminase (ALT): 0-50 u/L
3. Albumin (serum)
   a. Newborn: 2.9 to 5.4 g/dl
   b. Infant: 4.4 to 5.4 g/dl
   c. Child: 4.0 to 5.8 g/dl
4. Albumin in meconium: negative
5. Alcohol (serum): negative; toxic level: greater than 300 mg/dl
6. Alpha fetoprotein level: less than or equal to 50 ng/ml
7. Ammonia (serum)
   a. Newborn: 64 to 107 mcg/dl
   b. Child: 29 to 70 mcg/dl (29 to 7 μmol/L) (SI units)
8. Amylase dehydrogenase (serum)—child: 45 to 200 dye units/dl
9. Arterial blood gases
   a. Partial pressure of oxygen (Po_2): 75 to 100 mm Hg
   b. Partial pressure of carbon dioxide (Pco_2)
      i. Infant: 27 to 40 mm Hg
      ii. All other ages: 35 to 45 mm Hg

   c. pH
      i. Premature infant (cord): 7.15 to 7.35
      ii. Premature infant (age 48 hours): 7.35 to 7.5
      iii. Newborn: 7.27 to 7.47
      iv. Infant: 7.35 to 7.45
      v. Child: 7.35 to 7.45
10. Aspartate transaminase (AST)
    a. Birth to 1 year: not determined
    b. 2 to 18 years: 2 to 4 μ/L
11. Bilirubin
    a. Total
       i. Newborn: 2.0 to 6.0 mg/dl
       ii. Age 48 hours: 6.0 to 7.0 mg/dl
       iii. Age 5 days: 4.0 to 12.0 mg/dl
       iv. Age 1 month to adult: 0.3 to 1.2 mg/dl
    b. Indirect (unconjugated)—age 1 month to adult: 0.3 to 1.1 mg/dl
    c. Direct (conjugated)—age 1 month to adult: 0.1 to 0.4 mg/dl
12. Bleeding time
    a. Normal time: 2 to 7 minutes
    b. Borderline time: 7 to 11 minutes
13. Blood urea nitrogen (BUN) (serum)
    a. Newborn: 8 to 18 mg/dl
    b. Infant or child: 5 to 18 mg/dl
    c. Adolescent: 8 to 17 mg/dl
14. Calcium (serum)
    a. Premature infant: 6 to 10 mg/dl
    b. Full-term infant: 7.5 to 11 mg/dl
    c. Child: 8.8 to 10.8 mg/dl
    d. Adolescent: 8.4 to 10.2 mg/dl
15. Carotene (serum)—child: 40 to 130 mcg/dl
16. Catecholamines
    a. Values for child lower than those for adult
    b. Total
       i. Random urine: 0 to 14 mcg/dl
       ii. 24-hour urine: less than 100 g/24 hr
    c. Epinephrine: less than 10 ng/24 hr
    d. Norepinephrine: less than 100 ng/24 hr
    e. Metanephrines: less than 100 ng/24 hr

17. Cerebrospinal fluid (CSF)
    a. Specific gravity: 1.007 to 1.009
    b. Glucose
        i. Infant or child: 60 to 80 mg/dl
        ii. All other ages: 40 to 80 mg/dl
    c. Protein
        i. Newborn: 45 to 100 mg/dl
        ii. Child: 10 to 20 mg/dl
        iii. Adolescent: 15 to 40 mg/dl
    d. Cell count
        i. Neonate: 0.5 polymorphonuclear cells; 0 to 5 mononuclear cells; 0 to 5 red blood cells (RBCs)/mm^3
        ii. All other ages: 0 polymorphonuclear cells; 0 to 5 mononuclear cells; 0 to 5 RBCs/mm^3
18. Cholesterol (serum)
    a. Age 1 to 4 years: less than or equal to 210 mg/dl
    b. Age 5 to 14 years: less than or equal to 220 mg/dl
    c. Age 15 to 20 years: less than or equal to 235 mg/dl
19. Copper (Cu) (serum)
    a. Newborn: 20 to 70 mcg/dl
    b. Child: 30 to 190 mcg/dl
    c. Adolescent: 90 to 240 mcg/dl
20. C-reactive protein (CRP) (serum)—child: less than 10 mg/L
21. Creatine phosphokinase (CPK)
    a. Infant: 20 to 31 units/L
    b. Infant to adolescent: 15 to 50 units/L
22. Creatinine (serum)
    a. Cord: 0.6 to 1.2 mg/dl
    b. Newborn: 0.3 to 1.0 mg/dl
    c. Infant: 0.2 to 0.4 mg/dl
    d. Child: 0.3 to 0.7 mg/dl
    e. Adolescent: 0.5 to 1.0 mg/dl
23. Cortisol (plasma)—child
    a. At 8 am: 15 to 25 mcg/dl
    b. At 4 pm: 5 to 10 mcg/dl
24. Culture results—blood, throat, sputum, wound, skin, stool, urine: negative or no growth of pathogen

25. Electrolytes (serum)
    a. Sodium (Na^+)
       i. Premature infant: 132 to 140 mmol/L
       ii. Infant: 139 to 146 mmol/L
       iii. Child: 138 to 145 mmol/L
       iv. Adolescent: 136 to 146 mmol/L
    b. Potassium (K^+)
       i. Infant: 4.1 to 5.3 mmol/L
       ii. Child: 3.4 to 4.7 mmol/L
       iii. Adolescent: 3.5 to 5.1 mmol/L
    c. Chlorine (Cl^-): 98 to 106 mmol/L
    d. Carbon dioxide (CO_2)
       i. Infant: 27 to 41 mm Hg
       ii. Child (male): 35 to 48 mm Hg
       iii. Child (female): 32 to 45 mm Hg
26. Enzyme-linked immunosorbent assay (ELISA): negative
27. Epstein-Barr virus (EB) testing
    a. IgM viral capsid antigen (VCA): elevated during acute phase of illness
    b. IgG VCA: elevated during acute phase of illness
    c. Epstein Barr nuclear antigen (NA) EBNA: elevated following acute illness (6 to 12 weeks after acute stage)
28. Erythrocyte protoporphyrin concentration—1 to 2 years: 8 µg/dl of red blood cells
29. Erythrocyte sedimentation rate (ESR, sed rate)
    a. Newborn: 0 to 2 mm/hr
    b. Age 4 to 14 years: 0 to 10 mm/hr
30. Fasting blood glucose
    a. Newborn: 30 to 80 mg/dl
    b. Child: 60 to 100 mg/dl
31. Fecal occult blood: negative
32. Ferritin concentration (serum)—abnormal: less than 10 to 12 mcg/L
33. Ferritin determination (serum)
    a. Newborn: 20 to 200 ng/ml
    b. 1 month: 200 to 500 ng/ml
    c. 2 to 12 months: 30 to 200 ng/ml
    d. 1 to 16 years: 8 to 140 ng/ml

34. Fibrin degradation products (FDP) (serum)
    a. Adult: 2 to 10 mcg/ml
    b. Child: test not usually performed
35. Fibrinogen level (plasma)
    a. Newborn: 150 to 300 mg/dl
    b. Child: 200 to 400 mg/dl
36. Gastric pH: 1.5 to 3.5
37. Glucose (serum): 40 to 100 mg/dl
38. Glucose tolerance test (GTT) results (oral)—child 6 years or older:

Time (hr)	Whole Blood (mg/dl)	Serum (mg/dl)
{½}	<150	<160
1	<160	<170
2	<115	<125
3	60–100	70–110

39. Hematocrit (Hct)
    a. Newborn: 44% to 75%
    b. Infant: 28% to 42%
    c. Age 6 to 12 years: 35% to 45%
    d. Age 12 to 18 years (male): 37% to 49%
    e. Age 12 to 18 years (female): 36% to 46%
40. Hemoglobin (Hb)
    a. Age 1 to 3 days: 14.5 to 22.5 g/dl
    b. Age 2 months: 9.0 to 14.0 g/dl
    c. Age 6 to 12 years: 11.5 to 15.5 g/dl
    d. Age 12 to 18 years (male): 13.0 to 16.0 g/dl
    e. Age 12 to 18 years (female): 12.0 to 16.0 g/dl
41. Hemoglobin electrophoresis (hemoglobin F [Hb F])
    a. Newborn: Hb F, 50% to 80% of total Hb
    b. Infant: Hb F, 8% of total Hb
    c. Child: Hb F, 1% to 2% of total Hb after 6 months
42. Human immunodeficiency virus type 1 (HIV-1) (serum)—child: seronegative

43. Human leukocyte antigen (HLA)—identifies specific leukocyte antigens
44. Immunoglobulin (Ig) values (serum):

%	Total	NEW-BORN	3 MO	6 MO	1–3 YR	4–6 YR	6–16 YR
IgG	80	650–1250	275–750	200–1100	300–1400	550–1500	700–1650
IgA	15	0–12	5–55	10–90	20–150	50–175	50–225
IgM	4	5–30	15–70	10–80	20–230	20–100	22–260
IgD	0.2	—	—	—	—	—	—
IgE	0.0002	—	—	—	<10	<25	<62

45. Iron (serum): 50 to 120 mcg/dl
46. Iron concentration (serum): 30 to 70 mcg/g
47. Lactic dehydrogenase (LDH) (serum)
    a. Newborn: 300 to 1500 international units/L
    b. Child: 50 to 150 international units/L; 100 to 295 units/L
48. Low-density lipoprotein (LDL) cholesterol levels (ages 2 to 19): greater than 130 mg/dl (3.36 mmol/L) should be monitored; greater than 160 mg/dl (4.14 mmol/L) and parental risk factors indicate need for drug therapy; greater than 190 mg/dl (4.91 mmol/L) without parental risk factors indicates need for drug therapy
49. Lead (serum)—child: normal range, 10 to 20 mcg/dl
50. Lipase (serum)
    a. Infant: 9 to 105 units/L
    b. All other ages: 20 to 180 units/L
51. Magnesium (serum)
    a. Newborn: 1.4 to 2.9 mEq/L
    b. Child: 1.6 to 2.6 mEq/L
52. Microlymphocytotoxicity test—identifies specific leukocyte antigens
53. Osmolality (serum)—child: 270 to 290 mOsm/kg
54. Osmolality (urine)
    a. Newborn: 100 to 600 mOsm/L
    b. Child: 50 to 1200 mOsm/L; usual range, 300 to 900 mOsm/L
55. Ova and parasites (O and P) (feces)

    a. Child: negative
    b. Parasites most often found in stool: roundworms, ameba, hookworms, protozoa, tapeworms
56. Partial thromboplastin time (PTT) and activated partial thromboplastin time (APTT)
    a. Newborn to age 3 months: higher than adult times
    b. Child: higher than adult times
    c. Adult: PTT, 30 to 45 seconds; APTT, 35 to 45 seconds
57. Phosphorus (serum)
    a. Premature infant: 4.6 to 8.0 mg/dl
    b. Newborn: 5.0 to 7.8 mg/dl
58. Plasminogen (plasma)—adult: 2.5 to 5.2 units/ml; 20 mg/dl
59. Platelet count
    a. Newborn: 84,000 to 478,000/mcl
    b. All other ages: 150,000 to 400,000/mcl
60. Polymerase chain reaction (PCR): DNA-negative
61. Protein (serum)
    a. Premature infant: 4.2 to 7.6 g/dl
    b. Newborn: 4.6 to 7.4 g/dl
    c. Infant: 6.0 to 6.7 g/dl
    d. Child: 6.2 to 8.0 g/dl
62. Protein (urine)
    a. Values higher in children
    b. Random urine specimen: negative, 0 to 5 mg/dl; positive, 6 to 2000 mg/dl
    c. 24-hour urine specimen: 25 to 150 mg/24 hr
63. Prothrombin time (PT, pro time)
    a. Newborn: 12 to 21 seconds
    b. All other ages: 11 to 15 seconds
64. Red blood cells (RBCs)
    a. Infant (1 to 18 months): 2.7×10^6 to $5.4 \times 106/mm^3$
    b. Preschooler: $4.27 \times 10^6/mm^3$
    c. School-age: $4.31 \times 10^6/mm^3$
    d. Adolescent: $4.60 \times 10^6/mm^3$
65. Reticulocyte count
    a. Birth to 6 months: 3% to 7%
    b. Six months to 2 years: 0.3% to 2.2%

      c. All other ages: 0.5% to 1.5%

66. Serum glutamic-pyruvic transaminase (SGPT)

      a. Age 6 to 12 months: 16 to 36 international units/L

      b. Age 2 to 17 years: 622 international units/L

67. Serum glutamic-oxaloacetic transaminase (SGOT)

      a. Age 6 to 12 months: less than or equal to 40 international units/L

      b. Age 2 to 17 years: 10 to 30 international units/L

68. Southern blot test—detects mitochondrial deletions

69. Sweat test results: negative

70. Testosterone (total) (serum)

      a. 1 to 5 years

         i. Male: 0.3 to 30.0 ng/dl

         ii. Female: 2 to 20 ng/dl

71. Testosterone (free) (serum)

      a. 6 to 9 years

         i. Male: 0.1 to 3.2 pg/mL

         ii. Female: 0.1 to 0.9 pg/mL

72. Thyroid-stimulating hormone (TSH) (serum)—newborn: less than 7 mL/units/L

73. Toxoplasmosis, rubella, cytomegalovirus, and herpes simplex (TORCH) titer—infant under 2 months: negative

74. Transferrin (serum): 200 to 400 mg/dl

75. Triglycerides (serum)

      a. Infant: 5 to 40 mg/dl

      b. Child (5 to 11 years): 10 to 135 mg/dl

      c. Adolescent or young adult (12 to 29 years): 10 to 140 mg/dl

76. Uric acid (serum)

      a. Female: 2.0 to 6.0 mg/dl

      b. Male: 3.0 to 7.0 mg/dl

77. Urinalysis

      a. Specific gravity: 1.003 to 1.035

      b. pH

         i. Infant: 5.0 to 7.0

         ii. All other ages: 4.8 to 7.8

      c. Protein: negative

      d. Blood: negative

      e. Glucose: negative

      f. Ketones: negative

78. Urine, 24-hour
    Sodium
    a. 6 to 10 years
        i. Male: 41 to 115 mEq/24 hr
        ii. Female: 20 to 69 mEq/24 hr
    b. 10 to 14 years
        i. Male: 63 to 117 mEq/24 hr
        ii. Female: 48 to 168 mEq/24 hr
    Chloride
    a. Infant: 2 to 10 mEq/24 hr
    b. Child younger than 6 years: 15 to 40 mEq/24 hr
    c. 6 to 10 years
        i. Male: 36 to 110 mEq/24 hr
        ii. Female: 18 to 74 mEq/24 hr
    d. 10 to 14 years
        i. Male: 64 to 176 mEq/hr
        ii. Female: 36 to 173 mEq/hr
    Potassium
    a. Infant: 4.1 to 5.3 mEq/24 hr
    b. 6 to 10 years
        i. Male: 17 to 54 mEq/24 hr
        ii. Female: 8 to 37 mEq/24 hr
    c. 10 to 14 years
        i. Male: 22 to 57 mEq/24 hr
        ii. Female: 18 to 58 mEq/24 hr
    Calcium
    Infant/child: less than 6 mg/kg/d
    Magnesium
    1.3 to 2.3 mg/dl
79. Urine level of reducing substances
    a. Glucose: negative
    b. Galactose: negative
80. Urine phenylpyruvic acid: negative
81. Urine toxic screens
    a. Amphetamine: negative; toxic level: 1000 ng/ml (cutoff value)
    b. Cannabinoids (e.g., marijuana): negative; toxic level: 50 ng/ml (cutoff value)
    c. Cocaine: negative; toxic level: 1 to 215 ng/ml

    d. Methadone: negative; toxic level: 300 ng/ml (cutoff value)

    e. Opiates (e.g., morphine): negative; toxic level: 2000 ng/ml (cutoff value)

82. Western blot: negative

83. White blood cell (WBC) count
    a. Infant: 6000 to 17,500/mm^3
    b. Preschooler: 5500 to 15,500/mm^3
    c. School-aged child: 4500 to 13,500/mm^3
    d. Adolescent: 4500 to 11,000/mm^3

84. White blood cell differential:

Cell Type	Percentage of Total	Values (mcl/mm^3)
Neutrophils		
Total	61 (newborn)	—
	32 (1 yr)	—
	50–70 (>1 yr)	2500–7000
Segmented	50–65 (>1 yr)	2500–6500
Band	0–5 (>1 yr)	0–500
Eosinophils	1–3	100–300
Basophils	0.4–1.0	40–100
Monocytes	4–9 (1–12 yr)	—
	4–6 (>12 yr)	200–600
Lymphocytes	34 (newborn)	—
	60 (1 yr)	—
	42 (6 yr)	—
	38 (12 yr)	—
	25–35 (>12 yr)	1700–3500

REFERENCES

Kee JL: *Laboratory and diagnostic tests with nursing implications*, ed 4, East Norwalk, Conn, 1995, Appleton & Lange.

Malarkey LM, McMorrow MC: *Saunders nursing guide to laboratory and diagnostic tests*, St. Louis, 2005, WB Saunders.

National Institutes of Health Clinical Center: *Pediatric laboratory ranges, October 12, 2004* (website): http://clinicalcenter.nih.gov/ccc/pedweb/pedsstaff/pedlab.html. Accessed June 5, 2005.

Watson J, Jaffe M: *Nurse's manual of laboratory and diagnostic tests*, Philadelphia, 1995, FA Davis.

E

❖

Height and Weight Growth Curves

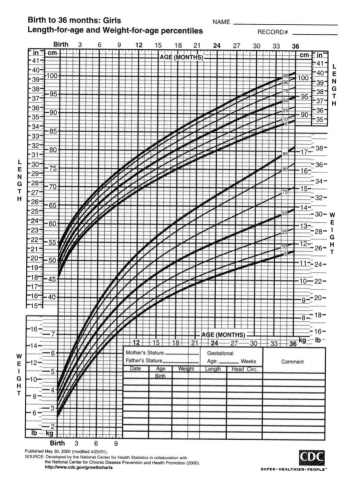

Figure E-1 Girls: birth to 36 months. Length and weight. These charts were developed by the National Center for Health Statistics in collaboration with the National Center for Chronic Disease Prevention and Health Promotion, 2000. The data on these charts are considered representative of the general United States population.

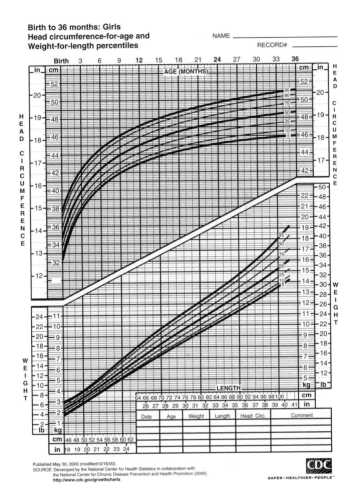

Figure E-2   Girls: birth to 36 months. Head circumference, length, and weight.

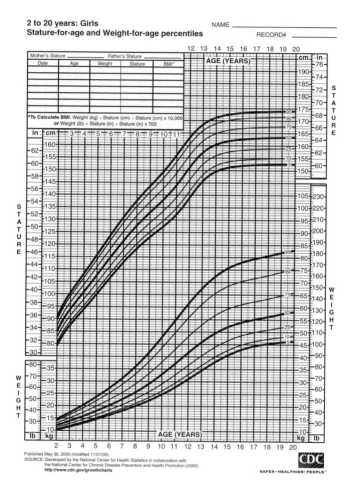

Figure E-3 Girls: 2 to 20 years. Stature and weight.

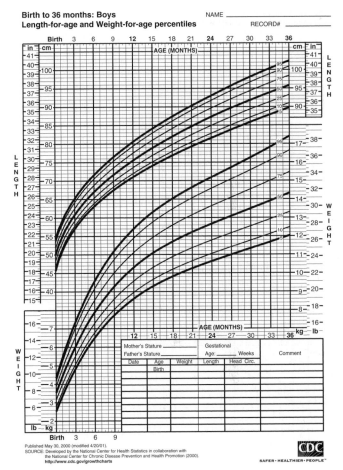

Figure E-4 Boys: birth to 36 months. Length and weight.

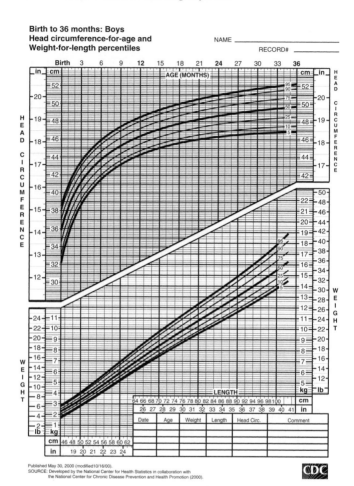

Birth to 36 months: Boys
Head circumference-for-age and
Weight-for-length percentiles

NAME _____

RECORD# _____

Published May 30, 2000 (modified10/16/00).
SOURCE: Developed by the National Center for Health Statistics in collaboration with
the National Center for Chronic Disease Prevention and Health Promotion (2000).

Figure E-5 Boys: birth to 36 months. Head circumference, length, and weight.

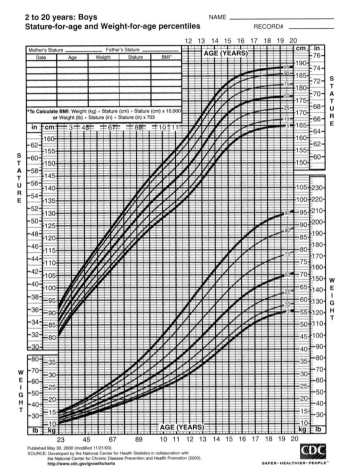

Figure E-6   Boys: 2 to 20 years. Stature and weight.

F

❖

Psychosocial Interventions

PREPARATION FOR PROCEDURES OR SURGERY

1. Prepare child and parents for procedure or surgery.
   a. Provide age-appropriate explanations.
      i. For younger children, use of sensory materials such as graphics (e.g., pictures) or props (e.g., bandages, surgical mask) enhances child's comprehension.
      ii. For older children, use of illustrations such as films, pictures (e.g., anatomic figures), computer simulations, and videos is helpful to supplement explanation.
   b. Explain procedure or surgery and preoperative routine in terms of sequence of events to occur, including sensory information (e.g., mouth will feel dry, child will feel sleepy).
   c. For younger children, encourage preprocedural play such as using medical equipment, doll, or stuffed animal as means of explaining procedure or surgery.
   d. Use age-appropriate means for explaining body changes following procedure or surgery and for eliciting concerns from child.
   e. Provide and reinforce information for parents about child's condition and treatment to help them answer their child's questions or relieve their own anxiety.
   f. Assure child that procedure is not being done because child is "bad."
   g. Use of distraction such as play, use of dolls, humor may be helpful.

2. Prepare child and parents emotionally for surgery.
   a. Provide understandable explanations in lay terms.
   b. Use active listening to elicit concerns.
   c. Encourage expression of feelings (e.g., guilt, anger, anxiety, feeling of being overwhelmed).
   d. Encourage expression of fears concerning child's well-being.
   e. Provide anticipatory information about emotional responses to surgery.
   f. Encourage parents to room in and participate in child's care as means of promoting security and decreasing anxiety.
   g. Encourage parental participation during selected procedures; some procedures can be very traumatic for parents and convey erroneous message to younger child that parents cannot "protect" child from harm.
   h. Encourage parental participation during induction of anesthesia and during recovery (if applicable).
   i. Provide for parents' physical comforts (e.g., sleeping and hygiene).
   j. Encourage use of preexisting support systems such as family members, close friends, and clergy.
   k. Encourage incorporation of some home routines—such as use of child's blanket, praying, and storytelling—into hospital routine.
   l. Assist parents in providing support and information to siblings while child is hospitalized.
   m. If needed, provide information to parents about addressing sibling needs such as by disclosing information about child's clinical status, maintaining household routines, arranging for family members or friends to supplement parents' caretaking activities, and communicating with school personnel.
3. Assist and support child during preoperative laboratory and diagnostic tests.
   a. Prepare or provide information about upcoming procedures (e.g., complete blood count, urinalysis, laboratory and diagnostic tests).

   b. Assist in collection of preoperative laboratory and diag-
      nostic data with sensitivity to the child's emotional
      responses of anxiety, fear, and need for modesty.
   c. Prepare child for surgery by obtaining nursing assess-
      ment data such as evaluation of body systems and
      nursing history.
   d. Monitor child's reactions to presurgical or preprocedural
      preparations.
4. Monitor child's baseline status before surgery or procedure.
   a. Vital signs
   b. Body system assessment (refer to Nursing Assessment in
      Appendix A)

SUPPORTIVE CARE

1. Alleviate anxiety caused by various aspects of hospital
   experience, including invasive procedures for diagnostic
   tests, pain, threatening and confusing hospital environment,
   unfamiliar hospital personnel, knowledge deficit pertaining
   to hospital routines and treatments, and age-related fears.
   a. Provide therapeutic play and/or explanations during all
      phases of illness and for each new procedure based on
      child's developmental level (see the previous section,
      Preparation for Procedures or Surgery, for additional
      information).
   b. Explain each procedure or hospital routine that is
      appropriate to the child's and parents' cognitive levels;
      allow enough time for child and parents to ask questions
      and express anxieties.
   c. Suggest ways for parents to support their child during
      hospitalization and procedures (e.g., holding child after
      procedure).
   d. Consult parents and child about preferences among
      "quiet" toys and activities during acute phase of illness;
      encourage parents, child life specialists, and volunteers to
      play with child, allowing for rest periods and then passive
      participation (see Appendix B).
   e. Encourage and promote socialization with peers as
      means to cope adaptively with effects of disease.
2. Provide emotional and other support to parents.

   a. Provide and reinforce explanations about hospital experience.

   b. Encourage use of preexisting support systems (e.g., relatives, friends, clergy).

   c. Encourage expression of feelings using active listening techniques.

   d. Provide for physical comforts (e.g., arrangements for sleeping, bathing).

   e. Refer to social services if appropriate for in-hospital support and community-based resources following discharge.

   f. Refer to in-hospital parents support group; encourage parents to network with other parents in hospital for support.

3. Provide comfort measures to ease child's anxiety and discomfort during hospitalization.

   a. Teach parents how to hold and comfort child who has intravenous support and attachments to other medical equipment.

   b. Encourage parents to participate in aspects of child's care such as bathing and feeding; however, if parents are uncomfortable or otherwise unable to provide care, they should not feel pressured to do so.

   c. Until child's condition stabilizes or improves, keep stimulation to a minimum; arrange procedures or treatments so as to minimize interruptions, especially at night.

   d. Teach parents nonpharmacologic pain relief measures to use with child (see Appendix I).

4. Provide developmentally appropriate visual, auditory, and tactile stimulation (see Appendix B) as a means of providing comfort and support and alleviating anxiety).

5. Provide consistent nursing care to promote trust and to alleviate anxiety.

6. Encourage use of recreational and diversional activities to alleviate anxiety (see Appendix B).

REFERENCES

Bar-Mor G: Preparation of children for surgery and invasive procedures: Milestones on the way to success, *J Pediatr Nurs* 12(4):252, 1997.

Brewer S et al: Pediatric anxiety: Child life intervention in day surgery, *J Pediatr Nurs* 21(1):13, 2006.

Clatworthy S, Simon K, Tiedeman ME: Child drawing: Hospital—An instrument designed to measure the emotional status of hospitalized school-aged children, *J Pediatr Nurs* 14(1):2, 1999.

Cote CJ: Preoperative preparation, premedication and induction of the pediatric patient, *Curr Rev Nurse Anesth* 25(19):215, 2003.

Justus R et al: Preparing children and families for surgery: Mount Sinai's multidisciplinary perspective, *Pediatr Nurs* 32(1):35, 2006.

LaMontagne LL, Hepworth JT, Cohen F: Effects of surgery type and attention focus on children's coping, *Nurs Research* 49(5):245, 2000.

LaMontagne LL et al: Children's preoperative coping and its effects on postoperative anxiety and return to normal activity, *Nurs Research* 45(3):141, 1996.

Tiedeman ME, Clatworthy S: Anxiety responses of 5 to 11 year old children during and after hospitalization, *J Pediatr Nurs* 12(2):334, 1990.

Vagnoli L et al: Clown doctors as a treatment for preoperative anxiety in children: A randomized prospective study, *Pediatrics 116(4):563, 2005* (website): www.pediatrics.org/cgi/content/full/116/4/e563. Accessed July 4, 2006.

❖

Community Services

SPECIAL EDUCATION

Special education refers to the educational services and support provided to children and youths with disabilities. As described later, service systems in education, developmental disabilities, rehabilitation, social services, and job development have been created to promote improved educational and adult outcomes for infants, children, and youths with disabilities. Until recently, the emphasis of special education programs was on providing services in segregated settings that focused on limited objectives with a deficit-oriented approach. Best practice approaches foster the provision of services and supports within inclusive general education settings. That is, students who need special education services are taught in general education classrooms with students who do not have disabilities rather than only with other students in special education.

In educational settings, the mechanism for developing a plan to ensure that students achieve their educational, social, health-related, vocational, and community life goals is described. The individualized education plan for students in the elementary and middle grades and the individualized transition plan for students 14 to 21 years of age describe the processes used to assist students with disabilities to achieve their educational goals. Early intervention refers to the system of services available to infants and toddlers who have or are at risk for disabilities.

EARLY INTERVENTION

The early intervention (EI) system was initially authorized in 1986 in the Education of the Handicapped Act amendments

(Public Law [PL] 99–457) and was reauthorized with subsequent amendments, most recently in the Individuals with Disabilities Education Improvement Act (IDEA) (PL 108–446) in 2004.

EI services are provided to infants and toddlers from birth to 3 years of age. Infants and toddlers who qualify for EI services are those who (1) experience a delay in physical, cognitive, communication, psychosocial, or adaptive development; (2) have a physical or mental diagnosis likely to result in a developmental delay; (3) are considered to be at risk for a developmental delay; and (4) are developmentally delayed children 3 to 5 years of age who are enrolled in EI and would benefit by continuing in preschool readiness programs/special education programs. Examples of children eligible for EI are those born prematurely; those with Down syndrome or other genetic disorders, mental retardation, or low birth weight; those exposed in utero to illicit substances and alcohol; those born small or large for gestational age; and those with visual and/or hearing impairments. The goals of EI are to promote the infant's optimal growth and development and to provide services and support to families to promote their involvement in assisting their child to reach his or her optimal function. EI has been demonstrated to enhance neurodevelopmental outcomes for infants and toddlers. Several types of EI programs are available. An EI program may be center based or home based or a combination of both. Center-based programs are situated in locations in the community where services are rendered. EI services also may be provided in the family's home.

Infants and toddlers who are at risk for or who have been diagnosed with disabilities are referred to EI services. Eligibility is assessed by an interdisciplinary team of professionals that includes but is not limited to a pediatrician, psychologist, nurse, occupational and physical therapists, speech and language specialist, audiologist, registered dietitian, and family therapist. Once eligibility has been determined, an individualized family service plan (IFSP) is developed that is family centered and is based on family priorities. The IFSP specifies the necessary services and supports that will assist the child and family in meeting their goals. The IFSP is evaluated annually and is reviewed by parents every 6 months (more often if needed). Services are provided at either no cost or are based on a sliding scale determined by the state. Services should be provided in the most inclusive settings possible. EI services can be initiated before the assessment process is completed. Parental consent must be obtained before implementing the IFSP. Infants and toddlers are referred to EI services for the following services based on the IFSP:

1. Case management/service coordination
2. Assistive technology devices and services
3. Speech and language therapy
4. Audiology
5. Vision services
6. Physical therapy
7. Occupational therapy
8. Psychologic evaluation and therapy
9. Family support services, including counseling, training, and in-home visits
10. Diagnostic/evaluation medical services
11. Health services to support the child's participation in EI

INDIVIDUALIZED EDUCATION PROGRAM

1. The individualized education program (IEP) is the written plan for a child with a disability as determined by an interdisciplinary process involving educational personnel with expertise in special education and related services. IEPs are written for students who receive special education services and are reviewed by the IEP team, which includes a general education teacher, on an annual basis. Parental requests for multiyear reviews can be made, and parents may request changes to the plan. The IEP contains information about the extent to which the child's disability affects his or her educational progress and participation in school activities and about the special education and related services, supplementary aids and services, and program modifications and/or supports that will be provided in as inclusive a setting as possible for the child to meet IEP goals.
2. According to the provisions of IDEA, the child's IEP team consists of the following individuals:

    a. The child's parents

    b. At least one regular teacher (if the child is in general education)

    c. At least one special education teacher

    d. Educational representative from the school (e.g., school administrator) who has supervisory authority to ensure that IEP services will be provided and is knowledgeable about the general education program and school resources

    e. Educational personnel who can provide the findings and interpret the evaluations (e.g., school counselor, psychologist)

    f. Other experts, such as related services personnel

    g. The child, as appropriate

3. Beginning at 16 years of age or earlier, with an annual update thereafter, the IEP must contain statements of appropriate postsecondary goals related to education, training, employment and, when appropriate, independent living skills:

    a. Identification of a coordinated set of activities that are results oriented and are reviewed annually to promote the movement of the student from school to postschool activities

    b. Activities that are focused on academic and functional achievement and include postsecondary education, vocational training, integrated/supported employment, continuing adult education, adult services, and independent living/community participation

4. Students are to be included in IEP meetings if the purpose is to discuss transition goals and services.

5. If the agency does not provide a transition service specified in the IEP, then the IEP team meets to either revise the IEP or to generate new strategies to achieve the objective (the agency is not relieved of responsibility to provide services identified in the IEP).

6. One year before the student reaches the age of majority (varies according to state), the student and family are informed that IDEA legal rights are transferred to the youth.

INDIVIDUALIZED HEALTH PLAN (IHP)

The individualized health plan (IHP) is the nursing plan of care for students with chronic illnesses/disabilities. Unlike the IEP, which is developed by a team of educational and interdisciplinary personnel, the IHP is developed, implemented and evaluated by the school nurse. The IHP serves as the template for the provision of nursing services to students with health needs in the school setting, depending on the individual needs of the student. The nurse may work closely with other educational personnel in implementing the IHP. For example, if a student has a shunt, the nurse may instruct the student's teacher on the signs and symptoms of increased intracranial pressure, which should be promptly reported to the school nurse.

STATE CHILDREN'S HEALTH INSURANCE PROGRAM

In 1997, with the passage of the Balanced Budget Act, Congress expanded the Medicaid program for children. This new legislation established the State Children's Health Insurance Program (SCHIP), which made it possible for states to provide health insurance coverage to uninsured children whose family income is below the financial eligibility requirements for Medicaid (up to 200% of the federal poverty level). Under this new program, the federal government provides states $4 billion annually to help with the costs of health insurance for eligible children. Each state has the flexibility to determine eligibility criteria within the following broad guidelines: (1) the individual is not currently eligible for Medicaid insurance, (2) the individual is under 19 years of age, and (3) family income is at or below 200% of the federal poverty level ($36,000 for family of four). The type of health services available for eligible children are (1) physician visits, (2) hospitalizations, (3) immunizations, (4) emergency department visits, and (5) dental benefits (an optional benefit, although all states offer it). It is important that the parents and child review and understand the benefits available through the state's SCHIP. For information on specific state programs, see the following website: www.statelocalgov. net/index.cfm

EARLY AND PERIODIC SCREENING, DIAGNOSIS, AND TREATMENT PROGRAM

The Early and Periodic Screening, Diagnosis, and Treatment Program (EPSDTP) is a federally funded program (Medicaid) that is administered by each state to enable eligible poor children to receive an array of preventive health care, diagnostic, and treatment services. The goal of the program is to ensure that eligible children receive the necessary pediatric health care services to prevent childhood illnesses and disabilities. Each state is responsible for administering its own EPSDTP but must offer the assortment of services specified by federal regulations. The state EPSDTP does not provide services directly but is responsible for reimbursement and for ensuring that an adequate number of providers are available to supply timely, accessible, and comprehensive services. This program is for children from birth through 18 years of age, whose family incomes are up to 200% of the federal poverty level. Services include comprehensive health, mental, and developmental history taking; physical examination (unclothed); immunizations; and dental, vision, and hearing screening.

TITLE V PROGRAM FOR CHILDREN WITH SPECIAL HEALTH CARE NEEDS

The Title V Program for Children with Special Health Care Needs is a publicly funded health care program for eligible children and youths with special health care needs. This program was originally enacted in 1935 as Title V of the Social Security Act. Funded by federal, state, and local governments, this program provides health care, related services, and case management services to children with special health care needs whose condition meets the medical eligibility requirements and whose family income meets the financial eligibility requirements. The age range of eligibility is from birth through 21 years of age. State programs are responsible for ensuring the availability of adequate numbers of professionals who meet the service standards set by program guidelines. Services received by children with special health care needs include long-term specialty care services provided by an interdisciplinary team of professionals (physicians, registered nurses, social workers, nutritionists), medications, hospitalizations, case management, assistive technology, and necessary medical equipment and supplies such as wheelchairs, and suction machines.

SPECIAL SUPPLEMENTAL NUTRITION PROGRAM FOR WOMEN, INFANTS, AND CHILDREN

Created in 1972, the Special Supplemental Nutrition Program for Women, Infants, and Children (WIC) is designed to provide nutritious foods, nutritional education, and referrals for eligible individuals to community programs. Eligible low-income individuals (family income of no more than 185% of the federal poverty level) include (1) women who are pregnant (and up to 6 weeks following pregnancy or end of pregnancy), (2) women who are breast-feeding their infants up to 1 year of age, (3) nonbreast-feeding women up to 6 months after birth of infant or end of pregnancy, (4) infants up to 1 year of age, and (5) children up to 5 years of age. This nonentitlement program is administered by the U.S. Department of Agriculture and is provided through a number of clinical and community settings that include hospitals, community health departments, schools, public housing settings, Indian Health Services facilitates, migrant health services, and mobile clinics. The annual funds budgeted for the program are not sufficient to cover services for all eligible populations. Services provided by WIC include the following:

1. Coupon vouchers for nutritious foods such as milk, juice, eggs, and cheese that can be redeemed at local grocery stores
2. Classes on healthy eating and health behaviors
3. Breast-feeding classes
4. Referrals to other community-based programs for health and social services

HEAD START AND EARLY HEAD START PROGRAMS

The Head Start preschool program is a federally funded developmental and family support program for low-income individuals (family income of less than $15,000/yr) and serves preschool children 3 to 5 years of age and their families. More than 20 million children have participated in the Head Start program since its inception in 1965 as an initiative of President Johnson's War on Poverty. The goal of Head Start is to better prepare low-income preschool children for elementary school by providing them with enriched learning and social opportunities and health care. An additional goal is to enable parents to learn the child care skills that will permit them to obtain employment in Head Start. Twenty-seven percent of Head Start staff are current or former parents of children in Head Start. Currently, about 909,000 ethnically and racially diverse children (black, 30.7%; white, 39.8%; Hispanic, 34%; American Indian/Alaska Native: 4.2%; Asian, 1.8%; Hawaiian/Pacific Islander: 0.9%; Bi-Racial/Multi-Racial: 6.4%; Unspecified/Other: 16.2%) are enrolled in Head Start. In addition, 12.1% of children enrolled in Head Start have disabilities. Eighty-seven percent receive medical and dental services through the Medicaid/EPSDT program. The Head Start program provides a range of services to preschool children, including child-centered early childhood development and education services based on the child's learning and development needs. These programs involve indoor and outdoor play activities such as painting, dancing, game playing, storytelling, and learning projects. There are also many educational and support programs for parents. Head Start staff make home visits to provide additional instruction and support. Parents play an active role in Head Start programs as volunteers, which enables them to gain work experience for employment. The Early Head Start program, similar in purpose to the Head Start program, began in 1995 and currently serves 62,000 infants and toddlers 3 years of age and younger.

The Head Start program is administered by the Head Start Bureau of the U.S. Department of Health and Human Services. Federal funding for local programs is awarded to local public agencies, schools, and nonprofit and for-profit organizations. Eighty percent of funding comes from the federal government; the remaining funds are provided by local communities. Services provided by Head Start include the following:

1. Preschool program
2. Health care, including medical, dental, mental health, and nutritional services
3. Referral to community-based social service agencies

SUPPLEMENTAL SECURITY INCOME PROGRAM

The Social Security Administration (SSA) administers the Supplemental Security Income (SSI) program. Eligible children with disabilities are provided monthly SSI payments. Eligibility criteria include the following: (1) family income below a designated level; (2) U.S. residency, U.S. citizenship or, for noncitizens, a connection with military service or status as a designated refugee or as an individual granted asylum; (3) blindness; (4) marked and severe functional limitation resulting from a physical or mental condition or a combination of conditions; (5) persistence of the condition for longer than 1 year or an expectation that the condition will cause the child's death; (6) family income of less than $500/mo for the child; and (7) resources of less than $2000 for the child.

Eligibility is determined by state Disability Determination Services (DDSs) contracted by the SSA. The DDS evaluation team reviews the assessment data from doctors, teachers, counselors, therapists, and social workers regarding the extent to which the child's disability affects the child's level of functioning. All eligibility determinations are based on the written report and on the child's medical records. No in-person interviews or evaluations are conducted. The disability evaluation specialist determines whether the child's disability corresponds to one of the 100 SSA listings of physical or mental impairments or "medically equal" or "functionally equal" impairment.

Many programs specifically targeted adolescents and young adults who want to work or continue their education and still receive their SSI benefits. These programs include the *Earned Income Exclusion, Students Earned Income Exclusion, Impairment Related Work Expenses Plan for Achieving Self-Support (PASS)* and *The Ticket to Work and Work Incentive Program of 1999.* For additional information, see the following website: www.ssa.gov An SSA representative can be contacted directly at 800–772–1213 between 7 am and 7 pm. The TTY number is 800–325–0778. The SSA recommends making phone calls after the beginning of the week and after the beginning of each month.

REFERENCES

American Academy of Pediatrics: State insurance program (SCHIP), Medicaid provisions of the Balanced Budget Act of 1997(PL 105–33), *American Academy of Pediatrics* (serial online): www.aap.org/advocacy/schippro.htm. Accessed November 12, 2002.

Education of the Handicapped Act Amendments of 1986 (PL 99–457), US Code, vol 20, secs 1400 et seq (1986).

Individuals with Disabilities Education Act (IDEA) of 1990 (PL 101–476), US Code, vol 20, secs 1401 et seq (1990).

Individuals with Disabilities Education Act (IDEA) of 1991 (PL 102–119), US Code, vol 20, secs 1400 et seq (1991).

Individuals with Disabilities Education Act (IDEA) (PL 105–17), June 4, 1997.

Individuals with Disabilities Education Improvement Act of 2004 (PL 108–446), US Code, vol 20, secs.

Los Angeles Medical Home Project for Children With Special Health Care Needs (website): http://mchneighborhood.ichp.ufl.edu/medicalhomela/LA%20medical%20Home.htm. Accessed June 28, 2007.

Maternal and Child Health Library: Knowledge path: Early and Periodic Screening, Diagnostic, and Treatment (EPSDT) Services, *MCH Library* (serial online): www.mchlibrary.info/KnowledgePaths/kp_EPSDT.html. Accessed January 19, 2006.

Porter S et al, editors: *Children and youth assisted by medical technology in educational settings: guidelines for care* Baltimore, 1997, Paul H. Brookes.

Social Security Administration: Understanding Supplemental Security Income SSI Work Incentives, *SocialSecurityOnline* (serial online): www.ssa.gov/notices/supplemental-security-income/text-work-ussi.htm. Accessed June 28, 2007.

U.S. Department of Health and Human Services: About Head Start, *Administration for Children & Families* (serial online): www2.acf.dhhs.gov/programs/hsb/about/#history. Accessed January 19, 2006.

U.S. Department of Health and Human Services: State children's health insurance program, Centers for Medicaid and Medicare Services (serial online): www.cms.hhs.gov/home/schip.asp. Accessed January 18, 2006.

United States Department of Agriculture: About WIC, WIC at a glance, *Food & Nutrition Service* (serial online): www.fns.usda.gov/wic/aboutwic/wicataglance.htm. Accessed January 19, 2006.

U.S Department of Health & Human Services, Administration for Children & Families: Head Start Program fact sheet, fiscal year 2007, *Office of Head Start* (serial online): www.acf.hhs.gov/programs/hsb/research/2007.htm. Accessed July 3, 2007.

H

❖

Pediatric Palliative Care

Significant advances in health care, standards of living, technology, and clinical practices have resulted in improvements in child mortality rates over the past century. Nonetheless, every year, as evidenced by the statistic above, thousands of parents lose children to prematurity, injuries, cancer, heart disease, and other illness. Thousands of others, including grandparents, siblings, other family members, friends, schoolmates, and professional care givers, are affected by these deaths as well. Because childhood death has become an uncommon occurrence, when it does occur it is particularly tragic.

Pediatric palliative care is comprehensive care for infants and children who are not going to get better. This care is child-centered but also attends to the needs of the entire family. The goal is to enhance the child's time on earth, maintaining dignity and supporting the family's experience with empathy and cultural sensitivity.

THE PALLIATIVE CARE TEAM

A variety of people may be members of the interdisciplinary pediatric palliative care team. The child and the family are included as members of the team. Professional members may include doctors (primary providers and specialists), nurses and nursing assistants, pharmacists, social workers, dietitians, volunteers and respite workers, pastoral caregivers or chaplains, child life therapists, bereavement counselors, teachers, psychologists, and physical, occupational, and speech therapists.

PRECEPTS OF PEDIATRIC PALLIATIVE CARE

Last Acts, a national coalition to improve care and caring near the end of life, developed precepts of palliative care for children, adolescents, and their families. When the need for palliative care is identified, the primary care provider or the specialty care provider initiates discussions about the trajectory of the illness and about advanced planning. Specific areas that should be addressed include assessment and management of pain and other symptoms, emotional and spiritual support, and practice concerns including the following:

1. Respecting patient goals, preferences, and choices
2. Comprehensive caring
3. Using the strength of interdisciplinary resources
4. Acknowledging and addressing caregiver concerns
5. Building systems and mechanisms of support

ASSESSMENT AND MANAGEMENT OF PAIN AND OTHER SYMPTOMS

A high priority is placed on physical comfort. In addition to pain, other symptoms include anxiety and fear, depression, agitation, disordered sleep, feeding problems, gastrointestinal (GI) symptoms, respiratory symptoms, urinary symptoms, and skin problems. Supportive care for several emergencies is also described.

1. Pain
   a. Refer to Appendix I for assessment.
   b. Whenever possible, medications should be given orally. Alternative routes include intravenous (IV), subcutaneous (subQ), transmucosal, rectal, nasal, epidural, and intrathecal.
   c. Opioids should be given around the clock to treat moderate to severe pain. Additional doses may be prescribed for breakthrough pain.
   d. Adjuvants may be necessary to manage specific types of pain.
2. Anxiety and fear
   a. Anxiety in children is based on previous experiences. It is important to explore fears, perceptions, and understanding with the child and the family.

    b. Identify the child's coping and communication styles.

    c. Child-life therapy may be helpful in discussing diagnosis, treatment, and prognosis with the child. The therapist may participate in the discussion or guide the parents in how to discuss these topics with the child themselves.

    d. The mainstay for the pharmacologic management of anxiety in children is the use of benzodiazepines.

3. Depression

    a. Depression is probably underrecognized in children.

    b. A referral to a psychologist or psychiatrist may be needed.

    c. Pharmacologic management may include selective serotonin reuptake inhibitors (SSRIs) or tricyclic anti-depressants.

4. Agitation

    a. Agitation is often a multifactorial symptom. Causes include environmental factors, combinations of medications, pain, dyspnea or infections (e.g., respiratory, urinary tract).

    b. Assess for organic causes of agitation (infection and pain).

    c. Assess environment for excessive stimuli (e.g., noise, light, and people).

    d. Pharmacologic management includes haloperidol, benzdiazepines, levomepromazine, and phenobarbital.

5. Disordered sleep

    a. Disordered sleep may also be multifactorial.

    b. If possible, sedative medications should be given at night.

    c. Maintain appropriate day-night orientation.

    d. Medications may be used to regulate the sleep-wake cycle.

6. Feeding problems

    a. May be related to GI symptoms (see following Point 7), oral thrush, metallic or altered taste related to chemotherapy, xerostomia from radiation therapy, and untreated nausea.

    b. Assess the child's and the family's values regarding food. To be forced to eat when not hungry can be as distressing as being denied food when hungry.

    c. Several small meals per day may be more appropriate than a few large meals per day.

    d. Allow the child as much freedom as possible in choosing the kinds of foods taken orally.

    e. Even though artificial feedings via nasogastric or gastrostomy tubes are available, in the terminal stages it is rarely in the child's best interest for life to be prolonged in this manner. Anorexia is a natural progression of disease.

7. GI symptoms

    a. Refer to Appendix A for GI assessment.

    b. GI symptoms may be related to a specific disease process or side-effects of medications.

    c. Nausea and vomiting: medications should be chosen based on mechanism of action and the cause of the nausea and vomiting.

    d. Constipation: opioids may contribute to constipation. Dietary measures and increased fluids help to relieve constipation. If necessary, the combination of a gentle laxative and a stool softener are usually effective. An enema may be necessary to evacuate the bowel before starting a laxative regimen.

    e. Irreversible bowel obstruction: pharmacologic bowel paralysis is warranted in cases of irreversible bowel obstruction and nausea and vomiting associated with GI dysmotility.

    f. Diarrhea: uncontrolled diarrhea can result in significant skin breakdown and increase the risk for sepsis. Opioid derivatives are effective in reducing diarrhea.

    g. Oral hygiene: ice chips, wet sponges, and glycerin swabs can be use to keep the oral mucosa moist. If the child does not have impaired swallowing or esophageal ulcerations, pineapple chunks or ascorbic acid dissolved on the tongue can help the mouth feel fresh.

8. Respiratory symptoms

    a. Refer to Appendix A for respiratory assessment.

    b. Reposition child as needed.

    c. Improve airflow in room (e.g., open window) and minimize crowding to relieve air hunger.

   d. Dyspnea: oxygen may be helpful if dyspnea is related to hypoxia. Face masks may be uncomfortable and may contribute to a feeling of suffocation.

   e. Nebulized air, bronchodilators, and chest physiotherapy may be helpful.

   f. Noisy breathing with wet secretions at the end of life (the death rattle) can be distressing for the family. The use of anticholinergic agents may be helpful.

9. Urinary symptoms

   a. Refer to Appendix A for renal assessment.

   b. Decreased urine output and renal failure may be associated with the natural progress of disease.

   c. Urinary retention may be due to opioids or constipation.

   d. Incontinence may be due to retention with overflow.

   e. Bladder spasms may be related to mechanical irritation or neurogenic bladder.

   f. Intermittent or indwelling catheterization may be necessary.

   g. Pain related to renal or ureteral obstruction can be relieved with urinary diversion techniques.

   h. Pain not related to obstruction should be treated with opioids or antispasmotics.

10. Skin problems

   a. Pruritus—medications that cause itching and rashes may be treated with emollients, humidified air, and topical or systemic medications.

   b. Pressure sores—require meticulous skin hygiene, frequent repositioning, and avoiding hard surfaces and shearing forces on body parts. If bed sores are present, the goal of care is to promote healing.

11. Emergencies

   a. Increased intracranial pressure

      i. Assessment: headaches, nausea and vomiting, made worse by lying down, most severe in the morning, papilledema, increased head circumference, altered level of consciousness (LOC), Cushing's triad (increased respiratory rate, increased blood pressure, and decreased heart rate), and seizures

      ii. May be treated with high-dose dexamethasone, comfort measures, pain management, limited fluids, radiotherapy (palliative), and ventricular-peritoneal shunt (palliative)

  b. Spinal cord compression

      i. Assessment: leg, neck, and back pain, extreme weakness or paralysis, ataxia, sensory or autonomic dysfunction

      ii. May be treated with high-dose dexamethasone, comfort measures, pain management, radiotherapy, and surgery, if benefit of surgery outweighs the potential of prolonged hospitalization

  c. Obstruction of the superior vena cava

      i. Assessment: dyspnea, cyanosis, fullness in head and headache, worse when lying down, increased by Valsalva maneuvers, facial fullness and plethora, enlarged cervical lymph nodes, distended, nonpulsatile jugular veins, wheezing and decreased breath sounds, and superficial veins over upper thorax

      ii. Tumors may be treated by clots by thrombolysis followed by anticoagulants—high-dose steroids followed by radiotherapy. Clot—thrombolysis followed by anticoagulants

  d. Intractable seizures

      i. Often increase in frequency and severity as terminal phase is reached.

      ii. May be treated with phenobarbital, midazolam, or both, rectal diazepam for breakthrough seizures. As death approaches, it may not be appropriate to treat minor seizures and those of short duration. Inform and reassure parents that seizures lasting 5 to 10 minutes cause little harm.

  e. Hemorrhage

      i. Occurs rarely

      ii. If a large hemorrhage is an expected terminal event, it may be helpful to have a supply of green, black, or red towels available at the bedside. These towel colors help to reduce the visual impact of the bleeding

CULTURAL CONSIDERATIONS

The importance of providing culturally competent care has come to light as diversity within, and among groups has been recognized. The first step to cultural competence is understanding one's own perspectives. In addition, it is essential never to make assumptions about individuals based on their cultural affiliations. The Oncology Nurses Society has developed a Multicultural Tool Kit to help nurses provide culturally competent care (www.ons.org/clinical/special/toolkit.shtml).

SPIRITUAL CONCERNS

Spirituality is a search for meaning in life and a desire for connectedness to the universe. Religious beliefs may or may not be bound to a person's spirituality. The understanding of death and spirituality are developmentally defined concepts. The interventions may be applicable for surviving siblings and children who have experienced loss of a parent or other family member, as well as for the dying child.

An important part of culture, especially in relation to palliative care, is spirituality. The B-E-L-I-E-F model for spiritual assessment, adapted for palliative care, is outlined in Box H-1. The child and the family may have a personal spiritual advisor whom they wish to have involved in the care. With the family's permission, explain the child's illness to the spiritual advisors. Families may need time to reflect on the meaning of the illness and possibility of death.

CONCEPT OF DEATH
Newborns to 2 to 3 years
Perceptions

Infants and very young children up to the age of 2 to 3 years have no concept of death. Children in this age group may sense something is wrong as they receive cues and sense tension in people around them. They sense the absence of a significant person and the presence of new people in their environment. There may be signs of irritability and changes in eating, crying,

BOX H-1

B-E-L-I-E-F Model for Spiritual Assessment in Pediatric Palliative Care

Belief system
- Does your family belong to a specific religious group?
- What is the extent of your involvement with this group?
- Does your child actively participate in this group?

Ethics or values
- What ethics or values are important in your family life?

Lifestyle
- Does your family have special prayers or rituals that you practice in your daily life?
- Does your family observe any dietary restrictions?

Involvement in a spiritual community
- Does your family belong to any spiritual or support groups?
- Would you like the palliative care team to have contact information for an individual in your faith or spiritual community?

Education
- Does your child receive religious education?
- How should we incorporate your and your child's spiritual beliefs into your child's care?

Future events
- Are there any rites of passage that are to occur in your family in the near future?
- What roles will members of your faith or spiritual community play in the spiritual care of your child?

Adapted from McEvoy M: An added dimension to the pediatric health maintenance visit: The spiritual history, *J Pediatr Health Care* 14(5): 216, 2000.

and bowel and bladder habits. Their spiritual development includes faith that is reflected in trust and hope in others. There is a need for sense of self-worth and love.

Interventions
1. Maintain normal routines and structure whenever possible.
2. Provide verbal and physical affection and comfort.

3. Provide a warm, familiar, loving caretaking when parents are not available.
4. Provide transitional objects such as favorite toys.

Age 3 to 6 years
Perceptions
In early childhood, the children believe death is reversible, similar to going to sleep or a parent going to work. Children in this age group believe that people who die will come back. "Magical thinking" is characteristic of this group. Children believe that their thoughts, actions, and words cause death or can bring back the deceased. They may also view death as a punishment for bad behavior. These children continue to be greatly influenced by their parents' emotional state. Abstract concepts, such as heaven, are difficult at this stage of development. Regressive behaviors are common. Verbal expression may be limited; therefore, acting out of feelings is common. There may be an increase in aggression and irritability. As they try to make sense of loss, 3- to 6-year-olds may ask the same questions repeatedly. They may exhibit somatic symptoms, use play as an escape mechanism, and connect events that do not belong in connection. Sadness may be transient. Anxiety may be limited because of the belief that the deceased can come back. At this stage of development, participation in rituals, if rituals are part of the family's practice, becomes important.

Interventions
1. Maintain normal routines and structure whenever possible.
2. Provide opportunities to express feelings through drawing and play.
3. Help the child to identify and verbalize feelings, fears, and reactions.
4. Honesty is important; if you do not have an answer to a question, tell the child you do not have an answer.
5. Use specific, concrete language when giving explanations. Avoid the use of euphemisms and clichés.
6. Gently confront magical thinking. Make sure the child does not feel responsible for the death.
7. Be tolerant of regressive behavior.

Age 6 to 9 years
Perceptions
Children at this stage of development may or may not begin to understand the finality of death. Children in this age group view death as a taker or spirit that comes and gets you. There may be fear that death is contagious and that other loved ones will die as well. These children are fascinated with the physiology and details of death. There is a fascination with issue of mutilation and an interest in the appearance of the body. There may be a connection to death and violence. The child may ask who killed the deceased. Many have concerns about how the deceased will eat, breathe, and so forth. Children may ask concrete questions, and yet have trouble expressing their feelings verbally. There may be increased aggression, defense against feeling helpless, and somatic complaints. Abstract concepts, such as heaven, may continue to be difficult. Faith concerns revolve around right and wrong. Rituals become part of personal identity.

Interventions
1. Talk with the child, ask questions, identify fears, help him or her to share bad dreams, and reassure the child that he or she is in no way responsible for death.
2. Normalize feelings and fears.
3. Address distortions and perceptions.
4. Honesty is important; if you do not have an answer to a question, tell the child you do not have an answer.
5. Provide opportunities for play and drawing.
6. Use specific, concrete language when giving explanations. Avoid the use of euphemisms and clichés.

Age 9 to 13 years
Perceptions
At this stage of development, the understanding of the concept of death is nearer to that of an adult. There is a greater awareness of the finality of death. Children in the age group are concerned with how their world will change (if a loved one dies) and worry about how loved ones will cope without them (if the child is the one who is dying). They exhibit a fragile independence, with fewer questions and a reluctance to

open up to others. There may be disruption in peer relationships, increased anger and guilt, and somatic symptoms. These children may be self-conscious about their fears. Faith remains concerned with right and wrong. There may be a greater interest in rituals and other spiritual aspects of life.

Interventions
1. Encourage discussion regarding concerns and feelings.
2. Provide opportunities for and encourage expressive activities such as writing or drawing.
3. Address tendencies to act out.
4. Allow for regressive behavior.
5. Honesty is important; if you do not have an answer to a question, tell the child you do not have an answer.
6. Avoid clichés.

Age 13 to 18 years
Perceptions
Most adolescents will have adult understanding about death. Death is viewed as the enemy. Normal maturational changes in the adolescent's body represent growth and life. Death is a contrast. A sense of future is a normal part of the adolescent's psychology. This age group may intellectualize or romanticize death. Indifference may be used as a protective coping mechanism. Adolescents prefer to grieve with their peer group rather than with adults. They may need permission to grieve. Thoughts of suicide are not uncommon. Adolescents may repress sadness, feel anger, and be depressed. Escapism is exhibited in driving fast, drug and alcohol use, or acting out sexually. They may have somatic complaints. Questioning religious and spiritual beliefs is common. There is an evolution of the adolescent's relationship with a higher power. The search for meaning, purpose, hope, and value of life begins during this stage of development.

Interventions
1. Do not assume that adolescents can handle death-related issues on their own.
2. Be available, but allow space, do not push.
3. Peer support groups may be helpful.
4. Give permission to regress.

5. Honesty is important; if you do not have an answer to a question, tell the adolescent you do not have an answer.
6. Help control impulse toward reckless behavior.
7. Deromanticize death.
8. Avoid clichés.

Bereavement Care

An important component of spiritual and emotional care of the family is bereavement care. The loss of a child can be at times a personal, emotional and spiritual crisis. Grief proceeds through a series of overlapping phases that may ebb and flow. Generally the first phase is characterized by shock and denial. A sense of emotional numbness is common. Next there is cognitive and emotional acknowledgment of the reality of the loss. This is a period of intense preoccupation with the loss. Family members may exhibit behavioral, cognitive, social, and somatic manifestations of distress. Most parents do not ever "get over" the loss of the child, but they learn to adjust. The loss becomes integrated into their everyday lives. Signs of healing and resolution of grief include resumption of everyday functioning, deriving pleasure from life, and establishing new relationships. This is the final phase of grief. Siblings may feel separated from their grieving parents. A surviving child may try to take on the family role of the deceased child (the "good" child, the athlete, etc.). Siblings need reassurance that they are loved for themselves.

Advanced Planning

Advanced planning helps patients and families express their wishes about what to do as serious and life-threatening problems arise. Team members who are responsible for helping families with advanced planning must be familiar with relevant local, state, and federal laws such as those regarding do-not-resuscitate orders and surrogate decision making. The focus of advance planning is to identify decision makers, to discuss illness trajectory, to identify the goals of care, and to think about issues regarding care or concerns near the end of life. Once the decision makers are identified, they are included in the process of advanced planning. Next, family and child understanding of the illness and the prognosis are explored. Misperceptions are clarified, and impending death is explained in a manner that the family and the child can understand. The third step in the advanced planning process is to determine the goals of care. These goals may be curative, uncertain, or primarily focus on providing comfort. Shared decisions about the future or continued use of life-sustaining technology and aggressive medical interventions are made. These decisions are generally made by the patients and families. The family's values may be different from those of the primary health team, and they should be respected. If these decisions seem inconsistent with the presumed understanding of the illness and prognosis, or if the family does not understand the outcomes of their decisions, continued review and discussion of available options is reasonable. An ethicist may be helpful in mediating conflict between families and the health care team.

Practical Concerns

Practical concerns include communication, desired location of palliative care, needs for specific equipment to meet the child's functional status, creating and disseminating plans of care to all appropriated environments, and financial concerns. A care coordinator should be designated and a method of contacting the coordinator should be available. Anticipation of equipment needs and ordering in advance may prevent a costly and unwanted hospitalization. If the child continues to go to school, the care coordinator or another team member should visit the school to provide education and support. Finally, discuss potential financial burdens of care with the family. Social services and financial counselors can be invaluable in helping reduce the strain of financial concerns.

Ethical Concerns

The goals of palliative care are based on the ethical principles of beneficence, nonmaleficence, and autonomy. Beneficence demands that health care professionals provide care that promotes the well-being of patients and their families. Nonmaleficence demands that professionals avoid doing harm to patients. In terms of palliative care, it is important to recognize that continued aggressive curative therapies may cause more harm than benefit. Autonomy demands respect for parents' moral right to participate in the medical decisions for their minor children who are not mentally competent, to respect the decisions of minor children who have functional capacity to make their own decisions, and to respect minor children who are developing autonomy by obtaining assent for treatment.

REFERENCES

American Academy of Pediatrics, Committee on Bioethics: Guidelines on forgoing life-sustaining medical treatment, *Pediatrics* 93(3):532, 1994.

Bowden VR et al: Precepts of palliative care for children, adolescents, and their families, *Society of Pediatric Nurses*, (serial online): www.pedsnurses.org/pdfs/last_acts_precepts[1].pdf. Accessed March 14, 2006.

Carter BS, Levetown M: *Palliative care for infants, children, and adolescents: A practical guide*, Baltimore, MD, 2004, Johns Hopkins University Press.

Field MJ, Behrman RE: *When children die: Improving palliative and end-of-life care for children and their families*, Washington, DC, 2002, National Academies Press.

Ginzburg K, Geron Y, Solomon Z: Patterns complicating grief among bereaved parents, *Omega* 45(2):119, 2002.

Haut C: Oncological emergencies in the pediatric intensive care unit, *AACN Clin Issues* 16(2):232, 2005.

Himelstein BP et al: Pediatric palliative care, *New Engl J Med* 350(17):1752, 2004.

Hospice of Southeastern Connecticut: *Children's understanding of death* (website): www.hospicenet.org/html/understanding.html. Accessed March 14, 2006.

Murphy K: Recognizing depression in children, *Nurse Pract* 29(9):18, 2004.

Robert Wood Johnson Foundation: A record of accomplishment in end-of-life care, *Robert Wood Johnson Foundation* (serial online): www.rwjf.org/newsroom/featureDetail.jsp?featureID=886&type=3. Accessed April 19, 2007.

Turkoski BB: When a child's treatment decisions conflict with the parents', *Home Healthcare Nurse* 23(2):123, 2005.

I

❖

Pain in Children

DEFINITIONS

The International Association for the Study of Pain defines pain as "an unpleasant sensory and emotional experience associated with actual or potential tissue damage, or described in terms of such damage." McCaffrey and Beebe (1994) state that "pain is whatever the person experiencing it says it is, existing whenever the experiencing person says it does." This definition does not necessarily imply that the child must verbalize pain. Pain may also be expressed through crying, vocalizations, or other behavioral manifestations.

PHYSIOLOGY

Pain is a complex physiologic process that can be divided into three neurochemical events: transduction, transmission, and modulation.

Transduction occurs at the site of initiation of pain. Pain receptors (nociceptors) in the periphery are stimulated by a mechanical, thermal, or chemical event. This stimulus results in the release of pain-producing substances.

Transmission of the impulse continues as it travels into the dorsal horn of the spinal cord via large, thinly myelinated A-delta fibers and small, unmyelinated C fibers. From here the impulse is carried via the anterolateral pathway on to the thalamus and then to the cortex. It is in the cortex that the impulse is perceived as pain. Many factors, including culture, past experience, the meaning of the pain, and emotional state, contribute to the individual's perception of pain. Both transduction and transmission occur in afferent pathways.

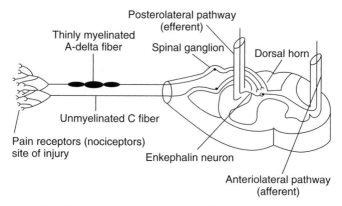

Figure I-1 Transduction, transmission, and modulation of pain.

Modulation of pain occurs in the brain at the level of the periaqueductal gray matter and the medulla oblongata, as well as in the dorsal horn of the spinal cord, as endogenous opioids (enkephalins) are released in the posterolateral pathway, an efferent pathway.

Figure I-1 shows transduction, transmission, and modulation of pain in the dorsal horn.

NATURE OF PAIN

Table I-1 provides a brief overview of the types of pain with descriptions and examples of each.

PAIN ASSESSMENT

Self-report is the most accurate means of obtaining information regarding the location and intensity of the child's pain. Input from the family is very important and may be necessary if the child is unwilling or unable to report for himself or herself. Obtaining a pain history is helpful in developing a plan of care for the child. Ask questions regarding the child's previous experience with painful events, including how the child responds to pain and what methods of pain management have been successful in the past. Also learn what word the child uses to describe

TABLE I-1
Nature of Pain

Type	Description	Examples
Acute	Brief; associated with tissue damage or inflammation; intensity steadily diminishes over days to weeks	Surgical pain, burns, fractures
Chronic persistent	Persistent or near-persistent pain over a period of 3 months or longer	Arthritis, sickle cell crisis
Recurrent	Repetitive painful episode alternating with pain-free intervals	Headache; abdominal, chest, or limb pain
Neuropathic	Persistent pain related to persistent or abnormal excitability in the peripheral or central nervous system with no ongoing tissue injury; often described as "burning," "strange," or "pins and needles"	Amputation pain syndromes, plexus injuries, reflex sympathetic dystrophy
Psychogenic	Persistent pain that is a manifestation of a psychiatric disease	Somatization disorder, somatoform pain disorder, conversion disorder

pain (e.g., "boo-boo," "owie"). The pain assessment should be tailored to the child's developmental level.

Physiologic signs are neither specific nor sensitive indicators of pain but may be used as an adjunct to behavioral assessment and self-report in all age groups. Assess behavioral manifestations with caution, because many children will play, watch television, or sleep as a means of coping with pain. If the child is receiving sedatives in addition to analgesics, behavioral response to pain may be blunted.

Neonates and Infants (Birth to 1 Year)

Use of behavioral indexes is the best method of assessing pain in neonates. Facial grimaces, alterations in tone and activity, and crying are the most often used indicators of pain in this age group. Premature and critically ill neonates may not respond as vigorously to pain as healthy, full-term neonates. This lack of response does not indicate a lack of perception.

Behavioral indexes are also the most useful indicators of pain for infants beyond the neonatal period. In addition to facial grimaces, alterations in tone and activity, and crying, these infants demonstrate deliberate withdrawal from the painful stimulus and a wide variety of vocalizations.

Toddlers (1 to 3 Years)

Behavioral responses also continue to be the standard for pain assessment in toddlers. However, their behavioral repertoire is expanded to include rubbing the site of pain and aggressive behavior (biting, hitting, and kicking). Some toddlers are capable of verbalizing where something hurts, but they cannot describe the intensity of the pain.

Preschoolers (3 to 5 Years)

By age 3 to 4 years, most children can begin to use self-report tools such as the Oucher Scale (Figure I-2) or the Wong-Baker FACES Pain Rating Scale (Figure I-3). These tools provide the most accurate measure of a child's pain. Preschoolers are better able to describe the intensity of their pain. This age group may also display aggressive behavior in response to pain.

School-Aged Children (5 to 13 Years)

The Oucher Scale is also useful for school-aged children. Children in this age group may use either the faces shown on the scale or the numeric values. By age 7 or 8 many children can use a numeric scale. These children should have an under-

OUCHER

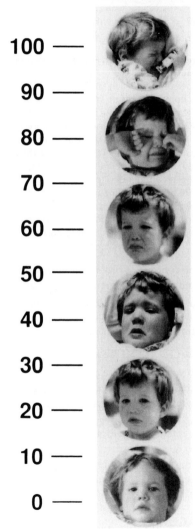

Figure I-2   The Caucasian Oucher Scale, developed and copyrighted by Judith E. Beyer, RN, PhD, 1983. This tool is also available in Hispanic and African American versions.

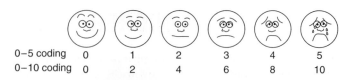

0–5 coding	0	1	2	3	4	5
0–10 coding	0	2	4	6	8	10

Figure I-3   Wong-Baker FACES Pain Rating Scale.

English instructions:

Explain to the person that "Each face is for a person who feels happy because he has no pain (hurt) or sad because he has some or a lot of pain. **Face 0** is very happy because he doesn't hurt at all. **Face 1** hurts just a little bit. **Face 2** hurts a little more. **Face 3** hurts even more. **Face 4** hurts a whole lot. **Face 5** hurts as much as you can imagine, although you don't have to be crying to feel this bad." Ask the person to choose the face that best describes how he or she is feeling.

Rating scale is recommended for persons age 3 years and older.

Brief word instructions: Point to each face, using the words to describe the pain intensity. Ask the child to choose face that best describes his or her own pain, and record the appropriate number. (From Hockenberry MJ, Wilson D: *Wong's nursing care of infants and children*, ed. 8, St. Louis, 2007, Mosby.)

standing of the concept of order and number. Children in this age group can describe the intensity and location of their pain in greater detail. They may tend to act brave, demonstrating less overt behavior patterns, such as clenching their fists and teeth or remaining very still or rigid.

Adolescents (13 to 19 Years)

Any of the tools described here are useful for adolescents. They can also respond to being asked, "On a scale of 0 to 10, with 0 being no pain and 10 being the worst pain you have ever had, what is your pain now?" Adolescents are capable of describing the intensity, the location, and the duration of their pain. They also display a variety of behavioral responses including mood swings and regression to an earlier developmental stage. Adolescents tend to dismiss their pain and refuse intervention in the presence of their peers.

PAIN MANAGEMENT

Pain management is, ideally, a multidisciplinary effort. The pain management "team" may include any or all of the following professionals: nurse, physician, child life specialist, respiratory therapist, occupational therapist, physical therapist, and chaplain, along with the child and the family. Strategies for pain management should include both pharmacologic and non-pharmacologic approaches. The following sections describe both types of management strategies.

Pharmacologic Management

Acute pain is managed with opioid and nonopioid analgesics. Table I-2 provides a list of selected medications used for the management of acute pain in the pediatric population. Patient-controlled analgesia and epidural analgesia are described in the following sections.

Because intramuscular injections are painful and frightening for children, this route of administration should be reserved for exceptional circumstances.

Patient-Controlled Analgesia

Patient-controlled analgesia (PCA) is a method of intravenous administration of small boluses of opiates and is often used in the treatment of postoperative pain. The child uses a hand-operated device to signal the PCA pump to deliver a bolus dose of the medication. The pump will deliver the medication directly into the child's intravenous line provided that a set period of time ("lockout interval") has passed since the previous dose was administered. In addition to the boluses, many PCA pumps have the capability to deliver a background or continuous infusion of the opiate. Delivery of a continuous infusion helps maintain a steady therapeutic drug level even when the child is sleeping.

The child must have the cognitive ability to understand the principles of PCA. By the age of 7 years, most children can use PCA without difficulty. Each individual child's developmental level must be assessed before initiation of this method of drug administration. Teaching the child about PCA preoperatively is helpful.

Benefits of PCA include elimination of delay in analgesic administration, high levels of client satisfaction, usefulness for all types of acute pain, potential reduction in total medication requirement, and reduction in nursing staff workload.

TABLE I-2
Selected Medications Used to Manage Acute Pain in the Pediatric Population

Drug	Dose (mg/kg)*	Route	Frequency	Comments
Opioids				
Morphine	0.3	PO	Every 3–4 hr	The standard for opioid therapy, most commonly used opioid in neonates
	0.1	IV	Every 3–4 hr	
Codeine	1	PO	Every 3–4 hr	Not recommended for parenteral use; decreased incremental analgesic effect with doses higher than 65 mg
Hydromorphone	0.06	PO	Every 3–4 hr	—
	0.015	IV	Every 3–4 hr	—
Hydrocodone	0.2	PO	Every 3–4 hr	Doses of aspirin and acetaminophen in combination products must be adjusted as appropriate for body weight
Meperidine	0.75	IV	Every 3–4 hr	Reserved for very brief courses of opioid (Demerol) use in clients who have demonstrated allergy to morphine or hydromorphone; accumulation of the metabolite normeperidine may result in seizures

Methadone	0.2	PO	Every 6–8 hr	—
	0.1	IV	Every 6–8 hr	—
Oxycodone	0.2	PO	Every 3–4 hr	Doses of aspirin and acetaminophen in combination products must be adjusted as appropriate for body weight
Nonopioids				
Acetaminophen	10–15	PO or PR	Every 4 hr	No antiinflammatory activity
Nonsteroidal antiinflammatory drugs (NSAIDs)				
Aspirin	10–15	PO	Every 4 hr	Inhibits platelet aggregation; may cause postoperative bleeding; do not administer salicylates to children with suspected or confirmed viral infection (e.g., chickenpox)
Choline	25	PO	Twice a day	May have minimal antiplatelet activity; magnesium oral liquid available; do not administer salicylates to children with suspected or confirmed viral infection (e.g., chickenpox)

Continued

TABLE I-2
Selected Medications Used to Manage Acute Pain in the Pediatric Population—cont'd

Drug	Dose (mg/kg)*	Route	Frequency	Comments
Ibuprofen	10	PO	Every 6–8 hr	Oral suspension available
Naproxen	5	PO	Every 12 hr	Oral liquid available
Ketoralac	0.5	IV	Every 6–8 hr	The only parenteral NSAID; has not been approved for use in the pediatric population; there are presently ongoing clinical trials regarding the use of the IM preparation as an IV preparation in the pediatric and adult populations

IM, Intramuscular (route); *IV*, intravenous (route); *PO*, by mouth; *PR*, by rectum.
*Recommended dose for children weighing less than 50 kg.

Complications are the same as those for other methods of opiate administration—respiratory depression, urinary retention, pruritus, nausea, and vomiting.

Epidural Analgesia

Epidural analgesia may be used in children who have undergone any of a variety of surgeries, including thoracic, abdominal, and genitourinary tract procedures. The epidural catheter is placed by an anesthesiologist and provides access for continuous opiate infusion or delivery of boluses of opiates and/or local anesthetics.

Compared with traditional intravenous or PCA administration of opiates, smaller doses of opiate given via an epidural catheter provide adequate pain control with less sedation. Because of the increased comfort level, the child is better able to participate in postoperative care. Additional benefits include earlier ambulation and increased ability to deep breathe. Potential side effects of epidural analgesia include respiratory depression, urinary retention, pruritus, infection, spinal headache, nausea, and vomiting.

Nonpharmacologic Management

Behavioral and other nonpharmacologic techniques may be used in conjunction with pharmacologic management of acute pain. Table I-3 lists selected nonpharmacologic pain management strategies. These techniques often allow for a reduction in the amount of analgesic used. It is important to assess the child's individual response to any strategy. Involving families in these strategies often enhances their success.

PROCEDURAL PAIN

Invasive procedures are essential in diagnosis and treatment for many hospitalized children. These procedures include venipuncture, intravenous catheter insertion, circumcision, cardiac catheterization, chest tube insertion, central line insertion, bone marrow aspiration, and biopsy. Some dressing changes may also cause significant pain and stress in children.

The child and the family should be adequately prepared for the procedure. The type of preparation should be based on the child's developmental level. Be aware of the environment in

TABLE I-3
Nonpharmacologic Pain Management Techniques

Age Group	Techniques
Neonates	Pacifiers
	Music (fetal heart sounds)
	Swaddling, blanket nests, or boundaries
	Speaking in quiet tones
	Minimization of noxious stimuli: frequent handling, noise, bright lights (premature neonates may be overwhelmed by increased sensory stimuli)
Infants	Visual stimuli
	Speaking in quiet tones
	Pacifiers
	Rocking
	Swaddling (for younger infants)
	Music
	Cutaneous stimulation: transcutaneous electric nerve stimulation, heat, cold, massage
Toddlers	Magic wands
	Kaleidoscopes
	Pop-up books
	Music
	Controlled breathing—blowing bubbles
	Cutaneous stimulation
Preschoolers	Magic wands
	Kaleidoscopes
	Pop-up books
	Finding hidden picture *(Where's Waldo?)*
	Listening to music or a story through a headset
	Video watching
	Emotive imagery—using a child's favorite superhero to "fight" the pain
	Controlled breathing
	Behavioral rehearsal—becoming familiar with a procedure through play
	Cutaneous stimulation

TABLE I-3
Nonpharmacologic Pain Management Techniques—cont'd

Age Group	Techniques
School-aged children	Imagery Listening to music or a story through a headset Video watching Controlled breathing Behavioral rehearsal Cutaneous stimulation Modeling—observing another child during a procedure; the child models or demonstrates behavior that assists in mastering the procedure (can be live or on videotape)
Adolescents	Imagery Music Controlled breathing Video watching Cutaneous stimulation Modeling

which the procedure is to be performed. Minimize noise, provide adequate lighting, and ensure privacy. The child's room and bed are considered safe places. Procedures should not be performed in the room or the bed unless absolutely necessary.

Allow a family member (ideally, mother and/or father, if present) to be with the child before, during, and after the procedure. The family member should be prepared for his or her role, which usually involves assisting in nonpharmacologic pain relief measures.

If anxiolytics are used to reduce anxiety associated with procedures, it is important to remember that these medications will blunt the child's response to pain but will not provide pain relief.

A key principle in the management of procedural pain is the provision of maximal treatment for the pain and anxiety of a first procedure, particularly if the child must undergo repeated procedures. This helps to reduce the development of anticipatory anxiety before subsequent procedures.

REFERENCES

International Association for the Study of Pain, Subcommittee on Taxonomy: Pain terms: A list with definitions and notes usage, *Pain* 6 (249), 1979.

James SR, Ashwill JW: *Nursing care of children: Principles & practice*, ed 3, Philadelphia, 2007, WB Saunders.

McCaffrey M, Beebe A: *Pain: Clinical manual for nursing practice*, St. Louis, 1994, Mosby.

Oakes LL: Assessment and management of pain in the critically ill pediatric patient, *Crit Care Nurs Clin North Am* 13(2):281, 2001.

Rodriguez E, Jordan R: Contemporary trend in pediatric sedation and analgesia, *Emerg Med Clin North Am* 20(2):199, 2002.

Index

Page reference followed by *b* indicates box; *f* indicates illustration; *t* indicates table.